HANDBOOK OF BALANCE FUNCTION TESTING

Handbook of Balance Function Testing

Gary P. Jacobson, Ph.D.
Director, Division of Audiology
Department of Otolaryngology
Henry Ford Hospital
Detroit, Michigan

Craig W. Newman, Ph.D.
Division of Audiology
Department of Otolaryngology
Henry Ford Hospital
Detroit, Michigan

Jack M. Kartush, M.D.
Michigan Ear Institute
Farmington Hills, Michigan

THOMSON
DELMAR LEARNING

Australia Canada Mexico Singapore Spain United Kingdom United States

COPYRIGHT © 1997 Delmar.
Thomson Learning™ is a trademark used herein under license.

Printed in the United States of America
    9 10 XXX 05 04

For more information, contact Thomson Delmar Learning 5 Maxwell Dr. Clifton Park, NY 12065 or find us on the World Wide Web at http://www.delmarlearning.com

Library of Congress Cataloging-in-Publication Data:
ISBN: 1-5659-3907-7

To our families, who kept us connected to the "real world" during the course of this project, and to our teachers, who taught us how to write, how to think, and how to ask questions.

CONTRIBUTORS

Dennis I. Bojrab, M.D.
Ear Consultants of Michigan
Royal Oak, Michigan
Assistant Clinical Professor
Wayne State University
Detroit, Michigan

Thomas Brandt, M.D.
Professor, Chairman of Neurology
Department of Neurology
Ludwig-Maximilians University
Munich, Germany

James R. Carl, M.D.
Assistant Professor of Ophthalmology and
    Neurology
University of Pittsburgh School of Medicine
Pittsburgh, Pennsylvania

Josef Elidan, M.D.
Professor and Chairman
Department of Otolaryngology/Head and
    Neck Surgery
Hadassah University Hospital
Jerusalem, Israel

Joseph M.R. Furman, M.D., Ph.D.
Associate Professor
Departments of Otolaryngology, Neurology,
    and Electrical Engineering
University of Pittsburgh School of Medicine
Director, Division of Balance Disorders
Montefiore University Hospital
The Eye and Ear Institute Pavillion
Pittsburgh, Pennsylvania

Timothy C. Hain, M.D.
Associate Professor
Northwestern University Medical School
Director of Vestibular Laboratory
Northwestern Memorial Hospital
Chicago, Illinois

James W. Hall III, Ph.D.
Associate Professor and Director of
    Audiology
Division of Hearing and Speech Sciences
Department of Otolaryngology
Vanderbilt University School of Medicine
Vanderbilt Balance and Hearing Center
Nashville, Tennessee

Susan J. Herdman, Ph.D., P.T.
Assistant Professor
Department of Otolaryngology-Head and
    Neck Surgery
The Johns Hopkins University
Baltimore, Maryland

Larry Hoffman, Ph.D.
Assistant Professor
Division of Head and Neck Surgery
UCLA School of Medicine
Los Angeles, California

Vicente Honrubia, M.D.
Professor, Head and Neck Surgery
    (Otolaryngology)
Director, Victor Goodhill Ear Center
UCLA School of Medicine
Los Angeles, California

Gary P. Jacobson, Ph.D.
Director, Division of Audiology
Department of Otolaryngology
Henry Ford Hospital
Detroit, Michigan

Jack M. Kartush, M.D.
Michigan Ear Institute
Farmington Hills, Michigan

Michael J. LaRouere, M.D.
Attending Physician
Michigan Ear Institute
Providence Hospital
Farmington Hills, Michigan

Lewis M. Nashner, Sc.D.
Adjunct Professor of Physiology
Oregon Health Sciences University
Adjunct Senior Scientist
R.S. Dow Neurobiological Sciences Institute
Good Samaritan Hospital
Portland, Oregon

Craig W. Newman, Ph.D.
Division of Audiology
Department of Otolaryngology
Henry Ford Hospital
Detroit, Michigan

Edward L. Peterson, Ph.D.
Section Head of Biostatistics
Henry Ford Hospital
Detroit, Michigan

Mitchell K. Schwaber, M.D.
Assistant Professor
Department of Otolaryngology
Vanderbilt University Medical Center
Nashville, Tennessee

Michael D. Seidman, M.D.
Department of Otolaryngology
Henry Ford Hospital
Detroit, Michigan

Haim Sohmer, Ph.D.
Department of Physiology
Hebrew University—Hadassah Medical
  School
Jerusalem, Israel

Charles W. Stockwell, Ph.D.
Director, Vestibular Laboratory
Providence Hospital
Southfield, Michigan

PREFACE

The idea for this book started 10 years ago when, frustrated by being unable to locate a concise source that described the whole of balance function testing, two of the editors (G.P.J. and C.W.N.) pondered the idea of writing a text on the subject. We discussed these thoughts with a number of our colleagues who had themselves either written or edited texts. Although they saw the need for such a book, their responses were far from encouraging because of the amount of time and energy required to complete such a project.

Some 10 years later, still frustrated by the fact that a comprehensive text on balance function testing was not available, the same editors again approached the subject with caution. At present, the clinician interested in understanding the anatomy and physiology of the balance system and the evaluation of the same may find this information distributed throughout a number of excellent texts. However, while these volumes are excellent resources, none of these books by themselves are designed for the practitioner who must carry out the task of preparing a patient for testing, conducting the examination, and interpreting the data. Also, the area of balance function testing has become quite complex over the past 10 years. Now more than ever, sophisticated balance function assessment procedures have found their way into many clinical practices. When we entered the field, electronystagmo-graphy (ENG) was the only vestibular function test battery routinely used for clinical purposes. Within the more recent past, rotational testing and computerized dynamic posturography (CDP) have been added to the clinician's armamentarium.

Fortunately, B.C. Decker/Mosby-Year Book was genuinely enthusiastic and willing to take on this project. We then recruited a neurotology colleague (J.K.) and made our commitment to the publisher. We managed to enlist the services of a number of nationally and internationally known experts in the area of balance function testing and correlated areas to participate in this project. Writing a chapter is a time-consuming and formidable task. We are grateful to our contributors for their enthusiasm and commitment in helping us to complete this work.

The present text has been designed to serve as a resource "handbook" for clinicians and technicians who assess patients with balance system disorders. Part I provides a historical framework for understanding the evolution of balance function testing. Part II begins with a comprehensive overview of the anatomy and physiology of the vestibular system and the underlying principles of electro-oculography. These chapters set the stage for the remainder of the section, which focuses on the subtests comprising the ENG test battery. Parts III and IV provide the reader with a comprehensive description of rotational and CDP test techniques. In Part V, "special issues" associated with balance function testing are addressed. In addition to information regarding the medical and surgical management of vertiginous patients, a variety of topics are discussed, including intraoperative monitoring during vestibular surgery, assessment of balance function handicap, balance rehabilitation, and vestibular evoked potentials. The latter chapters represent the most current information relating to these adjunct areas.

In putting this handbook together, our goal has been to provide a comprehensive, readable, and practical description of all balance function tests and their interpretation. It is up to the reader to judge the extent to which we have accomplished our goal.

GARY P. JACOBSON, PH.D.
CRAIG W. NEWMAN, PH.D.
JACK M. KARTUSH, M.D.

CONTENTS

PART III: ROTATIONAL TESTING   *235*

PART IV: POSTUROGRAPHIC TESTING   *259*

PART V: SPECIAL ISSUES   *335*

PART I

Introduction

CHAPTER 1

An Historical Perspective on Balance Function Testing

Joseph M. R. Furman, M.D., Ph.D.

Ideas regarding vestibular function have been developing since the late eighteenth century. Scientists such as Erasmus Darwin, Pierre Flourens, J. E. Purkyně, and Hermann Helmholtz are examples of leaders in the early thinking about vestibular and ocular motor function.[2, 5, 13, 15] In 1873 and 1874, three researchers, including Ernst Mach, Joseph Breuer, and Alexander Crum-Brown, published papers almost simultaneously regarding theories of motion perception.[6] One of the outgrowths of the work of these and other great thinkers was the field of vestibular and ocular motor assessment.

The history of vestibular physiology has been thoroughly described by Pappas,[13] as seen through the eyes of Robert Barany, who, in the early 20th century, made major contributions to the medical understanding of the human vestibular mechanism and labyrinthine nystagmus. For his contributions to vestibular physiology, Barany received the Nobel Prize in 1915. Barany developed the convection theory underlying the response to caloric stimulation. He also investigated rotational testing and devised the rotating chair. Barany's method of rotation included rotating a patient ten times in 20 seconds (an average of 180°/sec) and then abruptly stopping the rotation and observing postrotational nystagmus. In addition to caloric and rotational testing, galvanic testing was also employed in the early twentieth century. Whereas caloric and rotational testing have become the mainstay of vestibular assessment, galvanic testing has not proved to be as useful. Also to Barany's credit was an investigation of postural instability produced by vestibular lesions, which predates current assessment of upright stance using dynamic posturography.

These three broad categories of vestibular assessment—caloric testing, rotational testing, and posturography testing—are the techniques found today in many university facilities. Of the three, caloric testing remains the mainstay of vestibular assessment because it provides the ability to test each ear separately. Rotational testing, although it stimulates both labyrinths simultaneously, remains popular because it is precise, can be repeated without much patient discomfort, and can be used to assess visual-vestibular interaction. Posturography is still developing and is growing in clinical use. Each of these three modern practices has had somewhat of a different genesis, though each is built on underlying principles developed in the eighteenth, nineteenth, and early twentieth centuries. Modern methods of recording responses such as eye movement, postural sway, and evoked potentials, together with the advent of computers has altered the precise manner in which testing is performed.

The development of electronystagmography, which is the use of electro-oculography to record nystagmus, was described for the first time in North America in 1929 by I. L. Meyers[8] and has had a profound influence on vestibular assessment using both caloric stimulation and rotational stimulation. Subsequent work by O. H. Mowrer et al.[9] determined that the basis of electro-oculography was the corneoretinal dipole potential. The advent of objective eye movement recording using electro-oculography allowed subjects' responses to be recorded both in the light and in the dark; for rotational testing, responses could be recorded *during* the stimulus.

Although caloric testing is the most common method of vestibular assessment, there are many variations in how this test is performed (see Chapters 8 and 9). As yet there is no accepted standard of practice, although the alternate binaural bithermal method introduced by Fitzgerald and Hallpike in 1942[4] is the most commonly used. The advent of computers has allowed caloric responses to be analyzed by automation but has not altered testing procedures.

The type of rotational testing introduced by Barany used an impulsive stimulus: that is, an abrupt, short-lived acceleratory stimulus. This stimulus had the advantage that it could be delivered by hand and the patient's response could be observed with the naked eye while the patient was still. Van Egmond and associates[14] introduced the term "cupulogram" for the plot of postrotatory sensation and nystagmus duration versus the magnitude of the impulses used because impulsive stimulation was thought to impart a brief displacement of the semicircular canal cupula. Impulsive testing is still used today in many laboratories that perform rotational testing because it has the advantage of producing an abrupt, high-intensity, unidirectional acceleratory stimulus. Because of its high intensity, such a stimulus is especially useful in measuring the responses of patients with bilaterally reduced vestibular function.[1]

Other types of rotational stimuli have been studied, and some are used regularly by many laboratories (see Chapter 10). Constant acceleration testing has not proved to be particularly useful. Sinusoidal rotation initially was performed using a torsion swing chair, which provides a damped sinusoidal oscillation. More recently, computer-controlled turntables deliver sinusoidal stimuli of precise frequency and amplitude.[1, 3, 7, 12] Like caloric testing, there is no established rotational test battery, although many laboratories use a combination of impulsive testing and sinusoidal testing at various frequencies and amplitudes.

Dynamic posturography testing is still a field undergoing development. In many laboratories, it is performed using a technique originated by Lewis Nashner, who in the early 1970s developed a method that attempted to isolate the influence of the vestibular labyrinth on the postural control system[10, 11] (see Chapters 12 to 14). Although both caloric and rotational testing assess the vestibulo-ocular system, posturography testing has the potential to add unique information to balance function assessment regarding the influence of vestibular lesions on upright postural control. Moreover, dynamic posturography has the potential to address "balance" in the broader sense of standing and walking. As compared with rotational testing, and certainly as compared with caloric testing, posturography testing is not nearly as well developed and formalized. Further experience and research will determine the ultimate role of posturography in balance function assessment.

There are several tests of ocular motor function and vestibulo-ocular function that, together with caloric testing, have evolved into current-day "electronystagmography." Whereas *electro-oculography* is the method of using the corneoretinal dipole potential to assess eye position, *electronystagmography* has come to mean the combination of caloric testing and other stimuli that may produce *nystagmus*. These stimuli include removing visual fixation, gazing from the primary position, and changing a patient's orientation with respect to gravity (that is, positional testing, discussed in Chapter 7). Additionally, assessment of ocular motor function directly by measurement of saccades, ocular pursuit, and optokinetic nystagmus has become an integral part of electronystagmography. This is appropriate because the vestibulo-ocular reflex is an indirect method of assessment of vestibular function, and abnormalities of the ocular motor system, per se, may obscure a vestibular abnormality.

Ocular motor testing has developed somewhat separately from balance function testing into a method of assessing neurologic function. Typically, when coupled with other vestibular tests, oculomotor testing is performed only as a screening battery. However, when performed properly using computer methods and interpreted by experienced observers, ocular motor testing provides information that is often useful independent of vestibular system assessment (see Chapters 3–6). The newer special issues in balance function testing include intraoperative monitoring (see Chapter 16) and others still in the developmental phase, such as vestibular evoked potentials (see Chapter 19).

Two current issues in the area of management of persons with balance function impairment include the *handicap* caused by balance disorders and the *rehabilitation* of the patient with balance disorders (see Chapters 17 and 18). Although the efficacy of physical therapy for patients with balance disorders has not been formally established, there is much clinical literature to suggest that it is indeed useful. The broad array of interdisciplinary backgrounds focused on testing and treatment of balance disorders is indicative of the fact that balance function assessment is a complex endeavor and a progressive, growing field of knowledge.

REFERENCES

1. Baloh RW, Honrubia V: *Clinical Neurophysiology of the Vestibular System.* Philadelphia, FA Davis, 1979.
2. Cohen B: The roots of vestibular and oculomotor research. *Hum Neurobiol* 1984; 3:121–128.
3. Cramer RL, Dowd PJ, Helms DB: Vestibular responses to oscillations about the yaw axis. *Aerospace Med* 1963; 34:1031.
4. Fitzgerald G, Hallpike CS: Studies in human vestibular function: Observations on the directional preponderance ("Nystagmusbereitschaft") of caloric nystagmus resulting from cerebral lesions. *Brain* 1942; 65:115–137.
5. Grusser OJ: J. E. Purkyne's contributions to the physiology of the visual, the vestibular and the oculomotor systems. *Hum Neurobiol* 1984; 3:129–144.
6. Henn V: E. Mach on the analysis of motion sensation. *Hum Neurobiol* 1984; 3:145–148.
7. Mathog RH: Testing of the vestibular system by sinusoidal angular acceleration. *Acta Otolaryngol* 1972; 74:96.
8. Meyers IL: Electronystagmography. *Arch Neurol Psychiatr* 1929; 21:901–918.
9. Mowrer OH, Ruch TC, Miller NE: The corneoretinal potential difference as the basis of the galvanometric method of recording eye movements. *Am J Physiol* 1935–1936; 14:423–428.
10. Nashner LM: A model describing vestibular detection of body sway motion. *Acta Otolaryngol* 1971; 72:429–436.
11. Nashner LM: Vestibular postural control model. *Kybernetick* 1972; 10:106–110.
12. Niven JJ, Hinson C, Correlia MJ: An experimental approach to the dynamics of the vestibular mechanisms, in *Symposium on the Role of the Vestibular Organs in the Exploration of Space.* NASA Publication No SP-77:43. Pensacola, Fla, National Aeronautics and Space Administration, 1965.
13. Pappas DG: Barany's history of vestibular physiology. *Ann Otol Rhinol Laryngol* 1984; 93:1–16.
14. Van Egmond AAJ, Groen JJ, Jongkees LBW: The turning test with small regulable stimuli. I: Method of examination: Cupulometria. *J Laryngol Otol* 1948; 2:63.
15. Westheimer G: Helmholtz on eye movements. *Hum Neurobiol* 1984; 3:149–152.

PART II

Electronystagmography

CHAPTER 2

Practical Anatomy and Physiology of the Vestibular System

Vicente Honrubia, M.D., and Larry F. Hoffman, Ph.D.

OVERVIEW OF VESTIBULAR FUNCTION

The vestibular system plays a central role in the maintenance of equilibrium and gaze stability. The vestibular sensory organs transduce the forces associated with head acceleration and gravity into a biological signal. This signal is utilized by control centers within the central nervous system (CNS) to develop a subjective sensation of head position in relation to the environment, and to produce motor reflexes that facilitate vision and locomotion. In this function, the vestibular system represents one of the elements involved in a larger task that is better described as *orientation*, a function that requires the interaction of the vestibular system together with other systems to make navigation within the environment possible.

The importance of vestibular function in the broader context of animal orientation and navigation is illustrated through a brief discussion of the phylogenetic representation of vestibular receptors.[16] The appearance of the vestibular receptors paralleled the ability of most primitive forms of life to move in their environment. These rudimentary vestibular receptors are referred to generally as *statocysts*, although they may appear in a variety of forms. An illustrative example of the introduction of statocysts to facilitate navigation is in the aquatic tunicate *Ciona intestinalis*, an animal that is free-swimming in the tadpole larval form but metamorphoses into a sessile adult form. In this animal, statocysts are found only premetamorphically but are lost in the postmetamorphic form.

The interaction between vestibular and other sensory systems subserving navigation is also found in phylogenetically primitive animals. For example, in the invertebrate *Hermissenda*, with only rudimentary vestibular and visual receptors, the two systems fully interact to control locomotor behavior.[48] Afferent signals from photoreceptors in the eye and from hair cells in the statocyst converge on interneurons in the cerebropleural ganglia, which project to putative motor neurons in each pedal ganglion to effect turning of the animals toward light. Such sensory interaction forms the rudiment of that found in humans, where gaze stabilization is achieved through the interaction of vestibular, neck proprioceptive, and visual inputs. For this oculomotor behavior the interaction can be synergistic or antagonistic. For example, when head movements lie in a direction opposite to that required to maintain the desired gaze position, the visual and vestibular reflexes work in concert to facilitate behavior. On the other hand, when the head is being turned to follow a moving object (such as a flying bird or speeding auto), the visual reflex overrides the vestibular signals that would otherwise lead to conflicting oculomotor behavior, producing blurred vision and, most likely, disorientation.

The diagram in Figure 2–1 schematizes the convergence and interaction of different sensory systems subserving the ultimate goal of appropriate orientation within the environment. Each receptor system provides information to a first line of individual processors. These messages then converge upon a common central processor to provide the signals effecting eye movements and postural reflexes. This common central processor is believed to be a distributed property of the CNS but, as will be shown later, the vestibular nuclei are a major component of this processor. An important aspect of the functional organization of this orientation system is the operation of adaptive feedback loops in a manner similar to that involved in other aspects of brain function and behavior.[66] These loops provide the central processor with

information from across sensory modalities to perform automated tasks, such as the repetitive execution of an athletic skill, or navigation and locomotion as in the examples mentioned earlier. Adaptive mechanisms are also important in selecting orienting strategies, such as maintaining equilibrium after a shift in one's center of gravity by moving—individually or in concert—the knees, hips, or arms.[99] Indeed, it can be thought that even the simplest and most natural tasks, such as standing and walking, result from learned experiences involving multiple sensory interactions.

The importance of adaptation within the vestibulo-ocular reflex (VOR) is apparent when one considers that the amplitude of eye movement elicited by the VOR changes by several percent whenever magnifying or minifying spectacles are used. An extreme example of such adaptation is the complete direction reversal of the VOR reflex that occurs after one wears glasses with reversing prisms for several days (that is, the eyes will move in the same direction as that of the head instead of the opposite direction).[96] The neuroanatomic and physiologic substrate for this capability is only partly understood, but the clinical im-

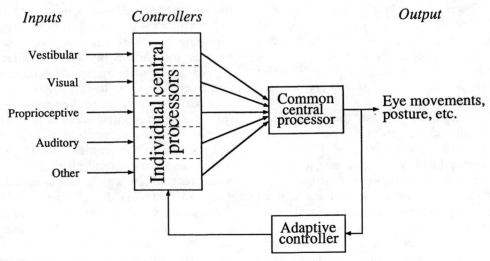

FIG 2–1.
Schematic diagram illustrating the organization of central nervous system integration of the polymodal sensory inputs with the motor outputs commonly associated with the activation of vestibular receptors.

portance of adaptive mechanisms is clear: clinical findings may be the direct reflection of the system's adaptation to a pathologic perturbation. Modern approaches to the evaluation of vestibular function must consider the multiplicity of functional and anatomic correlates. These considerations are also pertinent to pathologic conditions.

What are the strategies that patients use to compensate for loss of vestibular function? Why do some patients continue to complain of dizziness for months after such lesions, whereas others recover rapidly? Understanding the adaptive mechanisms is fundamental to understanding patient symptoms (which can be interpreted as a reflection of the failure to develop coping strategies) and for the design of rehabilitation programs.

Vestibular Reflexes

The basic elements of a vestibular reflex are the receptors transducing head movements (hair cells), and a three-neuron arc consisting of a primary afferent bipolar neuron, a central processor interneuron, and an effector neuron (Fig 2–2). Comparable three-neuron reflex arcs have wide distribution in the animal kingdom. For example, they have been identified in the phylum *Mollusca*, among which the class *Cephalopoda* has contributed to many classic anatomic and physiologic studies of gravitational reflexes.[16] An important three-neuron vestibular reflex involved in the stabilization of gaze is the VOR effected by stimulation of the horizontal semicircular canals. This reflex involves clockwise (as viewed from above the rotating subject) angular acceleration in the plane of the horizontal semicircular canals, resulting in increased activity in afferent neurons innervating the crista ampullaris of the right horizontal semicircular canal. These signals are carried to the vestibular nuclei situated in the dorsolateral medulla of the brain stem.

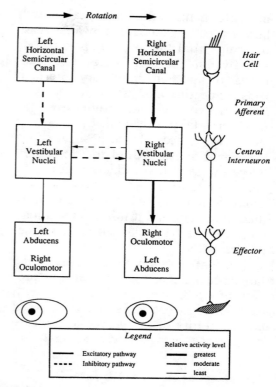

FIG 2–2.
Schematic diagram illustrating organization of the horizontal vestibulo-ocular reflex. At right is shown the neural components at each stage of the simplest three-neuron (that is, primary afferent neuron to effector motoneuron) pathway of the reflex.

Central processor neurons in the vestibular nuclei then transmit the signal to effector neurons in the left abducens and right oculomotor nuclei. Excitation of these effector (motor) neurons leads to contraction of the left lateral rectus and right medial rectus muscles, initiating compensatory deviation of the eyes to the left.

A very important aspect of vestibular function is the organization of participating structures into conjugate pairs on each side of the neuraxis, such that they react reciprocally to the acceleration stimuli. The reciprocal nature of activity in primary afferent neurons innervating the horizontal semicircular canal cristae is based on the presence of a level of spontaneous activity even when the system is at rest. During the head rotation described earlier, the increase in firing in the right horizontal ampullary nerve is accompanied by a decrease in firing (from the level of spontaneous activity) in the left horizontal canal nerve. In addition, inhibitory interneurons connecting the vestibular nuclei receive primary afferent activity from the ipsilateral labyrinth, and, by means of these two classes of neurons, the afferent signal arriving from the ampullary nerve exerts a dual influence on the effector system: it excites the agonist group of muscles (left lateral and right medial rectus), and it inhibits the antagonist muscle (right lateral and left medial rectus).

The control of motor responses by the labyrinth is, therefore, a two-way process of excitation and inhibition with each having two modes of action, based on the ability of the nerves to increase or decrease their activity (see Fig 2–2).

Function of the Vestibular Reflexes

At least three major functional roles for vestibular reflexes can be identified. The first is to maintain posture. If the pull of gravity on the body were unopposed by forces developed in the muscles, the body would collapse. Reflexes in this category are dependent on the function of the maculae and proprioceptive systems, but not on that of the semicircular canals. The second role is to produce "kinetic" or transitory contractions of muscles for maintenance of equilibrium and ocular stability during movement. This category includes reflexes arising from both the semicircular canals during angular acceleration and the otolithic organs during linear acceleration. Most natural head movements contain both types of acceleration and the vestibular reflexes act in concert to maintain equilibrium. A third role of vestibular reflex activity is to help maintain muscular tone, a role in which both maculae and cristae participate. The labyrinthine contribution to musculoskeletal tone can be demonstrated by the change of posture that follows unilateral labyrinthectomy in healthy animals. Tone is increased in the extensor muscles of the contralateral extremities and decreased in the ipsilateral extensor muscles.

Clinical Evaluation of Vestibular Function

Until recently, clinical vestibular tests were primarily system-oriented; that is, they attempted to isolate the vestibular system from other systems. This approach had its limitations because oculomotor and postural control are complex functions that require coordinated interaction of multiple sensory and motor systems. During the past decade, new methods have been developed to analyze objectively all the systems that control eye movements and posture. A large number of observations are being made that are producing an integrated and expanding picture of vestibular pathophysiology. This technology has created renewed interest in vestibular testing in different fields of medicine (such as otolaryngology, neurology, rehabilitation, ophthalmology, and psychology) because of its importance for evaluation not only of inner ear disorders but also of various neurologic conditions.

Most of the methods for evaluation of vestibular function are based on the measurements of reflex responses, and in order to interpret the results of clinical vestibular testing, one must have an understanding of the normal physiology of the vestibular reflexes. The *vestibulo-ocular reflexes*, in particular, will be reviewed extensively. The neurons in this reflex connect the labyrinthine receptor organs with the 12 extraocular muscles of the eyes; therefore, it is theoretically possible, through the measurement of eye movements, to correlate vestibular lesions with impairment of the organs' reflex functions. Although experimental investigations of vestibulo-ocular reflexes were initiated in the first quarter of this century, the contribution of each receptor organ and neural connection to the production of eye movements is still not completely known. The afferent signals from different vestibular receptors to each of the eye muscles overlap, and the central neural pathways lie so close to each other that it is often difficult to identify the receptor or pathway responsible for the deterioration of reflex function.

Measurements of subjective sensation of motion as a basis for the evaluation of vestibular function are, for the most part, experimentally at variance with those of other systems (such as hearing and vision). Within the range of most natural head movements, subjects refer to the sensation of motion in terms of the velocity of the motion, even though the vestibular receptors are sensors of accelerations. As will be shown later, the responses of most vestibular nerve fibers to the same type of stimuli reflect the time course of head velocity. In spite of the importance of the vestibular sys-

tem to the appreciation of a subject's motion in relation to objects and of objects in relation to individuals, there are no well-accepted methods for clinical evaluation of the sensations. Earlier attempts such as cupulometry were not successful, and there have been no further studies in this area.

ANATOMY

The Ear

The ear is a compound organ sensitive to sound and the forces associated with linear and angular acceleration. It is divided into three anatomic parts: the external, middle, and inner ear. Except for the auricle and the soft tissue (skin and cartilage) portion of the external auditory canal, the ear is enclosed within the temporal bone of the skull.

The cross-section of the temporal bone in Figure 2–3 illustrates the relationship between the three parts of the ear. Although the external and middle

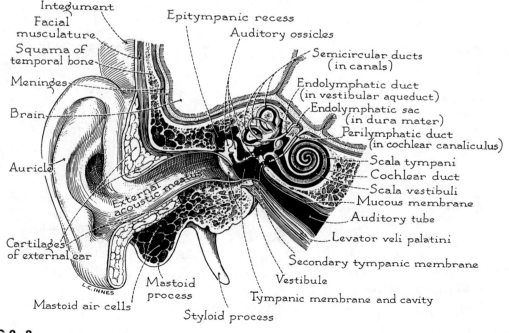

Integument
Facial musculature
Squama of temporal bone
Meninges
Brain
Auricle
External acoustic meatus
Cartilages of external ear
L.C. INNES
Mastoid air cells
Mastoid process
Styloid process

Epitympanic recess
Auditory ossicles
Semicircular ducts (in canals)
Endolymphatic duct (in vestibular aqueduct)
Endolymphatic sac (in dura mater)
Perilymphatic duct (in cochlear canaliculus)
Scala tympani
Cochlear duct
Scala vestibuli
Mucous membrane
Auditory tube
Levator veli palatini
Secondary tympanic membrane
Vestibule
Tympanic membrane and cavity

FIG 2–3.
Cross-section of ear, illustrating the gross anatomy of the external, middle, and inner ear. *(From Anson BJ, Donaldson JA: Surgical Anatomy of the Temporal Bone and Ear. Philadelphia, WB Saunders, 1973. Used by permission.)*

ear contribute primarily to auditory function with no direct bearing on vestibular function, an appreciation of their structure and development, particularly that of the middle ear, is important for understanding diseases involving the inner ear.[79] For example, infection arising in the middle ear can spread directly through its medial wall into the inner ear, or it can enter the intracranial cavity by breaking through the roof of the epitympanic recess (see Fig 2–3). Passageways interconnect the epitympanic recess and air cells throughout the temporal bone, so that infection beginning in the middle ear can spread to the vessels and nerves passing through the temporal bone.

squamous, mastoid, petrous, and tympanic (Figs 2–4 and 2–5). The tympanic portion, the smallest, forms the anterior, inferior, and part of the posterior wall of the external auditory canal (or external acoustic meatus in Figs 2–4 and 2–5). The petrous portion or pyramid contains the sense organs of the inner ear (see Fig 2–5). The seventh and eighth cranial nerves enter the petrous portion through the internal auditory canal; the facial nerve exits by way of the stylomastoid foramen of the mastoid portion (see Fig 2–5). The internal carotid artery and internal jugular vein enter the skull through the temporal bone, their bony canals forming part of the anteroinferior wall of the middle ear.

Temporal Bone

The temporal bone contributes to the base and lateral wall of the skull and forms part of the middle and posterior fossae.[5] It is divided into four parts: the

Facial Nerve

Within the temporal bone course the peripheral segments of the facial nerve. It arises at the inferior border of the

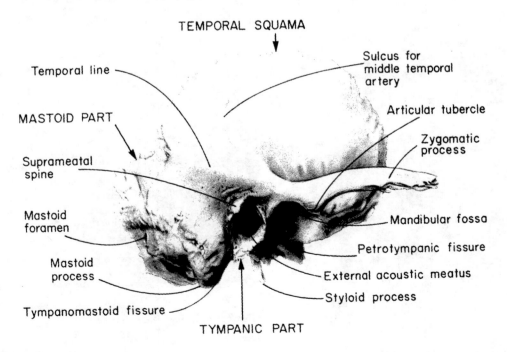

TEMPORAL SQUAMA

Temporal line

Sulcus for middle temporal artery

MASTOID PART

Articular tubercle

Zygomatic process

Suprameatal spine

Mastoid foramen

Mandibular fossa

Petrotympanic fissure

Mastoid process

External acoustic meatus

Styloid process

Tympanomastoid fissure

TYMPANIC PART

FIG 2–4.
Lateral view of the temporal bone. In this view, the squamous, mastoid, and tympanic portions of the temporal bone can be visualized. *(From Anson BJ, Donaldson JA: Surgical Anatomy of the Temporal Bone and Ear. Philadelphia, WB Saunders, 1973. Used by permission.)*

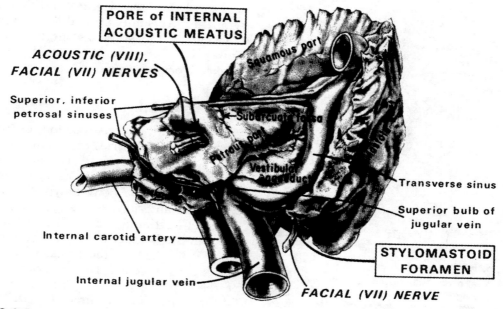

FIG. 2–5.

Medial view of the temporal bone. In this view, the squamous, mastoid, and petrous portions of the temporal bone can be visualized. *(From Anson BJ, Donaldson JA, Warpeha RL and Resnick MJ:* The facial Nerve, Sheath and Blood Supply in relation to the Surgery of Decompression. *Ann Otol Rhinol Laryngol 1970;79:710-27. Used by permission)*

pons and proceeds to the internal auditory canal on the superior surface of the cochlear nerve. Within the temporal bone, four portions of the facial nerve can be classified: the canal (or meatal) segment (7 to 8 mm); the labyrinthine segment (3 to 4 mm); the tympanic (or horizontal) segment (12 to 13 mm); and the mastoid (or vertical) segment (15 to 29 mm) (Fig 2–6).

The canal segment runs in close company with the vestibular and cochlear divisions of the eighth cranial nerve, while in its remaining segments the facial nerve lies separately within a bony canal, termed the facial or fallopian canal. The labyrinthine segment runs at nearly a right angle to the petrous pyramid, superior to the cochlea and vestibule, to reach the geniculate ganglion. At the geniculate ganglion, the nerve takes a sharp turn posteriorly, marking the beginning of the tympanic segment. The tympanic segment passes along the medial wall of the tympanic cavity su-

perior to the oval window and inferior to the horizontal semicircular canal. At the sinus tympani, the nerve bends inferiorly, marking the beginning of the mastoid segment.

Three major branches of the facial nerve lie within the temporal bone: the greater superficial petrosal nerve arising from the geniculate ganglion, the nerve to the stapedius muscle arising from the mastoid segment as it crosses the middle ear, and the chorda tympani leaving the facial nerve approximately 5 mm above the stylomastoid foramen.[18] The greater superficial petrosal nerve is composed of fibers of parasympathetic neurons originating in the superior salivatory nucleus that innervate the lacrimal glands and seromucinous glands of the nasal cavity. Additionally, this nerve carries fibers of afferent cutaneous sensory neurons that innervate parts of the external auditory canal, tympanic membrane, and middle ear, whose cell bodies are in the nucleus of the solitary

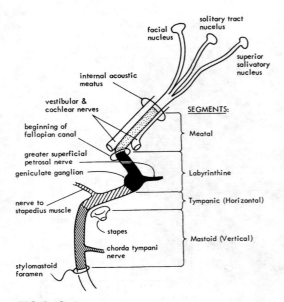

FIG 2–6.
The facial nerve, with its various parts and components, along its trajectory within the temporal bone. *(From Baloh RW, Honrubia V: Clinical Neurophysiology of the Vestibular System, ed 2. Philadelphia, FA Davis, 1990. Used by permission.)*

tract. The nerve to the stapedius muscle and the main facial nerve trunk are motor nerves originating from the facial nucleus in the caudal pons. The chorda tympani, like the greater superficial petrosal, is a mixed nerve containing (1) parasympathetic efferent fibers from the superior salivatory nucleus destined for the sublingual glands, and (2) afferent taste fibers from the anterior two-thirds of the tongue whose cell bodies are in the nucleus of the solitary tract.

Knowledge of the structure and function of each division of the facial nerve allows the clinician to localize disease affecting the nerve within the temporal bone. Lesions in the internal auditory canal commonly involve both the seventh and eighth cranial nerves. Lesions of the labyrinthine segment of the facial nerve above the geniculate ganglion impair ipsilateral (1) lacrimation, (2) stapedius reflex activity, (3) taste on the anterior two-thirds of the tongue, and (4) strength of the facial musculature. A lesion of the tympanic segment central to the nerve of the stapedius muscle affects only stapedius reflex activity, taste

as in (3), and facial musculature strength, and a lesion of the mastoid segment before the origin of the chorda tympani affects only (3) and (4). Finally a lesion at the stylomastoid foramen causes only ipsilateral facial muscle weakness or paralysis.

Bony Labyrinth

Within the petrous portion of the temporal bone, a series of hollow channels, the bony labyrinth, contains the auditory and vestibular sensory organs (see Fig 2–3). The bony labyrinth consists of an anterior cochlear part and a posterior vestibular part.[5] The *vestibule* is a central chamber (about 4 mm in diameter) marked by the recesses of the utricle and saccule. The superior and posterolateral walls of the vestibule contain openings for the three *semicircular canals*, and anteriorly is continuous with the scala vestibuli of the snail-shaped cochlea.

Medial to the bony labyrinth is the internal auditory canal, a cul-de-sac housing the seventh and eighth cranial nerves and internal auditory artery. The aperture on the cranial side is located at approximately the center of the posterior face of the pyramid of the temporal bone (see Fig 2–5). Two other important orifices are in this vicinity. Halfway between the canal and the sigmoid sinus, the slitlike aperture of the vestibular aqueduct contains the endolymphatic sac, a structure important in the exchange of endolymph. The second opening is that of the cochlear aqueduct at the same level as the internal auditory canal but on the inferior side of the pyramid (not visible in Fig 2–5). The labyrinthine opening of this channel is located in the scala tympani, providing a connection between the subarachnoid and the perilymphatic spaces.

Membranous Labyrinth

The membranous labyrinth is enclosed within the channels of the bony labyrinth (Fig 2–7,A). The space be-

A

B

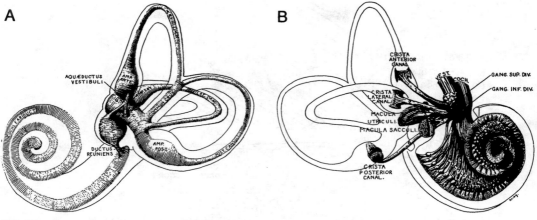

FIG 2–7.
The membranous labyrinth. **A,** this medial view of the exterior of the membranous labyrinth is indicated by the "shaded" system of conduits; the portions housing the five vestibular receptors are labeled. The inner wall of the bony labyrinth is indicated by the line around the membranous labyrinth. Also shown are the conduits providing communication between various portions of the membranous labyrinth (such as the *ductus reuniens*). **B,** the wall of the membranous labyrinth has been removed in this lateral view, exposing the five vestibular receptors. Also shown are the divisions of the eighth cranial nerve (*vest.,* vestibular; and *coch.,* cochlear), and the superior and inferior divisions of Scarpa's ganglion (*gang. sup. div.* and *gang. inf. div.,* respectively), which reside within the internal auditory canal. *1,* anterior canal nerve; *2,* horizontal canal nerve; *3,* utricular nerve; *4,* portion of superior vestibular nerve that innervates the saccule; *5,* main saccular nerve, from posterior vestibular nerve; *6,* posterior canal nerve.

tween the periostium of the bony labyrinth and the membranous labyrinth contains *perilymphatic fluid* (also known as *perilymph*) and a supportive network of connective tissue and blood vessels. The spaces within the membranous labyrinth contain *endolymphatic fluid* (also known as *endolymph*). The membranous labyrinth and endolymphatic system develops in the embryo as an invagination of the germinal ectodermal layer.[4] Starting as a simple fold, it soon becomes a closed cavity, the otocyst, isolated from the original ectoderm. By the end of the 7th week, the endolymphatic duct system is lodged in mesenchymal tissue, and by the 14th week, it attains the size that it will have in the adult ear. By successive infolding of the wall of that otocyst, three main areas are formed: the endolymphatic duct and sac; the utricle and semicircular canals; and, last, the saccule and cochlear duct. The membranous cochlea holds the organ of Corti for the transduction of sound energy. The utricle, saccule, and semicircular canals (the receptor organs

for the sense of position and motion) constitute the membranous labyrinth proper (Fig 2–7,B) and transduce the forces associated with head acceleration. Finally, the endolymphatic duct provides a channel for the exchange of endolymph and to balance the pressure between the endolymphatic and subarachnoid spaces.

Labyrinthine Fluids

The fluid-containing spaces of the labyrinth are illustrated in Figure 2–8. Perilymph is, in part, a filtration product of cerebrospinal fluid and, in part, a filtrate from the vasculature of the inner ear.[122] Endolymph, on the other hand, is the product of secretory cells in the stria vascularis of the cochlea and dark cells of the vestibular labyrinth.[73, 122] Resorption of endolymph is generally agreed to take place in the endolymphatic sac. Evidence for this comes from experiments in which dye and pigment injected into the cochleae of animals has been observed to accumulate in the endolym-

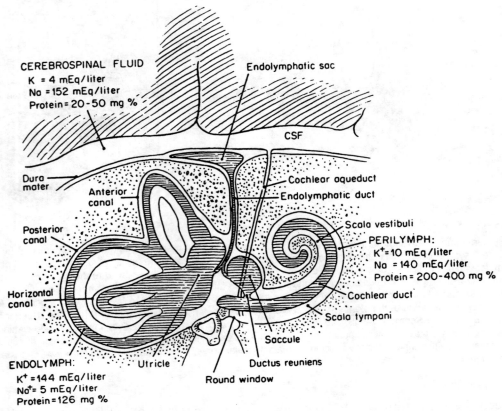

FIG 2–8.
Cross section of the inner ear. This diagram illustrates the fluid channels of the inner ear, and the difference in composition between *endolymph* and *perilymph*. *(From Baloh RW, Honrubia V: Clinical Neurophysiology of the Vestibular System, ed 2. Philadelphia, FA Davis, 1990. Used by permission.)*

phatic sac. Electron microscope studies of the membrane that lines the sac reveal active pinocytotic activity.[85] Furthermore, destruction of the epithelium lining the endolymphatic sac or occlusion of the duct results in an increase in endolymphatic volume in experimental animals.[74] The first change is a distension of cochlear and saccular membranes, which may completely fill the perilymphatic space. The anatomic changes resulting from this experiment are comparable to those found in the temporal bones of patients with Meniere's syndrome (either idiopathic or secondary to known inflammatory disease).

The chemical composition of the fluids filling the inner ear are similar to those of extracellular and intracellular fluids throughout the body. The endolymphatic system contains intracellular-like fluids with high potassium and low sodium concentrations, whereas the perilymphatic fluid resembles extracellular fluid with low potassium and high sodium concentrations.[122] The relationship between electrolytes and protein concentration in the different fluid compartments is shown in Figure 2–8.

THE HAIR CELL

Phylogeny

The basic element of the labyrinthine receptor organs that transduces mechanical force to nerve action potentials— the *hair cell*—is already developed in the statocysts of invertebrates.[16] These transducer cells are surrounded by supporting cells in specialized epithelial areas. These cells are characterized by ciliary bundles, comprised of one kinocilium and multiple stereocilia, protruding from their apical surface (Fig 2–9). The basal portion of the cell makes contact with terminals of afferent and efferent nerve fibers. The former carry information from the receptor to the CNS, and the latter provide feedback to the receptor cells from the CNS.

Two types of hair cells are found in birds and mammals (see Fig 2–9). *Type I* cells are globular or flask-shaped with a single, large, chalice-like terminal of a primary afferent neuron surrounding the base (the *calyx* type of primary afferent terminal). The afferent fibers inner-

vating these hair cells are among the largest in the nervous system (up to 20 μm in diameter). *Type II* cells, which are the only type of hair cells found in certain lower vertebrates (amphibians), are cylindrical with multiple bouton nerve terminals at their base.

The stereocilia are bound together at their top to the taller neighboring kinocilium. In experiments in which a force was applied directly to the cilia bundles of isolated hair cells, it was observed that the stereocilia and kinocilium move together with the rigidity of glass rods.[44] Recent findings indicate that the physical properties of the stereocilia can influence the function not

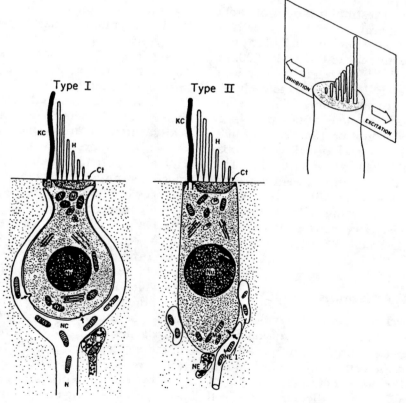

FIG 2–9.
Two types of hair cells found in the mammalian vestibular receptor neuroepithelium. These differ in gross morphology, as well as in the morphology of the afferent and efferent (no direct efferent contact upon type I cells) synapses. *KC*, kinocilium; *H*, hairs or stereocilia; *Ct*, cuticular plate; *M*, mitochondria; *Nu*, nucleus; *NC*, afferent neuron chalice; *NE 1*, afferent neuron bouton; *NE 2*, efferent neuron bouton. *Inset:* directional specificity of ciliary displacement to elicit excitation (depolarization) and inhibition (hyperpolarization) of the hair cell. *(From Baloh RW, Honrubia V: Clinical Neurophysiology of the Vestibular System, ed 2. Philadelphia, FA Davis, 1990. Used by permission.)*

only of individual hair cells, but also of whole receptor organs. For example, the length and stiffness of the cilia in the organ of Corti influence the motion of the overlying basilar membrane.[42] The stereocilia vary in length among hair cells of different organs, and even among hair cells at different loci within the same organ.[44, 76] In the frog crista there are two cilium patterns: the stereocilia of cells at the center are tall and thick and the kinocilia are relatively short, whereas stereocilia of cells at the periphery are thinner and the kinocilia are very long. The former are stiffer and have, presumably, a higher resonant frequency than the latter. Hair cells of mammalian vestibular receptors also have at least two stereocilia patterns.[6]

Within the vestibular labyrinth of one human temporal bone, the hair cells in the three cristae and two maculae number approximately 23,000 and 4,000, respectively,[117, 118] representing a ratio of approximately 1.4 hair cells to each primary afferent nerve fiber. These represent the full complement of hair cells to support labyrinthine function throughout life, as mammalian hair cells probably cannot regenerate after birth.[34] This contrasts the situation recently discovered for avian hair cells, where it was found that supporting cells can differentiate into sensory cells subsequent to hair cell destruction caused by acoustic trauma.[23, 120]

Hair Cell Activation

Stimulus Directionality

The adequate stimulus for hair cell activation is a force acting parallel to the top of the cell, resulting in bending of the hairs (see Fig 2–9, inset).[67] A force applied perpendicular to the cell surface (a compressional force) is ineffective in stimulating the hair cell. The stimulus is maximal when the force is directed along an axis that bisects the bundle of stereocilia and passes through the kinocilium. Deflection of the hairs

toward the kinocilium depolarizes the hair cell, while bending in the opposite direction hyperpolarizes the cell.[43] The effect is minimal when hair deflection is perpendicular to the axis of maximal excitation.

Physiology

Because the hair cells are embedded in the epithelium of the membranous labyrinth, their apical surface is in contact with the endolymph in the interior of the organ (high in potassium), while the basal surface is in contact with the perilymph that surrounds the organ (high in sodium). As with all living cells, the hair cell is selectively permeable, allowing some ions to enter while others are excluded. This selective permeability is achieved through the opening and closing of channels that allow only certain types of ions to cross the cell membrane. There is a voltage difference between the inside of the cell and the surrounding fluid, called the transmembrane potential. The cilia-bearing surface of the cell membrane is morphologically different from the rest, being thicker and more electron-dense, and is called the cuticular plate. During physiologic stimulation, ohmic resistance changes in proportion to the magnitude of hair deflection causing modulated changes in ionic conductance, resulting in current flow in a local circuit between the cuticular plate and other areas of the cell membrane (Fig 2–10). The voltage drop produced in the vicinity of the hair cells by the current flow is known as the *microphonic potential* (or, more generically, the receptor potential) of these receptor organs.[25, 67] In contrast to nerve action potentials, the hair cell microphonic potentials have no refractory period, following the frequency of the stimulation above several thousand hertz, and are highly resistant to anoxia. The electric currents associated with the receptor potentials act on the synaptic contacts between hair cells and nerve terminals by modulating the release of

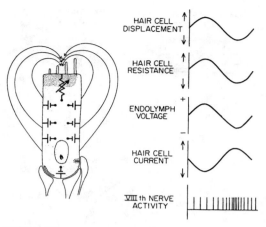

HAIR CELL DISPLACEMENT

HAIR CELL RESISTANCE

ENDOLYMPH VOLTAGE

HAIR CELL CURRENT

VIIIth NERVE ACTIVITY

FIG 2–10.

Schematized mechanism of hair cell activation. *Arrows* emanating from lateral aspect of hair cell illustrate the lines of current required that complete the local endolymph-perilymph circuit subsequent to stereocilia deflection. The *graphs at right* illustrate the modulation of each parameter subsequent to a sinusoidal stimulus eventually producing the modulation of the frequency of action potentials in the eighth cranial nerve. *(From Baloh RW, Honrubia V: Clinical Neurophysiology of the Vestibular System, ed 2. Philadelphia, FA Davis, 1990. Used by permission.)*

chemical transmitters which, in turn, modulate the firing of action potentials by primary afferent neurons.

Some hair cells may actively participate in the mechanotransduction process. This has been best studied in the cochlea, where the outer hair cells, which contain several contractile proteins, have been found to vary their length under direct electrical stimulation.[15] Therefore, the physiologic properties of the stereocilia of cochlear hair cells may be influenced by electrical currents of neighboring physiologically activated cells. Likewise, their mechanical properties could be affected by postsynaptic potentials from efferent neurons innervating the receptor.[97] The stereocilia of the vestibular hair cells contain actin molecules and undergo an active change in stiffness under conditions that elicit activity in muscle cells, such as experimentally changing the concentration of calcium ions.[104] It is logical to expect that anatomic differences in stereocilia reflect important differences in the process of transducing head motion information into neural signals.[139]

One of the most important findings concerning hair cell function was the discovery by Hoagland in the 1930s that afferent neurons from the lateral line organs of fish generated continuous spontaneous activity.[60] This observation has subsequently been confirmed in all other sensory systems and represents a fundamental discovery in sensory physiology. Although the mechanism responsible for this spontaneous firing of action potentials is not explicitly known, there is evidence indicating that spontaneous activity in vestibular afferents of bullfrogs is neurotransmitter mediated,[3] suggesting that neurotransmitter is steadily diffusing across the hair cell–afferent neuron synapse. As indicated earlier, bending of the hairs toward the kinocilium results in an increase of the firing rate, and bending of the hairs away from the kinocilium results in a decrease. The spontaneous firing rate varies among different animal species and among different sensory receptors. It is thought to be greatest in the afferent neurons of the semicircular canals of mammals (up to 90 spikes per second) and lowest in some of the acoustic nerve fibers innervating mammalian hair cells (1 to 2 spikes per second).[51, 72]

THE VESTIBULAR RECEPTORS

Basis for Stimulus Specificity of the Vestibular Receptor Organs

The cilia bundles of hair cells within the sensory neuroepithelium of the vestibular receptors project in and are coupled to an overlying gelatinous structure. This structure is called the *otolithic membrane* for the macula of the utricle and saccule, and the *cupula* for the cristae of the semicircular canals (Figs 2–11, A and C). For both type of sensory organs, the neuroepithelium is rigidly coupled to and moves with the head, while the otolithic membranes

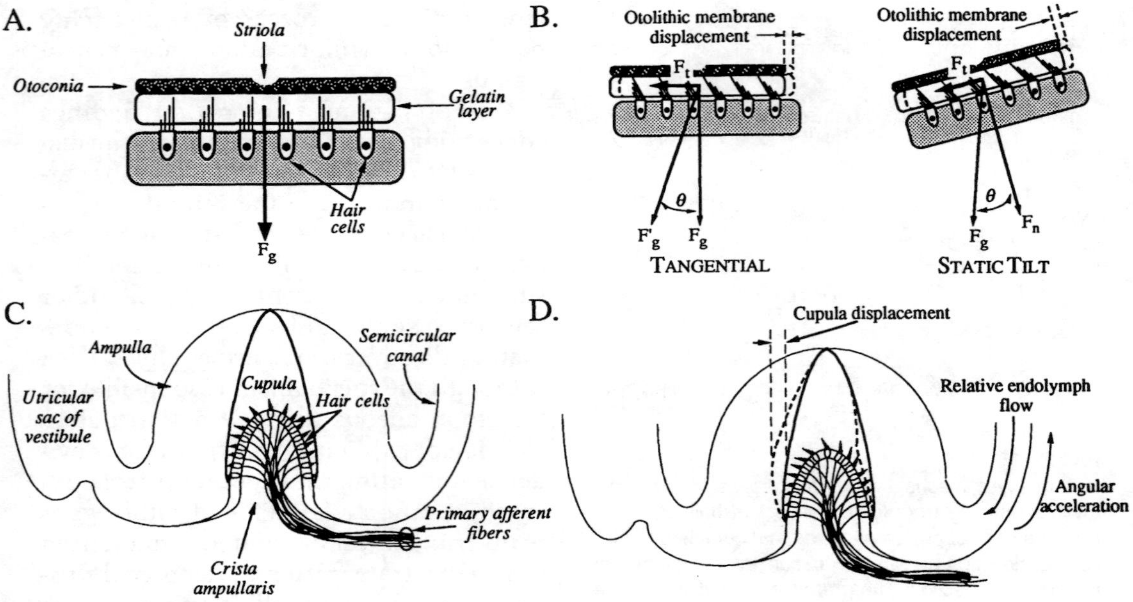

A.

B.

C.

D.

FIG 2–11.
Diagram of the primary anatomic features of the utricular macula **(A)** and the semicircular canal and crista **(C)**. The macula of the saccule differs in that the hair cells exhibit the opposite polarization relationship between striola and kinocilia. A schematized version of the displacement of the macula **(B)** and cupula **(D)** is also shown. Note the diaphragm-like displacement of the cupula subsequent to relative endolymph flow.

and cupulae are surrounded and affected by endolymph. The effective stimulus to the hair cells is the relative displacement of their cilia, which is produced when movement of the neuroepithelium occurs relative to the overlying structure. This condition is met during movements of the head, whereby endolymph, *not* being rigidly coupled to the head and exhibiting inertia, will resist that movement and likewise effect the otolithic membranes or cupulae (see Figs 2–11, B and D).

In the case of the macular organs, the otolithic membranes (comprised of the otoconia and gelatin layers, Fig 2–11, A) overlying the hair cells of the maculae have densities that are greater than that of the surrounding endolymph, and therefore exert a downward force on the sensory neuroepithelium as a result of Earth's gravity (F_g in Fig 2–11, A). During static tilt of the head (Fig 2–11, B, STATIC TILT), the weight of this membrane produces a shearing force (F_t) on the underlying hair cells that is proportional

to the sine of the angle θ between the line of the gravitational vector (F_g) and a line perpendicular to the plane of the macula (F_n in Fig 2–11,B). A comparable analysis may be applied to linear acceleration forces that are tangential to the plane of the macula (F_t in Fig 2–11,B, TANGENTIAL).

The hair cell cilia in the cristae of the semicircular canals are embedded in the cupula, a gelatinous substance having the same specific gravity as that of surrounding fluids (see Fig 2–11, C). Consequently, the cupula is effectively neutrally buoyant, and as such does not exert a force due to the earth's gravitational vector on the underlying crista and is not subject to displacement by relative changes in the line of gravitational force. The forces associated with angular head acceleration, however, do result in a displacement of the cupula, which stimulates the hair cells of the cristae in the same way that displacement of the otolith stimulates the macular hair cells (see Fig 2–11, D). Because the mechanical properties of the "support and coupling" structures differ in these two organs, the frequency ranges at which the cilia can be moved by applied forces also differ.

Semicircular Canals

Relationship Between Structure and Function

The semicircular canals are three membranous tubes with a cross-sectional diameter of, at maximum, 0.4 mm, each forming about two-thirds of a circle having a diameter of about 6.5 mm. They are aligned to form a coordinate system (Fig 2–12).[11, 12, 24] The plane of the horizontal semicircular canal makes a 30° angle with the horizontal plane; the other two canals are in vertical positions almost orthogonal to each other. The anterior canal is angled anterolaterally over the roof of the utri-

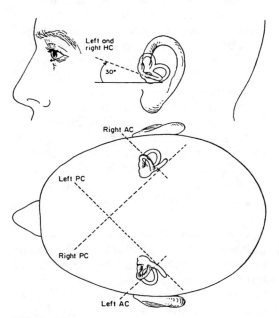

FIG 2–12.
Orientation of the semicircular canals of the human vestibular labyrinth. Note the angle of the plane of the horizontal semicircular canal relative to the eye and ear *(upper diagram)*, and that the primary planes of the anterior canal from one side and posterior canal from the opposite side are parallel, and as such act as conjugate pairs. *(From Baloh RW, Honrubia V: Clinical Neurophysiology of the Vestibular System, ed 2. Philadelphia, FA Davis, 1990. Used by permission.)*

cle, and the posterior canal is angled downward and laterally behind the utricle.The two vertical canals share a common opening on the posterior side of the utricle. Because the planes of the canals are not aligned perfectly, orthogonal natural angular head movements stimulate at least two canals and often all three.

At the anterior opening of the horizontal and anterior canals and the inferior opening of the posterior canal, each tube enlarges to form the ampulla. A crestlike septum—the crista—crosses each ampulla in a direction perpendicular to the longitudinal axis of the canals (see Fig 2–11, C). The cupula extends from the surface of the crista to the ceiling of the ampulla, forming what appears to be a water-tight seal.[112] In birds and lower mammals a higher proportion of type I hair cells are located in the ridge at the center of the crista, whereas type II hair cells predominate in the periphery.[37] In primates, type I hair cells predominate throughout the crista.[54]

The hair cells within each crista are oriented so that all their kinocilia point in the same direction. In the vertical (anterior and posterior) canals the kinocilia are directed toward the canal side of the ampulla, whereas in the horizontal canal they are directed toward the utricular side. The opposite morphologic polarization is the basis for the difference in directional sensitivity between the horizontal and vertical canals. The afferent nerve fibers of the horizontal canals are stimulated by endolymph movement in the utriculopetal (*toward* the utricle) direction and those of the vertical canals are stimulated by utriculofugal (*away* from the utricle) endolymph flow.

Dynamic Characteristics of Semicircular Canal Function—The Pendulum Model

The functional role of the semicircular canals was first linked to their gross and anatomic features by investigators in the late 1800s. Exposing the membranous labyrinth of the semicircular canals of pigeons, Ewald[36] applied positive and negative pressures to each canal membrane to cause ampullopetal and ampullofugal endolymph flow and made three important observations that became known as Ewald's laws of canal function: (1) the eye and head movements always occurred in the plane of the canal being stimulated and in the direction of endolymph flow; (2) ampullopetal endolymph flow in the horizontal canal caused a greater response (that is, induced movements) than did ampullofugal endolymph flow; and (3) ampullofugal endolymph flow in the vertical canals caused a greater response than did ampullopetal endolymph flow.

Steinhausen[128] and later Dohlman[30] first visualized the details of the movement of the cupula during endolymph flow, and observed the similarity between the cupular movement and that of a pendulum in a viscous medium. These observations led Steinhausen to model cupular kinematics accordingly, which has become known as the pendulum model of vestibular function. Although the large movements observed by Steinhausen and Dohlman were later realized to be artifactual, the basic principle has generally been upheld by more recent experimental and theoretical studies. Furthermore, physiologic verification of the model has been made by detailed study of the relationship between angular head acceleration and the transmission of action potentials in isolated ampullary nerve fibers (discussed later).

Biophysics of Cupula Displacement

On the basis of fluid mechanics, it can be argued that because of the configuration and dimensions of the canals, the endolymph movement can only occur along the cylindrical canalicular cavity. According to Newton's third principle, when an angular acceleration (and hence a force, $M\ddot{\theta}_h(t)$) is applied to the head, displacement of the cupula-endolymph system acting as a solid mass is opposed by three restraining forces: (1) an elastic force, $K\theta_c(t)$, due to the cupula's springlike properties; (2) the force due to the cupula-endolymph viscosity, $C\dot{\theta}_c(t)$; and (3) an inertial force, $M\ddot{\theta}_c(t)$, due to the fluid's mass. Cupular displacement can be described by the following equation, which is referred to as the equation of the pendulum model of semicircular canal function:

$$M\ddot{\theta}_c(t) + C\dot{\theta}_c(t) + K\theta_c(t) = M\ddot{\theta}_h(t) \quad (2-1)$$

The terms incorporated into equation 2-1 are: θ_c is the angular displacement of the cupula-endolymph system with respect to the wall of the canals; $\dot{\theta}_c$ and $\ddot{\theta}_c$ are the first (velocity) and second (acceleration) time derivatives of the cupular displacement; $\ddot{\theta}_h$ is the angular acceleration of the head; the coefficients M, C, and K all refer to the cupula-endolymph system, and represent the moment of inertia (M), the moment of viscous friction (C), and the moment of elasticity (K). There is always an equilibrium between the force applied to the fluid, $M\ddot{\theta}_h(t)$, and the various aspects of the cupula position and motion. The relationship between the time course of head acceleration, head velocity, and cupula displacement as predicted by the pendulum model for three different types of angular rotation stimuli commonly used in clinical vestibular testing is illustrated in Figure 2-13.

Constant Angular Acceleration.—The moment-to-moment fluid displacement following constant angular acceleration has an exponential time course that can be determined by a more detailed mathematical treatment of the pendulum model.[133, 135] The trajectory of the cupula as a function of time (*t*) following the application of a constant angular acceleration (α) stimulus is given by the following equation:

$$\theta_c(t) = \alpha \frac{M}{K}(1 - e^{-tK/C}) \quad (2-2)$$

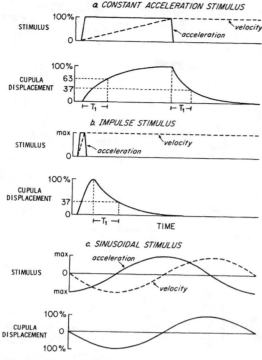

FIG 2–13.

Relationship between constant, impulse, and sinusoidal angular acceleration stimuli and the resultant cupular displacement, as predicted from the pendulum model. *(From Baloh RW, Honrubia V: Clinical Neurophysiology of the Vestibular System, ed 2. Philadelphia, FA Davis, 1990. Used by permission.)*

Accordingly, after a very long time the exponential term diminishes ($e^{-\infty} \rightarrow 0$) and the cupular deviation becomes proportional to the product of the acceleration magnitude (α) and the coefficient of proportionality M/K. Considering the exponential term $e^{-tK/C}$, it can be appreciated that when t is equal to C/K the exponential term has the value e^{-1}, or ≈ 0.37. The term within the parentheses on the right-hand side of equation (2–2) is now equal to 0.63. Consequently, measuring the time at which the response is 63% of the total provides an estimate of the value of C/K. This value is referred to in vestibular physiology as τ_1, the long time constant of the cupula. The high-frequency sensitivity of the cupula is determined by the so-called short time constant of the cupula, or τ_2, given by the ratio of the moment of inertia to the viscous friction coefficient ($\tau_2 = M/C$). The

product of the two terms as determined from equation 2–2, M/K · K/C, provides an estimate of τ_2.[135]

According to the pendulum model, not only is the deviation of the cupula driven by a constant acceleration stimulus dependent on the restraining elastic force of the cupula, but after the stimulus is terminated, the same force becomes a restoring drive and the cupula returns to the resting position. If the cupula was deviated an amount θ_c, the return to the resting position takes place according to the following equation:

$$\theta_c(t) = \theta_c \, e^{-tK/C} \qquad (2–3)$$

Thus the recovery process takes place with the same time constant $\tau_1 = C/K$ as that of the initial deviation. The deviation decays 63% for every interval of time (t) equal to τ_1, as shown graphically in Figure 2–13, *a*.

Impulse Angular Acceleration.—The displacement of the cupula following a brief impulse of angular acceleration is illustrated in Figure 2–13, *b*. This type of angular acceleration, although the least natural, is of great value in clinical vestibular testing. An impulse of acceleration is generated by changing the velocity of the head ($\Delta \dot{\theta}_h$) with the maximum acceleration possible. The maximum deviation of the cupula takes place almost immediately and is proportional to the magnitude of the "instantaneous" change in head velocity [$\theta_c(t) \approx \tau_2 \dot{\theta}_h$]. Of particular note, the cupular deviation thereafter decays exponentially with the same time course as that following the constant acceleration stimulus. That is, it takes one time constant (τ_1) to return 63% of the maximum deviation.

Sinusoidal Angular Acceleration.—Two types of measurements are typically used to quantify the response to sinusoidal stimulation: *gain* (that is, response *magnitude*) and *phase* (response *timing*, relative to the stimulus). In the case of cupular displacement illustrated in Figure 2–13, *c*, gain is defined as the ratio of the output (peak cupular displacement) to the input (peak head acceleration). The phase shift (in degrees, where 360° = one sinusoidal cycle = 1/cycle period) represents the timing between comparable points of the output (response) and the input (stimulus) waveforms. Such relationships are better described using *control systems analysis*. These analytical techniques incorporate the concept of the transfer function (T_f), defined as the ratio of the system's output (O) to the system's input (I). Using Laplace notation, this ratio may be expressed algebraically by $T_f(s) = O(s)/I(s)$. In the present context, the relationship between the output, cupular deviation ($\theta_c(t)$), and the input, ($\ddot{\theta}_h$), is given by the expression

$$\frac{\theta_c(t)}{\ddot{\theta}_h} = \frac{\tau_1\tau_2}{(\tau_1 s + 1)(\tau_2 s + 1)} \qquad (2\text{–}4)$$

where τ_1 and τ_2 are the long and short vestibular time constants, respectively. For many instances in vestibular physiology it is helpful to view the transfer function relative to stimulus *velocity*, where the input would be represented by the term $\dot{\theta}_h(t)$. Again, in the present context of a sinusoidal stimulus with angular frequency ω (in radians per second), equation (2–4) can be rewritten as

$$\frac{\theta_c(t)}{\dot{\theta}_h(t)} = \frac{\tau_1\tau_2\omega}{(\tau_1\omega + 1)(\tau_2\omega + 1)} \qquad (2\text{–}5)$$

The gain and phase relationship between the output and input as a function of stimulus frequency is commonly represented graphically by a *Bode plot* (Fig 2–14).

Some practical interpretations of the Bode plot for the equation of the pendulum model are as follows. For very low frequencies where ω $\ll 1/\tau_1$, the terms in the denominator of equation (2–5) approach 1, and the gain is determined by the product $\tau_1\tau_2\omega$. The gain, therefore, increases linearly as the frequency (ω) increases:

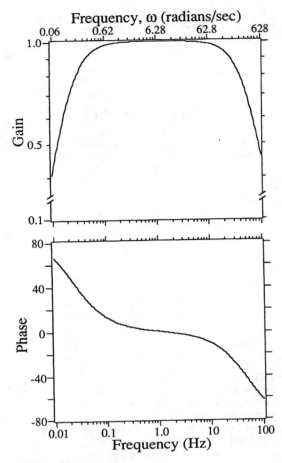

FIG 2–14.
Bode plots of normalized *gain* and *phase* as predicted by the equation of the pendulum model of semicircular canal function. Note the logarithmic scale for the abcissa and gain ordinate axes. The values for the two time constants of the equation are 7 and 0.003 seconds for τ_1 and τ_2, respectively.

$$\frac{\theta_c(t)}{\dot{\theta}_h(t)} \approx \tau_1\tau_2\omega \qquad (2\text{–}6)$$

For middle frequencies, when $1/\tau_1 < \omega < 1/\tau_2$, the gain is controlled by the first term in the denominator, or:

$$\frac{\theta_c(t)}{\dot{\theta}_h(t)} \approx \frac{\tau_1\tau_2\omega}{\tau_1\omega} \qquad (2\text{–}7)$$

$$\theta_c(t) \approx \tau_2\dot{\theta}_h(t)$$

Cupular deviation, therefore, is proportional to the velocity of the stimulus in this frequency range.

Finally, for very high frequencies ω >

$1/\tau_2$, the gain decreases as a function of frequency:

$$\frac{\theta_c(t)}{\dot{\theta}_h(t)} \approx \frac{1}{\omega} \qquad (2\text{–}8)$$

The phase relationship between the stimulus and response also varies with frequency (see Fig 2–14). At low frequencies, the response (θ_c) leads the stimulus ($\dot{\theta}_h$), reaching a maximum of 90° or a quarter cycle at very low frequencies ($\omega < 1/\tau_1$). In the middle-frequency region ($1/\tau_1 < \omega < 1/\tau_2$), the response and the stimulus are in phase. For very high frequencies ($\omega > 1/\tau_2$), the response lags behind the stimulus, reaching a maximum phase delay equivalent to another quarter cycle.

Innervation of the Crista Ampullaris

The transduction of head angular acceleration stimuli is communicated to the CNS by primary afferent neurons innervating hair cells within the neuroepithelium of the *crista ampullaris* (see Fig 2–11, C). These are true sensory bipolar neurons whose cell bodies are found in Scarpa's ganglion, from which a peripheral process projects to the receptor epithelia (see Fig 2–7, B) and a central process projects toward the CNS (for example, the vestibular nuclei, cerebellum, or reticular formation). These neurons, along with those innervating the macular receptors (discussed later), comprise the vestibular portion of the eighth cranial nerve, whereby Scarpa's ganglion is found within the internal auditory canal of the petrous portion of the temporal bone (see Fig 2–5). The patterns of primary afferent innervation within the cristae have been investigated with regard to the diameter and morphology of synaptic endings exhibited by the primary afferents.

In the vestibular nerve there is a unimodal distribution of primary afferent neurons with regard to axon and cell body diameter with a skewedness toward the smallest neurons (histograms in Fig 2–15). Additionally, fibers of various diameters are not equally distributed with respect to the region of the crista to which they project. Schematic sections through the base of human, monkey, and chinchilla cristae are shown in Figure 2–15. The largest-diameter fibers (>4.5 μm) innervate hair cells near the center of the crista, as illustrated by the greater density of "fibers" in the center region of the schematic. The smallest diameter fibers (<2.5 μm) are observed to predominate in the cristae periphery. Intermediate-sized fibers are distributed over the entire crista. Using precise methods for studying the number and diameters of fibers in the vestibular nerve, approximately the same diameter-dependent distribution of fibers is observed in the cristae of humans, squirrel monkeys and chinchillas, with the characteristic that their distribution corresponds to that proposed by the classical anatomists. Larger fibers (> 4 μm) represent about 10% of neurons, and smaller fibers (< 3 μm) about 30% of the population.

Classical morphologists observed that primary afferent neurons exhibited three types of endings within the cristae. The fibers with largest diameters had only calyces, or caliceal endings; small-diameter fibers had bouton endings; whereas intermediate-size fibers exhibited both types.[82] With recently developed techniques for labeling individual primary afferent neurons by intracellular injection of horseradish peroxidase, more detailed information has been obtained in the chinchilla regarding the innervation patterns associated with these different afferent ending morphologies and regions of the crista (Fig 2–16).[37] Afferent neurons with large axon diameters innervate only a few type I hair cells in the center of the crista with caliceal endings. Afferents with intermediate diameters have both bouton and caliceal endings (dimorphic) and are distributed more-or-less uniformly throughout the crista. Neurons with small axon diameters possess only

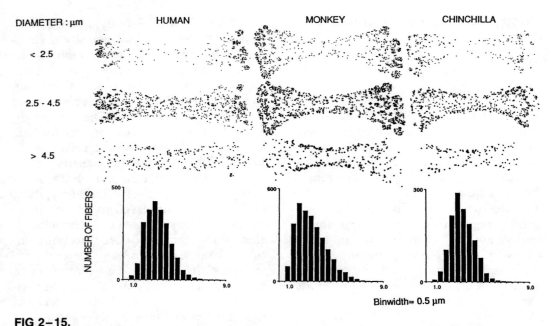

FIG 2–15.
Diameter-distribution of fibers to the human, monkey, and chinchilla cristae. The distribution of fibers within the three diameter categories shown at left (≤ 2.5 μm, between 2.5 and 4.5 μm, and > 4.5 μm) as they project across the topography of the cristae are shown in the crista cross-sections. In the three mammalian species, those fibers ≤ 2.5 μm are observed to be predominant in the lateral ends of the sections, whereas fibers > 4.5 μm are found predominantly in the central regions. Fibers of intermediate diameter are distributed across the entire section. The histograms in the *bottom row* of the figure demonstrate in greater detail the frequency of fibers of various diameters, and indicate that the diameter-dependent distribution of fibers projecting to the semicircular cristae exhibit a skewness toward small diameters. *(From Baloh RW, Honrubia V: Clinical Neurophysiology of the Vestibular System, ed 2. Philadelphia, FA Davis, 1990. Used by permission.)*

bouton endings and innervate multiple type II hair cells, predominantly in the perimeter crista regions (see Fig 2–16).

Response Characteristics of Canalicular Primary Afferent Neurons

Detailed measurement of afferent nerve activity from the crista of several animal species (including primates) revealed that the firing rate associated with physiologic rotatory stimulation follows qualitatively the prediction of the pendulum model of semicircular canal function.[8, 135] That is, the magnitude of change in frequency of action potentials for different stimuli has characteristics that are similar to the pendulum model's prediction of cupular deviation. For example, during sinusoidal head rotation, at the frequencies of natural head movements, the firing rates of most afferent neurons follow the time course of cu-

pular displacement shown in Figure 2–13, *c*. This sinusoidal change in firing frequency is superimposed on a rather high resting (or spontaneous) discharge (70 to 90 spikes per second in the monkey). In this range of stimulus frequencies (≈ 1.0 Hz), the peak firing rate occurs at the time of the peak angular head velocity. For sinusoidal rotation of small magnitude, the modulation is almost symmetrical about the baseline firing rate. For higher stimulus magnitudes, the responses become increasingly asymmetrical. For the largest stimulus magnitudes, the excitatory responses can increase up to about 400 spikes per second, but the growth of inhibitory response is limited to disappearance of spontaneous activity (that is, the decrease in firing from spontaneous levels during the inhibitory phase of the stimulus cannot, obviously, be less than 0 spikes per second). This asymmetry in afferent nerve re-

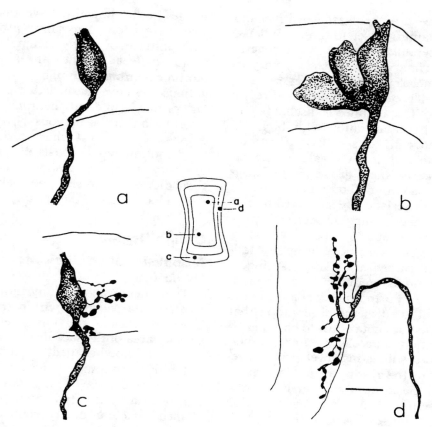

FIG 2–16.
Morphology and innervation loci of primary afferent neuron endings within the semicircular canal cristae of the chinchilla. The three broad classes of endings are demonstrated by these horseradish peroxidase–filled neurons. The *central diagram* illustrates the locus of innervation for the four neurons with the endings shown here. The *calyx* type of endings are found to innervate only type I hair cells with nerve chalices, but may be simple *(a)*, exhibiting only one calyx, or complex *(b)* and possess up to three calyces. Calyx-type afferents are found predominantly in the central region of the crista. The bouton type of endings exhibit multiple bouton terminals, innervating type II hair cells in the perimeter region of the crista. The dimorphic type of endings possess both calyces and boutons, and are found to innervate hair cells in all regions of the neuroepithelium. *(From Fernandez C, et al: The vestibular nerve of the chinchilla. I: Peripheral innervation patterns in the horizontal and superior semicircular canals. J Neurophysiol 1988; 60:167–181. Used by permission.)*

sponse to stimuli of large magnitude at least in part explains Ewald's second and third laws, discussed earlier, which were initially questioned because his "pneumatic hammer" produced a massive stimulus to the semicircular canals.[36]

Just as canalicular primary afferent neurons exhibit a continuous spectrum of axon diameters, these neurons also qualitatively exhibit a wide range of spontaneous firing rates and dynamic response characteristics. It has proved useful to divide them based on the regularity of their spontaneous discharge rate.[53, 55] This characteristic is represented by the coefficient of variation (CV) of spontaneous activity, defined as the ratio of standard deviation of the interspike interval to the mean interspike interval. Neurons with the most *irregular* baseline firing rate (that is, the highest values of CV, owing to the relatively greater interspike interval standard deviation) are, in general, the most sensitive and have high-frequency dynamics that indicate a response to cupular velocity as well as to cupular displacement. Neurons with the most regular firing rate are the least sensitive and have dynamics closer to those predicted by the pendulum model. As a general rule, a primary afferent's sensitivity to angular acceleration (in spikes per second per degree per second^2) is directly related to its spontaneous discharge CV; that is, irregular units, with high CV values, have higher sensitivity than regular units with low CV values. The exception is the small group (5%) of largest neurons with no bouton endings.

When the cristae are subjected to prolonged constant angular acceleration, a substantial proportion of nerve fibers undergo a slow decline in firing rate (adaptation) rather than maintaining a steady state as predicted by the pendulum model. Furthermore, adaptation is also manifested in the observation that firing rate does not return to baseline after cessation of acceleration but, rather, drops to a subresting level prior to returning to the resting rate.[52] A similar effect in the form of an overshooting of the baseline occurs after stimulation with an impulse of acceleration. Instead of the monotonic response predicted by the pendulum model (see Fig 2–13, *b*), the afferent nerve firing pattern exhibits a biphasic reaction with a prolonged secondary phase that slowly returns to baseline. Adaptation is more pronounced in irregular neurons. This adaptation behavior is probably due to hair cell transduction mechanisms.

Recently, it has been possible to study the correlation between anatomic and physiologic properties of individual primary afferent neurons by first recording the neuron's dynamic response to angular acceleration with a micropipette and then injecting it with horseradish peroxidase to study its morphology and anatomic connections. Initial studies in the bullfrog demonstrated that irregular neurons had thick axons and large somas that preferentially innervated the central ridge of the crista, whereas regular neurons had thin axons and small somas that predominantly innervated the periphery.[63, 65] Similar studies in the chinchilla have found specific correlation of dynamic properties with patterns of nerve terminals in the crista[7], at least for the caliceal and dimorphic neurons. Through these investigations, we have learned that canalicular primary afferent neurons convey information to the nervous system that emphasizes spectral characteristics of head motion on the basis of anatomic diversity of neuron's responses based on their differences in size and their innervation locus within the crista.

Otolith Organs

Biophysics of Otolithic Membrane Deviation

The membranous labyrinth forms two globular cavities within the vestibule: the utricle and the saccule. The sensory area of the sacculus—the macula—is a hood-shaped, differentiated patch of membrane in the medial wall of the saccular cavity, and is predominantly in a vertical position. The oval-shaped utricular cavity connects with the membranous semicircular canals by way of five openings. The macula of the utriculus is located next to the anterior opening of the horizontal semicircular canal and lies mostly in a horizontal position in a recess on the anterior wall of the utriculus. It communicates by the utricular duct with the endolymphatic duct at the same level, but by different openings from those of the saccular duct (see Fig 2–7,A). Thus, the endolymph in the superior or utricular part of the labyrinth is separated from that of the sacculus and cochlea by these tiny ducts. Each macula consists of a sensory neuroepithelium containing the receptor cells with a surface area less than 1 mm^2 that supports "a heavy load," the otolithic membrane (specific gravity, approximately 2.7). The otolith is composed of calcareous material embedded in a gelatinous matrix and has a mean thickness of 50 μm (see Fig 2–11, A). Even when the head is at rest, the calcareous material, because of its specific gravity, exerts a force (F_g) on the receptor. The distribution of F_g acting on the underlying sensory cells can be resolved into two vectors: one tangential (F_t), and the other normal to the surface of the receptor (F_g or F_n, depending on whether the linear acceleration is due to "tangential" forces or static tilt; see Fig 2–11, B). During static tilt, for example, the value of F_t is proportional to the sine of the angle tilt (θ), such that $F_t = F_g \sin\theta$, where F_g is equivalent to 1 g (earth gravity). During linear head acceleration, the instantaneous force acting upon the macula is the result of two vector forces: one in the direction opposite to that of head acceleration (F_t), and the other due to gravitational pull (F_g). Their interaction results in the vector force F'_g) as the apparent gravitational vector. Thus $F'_g = \sqrt{F_g{}^2 + F_t{}^2}$, and the apparent angle of gravity, θ, is given by $\theta = \arcsin F_t / F'_g$. In both cases, the sensory cells of the maculae transmit information on the displacement of the otolithic membrane to the CNS, where reflexes are initiated to contract muscles that dynamically oppose the forces acting on the head, and thus maintain equilibrium.

The calcareous material on the top of the otolith is called otoconia. The otoconia consists of small calcium carbonate crystals, ranging from 0.5 to 30 μm in diameter and having a density more than twice that of water. The striola is a distinctive curved zone running through the center of each macula. A higher proportion of type I hair cells are located near the striola than in the rest of the macula.[78] The hair cells on each side of the striola are oriented so that their kinocilia point in opposite directions. In the utriculus, the kinocilia face the striola as shown schematically in Figure 2–11, parts A and B; in the sacculus, they face away from it. As a consequence, displacement of the otolithic membrane of the macula in one direction has an opposite physiologic influence on the set of hair cells on each side of the striola. Furthermore, because of

the curvature of the striola, hair cells are oriented at different angles, making the macula multidirectionally sensitive. Because the maculae are located off-center from the major axis of the head, they are subjected to tangential and centrifugal forces during angular head movements.

As noted earlier, during head movement the calcified otolithic membrane is affected by the combined forces of applied linear acceleration and gravity and tends to move over the macula, which is mounted in the wall of the membranous labyrinth. The otolith is restrained in its motion by elastic, viscous, and inertial forces analogous to the forces associated with cupular movement. De Vries[28] measured the displacement of the large saccular otoliths of several fish and obtained estimates of the forces restraining the otoliths to the maculae. He proposed a model, analogous to the pendulum model, that describes the dynamics of otolith displacement as that of a heavily damped second-order lag system similar to that describing the dynamics of the crista. Displacements due to sinusoidal linear acceleration would be greatest at low frequencies. At higher frequencies, the otolith displacement decreases by one-half each time the frequency is doubled.

Innervation of the Maculae by Primary Afferent Neurons

As in the case of the cristae, there is a unimodal distribution of nerve fiber diameters supplying each of the maculae. Large-diameter fibers are concentrated near the striola, whereas the thinner fibers innervate the periphery. Intermediate-size fibers are more or less equally distributed over the entire macula. In the chinchilla, the same three types of nerve terminals seen in the cristae are also seen in the maculae.[41] Calyx units are limited to the striolar region, but even there dimorphic units outnumber caliceal units by about three to one.[41] Dimorphic units in the striolar region contacted fewer hair cells on average than those in the peripheral extrastriola region (Fig 2–17). For example, striolar dimorphic units contacted from 5 to 20 type II hair cells, whereas extrastriolar dimorphic units contacted from 10 to 40. Dimorphic units in the utricular macula averaged twice as many boutons as dimorphic units in the cristae of the chinchilla.

Response Characteristics of Primary Afferent Neurons

The nerve fibers innervating the maculae are activated by linear acceleration and by changes in the position of the head in space. Each neuron has a characteristic functional polarization vector that defines the axis of its greatest sensitivity. It is as though the terminal fibers of each afferent neuron are stimulated only by hair cells with kinocilia oriented in a given direction in space, forming one functional neuronal unit. The combined polarization vectors of neurons from both maculae cover all possible positions of the head in three-dimensional space. The majority of polarization vectors, however, are near the horizontal plane for the utricular macula and the sagittal plane for the saccular macula.[39] Diagrams of the functional polarization vectors determined by electrophysiological analysis in the squirrel monkey are remarkably similar to mor-

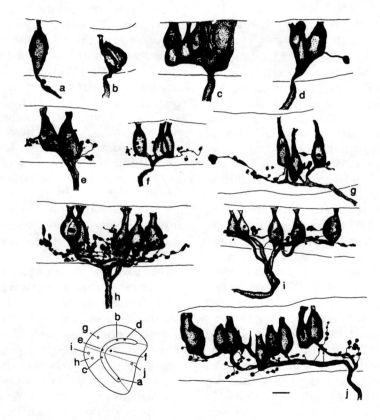

FIG 2–17.
Morphology and innervation loci of afferents innervating the utricular macula in the chinchilla. These horseradish peroxidase–filled afferent endings exhibit the same general classes (calyx, dimorphic, and bouton) described for the semicircular canal crista (see Fig 2–16). Some calyx-type afferent endings are more "complex" than those found in the cristae, exhibiting more than three calyces—as shown in *c*. The calyx-type afferent endings are found in the striolar region, whereas afferent endings of the dimorphic type are found throughout the utricular macula. Not shown in this diagram are the bouton type, which are found primarily in the perimeter regions of the macula. *(From Goldberg JM, et al: The vestibular nerve of the chinchilla. V: Relation between afferent discharge properties and peripheral innervation patterns in the utricular macula.* J Neurophysiol 1990; 63:791–804. Used by permission.)

phologic maps that plot the polarization of hair cells within each macula. None of the neuronal units exhibits a response to compressive forces; displacement of the cilia is the only adequate stimulus for the hair cell.[84]

With the subject in the normal upright position, gravity does not stimulate most of the neuronal units of the utricular macula (because it is orthogonal to most polarization vectors). The average resting discharge of the macular units in this position is approximately 65 spikes per second.[38] The macula is roughly divided into a medial and lateral section by the striola. Because, in the utricular macula, hair cell polarization (the direction of the kinocilia) is toward the striola, ipsilateral tilt results in an increase in the baseline firing of the units medial to the striola and a decreased firing of the units lateral to the striola. Owing to the curvature of the striola, many utricular primary afferents are also sensitive to forward and backward tilt.

Because the saccular macula is primarily in the sagittal plane when a subject is in the upright position, most of its functional polarization vectors are parallel to gravity. Though the polarization of hair cells relative to the striola is opposite that found in the utricle, the "push-pull" relationship of excitation and inhibition between hair cells juxtaposed across the striola also exists in the saccular macula. The saccular macula exhibits less curvature than the utricular macula, and most of its units have a preferred dorsoventral orientation. Saccular units at rest discharge at a rate essentially the same as that of utricular units.[38]

As in the case of the cristae, the spontaneous firing rate characterizes two broad classes of neuronal units in the maculae: regular and irregular.[40] The irregular firing units adapt rapidly when stimulated with constant linear acceleration, are more sensitive to small changes in linear acceleration, and have a wider frequency response than the regular units. During stimulation with static tilts, the regular units maintain a constant ratio between the applied force and the response. During stimulation with sinusoidal linear acceleration (back-and-forth linear displacement), their sensitivity is constant up to 0.1 Hz, but steadily declines at higher frequencies. These regular units, therefore, conform to many of the predictions of the DeVries[28] model of otolith function. In the chinchilla, regular units outnumber irregular units by approximately three to one.[49] The irregular units respond not only to otolith displacement, but also to the velocity of displacement. Following a change in head position in the excitatory direction of their polarization vector, they undergo an immediate increase in firing followed by a decline. This difference between the "presumed" displacement of the otolithic membrane and the afferent unit response may be related to mechanical linkage between the hair cell cilia and the membrane.[77]

As in the chinchilla crista, irregular units in the macula are more numerous in the striolar region, whereas regular units predominate in the periphery. Also as in the crista, caliceal units are always irregular and bouton units regular; dimorphic units can be either of these. Dimorphic units near the striola are typically irregular whereas those in the periphery exhibit regular spontaneous firing characteristics. Regular dimorphic units tend to innervate larger numbers of type II hair cells compared to irregular dimorphic units, but this is only a qualitative difference and some units innervating identical numbers of hair cells exhibit markedly different dynamic characteristics. Goldberg et al.[50] concluded that the response dynamics of both the canal and utricular afferents are primarily determined by transduction mechanisms that vary as one proceeds from central to peripheral zones and are not related to the discharge regularity or to the types and number of hair cells innervated.

CENTRAL PROCESSING

The Vestibular Nuclei

Vestibular signals originating in the two labyrinths first interact with signals from other sensory systems in the vestibular nuclei. Only a fraction of the neurons in the vestibular nuclei receive direct vestibular input, and most neurons receive afferent input from other sensory systems (such as visual or proprioceptive) or regions of the CNS (for example, the cerebellum, reticular formation, spinal cord, and contralateral vestibular nuclei).[109] Consequently, the output of neurons from the vestibular nuclei reflect the interaction of many systems.

Classification of Secondary Vestibular Neurons

Following stimulation of the vestibular nerve with a single brief electric pulse, two groups of secondary vestibular neurons have been identified based on their relationship to the whole nerve action potential recorded in the vestibular nuclei[110,125] (Fig 2–18). Some individual neurons respond with latencies between 0.5 and 1.0 ms (see Fig 2–18, B), suggesting that they receive monosynaptic input. Other neurons produced delayed action potentials (see Fig 2–18,C), suggesting that they are activated through multisynaptic connections. Only about 75% of neurons in the vestibular nuclei are activated by nerve stimulation, and approximately half of these are monosynaptically activated.[53,125] All monosynaptic connections are ipsilateral and excitatory. Among the monosynaptically activated neurons, about 37% respond to small electrical stimuli with very short latencies that activate only the thickest, most sensitive, irregular primary afferents. The rest of the neurons respond to larger electrical currents, suggesting that they receive a predominant input from thinner, regular afferents.

Physiologically, secondary vestibular neurons can be divided into two major groups[125]: type 1 neurons are excited; type 2 neurons are inhibited by ipsilateral rotation of the head. The former are activated by ipsilateral primary afferents, whereas the latter receive their input by way of commissural connections either from neurons in the reticular substance or directly from contralateral type 1 neurons. Type 1 neurons are excitatory, whereas type 2 neurons are always inhibitory. Contralateral labyrinthine stimulation excites type 2 neurons, and they, in turn, inhibit ipsilateral type 1 neurons. It follows that during head rotation, the activity of ipsilateral type 1 neurons is enhanced by excitation from the ipsilateral

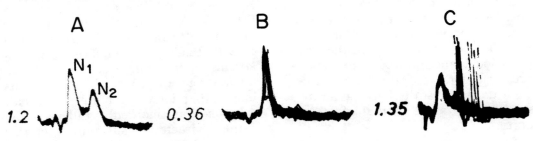

FIG 2–18.
Electrophysiologic recordings made in the vestibular nuclei subsequent to electric stimulation of the ipsilateral vestibular nerve. The traces shown here represent the superposition of approximately 20 responses. **A,** field potentials recorded from the medial vestibular nucleus, where N_1 and N_2 represent the response of monosynaptically activated and multisynaptically activated secondary vestibular neurons (vestibular nucleus neurons). **B,** response of a type 1 monosynaptically activated neuron, where all the spikes superimpose upon the N_1 field potential (only barely visible in this recording). **C,** for a multisynaptically activated neuron, the response latencies of individual action potentials (seen as the higher-amplitude spikes) can be seen to vary with respect to the superimposed N_2 potential (lower-amplitude deflection that preceeds the spikes). *(From Baloh RW, Honrubia V: Clinical Neurophysiology of the Vestibular System, ed 2. Philadelphia, FA Davis, 1990. Used by permission.)*

labyrinth and by decreased inhibition from neighboring type 2 neurons (whose input from the contralateral type 1 neurons has simultaneously decreased).

Organization of the Vestibulo-Ocular Reflexes

Much of our knowledge about the physiology of secondary vestibular neurons has come from studies of neurons that participate in the vestibulo-ocular reflexes. The basic organization of these reflexes is shown in Fig 2–19, A. Type 1 secondary neurons make direct contact with oculomotor neurons and provide axon collaterals to chains of interneurons (IN in Fig 2–19, A) located on the same side of the brain stem and cerebellum.[83] These interneurons, along with the commissural connections from the contralateral side, provide positive feedback to the secondary vestibular neurons.[125] While the response of the contralateral neurons during physiologic stimulation is opposite in sign to that of the ipsilateral neurons, the inhibitory interneurons convert the commissural pathway to a positive feedback loop. The net effect is to provide a temporal integration of signals from different vestibular receptors by sustaining the activity in the vestibular nuclei beyond that of the primary afferent signal, so-called *velocity storage*.[113] The effect of

velocity storage is graphically illustrated in Fig 2–19, B. Subsequent to an impulse of head acceleration the contraction of the eye muscles has a greater duration than that of canal neurons because the time constant of the signal to the oculomotor neurons (T_{COR}) is prolonged beyond that of the primary afferent response (T_1) because of feedback loops onto secondary vestibular neurons (Σ in Fig 2–19, B). This is due to the operation of interneurons in the feedback pathways, which can be viewed as valves controlling the spontaneous activity and dynamic properties of the secondary vestibular neurons (see Fig 2–19, A).

Many of the direct connections from the vestibular nuclei to the oculomotor neurons are part of a large fiber bundle, the medial longitudinal fasciculus (MLF), lying along the floor of the fourth ventricle. This fiber bundle extends from the cervical spinal cord to the reticular substance of the midbrain and thalamus, providing an interconnecting pathway between the vestibular and oculomotor complex in the rostral brain stem as well as connections to the abducens nuclei in the middle brain stem.[35] In addition to sending axons rostrally into the third and fourth nuclei, the MLF also sends collaterals into the reticular substance of the midbrain and thalamus.

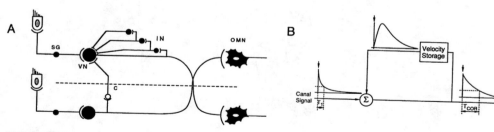

FIG 2–19.
Schematic representation of the anatomic and functional characteristics of the neural circuitry of the vestibulo-ocular reflex. **A,** anatomy of the components of the vestibulo-ocular reflex. The *dashed line* represents the brain stem midline. *SG,* Scarpa's ganglion; *VN,* vestibular nucleus neuron; *IN,* ipsilateral interneurons; *c,* commissural interneuron; *OMN,* oculomotor neuron; *filled neurons,* excitatory; *open neuron,* inhibitory. **B,** functional attributes of the neural circuitry shown in **A.** The dominant time constant of the reflex (T_{COR}) is prolonged compared to T_1 (representing the long time constant of the cupula as measured from the response of primary afferent neurons) by velocity storage within the positive feedback pathways (*IN* in **A**). *(From Baloh RW, Honrubia V: Clinical Neurophysiology of the Vestibular System, ed 2. Philadelphia, FA Davis, 1990. Used by permission.)*

Vestibulo-ocular Pathways

Semicircular Canal—Oculomotor Connections

Each semicircular canal is connected to the eye muscles in such a way that stimulation of a canal nerve results in eye movement approximately in the plane of that canal. For example, stimulation of the left posterior canal nerve excites the ipsilateral superior oblique and the contralateral inferior rectus muscles while inhibiting the ipsilateral inferior oblique and contralateral superior rectus. A disconjugate slow reflexive movement of the eyes is the result with a downward, counterclockwise rotatory movement in the plane of the left posterior canal in the ipsilateral eye and a vertical, downward movement of the contralateral eye. By systematically re-cording in different vestibular and oculomotor nuclei after stimulation of each semicircular canal, it has been possible to trace the main disynaptic excitatory and inhibitory pathways connecting the semicircular canals with the extraocular muscles (Fig 2–20).[131, 132] As a general rule, excitatory connections run in the contralateral MLF and inhibitory connections in the ipsilateral MLF.[103] The connections illustrated in Figure 2–20 are only part of the picture, however. Inasmuch as the planes of the semicircular canals are not exactly aligned with the planes of the three pairs of eye muscles, a spatial transformation from the canal to muscle coordinates must occur if eye movements are to compensate for head movements. In other words, it is not adequate to simply connect afferents from a single canal to a set of eye

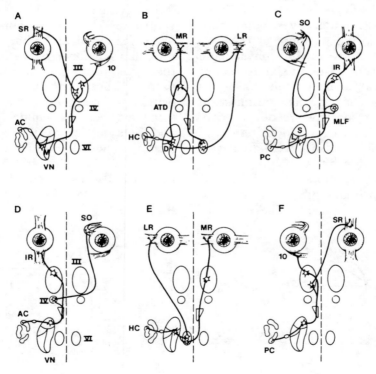

FIG 2–20.
Excitatory **(A–C)** and inhibitory **(D–F)** pathways between individual semicircular canal cristae and the extraocular muscles in the cat.[128, 129] *SR*, superior rectus; *IO*, inferior oblique; *MR*, medial rectus; *LR*, lateral rectus; *SO*, superior oblique; *IR*, inferior rectus; *AC*, anterior canal crista; *HC*, horizontal canal crista; *PC*, posterior crista; *VN*, vestibular nuclei; *S*, superior vestibular nucleus; *M*, medial vestibular nucleus; *L*, lateral vestibular nucleus; *D*, descending vestibular nucleus; *ATD*, ascending tract of Dieters; *VI*, abducens nucleus; *IV*, trochlear nucleus; *III*, oculomotor complex. *(From Baloh RW, Honrubia V: Clinical Neurophysiology of the Vestibular System, ed 2. Philadelphia, FA Davis, 1990. Used by permission.)*

muscles (as shown in Fig 2–20); other connections must also exist. Preliminary studies of labeled secondary vestibular neurons identified as part of the canal ocular reflex indicate that the spatial transformations occur through both a convergence of signals at the level of the vestibular nuclei and a divergence of signals at the level of the oculomotor nuclei.[94, 95, 105]

Otolith-Oculomotor Connections

The maculae project to all the extraocular eye muscles but the pathways are less clearly defined than are those from the semicircular canals due to anatomic differences between the organs. Owing to the differential orientation of kinocilia and stereocilia over the neuroepithelial surface of the maculae, activation by a discrete and unique stimulus vector is confined to a limited spatial area of the sensory surface. Considering the entire sensory surface, in which virtually all stimulus vectors (in the plane of the receptor) can be transduced, directional transformation between macular stimulus and eye movement represents a more complex situation than for the semicircular cristae, where the entire neuroepithelial surface is activated by a uniform stimulus vector. The latency of eye muscle activation after stimulation of the utricular and saccular nerves is similar to that recorded after semicircular canal nerve stimulation; disynaptic pathways also exist from the maculae to the extraocular muscles.[10, 33, 124] Because of the varied orientation of hair cells within the maculae, simultaneous electrical stimulation of all nerve fibers coming from one macular receptor organ produces a nonphysiologic excitation, and the induced eye movements fail to mimic the naturally occurring ones. Selective stimulation of different parts of the utriculus and sacculus results in mostly vertical and vertical-rotatory eye movements.[45, 129] As one would expect, stimulation on each side of the striola produces oppositely directed rotatory and vertical components.

Relationship Between Canal Afferent Signals and Eye Movements

The semicircular canal ocular reflexes produce eye movements that compensate for head rotations. The various transformations involved in this process for rotations in the horizontal plane are illustrated in Figure 2–21.[8] The natural stimulus for the semicircular canals is head angular acceleration (see Fig 2–21, *b,*). However, during sinusoidal rotation at the frequencies of natural head movements, due to the visco-elastic properties of the canal-cupula complex (as described by the pendulum model), the vestibular nerve firing rate (see Fig 2–21, *e*) is in phase with head velocity rather than head acceleration. Thus, the equivalent of one step of mathematical integration (a 90° phase shift) has occurred. The normal reflex response produces a compensatory eye movement equal and opposite to that of head movement (compare *a* and *g* in Fig 2–21). This eye movement results from activation of, among others, the abducens nerve to the left lateral rectus muscle (see Fig 2–21, *f*) during ampullopetal stimulation of the right cupula-vestibular nerve (see Fig 2–21, *d* and *e*). However, the recorded activity in the abducens nerve lags behind the activity in the vestibular nerve by an additional 90° delay. This raises a key question first addressed by Skavenski and Robinson[127]: What produces the phase shift between the firing rates of the vestibular and abducens nerves (between Fig 2–21, *e* and *f*)? To answer the question, they introduced the concept of an oculomotor integrator, a hypothetical neural network that integrates, in a mathematical sense, velocity coded signals (such as those originating in the vestibular end organ) to position coded signals required by the oculomotor neurons. Although the concept of neural integration

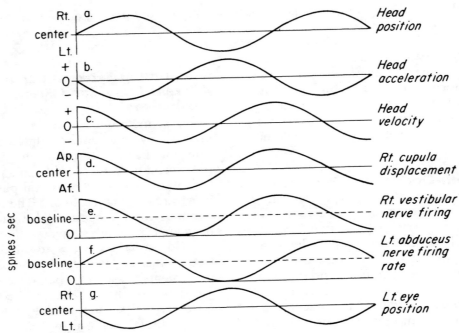

FIG 2–21.
Transformation of signals from sinusoidal changing head position *(a)* through the completely compensatory (that is, equal and opposite) eye position. *Rt.,* right; *Lt.,* left; *Ap.,* ampullopetal; *Af.,* ampullofugal. *(From Baloh RW, Honrubia V: Clinical Neurophysiology of the Vestibular System, ed 2. Philadelphia, FA Davis, 1990. Used by permission.)*

is now generally accepted, specific details are still debated. Some feel it is "localized" in a region of the brain stem[17, 20] or cerebellum,[19] but others consider it "a distributed property" of the feedback pathways shown in Figure 2–19, A. Galiana and Outerbridge[46] developed a mathematical model to show how these feedback pathways, particularly those by way of the commissural connections, could produce the necessary integration.

Although the VOR operates as an integrating angular accelerometer (that is, velocity detector) for frequencies greater than 0.1 Hz, at lower frequencies there is a progressive phase lead of eye velocity relative to head velocity reaching a maximum of 90° at about 0.001 Hz. In other words, the VOR response reflects the vestibular nerve output in phase with the natural stimulus angular acceleration. Velocity storage within the central VOR feedback pathways improves the low-frequency phase deficit of incoming primary afferent signals but does not correct it completely. As will be shown later, this low-frequency phase shift of the VOR is of little functional significance, inasmuch as natural head movements stimulate visual and vestibular reflexes and the combined responses from these two systems are perfectly compensatory at low frequencies. It does have important implications for clinical testing, however, because an increase in the low-frequency phase lead is a nonspecific sign of damage to the canal ocular reflex.

Neural Mechanisms for the Production of Nystagmus

The understanding of the neural mechanisms of eye movement responses is important for the evaluation of patients. Nystagmus production is a complex phenomenon that involves many neuronal centers and the changes in nystagmus characteristics are often of diagnostic value.

Secondary Vestibular Neurons.— Type 1 secondary vestibular neurons identified as part of the horizontal VOR show several patterns of discharge during vestibular stimulation. Some neurons exhibit firing characteristics similar to the vestibular nerve, reflecting head velocity. Other neurons discharge in patterns that exhibit components of eye position in addition to head velocity. Though the matter is subject to some debate, when utilizing stimuli that evoke a VOR response consisting of nystagmus, most secondary vestibular neurons pause their discharge with the onset of the nystagmus fast component (Fig 2–22). In fact, Berthoz et al.[9] reported that all secondary neurons identified as part of the horizontal vestibulo-ocular reflex in the alert cat paused during fast components.

Burst Neurons.—Two groups of neurons participating in the production of

fast components, located in the reticular formation in the paramedian pons and mesencephalon, are specialized to fire before the onset of rapid eye movements (saccades or nystagmus quick phases). The neurons fire with a high-frequency burst proportional to the velocity of the eye during the rapid eye movement. The excitatory burst neurons (EBNs) are responsible for the volley of excitatory activity to abducens motorneurons during an agonist fast component. Through a pathway that includes type 2 secondary vestibular neurons, EBNs also are the source of the pause in type 1 secondary vestibular neuron firing. The inhibitory burst neurons *(IBNs)*, on the other hand, provide the discharge volley responsible for the pause in contralateral abducens motorneurons during an ipsilateral fast component.

Pause Neurons.—The pause group of neurons, located in the reticular forma-

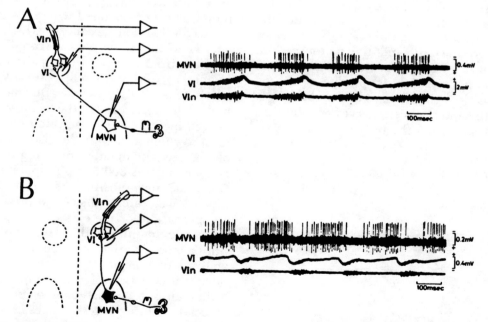

FIG 2–22.
Patterns of discharge of excitatory **(A)** and inhibitory **(B)** premotor type 1 neurons within the medial vestibular nucleus *(MVN)* as they relate to other electrophysiological correlates of vestibular nystagmus. Following the diagram of the experimental recording sites at *left*, the recordings from these sites are shown at *right*: *VI*, the field potential within the abducens nucleus; *VIn*, the whole-nerve recordings from the abducens nerve. *(Adapted from Shimazu H: Neuronal organization of the premotor system controlling eye movements and vestibular nystagmus. Adv Neurol 1983; 39:565–588.)*

tion near the midline at the level of the abducens, interrupt their background activity before rapid eye movements in all directions. These neurons fire at a remarkably regular baseline rate (about 200 spikes/sec in the monkey) and then abruptly pause just before the onset of rapid eye movements; they resume their regular firing at the end of the rapid eye movement. The connections of the burst and pause neurons with oculomotor neurons are summarized in Figure 2–23.

Oculomotor Neurons.—The relationship between the firing rate of oculomotor neurons and the movements of the eyes during each phase of nystagmus has been studied most extensively. During the production of agonist slow components (see Fig 2–22, A) the membrane potential is slowly depolarized by excitatory postsynaptic potentials arriving via the vestibulo-ocular pathways discussed in the previous sections. Toward the end of the slow component, the membrane potential rapidly becomes hyperpolarized, and the motor neuron abruptly terminates its discharge. This hyperpolarization is produced by the IBNs.[58, 59] The changes in membrane potential and abducens nerve firing rate are opposite when the neuron is participat-

ing antagonistically in the production of the slow component of nystagmus (see Fig 2–22, B). In this case, the sudden depolarization recorded intra-cellularly, and the burst of activity in the abducens nerve originates from the EBNs.

Measurement of the relationship between motor neuron firing rates and eye movements induced by vestibular or visual stimuli has shown that the motor neurons behave in the same way regardless of the nature of the stimulus.[115] Almost all oculomotor neurons exhibit a threshold above which they increase their firing rate roughly in proportion to the change in eye position in the orbit. A small percentage of the change in firing rate (approximately 20%) is proportional to the velocity of the eye movement. It is as though the firing rate of oculomotor neurons was designed to overcome both the elastic and the viscous forces (roughly in a 5:1 ratio) restraining the eye in the orbit. This relationship can be best appreciated by examining the rate of firing of an oculomotor neuron associated with a visually induced refixation saccade, in which the goal is to move the eyes as rapidly as possible from one position in the orbit to another, and to maintain the new position once it is reached. During the high velocity saccade, the oculomotor neuron increases its firing rate to a high level to compensate for the viscous drag of the eye ligaments (reaching firing rates as high as 800 to 1,000 spikes/sec). Once the new position is reached, a much lower rate of discharge produces compensation for the elastic restraining force and maintains the new position. Similar observation can be made by analysis of the motor neuron response during production of fast components. Equal amplitude fast components are associated with greater changes in firing rate if their velocity is greater (the nystagmus looks sharper). Although the reflex pathways for vestibular and visually induced eye movements involve different neuronal circuits, the motor neurons governing the extrinsic eye

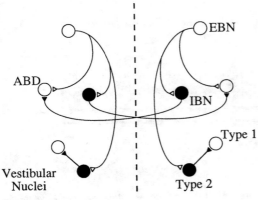

FIG 2–23.
Schematic wiring diagram of interneurons involved in the generation of nystagmus. *EBN*, excitatory burst neuron; *IBN*, inhibitory burst neuron; *ABD*, abducens neuron.

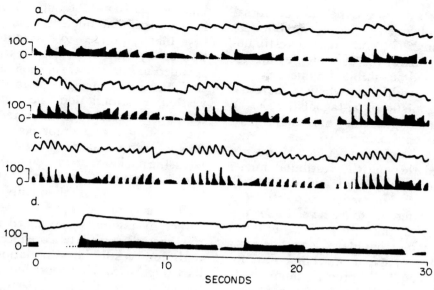

FIG 2–24.
Correlation between activity of a motoneuron in the abducens nucleus and eye movements of induced nystagmus in the cat. For each *pair* of traces, the *top trace* represents the eye movement recorded by electro-oculography, and the *bottom trace* represents the motoneuron's firing frequency. The recordings in *a, b,* and *c* were made during sinusoidal rotation at 0.1 Hz and peak velocities of 30, 60, and 120°/sec. The recordings in *d* represent spontaneous eye movements (that is saccades) during the 30-second recording epoch. *(From Baloh RW, Honrubia V: Clinical Neurophysiology of the Vestibular System, ed 2. Philadelphia, FA Davis, 1990. Used by permission.)*

muscles fire in the same manner regardless of the original sensory input (Fig 2–24)

Neural Mechanisms of Cervical-Vestibular Interaction

Ocular stability during most natural head movements results from a coordinated interaction of signals originating in the vestibular, visual, and neck receptors. The compensatory nature of neck-induced eye movements has been documented in many different animals. De Kleyn[27] showed that if one holds an animal's head stationary and displaces the body, a compensatory eye deviation occurs, which tends to preserve the relationship between gaze and the body axis. Nonfoveated animals, such as the rabbit, exhibit clear compensatory eye deviations because they possess almost no spontaneous eye movements.[22, 56] Cervico-ocular and VOR interaction is more difficult to study in humans because of the dominance of voluntary and visually controlled eye movements. Very few investigators have quantitatively assessed eye, head, and neck movement coordination in humans, and the clinical significance of lesions involving the cervico-ocular reflex pathways is uncertain.

Studies in animals have shown that the cervico-ocular reflex originates from nerve endings in the ligaments and capsules of the upper cervical articulations.[57, 93] The reflex can be induced by electrically stimulating the capsules of the upper cervical joints, the C-1 to C-3 dorsal roots, and the high cervical spinal cord. Reflexes are not induced by stimulating the superficial muscles or skin of the neck. Bilateral sectioning of the high cervical dorsal roots or the application of local anesthetic around the cervical articulations abolishes the cervico-ocular reflexes. Unilateral interruption of the neck ocular reflex pathways produces nystagmus in rabbits, cats, and monkeys when fixation is inhibited, although no consistent relationship exists between the side of dorsal root involvement and the direction of nystagmus.[26, 68] As with vestibulo-ocular reflexes, the eye muscles are either excited or inhibited by neck stimulation, depending on whether the muscle is agonistic or antagonistic for the required compensatory movement.

Electrophysiologic experiments suggest that the cervico-ocular reflexes are mediated through the vestibular nuclei (primarily the medial and descending nuclei).[57, 119] The precise projections of the neck afferents to each vestibular nucleus are only partially known, but it can be anticipated that inasmuch as the neck-induced eye movements compensate for displacement in the precise plane of body motion, the vestibular nuclei must contain a discreet topographic representation of cervical afferents in a manner similar to that of the vestibular afferents. Electrical stimulation of the high cervical dorsal roots in the cat produces evoked potentials in the contralateral vestibular nuclei[57] followed by excitation of the abducens nucleus ipsilateral to the neck stimulation and inhibition of the contralateral abducens nucleus. In addition, stimulation of the cervical dorsal roots enhances the amplitude of action potentials in the ipsilateral abducens nerve triggered by contralateral vestibular nerve stimulation and inhibits action potentials in the contralateral abducens nerve induced by ipsilateral vestibular nerve stimulation. Vestibulo-ocular and cervico-ocular reflex interaction, therefore, results from a convergence of neck and semicircular canal afferents on secondary vestibular neurons.

Neural Mechanisms of Visual-Vestibular Interaction

Shortly after it was demonstrated by Dichgans and co-workers[29] that neurons in the vestibular nuclei of goldfish responded to visual stimuli, similar observations were made by other investigators in a variety of animals and under a variety of experimental conditions.

Waespe and Henn[134] found that neurons in the vestibular nucleus of alert monkeys that responded to horizontal rotation of the animal in the dark also responded to horizontal rotation of the visual surround. During combined visual-vestibular stimulation, neurons were maximally excited (or inhibited) when the vestibular and optokinetic nystagmus were in the same direction (that is, when the background moved in the opposite direction of the monkey). If the optokinetic drum was mechanically coupled to the turntable so that both rotated together, nystagmus was reduced and neuronal activity was attenuated, compared with pure vestibular stimulation in the dark (Fig 2–25). These data indicate that the vestibular nuclei represent a major center for visual-vestibular interaction.

The mechanisms responsible for these effects are being elucidated. It is generally accepted that visual influences on vestibular-induced eye movement depend on the cooperation of two subsystems: the *smooth pursuit* and the *optokinetic* systems. The smooth pursuit system predominates in foveate animals, and subserves the tracking of small visual targets impinging on the retinal fovea. This system enables targets to be tracked at velocities as high as 100°/sec. The optokinetic system, on the other hand, is activated by full-field retinal stimulation. In lower animals it produces reflexive eye movements where eye velocities match that of the stimuli, which may reach 20 to 40°/sec for ipsilateral medially-directed (temporal-nasal) stimuli. The performance of the optokinetic system is somewhat worse for laterally directed stimuli. In primates, the two systems interact in such a way that the responses to visual field stimuli represent a combination of the two systems. The neural pathways for each system differ.

Afoveate Animals

In afoveate animals the subcortical, accessory optic system is the predomi-

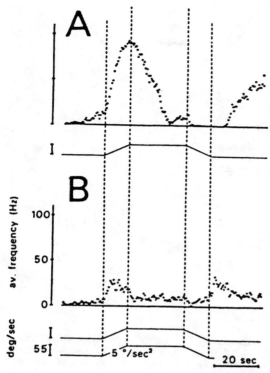

FIG 2–25.

Electrophysiologic recording of a type 1 neuron in the vestibular nuclei of a rhesus monkey during vestibular (**A**, turntable rotation in the dark) and combined visual-vestibular stimulation (**B**, optokinetic drum and turntable rotating together in the same direction). The combined visual and vestibular stimulation were conflicting in that the eye movements induced through optokinetic stimulation counteracted those induced through rotation (the latter of which are normally compensatory and opposite the direction of rotation). The profile of the stimuli are shown at the *bottom.* The response of the neuron during combined visual-vestibular stimulation is strongly attenuated. *(From Waespe W, Henn V: Motion information in the vestibular nuclei of alert monkeys: Visual and vestibular input vs. optomotor output. Prog Brain Res 1973; 50:683–693. Used by permission.)*

nate pathway for visual-vestibular interaction.[21, 111, 126] This system includes a group of nuclei at the mesodiencephalic border, which, like the lateral geniculate nucleus, receives direct projections from the contralateral retina. Unlike the lateral geniculate, however, neurons of the accessory optic system project directly to the brain stem and cerebellum. The most prominent cell group of the accessory optic system, the nucleus of the basal optic root, is identifiable in all

classes of vertebrates. Lázár[75] found that optokinetic responses are abolished in frogs after destruction of the basal optic root nuclei, whereas ablation of the lateral geniculate nuclei and optic tectum did not affect optokinetic responses. The electrophysiologic studies of Maekawa and colleagues demonstrated that the visual inputs to the flocculonodular node of the cerebellum in rabbits were accomplished through the accessory optic system.[88, 89] Furthermore, microelectrode recordings from neurons of the accessory optic nucleus in the rabbit as well as in the cat reveal units that exhibit a strong response to slow full-field retinal stimulation.[21, 62]

The principal anatomic pathways for visual-vestibular interaction in the rabbit as proposed by Ito[69] are shown in Figure 2–26. Retinal sensory information reaches the inferior olive by way of the accessory optic tract and the central tegmental tract. Neurons in the inferior olive activate Purkinje cells in the flocculus, nodulus, and adjacent parts of the cerebellum. These areas of the cerebellum also receive primary vestibular afferent fibers and secondary vestibular fibers originating mostly in the medial and descending vestibular nuclei. Outflow from the cerebellar Purkinje cells terminates at secondary vestibular neurons and runs in the adjacent reticular substance. Although Purkinje cell outflow to the vestibular nuclei is inhibitory, as with all Purkinje cell output, it ends on both excitatory and inhibitory vestibular neurons, thereby endowing it with the capability to enhance or inhibit the VOR. Several types of experimental data confirm the role of the flocculus in mediating visual-vestibular interaction in the rabbit. Electrical stimulation of the flocculus inhibits nystagmus induced by physiologic and electrical stimulation of the vestibular nerve.[70] The reflex contraction produced in agonist extra-ocular muscles by electrical stimulation of an isolated canal nerve is inhibited by prior stimulation of the flocculus, the accessory optic tract, or

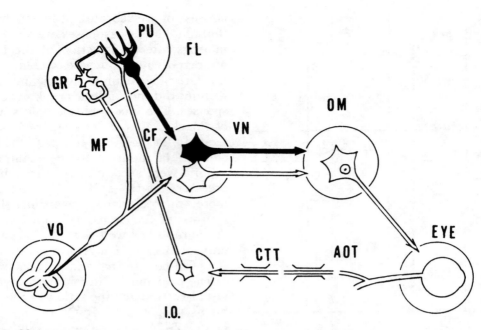

FIG 2–26.
Schematic diagram of the anatomic pathways subserving visual-vestibular interaction in the rabbit. *VO*, vestibular end organs; *VN*, vestibular nuclei; *OM*, oculomotor neurons; *AOT*, accessory optic tract; *CTT*, central tegmental tract; *I.O.*, inferior olive; *MF*, mossy fibers; *CF*, climbing fibers; *FL*, cerebellar flocculus; *GR*, granule cells; *PU*, Purkinje cells; *open neurons*, excitatory; *filled neurons*, inhibitory. *(From Ito M: Vestibulo-ocular reflex arc and flocculus, in Naunton RF (ed):* The Vestibular System. *New York, Academic Press, 1975. Used by permission.)*

the optic chiasm.[87] Finally, in animals with lesions of the flocculus or inferior olives, the vestibulo-ocular reflex cannot be modulated by visual stimulation.[64,70]

Foveate Animals

With the development of the fovea, cortical pathways become progressively more important in visual-vestibular interaction. Recent anatomic and physiologic studies in primates indicate that the visual signals reach the brain stem for interaction with vestibular signals by a complex cascade of interconnecting pathways. In contrast to the rabbit, neurons in the pretectal complex of the monkey receive predominate input from the visual cortex and respond equally well to small spots and to large random dot patterns moving through their receptive field.[61] There is, however, some specific pattern of activity which suggests that different nuclei contribute to one function more than others. Among this group of neurons the ones in the nu-

cleus of the optic tract (NOT) have the characteristics to be the relay pathway for the indirect visual pathway to the vestibular nuclei. They respond to ipsilateral directed movements of large to full fields.[98] Localized lesions in this nucleus and in the adjacent lateral temporal nuclei lead to deficits in the slow-rising phase of optokinetic responses of primates to ipsilateral stimuli and abolition of the optokinetic afternystagmus. This data suggests that these neurons are part of the direct visual input to the vestibular nuclei. However, the fast-rising component is unaffected as are the smooth pursuit responses.[71, 123] Neurons in these nuclei respond also to other signals, which suggests that they receive either direct or indirect cortical input. This nerve behavior does not depend exclusively on the visual subcortical pathway as in afoveated animals. The smooth-pursuit system depends on cortical pathways.

The striate cortex,[31] the superior

temporal sulcus (particularly the medial temporal and medial superior areas),[2, 90, 130, 138] and the posterior parietal cortex[116, 121] are the key cortical areas in the monkey for processing retinal motion information. These cortical centers project heavily to the dorsolateral pontine nucleus (DLPN), which is a primary source of afferents to the flocculus and vermal areas 6 and 7, two cerebellar areas involved in the regulation of eye movements.[91, 92] Neurons in the DLPN exhibit a directionally selective response to movement of discrete spots and large backgrounds, and microstimulation in the region of DLPN causes a short latency modification of the velocity of an ongoing smooth pursuit eye movement.[92]

In the monkey, lesions of the parietotemporal cortex,[86] DLPN,[92] and the flocculus[137] result in an impairment of (1) smooth pursuit, (2) the initial rapid rise in optokinetic nystagmus slow-phase velocity, and (3) visual vestibular interaction requiring the foveal pursuit pathway (for example, fixation suppression of vestibular nystagmus with a foveal target). By contrast, lesions of the pretectal nuclei (that is, the NOT) impair optokinetic nystagmus but not pursuit.

Organization of the Vestibulospinal Reflexes

It is helpful to consider the similarities and differences between the ocular and spinal vestibular reflexes as an introduction to the organization of vestibulospinal reflexes. The effector organs of the vestibulo-ocular reflexes are the extraocular muscles, and those of the vestibulospinal reflexes are the antigravity muscles—the extensors of the neck, trunk, and extremities. Comparable push-pull mechanisms exist for controlling the balance between the extensor and flexor skeletal muscles as for the eye muscles (see Fig 2–2). A major difference between the organization of ocular and spinal reflexes is the increased complexity of the spinal muscle re-

sponse, compared with the eye movements produced by an agonist and antagonist muscle. Even a simple movement about an extremity joint in a two-dimensional plane requires a complex pattern of contraction and relaxation in numerous muscles. Multiple agonist and antagonist muscles on both sides must receive appropriate signals to ensure a smooth, coordinated movement. Unfortunately, a simple recording technique does not exist for quantifying these complex skeletal muscle responses. These factors have hindered the mapping of connections between the labyrinthine receptors and individual skeletal muscles and have limited our understanding of the cellular basis for the vestibular contribution to postural reflexes.

Vestibulospinal Pathways

Secondary vestibular neurons influence neurons in the anterior horn of the spinal cord by means of three major pathways: (1) the lateral vestibulospinal tract; (2) the medial vestibulospinal tract; and (3) the reticulospinal tract. The first two arise directly from neurons in the vestibular nuclei, but the third arises from neurons in the reticular formation which are influenced by vestibular stimulation (as well as several other kinds of input). The cerebellum is highly interrelated with each of these pathways.

Lateral Vestibulospinal Tract

The vast majority of fibers in the lateral vestibulospinal tract, it is generally agreed, originate from neurons in the lateral vestibular nucleus (Fig 2–27).[14] A somatotopic pattern of projections originates in the lateral vestibular nucleus such that neurons in the rostroventral region supply the cervical spinal cord, whereas neurons in the dorsocaudal region innervate the lumbosacral spinal cord. Neurons in the intermediate region supply the thoracic spinal cord.

In the spinal cord, the fibers of the lateral vestibulospinal tract run ipsilat-

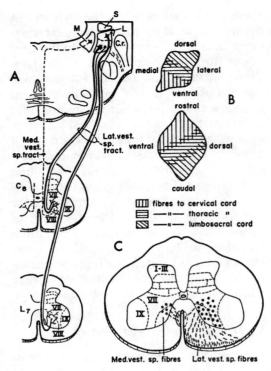

FIG 2–27.
Anatomy of the lateral and medial vestibulo-spinal tracts. *A,* sites of origin, trajectory of descending fibers in the spinal cord, and sites of termination within the laminae of the spinal cord grey matter. *S,* superior vestibular nucleus; *M,* medial vestibular nucleus; *L,* lateral vestibular nucleus; *C.r.,* restiform body. *B,* somatotopic organization of lateral vestibular nucleus with respect to the target regions of the spinal cord receiving lateral vestibulo-spinal tract neurons; *upper,* transverse section; *lower,* sagittal section. *C,* sites of termination within the spinal cord grey matter of vestibulo-spinal tract neurons. *(From Brodal A: Anatomical organization of cerebello-vestibulo-spinal pathways, in deReuck AVS, Knight J (eds):* CIBA Foundation Symposium: Myotatic, Kinesthetic, and Vestibular Mechanisms. *London, J & A Churchill, 1967, pp 148–218. Used by permission.)*

erally in the ventral half of the lateral funiculus and the lateral part of the ventral funiculus. The tract terminates throughout the length of the cord in the eighth lamina and the medial part of the seventh lamina, either directly onto dendrites of anterior horn cells or on interneurons that project to anterior horn cells of the axial and proximal limb musculature.[101] Some of the cells of the eighth lamina send their axons to the contralateral cord, probably accounting

for the bilateral effects that have been observed with stimulation of the lateral vestibular nucleus.

Medial Vestibulospinal Tract

The fibers of the medial vestibulospinal tract originate from neurons in the medial vestibular nucleus and enter the spinal cord in the descending medial longitudinal fasciculus (see Fig 2–27).[14] The fibers travel in the ventral funiculus as far as the midthoracic level. The majority end on interneurons in the seventh and eighth lamina of the cervical spinal cord.[100] No monosynaptic connections appear to exist between the medial vestibulospinal tract and cervical anterior horn cells.[47, 136]

Functionally, the medial vestibulospinal tract plays an important part in interaction of neck-vestibulo-ocular reflexes.

Reticulospinal Tract

The reticulospinal tract originates from neurons in the bulbar reticular formation.[106] The nuclei reticularis gigantocellularis and pontis caudalis provide most of the long fibers passing into the spinal cord, although the majority of neurons in the caudal reticular formation also contribute fibers. Both crossed and uncrossed fibers transverse the length of the spinal cord, terminating in the seventh and eighth laminae of the spinal cord.[102]

The vestibular nuclei are among many structures that project to the reticular formation. Axonal branches and collaterals of cells in all four main vestibular nuclei are distributed to the pontomedullary reticular formation. Only a small number of vestibular primary afferent fibers end in the reticular formation, so that the main vestibular influence on reticulospinal outflow is mediated by way of the secondary vestibular neurons.

Stimulation of the pontomedullary reticular formation in the regions where the long descending spinal projections originate results in an inhibition of both extensor and flexor motor neurons throughout the spinal cord.[80, 81]

The "spinal" cerebellum provides a major source of input to neurons whose axons form the lateral vestibulospinal and reticulospinal tracts. A somatotopic organization of projections to the lateral vestibular nucleus occurs in both the vermian cortex and fastigial nuclei of the cerebellum.[13, 108, 114] Direct projections connect the vermian cortex to the lateral vestibular nucleus, and indirect projections pass through the fastigial nuclei. The caudal part of the fastigial nucleus gives rise to a bundle of fibers that cross the midline (Russell's hook bundle), curving around the brachium conjunctivum before running to the contralateral lateral vestibular nucleus and dorsal lateral reticular formation. In addition, direct ipsilateral outflow passes from the fastigial nucleus to areas of the reticular formation that send long fibers to the spinal cord in the reticulospinal tract. The cerebellar-reticular pathways do not exhibit somatotopic organization.[108]

The cerebellar vermis and fastigial nuclei receive input from secondary vestibular neurons, the spinal cord, and the pontomedullary reticular formation. The result is a close-knit vestibular-reticular-cerebellar functional unit for the maintenance of equilibrium and locomotion.

Neural Mechanisms of the Vestibulospinal Reflexes

Studies of secondary vestibular neurons identified as part of the vestibulospinal pathways are few compared with those of neurons that are part of the vestibulo-ocular pathways. Duensing and Schaefer[32] identified four types of second-order otolith units based on their response to ipsilateral and contralateral tilts. Alpha neurons increased their firing rate with ipsilateral tilts and decreased their rate with contralateral tilts. Beta neurons showed the opposite response. Gamma and delta neurons in-

creased and decreased their discharge, respectively, regardless of the direction of head tilt. The great majority of the units were of the alpha or beta type (alpha units were twice as common as beta units). Adrian[1] first demonstrated that second-order otolith units that were activated by static head tilt were also activated by linear horizontal acceleration of the head in the opposite direction. Peterson et al.[107] studied the dynamic response of secondary vestibular neurons projecting to the spinal cord by way of the lateral vestibulospinal tract by applying sinusoidal polarizing currents to electrodes implanted close to the horizontal or anterior semicircular canal ampullae in decerebrate cats. They compared the activity in these secondary neurons with that of the neck muscle electromyogram. These secondary vestibulospinal neurons exhibited a range of behaviors, with some leading the applied stimulating waveform while others lagged the applied stimulating waveform, similar to the electromyographic activity recorded in the neck muscles. In other words, some of these units were in phase with head position rather than velocity, indicating that an integration of the peripheral afferent signal must have occurred at the level of the vestibular nuclei, just as it has been demonstrated to occur within the vestibulo-ocular reflex.

REFERENCES

1. Adrian ED: Discharges from vestibular receptors in the cat. *J Physiol* 1943; 101:389–407.

2. Albright TD. Direction and orientation selectivity of neurons in visual area MT of the macaque. *J Neurophysiol* 1984; 52:1106–1130.

3. Annoni J-M, Cochran SL, Precht W: Pharmacology of the vestibular hair cell-afferent fiber synapse in the frog. *J Neurosci* 1984; 4:2106–2116.

4. Anson BJ: Developmental anatomy of the ear, in Paparella MF, Shumrick DA, (eds): *Otolaryngology.* Philadelphia, WB Saunders, 1973.

5. Anson BJ, Donaldson JA: *Surgical Anatomy of the Temporal Bone and Ear.* Philadelphia, WB Saunders, 1973.

6. Bagger-Sjoback D, Takumida M: Geometrical array of the vestibular sensory hair bundle. *Acta Otolaryngol* 1988; 106:393–403.

7. Baird RA, Desmadryl G, Fernandez C, et al: The vestibular nerve in the chinchilla. II: Relation between afferent response properties and peripheral innervation patterns in the semicircular canals. *J Neurophysiol* 1988; 60:182–203.

8. Baloh RW, Honrubia V: *Clinical Neurophysiology of the Vestibular System.* Philadelphia, FA Davis, 1990.

9. Berthoz A, Droulez J, Vidal PP, et al: Neural correlates of horizontal vestibulo-ocular reflex cancellation during rapid eye movements in the cat. *J Physiol* 1989; (Lond) 419:717–751.

10. Blanks RHI, Anderson JH, Precht W: Response characteristics of semicircular canal and otolith systems in cat. II: Responses of trochlear motoneurons. *Exp Brain Res* 1978; 32:509–528.

11. Blanks RHI, Curthoys IS, Markham CH: Planar relationships of semicircular canals in the cat. *Am J Physiol* 1972; 223:55–62.

12. Blanks RHI, Curthoys IS, Markham CH: Planar relationships of semicircular canals in man. *Acta Otolaryngol* 1975; 80:185–196.

13. Brodal A: Anatomical organization of cerebello-vestibulo-spinal pathways, in De-Renck AVS, Knight J (eds): *CIBA Foundation Symposium: Myotatic, Kinesthetic and Vestibular Mechanisms.* London: Churchill Ltd, 1967, pp 148–169.

14. Brodal A: Anatomy of the vestibular nuclei and their connections, in Kornhuber HH (ed): *Handbook of Sensory Physiology.* VI/1: *The Vestibular System.* New York; Springer-Verlag, 1974, pp 239–351.

15. Brownell WE: Microscopic observation of cochlear hair cell motility. *Scan Electron Microsc* 1984; 3:1401–1406.

16. Budelmann BU: Morphological diversity of equilibrium receptor systems in aquatic invertebrates, in Atema J, Fay RR, Popper AN, et al. (eds): *Sensory Biology of Aquatic Animals.* New York, Springer-Verlag, 1988, pp 757–782.

17. Cannon SC, Robinson DA: Neural integrator failure from brain stem lesions in monkey. *Invest Ophthalmol Vis Sci* 1985; 26(suppl 3):47.

18. Carpenter MB: *Core Text of Neuroanatomy.* Baltimore, Williams & Williams, 1972.

19. Carpenter RHS: Cerebellectomy and the transfer function of the vestibuloocular reflex in the decerebrate cat. *Proc R Soc Lond [Biol]* 1972; 181:353–375.

20. Cheron G, Godaux E: Disabling of the oculomotor neural integrator by kainic acid injections in the prepositus-vestibular complex of the cat. *J Physiol* (Lond) 1987; 394:267–290.

21. Collewijn H: Direction-selective units in the rabbit's nucleus of the optic tract. *Brain Res* 1975; 100:489–508.

22. Collewijn H, Conijn P, Martins AJ, et al: Control of gaze in man: Synthesis of pursuit, optokinetic and vestibulo-ocular system, in Roucoux A, Crommelinck M (eds): *Physiological and Pathological Aspects of Eye Movements: Proceedings of a Workshop held at the Pont de'Oye Castle, Habay-la-Neuve, 1982.* The Hague, Dr. W Junk, Publishers for the Commission of the European Communities, 1982, pp 3–22.

23. Corwin JT, Cotanche DA: Regeneration of sensory hair cells after acoustic trauma. *Science* 1988; 240:1772–1774.

24. Curthoys IS, Blanks RHI, Markham CH: Semicircular canal functional anatomy in cat, guinea pig, and man. *Acta Otolaryngol* 1977; 83:258–265.

25. Dallos P: Membrane potential and response changes in mammalian cochlear hair cells during intracellular recording. *J Neurosci* 1985; 5:1609–1615.

26. de Jong PTVM, de Jong JMBV, Cohen B, et al: Ataxia and nystagmus induced by injection of local anesthetics in the neck. *Ann Neurol* 1977; 1:240–246.

27. De Kleyn A: Recherches quantitatives sur les positions compensatories l'oeil chez de lapin. *Arch Neerl Physiol* 1922; 7:138.

28. De Vries H: The mechanics of the labyrinth otoliths. *Acta Otolaryngol* 1950; 38:262–273.

29. Dichgans J, Schmidt CL, Graf W: Visual input improves the speedometer function of the vestibular nuclei in the goldfish. *Exp Brain Res* 1973; 18:319–322.

30. Dohlman G: On the mechanism of transformation into nystagmus on stimulation of the semicircular canals. *Acta Otolaryngol* 1938; 26:425–442.

31. Dow B: Functional classes of cells and their laminar distribution in monkey visual cortex. *J Neurophysiol* 1974; 37:927–946.

32. Duensing F, Schaefer KP: Uber die konvergenz verschiedener labyrintharer afferenzen auf einzelne neurone des vestibulariskerngebietes. *Arch Psychiatr Nervenkr* 1959; 199:345.

33. Eckmiller R: Concerning the linear acceleration input to the neural oculomotor control system in primates, in Roucoux A, Crommelinck M (eds): *Physiological and Pathological Aspects of Eye Movements: Proceedings of a Workshop held at the Pont de'Oye Castle, Habay-la-Neuve, 1982*. The Hague; Dr. W Junk, Publishers for the Commission of the European Communities, 1982, pp 131–137.

34. Engstrom H, Ades HW, Andersson A: *Structural Pattern on the Organ of Corti*. Baltimore, Williams & Wilkins, 1966.

35. Evinger LC, Fuchs AF, Baker R: Bilateral lesions of the medial longitudinal fasciculus in monkeys: Effects on the horizontal and vertical components of voluntary and vestibular induced eye movements. *Exp Brain Res* 1977; 28:1–20.

36. Ewald R: Physiologische Untersuchungen uber das Endorgan des Nervous Octavus. Weisbaden, Bergmann, 1892.

37. Fernandez C, Baird RA, Goldberg JM: The vestibular nerve of the chinchilla. I: Peripheral innervation patterns in the horizontal and superior semicircular canals. *J Neurophysiol* 1988; 60:167–181.

38. Fernandez C, Goldberg JM: Physiology of peripheral neurons innervating otolith organs of the squirrel monkey. I: Response to static tilts and to long-duration centrifugal forces. *J Neurophysiol* 1976; 39:970–984.

39. Fernandez C, Goldberg JM: Physiology of peripheral neurons innervating otolith organs of the squirrel monkey. II: Directional selectivity and force-response relations. *J Neurophysiol* 1976; 39:985–995.

40. Fernandez C, Goldberg JM: Physiology of peripheral neurons innervating otolith organs of the squirrel monkey. III: Response dynamics. *J Neurophysiol* 1976; 39:996–1008.

41. Fernandez C, Goldberg JM, Baird RA: The vestibular nerve of the chinchilla. III: Peripheral innervation patterns in the utricular macula. *J Neurophysiol* 1990; 63:767–780.

42. Flock A, Flock B, Ulfendahl M: Mechanisms of movement in outer hair cells and a possible structural basis. *Arch Otorhinolaryngol* 1986; 243:83–90.

43. Flock A, Jorgensen M, Russell I: The physiology of individual hair cells and their synapses, in Miller A (ed): *Basic Mechanisms in Hearing*. New York; Academic Press, 1973.

44. Flock A, Orman S: Micromechanical properties of sensory hairs on receptor cells of the inner ear. *Hear Res* 1983; 11:249–260.

45. Fluur E, Mellstrom A: The otolith organs and their influence on oculomotor movements. *Exp Neurol* 1971; 30:139–147.

46. Galiana HL, Outerbridge JS: A bilateral model for central neural pathways in vestibuloocular reflex. *J Neurophysiol* 1984; 51:210–241.

47. Gernandt BE: Vestibulo-spinal mechanisms, in Kornhuber HH (ed): *Handbook of Sensory Physiology. VI/1: The Vestibular System*. New York; Springer-Verlag, 1974.

48. Goh Y, Alkon DL: Sensory, interneuronal, and motor interactions within *Hermissenda* visual pathway. *J Neurophysiol* 1984; 52:156–169.

49. Goldberg JM, Desmadryl G, Baird RA, et al: The vestibular nerve of the chinchilla. IV: Discharge properties of utricular afferents. *J Neurophysiol* 1990; 63:781–790.

50. Goldberg JM, Desmadryl G, Baird RA, et al: The vestibular nerve of the chinchilla. V: Relation between afferent discharge properties and peripheral innervation patterns in the utricular macula. *J Neurophysiol* 1990; 63:791–804.

51. Goldberg JM, Fernandez C: Physiology of peripheral neurons innervating semicircular canals of the squirrel monkey. I: Resting discharge and response to constant angular accelerations. *J Neurophysiol* 1971; 34:635–660.

52. Goldberg JM, Fernandez C: Physiology of peripheral neurons innervating semicircular canals of the squirrel monkey. III: Variations among units in their discharge properties. *J Neurophysiol* 1971; 34:676–684.

53. Goldberg JM, Highstein SM, Moschovakis AK, et al: Inputs from regularly and irregularly discharging vestibular nerve afferents to secondary neurons in the vestibular nuclei of the squirrel monkey. I: An electrophysiological analysis. *J Neurophysiol* 1987; 58:700–718.

54. Goldberg JM, Lysakowski A, Fernandez C: Structure and function of vestibular nerve fibers in chinchilla and squirrel monkey. *Ann NY Acad Sci* (in press).

55. Goldberg JM, Smith CE, Fernandez C: Relation between discharge regularity and responses to externally applied galvanic currents in vestibular nerve afferents of the squirrel monkey. *J Neurophysiol* 1984; 51:1236–1256.

56. Gresty MA: A reexamination of "neck reflex" eye movements in the rabbit. *Acta Otolaryngol* 1976; 81:386–394.

57. Hikosaka D, Maeda M: Cervical effects on abducens motoneurons and their interaction with vestibuloocular reflex. *Exp Brain Res* 1973; 18:512–530.

58. Hikosaka O, Kawakami T: Inhibitory reticular neurons related to the quick phase of vestibular nystagmus—their location and projection. *Exp Brain Res* 1977; 27:377–396.

59. Hikosaka O, Maeda M, Nakao S, et al: Presynaptic impulses in the abducens nucleus and their relation to postsynaptic potentials in motoneurons during vestibular nystagmus. *Exp Brain Res* 1977; 27:355–376.

60. Hoagland H: Impulses from sensory nerves of catfish. *Proc Natl Acad Sci USA* 1932; 18:701–705.

61. Hoffmann KP, Distler C, Erickson RG, et al: Physiological and anatomical identification of the nucleus of the optic tract and dorsal terminal nucleus of the accessory optic tract in monkeys. *Exp Brain Res* 1988; 69:635–644.

62. Hoffmann KP, Schoppman A: Retinal input to direction selective cells in the nucleus tractus opticus of the cat. *Brain Res* 1975; 99:359–366.

63. Honrubia V, Hoffman LF, Sitko S, et al: Anatomic and physiological correlates in bullfrog vestibular nerve. *J Neurophysiol* 1989; 61:688–701.

64. Honrubia V, Koehn WW, Jenkins HA, et al: Effect of bilateral ablation of the vestibular cerebellum on visual-vestibular interaction. *Exp Neurol* 1982; 75:616–626.

65. Honrubia V, Sitko S, Kimm J, et al: Physiological and anatomical characteristics of primary vestibular afferent neurons in the bullfrog. *Int J Neurosci* 1981; 15:197–206.

66. Houk JC: Control strategies in physiological systems. *FASEB J* 1988; 2:97–108.

67. Hudspeth AJ: Mechanoelectrical transduction by hair cells in the acousticolateralis sensory system. *Ann Rev Neurosci* 1983; 6:187–215.

68. Igarashi M, Miyata H, Alford BR, et al: Nystagmus after experimental cervical lesions. *Laryngoscope* 1972; 82:1609–1621.

69. Ito M: The vestibulo-cerebellar relationships: Vestibulo-ocular reflex arc and flocculus, in Naunton RF (ed): *The Vestibular System.* New York; Academic Press, 1975, pp 129–146.

70. Ito M, Shiida T, Yaga N, et al: Visual influence on rabbit horizontal vestibuloocular reflex presumably effected via the cerebellar flocculus. *Brain Res* 1974; 65:170–174.

71. Kato I, Harada K, Hasegawa T, et al: Role of the nucleus of the optic tract in monkeys in relation to optokinetic nystagmus. *Brain Res* 1988; 364:12–22.

72. Kiang NYS: *Discharge Patterns of Single Fibers in the Cat's Auditory Nerve.* Cambridge, Mass, MIT Press, 1965.

73. Kimura RS: Distribution, structure and function of dark cells in the vestibular labyrinth. *Ann Otol Rhinol Laryngol* 1969; 78:542–561.

74. Kimura RS, Schuknecht H: Membranous hydrops in the inner ear of the guinea pig after obliteration of the endolymphatic sac. *Pract Otorhinolaryngol* 1965; 27:343–354.

75. Lázár G: Role of the accessory optic system in the optokinetic nystagmus of the frog. *Brain Behav Evol* 1973; 5:443–460.

76. Lewis ER: Inertial motion sensors, in Bolis I, Keynes RD, Maddrell HP (eds): *Comparative Physiology of Sensory Systems.* Cambridge, UK, Cambridge University Press, 1984, pp 587–610.

77. Lim DJ: Ultrastructure of the otolithic membrane and the cupula. *Adv Otorhinolaryngol* 1973; 19:35–49.

78. Lindeman HH: Studies on the morphology of the sensory regions of the vestibular apparatus. *Adv Anat Embryol Cell Biol* 1969; 42:1–113.

79. Lindsay JR: Petrous pyramid of the temporal bone: Pneumatization and roentgenologic appearance. *Arch Otolaryngol* 1940; 31:231–255.

80. Llinas R, Terzuolo CA: Mechanisms of supraspinal actions upon spinal cord activities. Reticular inhibitory mechanisms on alpha-extensor motoneurons. *J Neurophysiol* 1964; 27:579–591.

81. Llinas R, Terzuolo CA: Mechanisms of supraspinal actions upon spinal cord activities. Reticular inhibitory mechanisms upon flexor motoneurons. *J Neurophysiol* 1965; 28:413–422.

82. Lorente de No R: Etudes sur l'anatomie et la physiologie du labyrinthe de l'oreille et du VIIIe nerf. Deuxieme partie. *Trav Lab Rech Biol Univ Madrid* 1926; 24:53–153.

83. Lorente de No R: Anatomy of the eighth nerve. The central projection of the nerve endings of the internal ear. *Laryngoscope* 1933; 43:1–38.

84. Lowenstein O, Roberts TDM: The equilibrium function of the otolith organs of the thornback ray (*Raja clavata*). *J Physiol (Lond)* 1949; 110:392–415.

85. Lundquist P-G: The endolymphatic duct and sac in the guinea pig. *Acta Otolaryngol* [Suppl] 1965; 201:1–108.

86. Lynch JC, McLaren JW: The contribution of parieto-occipital association cortex to the control of slow eye movements, in Lennerstrand G, Zee DS, Keller EL (eds): *Functional Basis of Ocular Motility Disorders.* Oxford, UK, Pergamon Press, 1982; pp 501–510.

87. Maekawa K, Simpson JI: Climbing fiber activation of Purkinje cells in the flocculus by impulses transferred through the visual pathway. *Brain Res* 1972; 39:245–251.

88. Maekawa K, Takeda T: Mossy fiber responses evoked in the cerebellar flocculus of rabbits by stimulation of the optic pathway. *Brain Res* 1975; 98:590–595.

89. Maekawa K, Takeda T: Electrophysiological identification of the climbing and mossy fiber pathways from the rabbit's retina to the contralateral cerebellar flocculus. *Brain Res* 1976; 109:169–174.

90. Maunsell JHR, Van Essen DC: Functional properties of neurons in middle temporal visual area of the macaque monkey. I: Selectivity for stimulus direction, speed, and orientation. *J Neurophysiol* 1983; 49:1127–1147.

91. May JG, Anderson RA: Different patterns of cortico-pontine projections from separate cortical fields within the inferior parietal lobule and dorsal prelunate gyrus of the macaque. *Exp Brain Res* 1986; 63:265–278.

92. May JG, Keller EL, Suzuki DA: Smooth-pursuit eye movement deficits with chemical lesions in the dorsolateral pontine nucleus of the monkey. *J Neurophysiol* 1988; 59:952–977.

93. McCouch GP, Deering ID, Ling TH: Location of receptors for tonic neck reflexes. *J Neurophysiol* 1951; 14:191–195.

94. McCrea RA, Strassman A, Highstein SM: Anatomical and physiological characteristics of vestibular neurons mediating the vertical vestibulo-ocular reflex in the squirrel monkey. *J Comp Neur* 1987; 264:571–594.

95. McCrea RA, Strassman A, May E, et al: Anatomical and physiological characteristics of vestibular neurons mediating the horizontal vestibulo-ocular reflex in the squirrel monkey. *J Comp Neurol* 1987; 264:547–570.

96. Melvill Jones G: Adaptive modulation of VOR parameters by vision, In Berthoz A, Melvill Jones G (eds): *Reviews in Oculomotor Research*, vol 1; *Adaptive Mechanisms in Gaze Control.* Amsterdam, Elsevier, 1985, pp 21–50.

97. Mountain DC: Electromechanical properties of hair cells, in Altschuler RA, Bobbin RP, Hoffman DW (eds): *Neurobiology of Hearing: The Cochlea.* New York, Raven Press, 1986; pp 77–90.

98. Mustari MJ, Fuchs AF: Discharge patterns of neurons in the pretectal nucleus of the optic tract (NOT) in the behaving primate. *J Neurophysiol* 1990; 64:77–90.

99. Nashner LM: Strategies for organization of human posture, in Igarashi M, Black FO (eds): *Vestibular and Visual Control on Posture and Locomotor Equilibrium.* Basel, Karger, 1985, pp 1–8.

100. Nyberg-Hansen R: Origin and termination of fibers from the vestibular nuclei descending the medial longitudinal fasciculus. An experimental study with silver impregnation methods in the cat. *J Comp Neurol* 1964; 122:355–367.

101. Nyberg-Hansen R: Sites and mode of termination of fibers of the vestibulo-spinal tract in the cat. An experimental study with silver impregnation methods. *J Comp Neurol* 1964; 122:369–388.

102. Nyberg-Hansen R: Sites and mode of termination of reticulospinal fibers in the cat. An experimental study with silver impregnation methods. *J Comp Neurol* 1965; 124:71–99.

103. Ohgaki T, Curthoys IS, Markham CH: Morphology of physiologically identified second-order vestibular neurons in the cat with intracellularly injected HRP. *J Comp Neurol* 1988; 276:387–411.

104. Orman S, Flock A: Active control of sensory hair mechanics implied by susceptibility to media that induce contraction in muscle. *Hear Res* 1983; 11:261–266.

105. Perlmutter ST, Fukushima K, Peterson BW, et al: Spatial properties of second order vestibulo-ocular reflex neurons in the alert cat. *Abstr Soc Neurosci* 1988; 14:331.

106. Peterson BW: The reticulospinal system and its role in the control of movement, in Barnes CD (ed): *Brainstem Control of Spinal Cord Function.* New York, Academic Press, 1984, pp 28–86.

107. Peterson BW, Fukushima K, Hirai N, et al: Responses of vestibulospinal and reticulospinal neurons to sinusoidal vestibular stimulation. *J Neurophysiol* 1980; 43:1236–1250.

108. Pompeiano O: Cerebello-vestibular interrelations, in Kornhuber HH (ed): *Handbook of Sensory Physiology. VI/1: The Vestibular System.* New York, Springer-Verlag, 1974, pp 417–476.

109. Precht W: Vestibular mechanisms. *Ann Rev Neurosci* 1979; 2:265–289.

110. Precht W, Shimazu H: Functional connections of tonic and kinetic vestibular neurons

with primary vestibular afferents. *J Neurophysiol* 1965; 28:1014–1028.

111. Precht W, Strata P: On the pathway mediating optokinetic responses in the vestibular nuclear neurons. *Neuroscience* 1980; 5:777–787.

112. Ramprashad F, Landolt JP, Money KE, et al: Dimensional analysis and dynamic response characterization of mammalian peripheral vestibular structures. *Am J Anat* 1984; 169:295–313.

113. Raphan T, Matsuo V, Cohen B: Velocity storage in the vestibuloocular reflex arc (VOR). *Exp Brain Res* 1979; 35:229–248.

114. Roberts TDM: *Neurophysiology of Postural Mechanisms.* New York, Plenum, 1967.

115. Robinson DA: Oculomotor unit behavior in the monkey. *J Neurophysiol* 1970; 33:393–404.

116. Robinson DL, Goldberg ME, Stanton GB: Parietal association cortex in the primate: Sensory mechanisms and behavioral modulation. *J Neurophysiol* 1978; 41:910–932.

117. Rosenhall U: Mapping of the cristae ampullares in man. *Ann Otol Rhinol Laryngol* 1972; 81:882–889.

118. Rosenhall U: Vestibular macular mapping in man. *Ann Otol Rhinol Laryngol* 1972; 81:339–351.

119. Rubin AM, Young JH, Milne AC, et al: Vestibular-neck integration in the vestibular nuclei. *Brain Res* 1975; 96:99–102.

120. Ryals BM, Rubel EW: Hair cell regeneration after acoustic trauma in adult Coturnix quail. *Science* 1988; 240:1774–1776.

121. Sakata H, Sibutani H, Kawano K: Functional properties of visual tracking neurons in posterior parietal association cortex of the monkey. *J Neurophysiol* 1983; 49:1364–1380.

122. Salt AN, Konishi T: The cochlear fluids: Perilymph and endolymph, in Altschuler RA, Bobbin RP, Hoffman DW (eds): *Neurobiology of Hearing: The Cochlea.* New York, Raven Press, 1986; pp 109–122.

123. Schiff D, Cohen B, Raphan T: Nystagmus induced by stimulation of the nucleus of the optic tract in the monkey. *Exp Brain Res* 1988; 70:1–14.

124. Schwindt PC, Richter A, Precht W: Short latency utricular and canal input to ipsilateral abducens motoneurons. *Brain Res* 1973; 60:259–262.

125. Shimazu H: Neuronal organization of the premotor system controlling horizontal conjugate eye movements and vestibular nystagmus. *Adv Neurol* 1983; 39:565–588.

126. Simpson JI: The accessory optic system. *Ann Rev Neurosci* 1984; 7:13–41.

127. Skavenski AA, Robinson DA: Role of abducens neurons in vestibuloocular reflex. *J Neurophysiol* 1973; 36:724–737.

128. Steinhausen W: Uber Sichtbarmachung and Funktionsprufung der Cupula terminalis in den Bogengangs-ampullen der Labyrinths. *Arch Ges Physiol* 1927; 217:747.

129. Suzuki J-I, Tokumasu K, Goto K: Eye movements from single utricular nerve stimulation in the cat. *Acta Otolaryngol* 1969; 68:350–362.

130. Tanaka K, Hikosaka K, Saito H-A, et al: Analysis of local and wide-field movements in the superior temporal visual areas of the macaque monkey. *J Neurosci* 1986; 6:134–144.

131. Uchino Y, Hirai N, Suzuki S: Branching pattern and properties of vertical- and horizontal-related excitatory vestibuloocular neurons of the cat. *J Neurophysiol* 1982; 48:891–903.

132. Uchino Y, Suzuki S: Axon collaterals to the extraocular motoneuron pools of inhibitory vestibuloocular neurons activated from the anterior, posterior and horizontal semicircular canals in the cat. *Neurosci* Lett 1983; 37:129–135.

133. van Egmond AAJ, Groen JJ, Jongkees LBW: The mechanics of the semicircular canal. *J Physiol* 1949; 110:1–17.

134. Waespe W, Henn V: Gaze stabilization in the primate. The interaction of the vestibulo-ocular reflex, optokinetic nystagmus, and smooth pursuit. *Rev Physiol Biochem Pharmacol* 1987; 106:37–125.

135. Wilson VJ, Melvill Jones G: *Mammalian Vestibular Physiology.* New York, Plenum, 1979.

136. Wilson VJ, Wylie RM, Marco LA: Organization of the medial vestibular nucleus. *J Neurophysiol* 1968; 31:166–175.

137. Zee DS, Yamazaki A, Butler PH, et al: Effects of ablation of flocculus and paraflocculus on eye movements in primate. *J Neurophysiol* 1981; 46:878–899.

138. Zeki SM: The responses of cells in the anterior bank of the superior temporal sulcus in macaque monkeys. *J Physiol* (Lond) 1980; 308:85P.

139. Zenner HP, Zimmerman U, Gitter AH: Cell potential and motility of isolated mammalian vestibular sensory cells. *Hear Res* 1990; 50:289–294.

CHAPTER 3

Practical Anatomy and Physiology of the Ocular Motor System

James R. Carl, M.D.

TYPES OF EYE MOVEMENTS

The interpretation of eye movement records depends on an understanding of the underlying anatomy and physiology of the ocular motor system. The past 2 decades have brought tremendous advances in the knowledge of brain stem activity associated with eye movements, and a corresponding increase in the complexity of maps of neural pathways. While this new information adds to the ability of scientists and clinicians to understand and detect oculomotor and vestibular disorders, much of this detail is not necessary for routine evaluation of electronystagmography (ENG) recordings, and is well covered in more specialized sources.[6, 18] There are, however, some basic principles of organization that help make sense of this complex system and assist both in recording and interpreting eye movements. Because these organizational principles stem from the demands of the visual system and anatomy of eye muscles, these constraints are examined here first to set the stage for the underlying neurophysiology.

Conjugate Eye Movements Serving Foveal Vision

Two primary features of the human visual system determine the structure of all types of oculomotor control: the foveal region of high-resolution vision, and the two frontally directed eyes, which enhance depth perception. The human fovea consists of a small, 5° region of the retina where the light-transducing cells, primarily cones, are tightly packed, giving high resolution of images that fall on this region. The center of the fovea, the foveola, is a smaller 0.8° spot providing the best resolution of visual images.[23] For one to clearly see objects of interest in the visual environment the tiny foveola must be pointed at the object of regard. Because visual perception cannot be accomplished instantaneously, like a camera snapshot, the image must remain on the foveola; if it drifts away, visual clarity deteriorates. The rest of the retina, which loses resolution as images fall farther from the fovea, relays visual information that is largely used to assess changes in the environment that may require closer evaluation by moving the eye to point at the object of new interest, causing the image to fall on the foveola. Human foveal vision, therefore, places some specific demands on oculomotor function: the eye must be very accurately pointed, and the image must remain still, with no relative motion between image and eye. These requirements apply equally to both eyes, so the conjugate eye movements, or *versions*, that fulfill these visual needs move the eyes at the same time in the same direction. The visual axis, or direction in which the eye is pointing, can be changed by moving the eye in the orbit and by moving the head, carrying the eyes with it. *Gaze* refers to the combination of these and represents the line of sight with respect to objects in the environment. There are two classes of conjugate movements: movements to shift gaze, and movements to stabilize images. *Saccades*—rapid movements of both eyes simultaneously—exist primarily to change gaze angle, while the others hold images still on the fovea during the relative motion of eye and object. In Table 3–1 the classes of eye movements are summarized and some pertinent features of each type are listed.

Saccades

Saccades rapidly change the direction of the eye to acquire the image of an object of interest. Once a decision is made to look at a new object or in a new direction, these eye movements must be completed as quickly as possible in order to minimize the amount of time that the eye is in motion and vision is compromised. But accuracy is equally important, because an inaccurate saccade will require an additional, corrective saccade to get the eye on target, wasting extra time. Human saccadic eye movements represent a compromise between these competing demands. A long programming time, or latency, of about 200 ms allows a saccade to be generally quite accurate for movements of less than 10°, so that an extra corrective saccade is not required.[2] This requisite complex saccadic programming means that a decline in saccadic accuracy may be an early sign of brain stem or cerebellar abnormality. High eye speed and short duration of movement are generated during the saccade by maximally stimulating the appropriate eye muscles. Saccades thus place the highest demand on the ocular muscles; slowing of saccadic velocity is the first sign of many muscular or neurologic abnormalities. Saccades are also used to recenter the eye in the orbit when the vestibular or optokinetic response has carried the line of sight away from primary position.

Smooth Pursuit

Slow, smooth pursuit or tracking eye movements are required when an object of interest is moving in space relative to the head. The goal of pursuit movements is to match eye velocity to the angular velocity of the target so that the target image remains as steady as possi-

TABLE 3–1.

Classes of Eye Movements and Associated Features

	Purpose	Stimulus	Motion	Latency
Saccades	Shift gaze	Small object not in line of sight	Conjugate rapid	200
Pursuit	Stabilize image of moving object	Motion of small object	Conjugate slow and smooth	100
Fixation	Stabilize image of still object	Still object in line of sight	Small amplitude pursuit and saccades	
VOR	Stabilize images during head motion	Angular acceleration of head	Conjugate smooth opposite head	15
OKN	Stabilize images during sustained head rotation	Steady motion of entire field	Conjugate rapid and smooth alternating	75
Vergence	Align the eyes on object in depth	Double image or blur	Disconjugate very slow	150

ble on the fovea. To this end, this system is mostly sensitive to retinal-image motion caused by a still eye and a moving target (for example, when a seated person watches a bird flying by). Unless highly practiced, humans cannot make smooth-pursuit eye movements unless a moving image is present. Images drifting away from the fovea cause the eye to accelerate in the direction of the motion; that is, the eye speeds up to match the target's motion. If the image gets too far from the fovea, the saccadic system is invoked to generate a quick "catch-up" movement to again point the eye at the moving target so the pursuit system can attempt to match eye and target velocity. Most smooth-pursuit eye movements require occasional saccadic eye movements to re-center the image, because the pursuit system is not very accurate for targets moving above 10°/sec or for targets that suddenly change speed or direction. Smooth-pursuit eye movements have a latency of about 100 ms, so the response to a new stimulus occurs before a saccade, but the initial pursuit is quite sluggish, with a low acceleration of around 40°/sec².[5] The pursuit system compensates for this poor performance by attempting to predict the target motion and produce eye movements to match the expected target movement. This strategy is usually quite effective and allows the eyes to accurately follow objects moving in a regular fashion.[21]

Vestibular Eye Movements

Smooth eye movements generated by vestibular stimulation provide visual stabilization of the environment required during self motion. Any motion of head and body or head that moves the eyes in space causes the image of objects that are fixed in space to move on the retina. It is this relative movement between image and eye as a result of self motion that is probably the greatest continual threat to clear vision. People who have lost this reflexive visual stabilization as a result of vestibular disease may give dramatic testimony to its importance as they describe the need to be completely still in order to see clearly.[15] The vestibulo-ocular reflex (VOR) must respond quickly if it is to stabilize vision adequately; this is accomplished by a fairly direct three-neuron pathway with a very short latency of about 15 ms.[19] Most relative motion is created by head rotations, sensed by the six paired semicircular canals. Their signals are transformed by the vestibular nuclei and brain stem centers into an eye movement of equal and opposite velocity, thus stabilizing retinal images.[7] Linear or translational motion of the head may also disturb retinal images, but this disturbance depends on the distance to the object of interest.[28] Nearby objects require some eye movement to stabilize the object's retinal image visually, while distant objects do not. This type of motion is sensed by the otolith organs, and the corresponding eye movements are sometimes called linear or translational vestibular ocular reflex or otolith ocular reflex. This reflex is not typically tested in a clinical setting and does not produce much visual difficulty if absent.

Optokinetic Nystagmus

Optokinetic nystagmus (OKN) is a special repetitive eye movement with alternating fast saccadic eye movements in one direction and smooth movements in the opposite direction. The OKN movement serves as a "back-up" system to provide visual stabilization during sustained head rotations when the VOR response decays.[25] It may be generated in response to any visual stimulus that continually moves past the eyes in one direction. In the laboratory it is usually generated by asking the subject to view a rotating drum or long tape with stripes. More intense stimulation may be provided when the entire visual environment moves coherently in one direction, as when the subject is placed inside a rotating drum or when full-field projection is used. Optokinetic nystagmus has been studied extensively in lateral-eyed animals such as rabbits, in which the neural pathways and response characteristics qualify the eye movements as a separate type, but most pertinent features such as optokinetic afternystagmus and dependence on the vestibular nuclei are vestigial in humans, and human OKN is generated mostly by the smooth-pursuit and saccadic systems. The initial eye movement response to motion of the entire visual environment has characteristics slightly different from either smooth pursuit or OKN, and is called *ocular following.*[11] This response has the shortest latency of any visually guided eye movement, at 75 ms. The very low amplitudes and accelerations generated by the ocular following system require special techniques to demonstrate and are therefore not typically recorded during standard ENG examinations.

Fixation

A final oculomotor behavior of importance is *fixation*, or the maintenance of steady eyes without movement. Because no gross eye motion should be produced during this task, it is not often considered a type of eye movement. It is, however, an active process requiring continual correction of errors, usually by the use of tiny saccades and drifts of the eye to maintain correct eye position. Fixation has received little study in comparison with the other movements described, but there is probably a separate neural organization to deal with the need for continual fine corrections. Abnormalities of this process may be responsible for fixational instability and some types of nystagmus.[16] The corrective eye movements produced to maintain fixation are typically less than a degree in amplitude, and so are not seen with the normal resolution of eye-movement records from an ENG examination, but may be measurable when fixation is affected.

Disjunctive Movements Serving Binocular Vision

Binocular vision is the second feature of the human visual system that requires special eye movement control. For the eyes to provide useful stereo vision to enhance depth perception, both foveae must be pointed directly at the object of regard. In addition, visual images from the two eyes cannot be easily interpreted if they do not match. If the eyes do not point together, clear vision is lost and the highly disturbing symptom of diplopia is reported. The seriousness of this problem is underscored by the fact that when binocular oculomotor control is compromised, most people need to block the vision from one eye with a patch. Binocular vision thus requires highly coordinated eye movements from both eyes to ensure that matching images are provided at all times. The separation of the eyes also requires a change in the angle between the visual axes when one is viewing objects at different distances or undergoing self motion.

Vergence

In some circumstances the eyes move in an opposite but coordinated fashion. These disjunctive eye movements are called *convergence* when the eyes both move inward toward the nose to view nearby objects and *divergence* when the eyes move out to view more distant objects. Vergence movements are slow, smooth movements that may occur in response to separation of images from the two eyes (fusional) or to blurring of images (accomodative).[24] While pure vergence eye movements may occur, generally a saccade is also required, and the saccadic eye movement is often slightly disconjugate, with one eye moving farther than the other, thus changing the vergence angle and accomplishing much of the desired vergence during the saccade.[9]

COORDINATION AND CONTROL OF ACCURACY

The need for clear matching images for binocular vision places additional demands on ocular motor control which apply to all types of eye movements. The arrangement of the two eyes requires several special types of cooperation as well as adjustments for viewing distance. Continual threats to accuracy demand constant evaluation and compensation for appropriate eye movements to be maintained. The common measure of accuracy is the *gain*, the ratio of actual eye movement to desired eye movement. Multiple brain stem areas contribute to this vital component of quality control, ensuring cooperation and accuracy.

Cooperation of Types of Movement

Although often studied in isolation, various eye movements often occur simultaneously, allowing selection and observation of objects of interest—while walking, for example. The vestibular system is continually stimulated by the head motions during walking, while saccades change gaze and pursuit allows the eyes to follow objects. In some cases, the VOR must be "turned off" to allow for gaze changes instead of continuing to insist on stabilizing gaze. Pursuit movements, however, are greatly helped by the effective elimination of head movements so that only object motion must be accounted for in programming. The ability to switch systems off and on or to add the effects of all systems together is crucial for clear vision during complex behavior. In the laboratory or ENG testing situation, great care must be taken to create specific head motion, visual stimuli, and instructions to the patient in order to study these movements in isolation. Each type of eye movement uses different visual and physical stimuli to elicit and program eye motion, and the characteristics of ongoing control are also different, so it is not surprising that separate neural pathways are devoted to each system. The challenge to ocular motor control is to combine signals from each separate system into a single signal carrying all of the information in a cooperative fashion.

Hering's Law of Equal Innervation

For conjugate eye movements, each eye must undergo the same amount and direction of movement. This is accomplished by a neuronal calculation for a single eye; the same signal is then sent to the appropriate muscle pair for each eye. This neurally generated method of keeping the eyes moving together is described by Hering's law, and is the key to understanding the eye movements observed when one eye cannot respond properly because of neurologic or mechanical problems.[12] The level of innervation of an eye muscle can always be determined by examining the movement of the unaffected eye and remembering that the same signal was intended for each eye. This principle of equal innervation does not hold exactly, because the two involved muscles may have slightly different pulling directions or one may be injured; in either case, small adjustments to Hering's law will occur.

Ocular Torsion and Listing's Law

The eyes can physically rotate about the visual axis, creating torsional eye movements. Torsion movements cannot generally be created voluntarily, but they do occur during vestibular stimulation, albeit of low amplitude. Eye movements other than simple left-right or up-down create apparent rotations of the eye around the visual axis, called *induced torsion*. Clear binocular vision and vergence movements require matching torsion in each eye, so some cooperation must occur. Additional adjustments must be made to ensure that the amount of this induced torsion matches in each eye. Listing's law states that the torsional state of an eye is always as if the eye had reached its current position by a single rotation from primary position.[10] This constraint additionally means that the position of the eye can be described in only two dimensions, with the third dimension fixed by this neuronal regulation of torsional position.

Adjustments for Viewing Distance

Vestibular eye movements are affected by the separation of the eyes. The head normally rotates about an axis separate from and behind both eyes; consequently, a slightly larger compensatory movement is required when near objects are viewed. The gain must increase with convergence, by up to 50% or more for very close objects.[14] This increase is achieved, like all adjustments, without any conscious effort. The stimulus is probably the perceived distance of the viewed object, and the increase may occur even before the eyes converge. The translational VOR, the response to sideways movement of the head without rotation, likewise must change gain with convergence. The required eye movement for visual stabilization is inversely proportional to the viewing distance, so the adjustment is much greater than for the VOR.

Adaptation

The high level of accuracy demanded of eye movements is regularly threatened by a variety of factors: pathologic states of injury and disease, deterioration from aging, vestibular challenges from modern transportation, and visual challenges from spectacles.[20] All of these conditions may require a recalibration of some eye movements, particularly saccades and VOR, which occur without any feedback during the motion. When a saccade is launched by a neural program, the duration is too short to allow for visual assessment of the accuracy until the movement is completed. Adaptive regulation occurs for all eye movements and depends on brain stem circuits that monitor the accuracy of movements and can modify neural control signals. Weakness of an ocular muscle will cause each saccade in one direction to be too small and a corrective saccade to occur. The need for the corrective saccade is a signal that the initial saccade was not accurate. During VOR or pursuit eye movements, slip of the image on the retina means that the desired stabilization did not occur. This slip can serve as an error signal used to adjust the gains of the inaccurate movement in a process taking minutes to begin and improving for up to days. The cerebellum plays an important role in the continuous process of monitoring and adapting accuracy. Inaccurate movements and inability to adapt or correct gain are hallmarks of cerebellar lesions. Malfunctions of the adaptation process may account for some types of abnormal eye movements, such as periodic alternating nystagmus where the corrective process continually overshoots and an oscillation develops.[17]

OCULOMOTOR ANATOMY: THE FINAL COMMON PATHWAY

For each type of eye movement, separate regions of the brain transform the visual or physical stimulus into an appropriate neural command. While this initial processing is independent, all of the eye-movement systems depend on the same cranial nerves and ocular muscles to effect the specific type of eye motion desired. There are no separate muscle or nerve fibers to serve any single eye-movement system.[26] The brain stem cranial nerve nuclei, cranial nerves, and twelve extraocular muscles serve as a final common pathway for all eye movements. The anatomy of this final common path thus also places demands and constraints on the neurophysiology of eye movements.

Orbital Anatomy

The primary anatomic consideration for eye movements is the physical arrangement of the orbit and extraocular muscles. The eyeball is nearly a sphere, with the corneal bulge facing out of the orbit. The spherical scleral portion sits in a cushioning bed of fat in the orbit, connected by moderately redundant lengths of arteries, veins, and nerves. The eye is free to rotate in any direction about the effective center of the sphere, and for practical purposes, in the absence of orbital disease, all eye movements are rotations with the center of movement remaining fixed in the orbit. The range of eye rotation is limited by check ligaments attached to the globe. Figure 3–1, a magnetic resonance image of the orbits, demonstrates the relationship of the eyeball in the orbit and some of the attached extraocular muscles.

Viscoelastic Forces

The muscles and other tissues attached to the globe are responsible for the viscoelastic forces that resist eye movements. The elastic connective tissue around the eye creates a centering force that tends to move the eye back to a central position. These elastic forces must be countered by muscle tone to hold the eye in an eccentric position. The muscle tone needed is about proportional to the angular eccentricity of the eye position. Each eye movement caused by contraction of one muscle must be accompanied by a stretching of the antagonist muscle. This muscle stretching provides the greatest viscous resistance to rapid eye motion, and the muscle force needed to overcome it is about proportional to the angular velocity of the eye movement. The force needed for eye movement is therefore a combination of velocity-related forces to overcome viscous resistance and position-related forces to overcome elastic centering forces.

Extraocular Muscles

Six muscles, arranged roughly in three pairs, are attached to each eye. The four recti muscles (medial, lateral, superior, and inferior) run between the apex of the orbit and the front hemisphere of the eyeball; all rotate the eye toward the muscle. The oblique muscles both come from the front of the orbit near the rim to attach behind the equator to the rear hemisphere; they rotate the eye away from the muscle. The inferior oblique muscle does this directly,

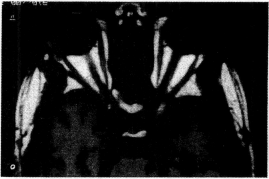 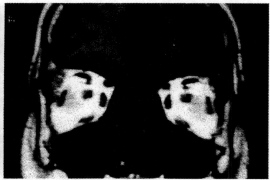

FIG 3–1.
Magnetic resonance imaging of the orbits. **A,** section through the horizontal recti and optic nerves. This section is the horizontal plane. **B,** frontal section just behind the eyeball. The muscles and optic nerves stand out as dark ovals as they are cut in cross-section. The inferior oblique muscle does not show up as it goes from the inferior orbital rim back to attach to the eye, in front of the plane of this section. A comparable schematic cross-section of the orbit is shown in Figure 3–2.

running between the inferior orbital rim and the underside of the globe. The superior oblique muscle achieves the same effect by using a long tendon that runs through a pulley or trochlea near the superior orbital rim and then back along the upper surface of the globe before attaching behind the equator. Contraction of each muscle causes the eye to rotate about a specific axis fixed within the orbit. The corresponding axes of the two muscles of each pair are close enough together that they may be combined and a single axis of rotation assigned to the pair. This axis goes through the center of the globe and is perpendicular to the plane containing the pair of muscles. The diagrams in Figure 3–2 indicate the axis of rotation of the two vertically acting muscle pairs. The axis for the horizontal recti muscles is vertical.

Axes of Ocular Rotations

Two key features to the scheme of ocular rotations are central to understanding the eye movements produced by the pull of each muscle. The first is that the axis of rotation of the eye produced by contraction of a single muscle (and the inverse produced by its partner) is essentially independent of the position of the eye.[22] The second is that these axes, particularly in the case of the oblique muscles, are not perpendicular to the visual axis, but are fixed with respect to the orbit.[29] The latter feature means that the movement of the visual axis as indicated by pupil movement, which has been a traditional way to describe eye movements, appears complex, with primary and secondary actions, and depends on eye position. Coordinate systems depending on the visual axis designate eye positions by horizontal, vertical, and torsional components.[1] These components are easy to recognize by noting the movement of the pupil, and are therefore most often used to describe eye movements. The disadvantage of this nomenclature is that the ocular muscles don't pull exactly in these directions. An upward movement of the pupil is caused by dif-

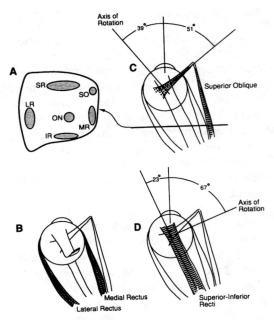

FIG 3–2.
Pulling directions and axis of rotation of extraocular muscles. **A,** schematic diagram of the location of the muscles just behind the eyeball, indicating the relative positions of the five muscles that attach to the apex of the orbit. *MR,* medial rectus; *LR,* lateral rectus; *SO,* superior oblique; *SR,* superior rectus; *IR,* inferior rectus; *ON,* optic nerve. The plane of this section is comparable to Figure 3–1, B and is shown in **C. B,** top view of lateral and medial rectus muscles responsible for horizontal rotations. The superior rectus muscle is stripped away to show the optic nerve. The plane of the section is comparable to that shown in Figure 3–1, A. **C,** similar view with superior oblique highlighted to illustrate the pulling direction of this muscle. The pulling direction and axis of rotation of the inferior oblique are very similar, as the muscle is under the eye but parallel to the portion of superior oblique attaching to the eye. The superior oblique attaches under the superior rectus. **D,** superior rectus is highlighted, showing the axis of rotation of this muscle and its partner, the inferior rectus, hidden directly beneath it.

ferent muscles when the eye is pointed medially compared to a lateral starting position, so there is no direct relationship between a vertical movement described in this fashion and the muscles that need to be stimulated. A coordinate system based on the visual axis is still the most commonly used in spite of this limitation. The recognition that eye movements occur as rotations about axes in three dimensions fixed in the orbit assists in understanding the relationship between the three-dimensional axes of the semicircular canals and the eye movements associated with stimulation of the canals. While a variety of axis systems may be used to describe movements of the eyes, all have in common the need for most real eye movements to involve all three pairs of muscles acting together. This coordinated behavior is then a requirement for the common final path for all eye movement systems.

Cranial Nerves and Nuclei

The twelve extraocular muscles are innervated by six cranial nerves: numbers III, IV, and VI on the left and right side. Each cranial nerve nucleus is located in the brain stem in a small region near the midbrain. The cranial nerves exit from the brain stem and follow separate but nearby routes to reach the extraocular muscles in the orbit. Lesions of a single cranial nerve cause characteristic abnormalities of eye movements and position. Diplopia is the most common complaint, but partial lesions may cause subtle symptoms only during saccadic or vestibular eye movements. Recognizing cranial nerve lesions is important because these symptoms may lead to an ENG investigation when the diagnosis of a cranial nerve palsy is not suspected. Observation of the patient for abnormal pupils, drooping eyelids, or ocular misalignment should be the first step in the ENG test. Although single cranial nerve lesions affect only one eye, the appropriate evaluation of ENG tracings will depend on knowing about significant muscle weakness. Weakness of a single muscle causes a deficiency in moving the eye in the direction of action of that muscle, creating diplopia. The increasing separation of visual axes of the two eyes and separation of images becomes greater as the eye moves farther in the direction of weak muscle action. When a patient complains of diplopia with greater image separation looking in one direction, the muscle responsible is the one that normally pulls the eye in the affected direction.

Oculomotor Nerve: Cranial Nerve III

The third cranial nerve, or oculomotor nerve, innervates the superior rectus, inferior rectus, medial rectus, and inferior oblique muscles. A complete lesion of this nerve allows only lateral movement of the eye and some torsion. The eye will typically be positioned slightly below and lateral to the primary position, "down and out". Because pupillomotor and eyelid muscles are innervated by the cranial nerve III, a lesion also causes ptosis, or eyelid drooping, and a large, unreactive pupil. Partial lesions may cause milder forms of the complete syndrome, or only some of the muscles may be affected and some of the signs present. Common causes of third-nerve palsies include ischemic lesions in diabetics and aneurysms of the posterior communicating artery.

Trochlear Nerve: Cranial Nerve IV

The fourth cranial nerve, or trochlear nerve, innervates only the superior oblique muscle. Because it is the only nerve to cross the midline, the nucleus is on the side opposite to the innervated muscle. Head trauma is the most common cause of a fourth-nerve palsy. Complaints due to paralysis of this nerve are usually limited to diplopia with vertical separation of images, particularly when looking down. Patients may also mention a twisting of images, a symptom that can also be caused by otolith or central vestibular problems. The superior oblique muscle normally contracts during head tilting toward the side of the muscle, so patients may adopt a head tilt away from the involved side to lessen the separation of images. Because the fourth cranial nerve is easily damaged in even mild head trauma, transient palsies are often seen following head injury.

Abducens Nerve: Cranial Nerve VI

The sixth cranial nerve, or abducens nerve, innervates the lateral rectus muscle. A lesion causes crossed eyes and double vision when looking toward the side of the affected nerve. Patients may adopt a head turn to keep gaze in the direction opposite the side of a lateral rectus muscle weakness. Mild weakness may show up as diplopia for distant objects only, as a slight crossing of the eyes is necessary when converging for near viewing. This nerve is also commonly affected by trauma, neurosurgery, and increased intracranial pressure. Because saccade velocities present the greatest challenge for muscle contraction, mild lesions of the sixth nerve will create abnormalities in several typical ENG tests in the affected eye only, giving low-velocity horizontal saccades towards the weak muscle and low-amplitude OKN for stripes moving to the opposite side.

Brain Stem Organization

The organization of cranial nerve nuclei in the brain stem is related to the pairing of right and left eye muscles. Because the left lateral rectus and right medial rectus must contract simultaneously for a leftward eye movement, these muscles are "yoked" and typically innervated as a pair. Physical and neural adaptations in the brain stem have developed to support this yoking of muscles in an efficient fashion. A lateral and medial recti yoked pair are connected by a nerve fiber tract called the medial longitudinal fasciculus, which crosses the midline and provides the neural substrate for the linking of this pair. The right inferior rectus and the left superior oblique both move the eye down when it is turned to the right, so they are similarly yoked. The crossing of the fourth cranial nerve after exiting from the brain stem allows the nuclei for this pair to be located on the same side of the brain stem, which assists in the pairing, and both are on the opposite side from the left posterior semicircular canal (SSC), which strongly activates the pair. The third cranial nerve nuclei are located just across the midline from each other, and have special-

ized regions or subnuclei to control the four muscles innervated by each nerve. The subnucleus for the superior rectus is located on the side opposite to the innervated muscle, unlike the others. This crossed representation means that the superior-inferior yoked muscle pairs have their nuclei on the same side of the brain stem. The general organization of the cranial nerve nuclei is for a yoked pair to be in close proximity on the same side of the brain stem or connected by a fiber tract, with each SSC from one ear activating the pair located on the opposite side. The axis of rotation of each yoked muscle pair and the connected SSC are nearly aligned so some primitive vestibular reflexes can operate in a direct fashion without major neural reorganization. The location of the brain stem and pairing of cranial nerve nuclei, and the relationship of semicircular canals and each pair, are illustrated in Figure 3–3. This organization probably developed to serve vestibular responses in animals without many visually guided movements, and humans have adapted the canal oriented design to also serve as the underlying plan for all eye movements.

Patterns of Neural Innervation

Experiments on monkeys have shown that all muscle fibers participate in all eye movements and that the muscle pulling force is proportional to the nerve firing rate.[27] The average firing rate of a nerve supplying a single muscle is therefore a close approximation to the force generated by the muscle. The position of the eye is the sum of the forces generated by the muscles pulling in opposite directions, with an increase usually seen in one and a complementary decrease in the opposed antagonist muscle. During a saccade, the agonist or pulling muscle must generate a maximal force to overcome the viscous stretching force of the antagonist muscle. At the end of a saccade away from the primary position, the eye is in a

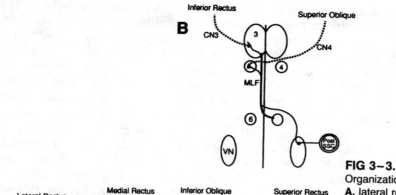

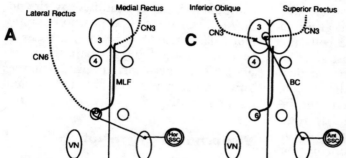

FIG 3–3.
Organization of cranial nerve nuclei. **A,** lateral rectus–medial rectus pairing with connections to the horizontal semicircular canal *(SSC)*. **B,** superior oblique–inferior rectus pairing with connections to the *posterior SSC.* **C,** superior rectus–inferior oblique pairing with connections to the *anterior SSC.* *CN,* cranial nerve; *3, 4,* and *6,* third, fourth, and sixth cranial nerve nuclei; *MLF,* medial longitudinal fasiculus; *VN,* vestibular nucleus; *BN,* brachium conjunctivum.

more eccentric orbital position, and the muscle must have a slightly higher pulling force to maintain the new eye position. The necessary innervation for a saccade is therefore a brief "pulse" of maximal firing rate to rapidly move the eye, followed by a smaller "step" increase in the tonic firing rate to maintain the new eye position. The antagonist muscle receives a complementary brief complete inhibition during the rapid movement followed by a new, lower tonic firing rate. In the case of the agonist, the amount of increased innervation, the step, needed to hold the eye in the new more eccentric position is approximately the mathematical integral of the brief pulse of innervation. This is equivalent to the idea that the pulse of innervation is a command for high eye velocity, while the step is a command for maintaining the new eye position, since integrated velocity yields position. The velocity portion of the signal is needed to overcome viscous stretching forces, while the position portion is needed to match the elastic centering forces. These must both be present and are added to create the "pulse-step" of

saccadic innervation. The proportionality of the visco-elastic forces to velocity and position of the eye means that nerve firing rates in the brain stem can be taken as direct correlates of eye position, greatly simplifying the neural programming for eye movements. A pursuit movement is a constant velocity eye movement, so the required innervation consists of a constant signal or step of firing to overcome the velocity-related forces, and a gradually increasing ramp component to overcome the increasing elastic forces as the eye moves farther from primary position. The waveform of firing for pursuit is therefore a "step-ramp," with the ramp component equal to the integral of the ongoing step component. The pulse-step commands of saccades and other complicated waveforms can be generated as a simpler velocity command with a "neural integrator" (NI) supplying the position command. A similar integration is needed to convert the velocity signal carried by the SSC into a position signal for compensatory eye movements of the VOR. The brain stem location of the NI is probably distributed over several nuclei and has not been definitively determined, but recent experiments in monkeys suggest the nucleus prepositus hypoglossi and the nearby medial vestibular nucleus as important sites, with the cerebellum an important accessory. If the NI is malfunctioning, the step or position portion of the neural command is weak or absent, agonist muscle tone is too low, and the eye drifts back toward the center of the orbit, resulting in gaze-evoked nystagmus.[4] The high-frequency pulse required for high-velocity saccades is generated by a special group of cells called burst cells. These cells are located in clusters in the brain stem near centers for horizontal and vertical saccade generation. These cells are considered unstable and need to be continually inhibited when not in use during a saccade. Pause cells fire tonically to inhibit burst cells, and pause during saccades to allow the burst cells to create the needed high firing rates. Turning off the pause cells may be a key feature of the initiation of saccades, and abnormalities of the tonic pause cell inhibition may allow uncontrolled saccade ac-

tivity such as ocular flutter. The generation of a pulse-step command for a saccadic eye movement is illustrated in Figure 3–4. Individual nerve firings and overall firing rates are shown for pause cells, burst cells, NI, and the final summation found in the cranial nerve nuclei for an activated agonist and inhibited antagonist eye muscle. Saccadic, pursuit, and vestibular neural processing systems all supply velocity signals that may be added together, and the combined signal is modified by the addition of an integrated position component. This train of nerve impulses is then distributed by a brain stem network to the appropriate cranial nerves and creates eye movements by the final common pathway.

Visuospatial Organization

Horizontal eye movements are most commonly studied and recorded, for the practical reasons that they are easy to record, more is known about the underlying anatomy, and the left-right organization is simpler than the bilateral con-

FIG 3–4.
Pulse-step programming for saccades. Each portion of the Figure shows a schematic representation of the individual nerve firing shown below and average firing rate graphed above. Output of burst cells and neural integrator are added to obtain the agonist pulse-step of innervation which is sent to the left lateral rectus muscle in this example. The eye movement trace for the leftward saccade is shown in the upper right corner.

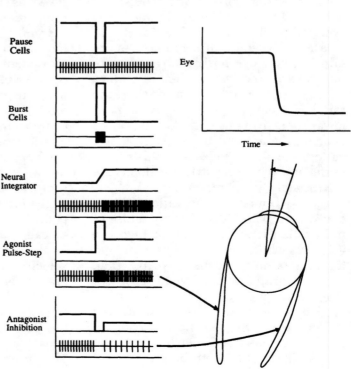

trol of vertical movements. Because oblique and vertical movements can be performed equally well and mixed with horizontal movements, there must be a mechanism for separating out the components to be sent to the pairs of extraocular muscles. The vestibular system has to perform this task in all three dimensions associated with the three pairs of semicircular canals, but the separation is done mechanically by the physical orientation of the canals. The underlying brain stem organization is probably related to the planes of the canals, with eye movements decomposed into canal-plane coordinates. Visually guided movements probably use the same organization with three pairs of centers for oculomotor control, one pair for each canal plane. The decomposition of a visual image that exists in two dimensions on the retina into the three-dimensional ocular rotations needed to point the eyes together is a particularly difficult task. The position of the eye in the orbit must also be taken into account to program the correct eye movement, and the details of this processing are not known. Localization of an object in space in craniotopic coordinates with respect to the head further requires the addition of eye position information to the retinotopic coordinates of retinal image information. Binocular vision has forced most human eye movements to take place in only two independent dimensions, with the third fixed. This collapsing of three dimensions into two dimensions for visually guided movements is probably accomplished by a tight coupling of the anterior-posterior canal "centers" so they act together as a single pair of "vertical" centers. This limitation makes less complicated the transformation from retinotopic coordinates of the image into the head–fixed eye rotations needed for the eyes to acquire the target. The programming of eye movements of a fixed size in spatial coordinates such as degrees into firing rates of nerves requires a spatiotemporal transformation. This may largely occur in the superior colliculus but probably involves multiple brain stem and cortical sites.

Supranuclear Centers for Eye Movement Control

Many cortical areas participate in the generation of eye movements in humans, but a few regions play a predominant role. A brief scheme will be presented, emphasizing areas that cause clear deficits in oculomotor control when a lesion is present. Visual information is initially processed in the primary visual cortex in the occipital lobes; passed through secondary visual centers in occipital, parietal, and temporal lobes; and then sent to higher cortical centers for selection and initiation of eye movements. Cortical signals generally descend to brain stem regions for further signal processing before entering the final common pathway. The cerebellum participates in the control of all eye movements, and plays a particularly important role in maintaining correct amplitudes and ensuring smooth, coordinated functioning. Cerebellar lesions tend to cause abnormalities of all types of eye movements, making them inaccurate and erratic, but do not generally abolish the movement. The parietal lobe interacts with many eye movements as it is involved with visual attention and selection of targets.

Saccades

Voluntary saccadic eye movements originate in the frontal eye fields (FEF) of the frontal lobes. Activation of one side produces saccades toward the other side, so rightward saccades are generated by left FEF activity.[3] Lesions of this area on one side, as may occur in stroke, cause a turning of the eyes toward the involved side due to a relative overaction of the opposite frontal eye field. This effect is temporary, indicating that other areas not usually active may take over the FEF function. Vertical saccades are generated by simultaneous bilateral activity of these regions. The basal ganglia are involved in modifying some types of saccadic eye movements, particularly those where the saccade is not a simple movement to a new target.[13] Patients with parkinsonism, a disorder of the basal ganglia, have trouble making saccades to remembered targets. The superior colluculi probably participate in the generation of most saccades and receive input from the contralateral frontal eye fields and basal ganglia. Signals from the superior colliculus are sent to the paramedian pontine reticular formation near the abducens nucleus for final assembly for horizontal saccades. The analogous structure for vertical saccades is the rostral interstitial nucleus of the medial longitudinal fasciculus and the nearby interstitial nucleus of Cajal, both near the oculomotor nucleus. The major brain stem areas of importance for generation of saccades are diagrammed in Figure 3–5.

Pursuit

Smooth-pursuit eye movements are largely generated in a negative feedback fashion based on eye and target speed mismatch, so the cortical areas of prime importance are those responsible for processing visual motion. In monkeys, the middle temporal visual area and associated cortex receive inputs from primary visual centers in the striate cortex of the occipital lobes and extract image motion information. Lesions of this region in monkeys causes a scotoma for motion, with poor or absent pursuit of moving images in specific parts of the

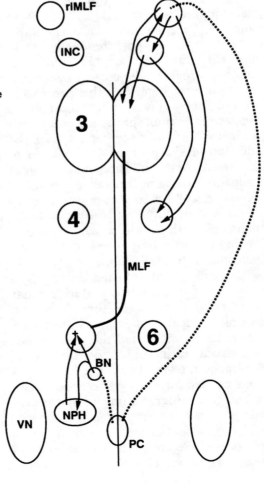

FIG 3–5.
Brain stem centers for saccade generation. Major centers and projections of brain stem regions involved in the generation of saccades are shown. Major structures include the third, fourth, and sixth cranial nerve nuclei, vestibular nuclei *(VN)*, and medial longitudinal fasiculus *(MLF)*. The region for horizontal saccade generation is near the sixth nerve nucleus and is collectively called the paramedian pontine reticular formation *(PPRF)*. Pause cells *(PC)* are located midline and have inhibitory projections (shown as dashed lines) to excitatory burst neurons *(BN)* in the PPRF for horizontal saccades and in the rostral interstitial nucleus of the medial longitudinal fasciculus *(riMLF)* for vertical saccades. For horizontal saccades, burst cell ouput is sent both directly to the sixth nerve nucleus and through the neural integrator, located in the nucleus prepositus hypoglossi *(NPH)*, and medial vestibular nucleus where the step of innervation is created by integrating burst cell firing. Similar processing for vertical saccades takes place in the riMLF and nearby interstitial nucleus of Cajal *(INC)*, both of them near and projecting to the third and fourth cranial nerve nuclei innervating vertically acting muscles. These areas have reciprocal connections across the midline via the posterior commisure mediating the necessary simultaneous involvement of both sides for most up or down saccades.

visual surround.[8] The homologous region in humans has not been specifically identified but probably lies near the junction of the temporal, parietal, and occipital lobes. Lesions of this area cause poor pursuit toward the side of the lesion, so a left-side lesion causes poor leftward pursuit and decreased OKN for leftward moving stripes. FEF and basal ganglia play much less important roles for smooth pursuit. The motion information from the middle temporal visual area goes primarily to the dorsolateral pontine nucleus on the same side for additional signal processing before distribution to the cranial nerve nuclei. Cerebellar control and modification are particularly important for smooth pursuit, as deterioration in pursuit performance is one of the earliest signs of cerebellar lesions.

REFERENCES

1. Alpern M: Kinematics of the eye, in Davson H (ed): *The Eye*, vol 3. New York, Academic Press, 1969, pp 13–25.

2. Becker W: Metrics, in Wurtz RH, Goldberg ME (eds): *The Neurobiology of Saccadic Eye Movements*. Amsterdam, Elsevier, 1989, pp 13–67.

3. Bruce CJ, Goldberg ME: Primate frontal eye fields. I: Single neurons discharging before saccades. *J Neurophysiol* 1985; 53:603–635.

4. Cannon SC, Robinson DA: Loss of the neural integrator of the oculomotor system from brain stem lesions in monkey. *J Neurophysiol* 1987; 57:1383–1409.

5. Carl JR, Gellman RS: Human smooth pursuit: Stimulus-dependent responses. *J Neurophysiol* 1987; 57:1446–1463.

6. Carpenter RHS: *Movements of the Eyes;* ed 2. London; Pion, 1988.

7. Cohen B: The vestibulo-ocular reflex arc, in Kornhuber HH (ed): *Handbook of Sensory Physiology*, vol VI. New York; Springer-Verlag, 1974, pp 477–540.

8. Dursteler MR, Wurtz RH: Pursuit and optokinetic deficits following chemical lesions of cortical areas MT and MST. *J Neurophysiol* 1988; 60:940–964.

9. Enright JT: Changes in vergence mediated by saccades. *J Physiol (Lond)* 1984; 350:9–31.

10. Ferman L, Collewijn H, Van den Berg AV: A direct test of Listing's law. I: Human ocular torsion measured in static tertiary positions. *Vision Res* 1987; 27:929–938.

11. Gellman RS, Carl JR, Miles FA: Short latency ocular-following responses in man. *Vis Neurosci* 1990; 5:107–122.

12. Hering E: in Bridgeman B, Stark L, (eds): *The Theory of Binocular Vision*. New York; Plenum, 1977.

13. Hikosaka O, Wurtz RH: Modification of saccadic eye movements by GABA-related substances. I: Effect of muscimol and bicuculline in monkey superior colliculus. *J Neurophysiol* 1985; 53:266–291.

14. Hine R, Thorn F: Compensatory eye movements during active head rotation for near targets: Effects of imagination, rapid head oscillation and vergence. *Vision Res* 1987; 27:1639–1657.

15. JC: Living without a balancing mechanism. *N Engl J Med* 1952; 246:458–460.

16. Kelly BJ, Rosenberg ML, Zee DS, et al: Unilateral pursuit-induced congenital nystagmus. *Neurology* 1989; 39:414–416.

17. Kornhuber HH: Nystagmus and related phenomena in man. An outline of otoneurology, in Kornhuber HH (ed): *Handbook of Sensory Physiology*, vol VI, *Vestibular System*, part 2. New York; Springer, 1974; pp 193–232.

18. Leigh RJ, Zee DS: *The Neurology of Eye Movements*, ed 2. Philadelphia, FA Davis, 1991.

19. Maas EF, Huebner WP, Seidmann SH, et al: Behavior of human horizontal vestibulo-ocular reflex in response to high-acceleration stimuli. *Brain Res* 1989; 499:153–156.

20. Melvill Jones G: Adaptive modulation of VOR parameters by vision, in Berthoz A, Melvill Jones G (eds): *Adaptive Mechanisms in Gaze Control*. Reviews in Oculomotor Research, vol 1. Amsterdam, Elsevier, 1985, pp 21–50.

21. Michael JA, Melvill Jones G: Dependence of visual tracking capability upon stimulus predictability. *Vision Res* 1966; 6:707–716.

22. Miller JM, Robinson DA: A model of the mechanics of binocular alignment. *Comput Biomed Res* 1984; 17:436–470.

23. Millodot M: Variation of visual acuity in the central region of the retina. *Br J Physiol Optics* 1972; 27:24–29.

24. Robinson DA: The mechanics of human vergence eye movements. *J Pediatr Ophthalmol Strabismus* 1966; 3:31–37.

25. Robinson DA: Linear addition of optokinetic and vestibular signals in the vestibular nucleus. *Exp Brain Res* 1977; 30:447–450.

26. Robinson DA: The functional behavior of the peripheral oculomotor apparatus: A review, in Kommerell G (ed): *Disorders of Ocular Motility. Neurophysiological and Clinical Aspects.* Munich, JF Bergman, 1978, pp 43–61.

27. Robinson DA, Keller EL: The behavior of eye movement motoneurons in the alert monkey. *Bibl Ophthalmol* 1972; 82:7–16.

28. Schwarz U, Busettini C, Miles FA: Ocular responses to linear motion are inversely proportional to viewing distance. *Science* 1989; 245:1394–1396.

29. von Noorden GK: *Binocular Vision and Ocular Motility,* ed 4. St Louis, CV Mosby, 1990.

CHAPTER 4

Principles and Techniques of Electro-oculography

James R. Carl, M.D.

A permanent record of eye movements is necessary for a detailed description and analysis of ocular motor functioning. Measurement of many of the important features of eye movements such as amplitude, latency, and velocity can be done accurately only when the motion of the eyes has been recorded. The key element of the record is the ability to determine the position of the eyes as a function of time, so the record is usually displayed on paper as a graph of eye position against time. Most methods of eye movement recording convert the eye position into a proportional voltage that can be analyzed electronically or converted into a graphical record by a chart recorder. Photographic or video methods are sometimes used, and each frame has to be analyzed for eye position so that a series of position versus time points can be plotted.

Electro-oculography (EOG) is the standard method by which eye movements are recorded in the clinical eye movement laboratory. The terms EOG and electronystagmography (ENG) test are often used interchangeably because for some time most recording of nystagmus and eye movements was by the EOG technique. Newer technology has begun to replace EOG methods in some instances and some laboratories, and most published research now uses more precise methods to measure eye movements. An understanding of the advantages and limitations of the various techniques of eye movement recording is therefore necessary, even if EOG is the only method used in a particular clinical ENG laboratory. In this chapter the practical use of EOG is given prominence, with a review of other relevant techniques provided toward the close of the chapter. The "electro" prefix in the term electronystagmography does imply the use of EOG method, but since ENG has become the standard term for the battery of tests of vestibular function, ENG is still used to describe the test even when other methods of eye movement recording are used.

PHYSICAL AND PHYSIOLOGICAL PRINCIPLES OF EOG

The advent of electronic amplification in the early part of the 1920s allowed researchers to discover that some types of nerve and muscle function were associated with tiny voltages. Recordings of heart muscle function by amplification of electrical signals quickly developed into the electrocardiogram, and similar but even smaller signals constituted the electroencephalogram of brain wave activity. Voltages measured on the face that varied with eye movement were recognized and are the basis for the EOG. The electrical signal recorded from eye movement differs from most of the others in that the eyeball acts like a small battery, with the cornea having a positive charge with respect to the retina. This corneoretinal potential remains effectively constant, and the voltage measured by skin electrodes near the eye varies because the "battery" is pointed in different directions as the eye moves.

Corneoretinal Potential

The corneoretinal potential is generated by metabolic activity of the retina, mostly by the retinal pigment epithelium. As with any battery, there must be a barrier or insulation between the positive and negative charges to maintain the potential difference, and the tight junctions between the pigment epithelial cells serve this function. The charge difference develops on either side of these cell junctions in the retina and is distributed throughout the eye by volume conduction. The potential is usually measured at the cornea for practical reasons and is about 1 mV. This baseline potential difference is altered by light stimulation of the retina, with about a twofold increase seen when light-adapted voltages are compared to dark-adapted ones. Because the voltage reflects metabolic activity of the retina, it is affected in some individuals by retinal disease. Measurement of this underlying battery potential is the basis for a test of retinal function also called an electro-oculogram. Voltage variations with light adaptation are a source of artifacts for eye movement recordings and must be taken into consideration during the ENG tests. Fortunately, these changes take place slowly over 5 to 10 minutes, so brief changes in the room illumination can be tolerated, while longer exposure to new light levels requires recalibration.

Figure 4–1 is a schematic illustration of how the movement of the eyeball "battery" causes a voltage variation at electrodes placed on the skin. To record

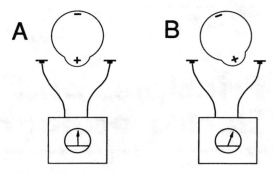

FIG 4–1.
Schematic diagrams of eyeball and electrodes. The electrodes measure skin potentials resulting from movement of the eye and the corneoretinal potential. **A,** the cornea at the front of the eye is positively charged with respect to the negatively charged retina. Voltage at the skin under the electrodes is symmetric, and no voltage difference is sensed when the eye views straight ahead. **B,** rotation of the eye brings the positively charged cornea nearer one electrode and the negatively charged retina nearer the other. The relative voltage difference created by eye movement provides the physical basis of electro-oculography.

these voltage changes a minute amount of current has to flow between the electrodes. The eye and skin complete an electric circuit with the electrodes and amplifiers. The measured voltage is affected by the resistance of this circuit, so the skin-to-electrode contact must maintain a constant resistance for an accurate measurement.

The separation of positive and negative potentials is called a dipole, and the orientation of this dipole with respect to the electrodes determines the voltage. Each of the two eyes creates its own dipole, and when the eyes look laterally, the positive pole of one eye moves nearer the negative pole of the other near the nose. These tend to cancel, so the potential at the electrodes on either side of the nose is about the same and near zero. Voltage measured by recording each eye alone is therefore due to the potential picked up by the lateral electrode compared to the near-zero potential near the nose (Fig 4–2). Bitemporal recordings with only the two lateral electrodes present larger signals, since eye movements to the side move

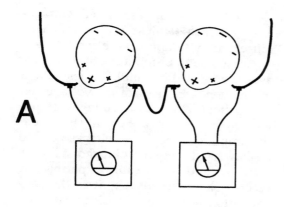

A

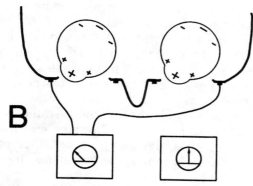

B

FIG 4–2.
Monocular **(A)** and bitemporal **(B)** recording. A, electrodes placed on either side of both eyes allow measurement of the movement of each eye separately. The potential sensed by the two electrodes near the nose is about the same because of volume conduction. This potential remains low because the more positively charged cornea of one eye is turned nearer to the more negatively charged retina of the other eye. B, bitemporal recordings generate larger differential voltages because as the eyes turn conjugately, one electrode is nearer the retina while the other is nearer the opposite cornea. Disconjugate eye movements are not sensed when bitemporal electrodes are used.

one positive pole nearer an electrode and a negative pole from the other eye nearer the other electrode. Bitemporal recordings are therefore more robust, but cannot sense disconjugate movements. Disconjugate eye movements must first be evaluated with careful inspection or with monocular EOG recordings. One convenient strategy is to place all four leads for monocular recording of both eyes. After eye move-

ment tests demonstrate conjugacy, the two bitemporal leads may be plugged into one horizontal channel and gain recalibrated.

Recording Artifacts

Muscle activity also produces some electrical voltages that can be measured by skin electrodes and represent a possible source of contamination of the EOG. Horizontal eye movements involve primarily eyeball movement with little lid motion, so the corneoretinal potential provides most of the measured voltage changes. Activation of the horizontal recti muscles has little effect at the skin. Vertical eye movements, however, may be heavily contaminated by eyelid artifacts, so measured skin voltages do not represent accurately the vertical motion of the eye.[7] Despite this difficulty, recordings of vertical signals are important as they do give some representation of vertical eye movement and they provide information about blinks and eyelid movements. Blink artifacts contaminate horizontal as well as vertical measurements, so recording them with vertically oriented electrodes allows recognition and avoids interpreting blinks or vertical eye movements as actual horizontal movements. Careful placement of electrodes can make the horizontal channel resistant to recording vertical information, but some "cross-talk" is inevitably present and simultaneous vertical recording assists in interpretation. Torsional eye movements are a twisting of the eye around the line of sight and are not sensed by the EOG technique because there is no relative movement of the corneoretinal potential with respect to the skin electrodes. Therefore it is possible for the clinician to observe some nystagmus during the examination that will not be present on the recording. Most of the EOG signal is due to movement of the corneoretinal dipole, but there are some distortions of the signal, particularly during saccades, that may be due to other factors or potentials present in periocular tissues.[4] These artifacts cannot be controlled, but their possible existence must be kept in mind during interpretation.

ELECTRO-OCULOGRAPHIC EQUIPMENT

Most laboratories use commercial equipment for amplifying and recording ENG data. Devices constructed specifically to amplify, filter, and record EOG signals are convenient and usually compact. However, some laboratories prefer to use separate instruments for each of these functions because of availability or increased flexibility. The electrodes placed on a patient create a possible shock hazard as they are designed to conduct electricity. Thus, all electronic equipment attached to patients should be properly isolated to prevent shocks, and most hospitals require regular inspections to assure the safety of the equipment. One-piece commercial equipment is usually adequately designed for safety, but the addition of any extra or alternative devices may create a possible hazard. All equipment electrically connected to the recording system is potentially connected to the patient through the electrodes and requires careful attention to proper isolation. Patients who have intracardiac catheters or pacemakers with wires extending through the skin should not undergo EOG testing, as these people are very sensitive to tiny currents.

Amplifiers

The electro-oculogram voltages generated by eye movements are very small, on the order of 20 µV per degree of eye movement. These voltages need to be amplified by a factor of about 10,000 so they can be used to drive chart recorders or to be digitized by computer equipment. In addition to eye movement voltages, the electrodes pick up unwanted voltages from other biological sources such as muscle activity and from electrical wiring in the room. Elimination of stray voltages is achieved by amplifier design and by frequency filtering of the voltage signal. Filters that block voltages of unwanted frequencies are usually built into the amplifier. The EOG voltages need to be converted into a graphical display for analysis and to create a permanent record. Chart recorders convert the voltages into traces on paper using an ink pen or thermal stylus. Recorders are often combined with the amplifiers in one piece of equipment having a single set of controls. When separate pieces of equipment are hooked together to amplify, filter, and record the EOG, each piece may have some of these controls. In this case it is best to leave all but one control of each type set at a fixed level. It is additionally important to know that the overall effect of passing signals through multiple pieces of equipment may be different, particularly in frequency response, from any of the individual settings.

Equipment for EOG should have multiple channels available for simultaneous recording. Three channels are desirable for recording the left and right eye horizontal movement independently as well as at least one vertical channel. More channels are useful to simultaneously record stimulus location and eye velocity. Differentiators are electronic devices that create a voltage proportional to the rate of change, or velocity, of an EOG position voltage. The velocity signal can be helpful in analyzing some fast eye movements, but the high-frequency noise levels in EOG recordings are differentiated into a much noisier velocity signal which generally precludes accurate assessment of slower eye velocities. Each channel of the amplification part of EOG equipment usually has four important controls: gain, offset, low-frequency response, and high-frequency response.

The gain of amplification is variable so that a specific eye movement, for example, a movement of 10°, with its associated EOG voltage, can be amplified to a predetermined voltage or to move the chart recorder stylus a specified distance (for example, 10 mm). Gain adjustment, sometimes labeled "sensitivity," allows a direct and simple method of relating the trace on the chart to eye movement. In the latter example, each millimeter on the chart paper represents 1° of eye movement. Gain may be increased so that the details of some eye movements may be examined, or decreased so that large eye movements do not create chart traces that go out of bounds. Gain settings are often controlled by two separate knobs: one coarse adjustment with fixed range settings, and one fine adjustment with variable control. Offset controls, sometimes called zero adjust, enable a specific eye position, usually straight ahead, to be represented by a fixed voltage, most often zero, which will center the recorder stylus. Because EOG voltages typically drift with time, readjustment of both gain and offset are usually necessary periodically during a recording session.

The EOG voltages measured at the electrodes on the face contain some small oscillations that are not related to eyeball movement and are considered "noise." One ubiquitous source of noise is the 60-Hz electomagnetic radiation broadcast by all of the electric wires present in the walls and electric power outlets. The EOG electrodes and wires act like antennas and pick up these 60-Hz waveforms. Differential input amplifiers are designed to eliminate the voltages common to both electrodes and amplify only the voltage difference between them. Since both electrodes pick up the same 60-Hz noise it is not amplified while the EOG signal is amplified. The ability of the amplifier to perform this separation is called common mode rejection and is specified by the manufacturer as a characteristic of the equipment. Voltage proportional to eye movement is considered "signal" and will always be contaminated by unwanted

noise. The ratio of these voltages is the "signal-to-noise" ratio and is one measure of the overall accuracy of the entire recording system.

Frequency Filters

The high-frequency and low-frequency filter controls eliminate noise and drift artifacts and can affect the accuracy of the recording. Unwanted noise voltage can often be separated from the desired eye movement voltages based on frequency. That is, most noise is of high frequency, whereas eye movements are of lower frequency. Electronic devices that pass the desired lower frequency voltages and attenuate the higher frequency noise voltages are low-pass filters. The transition from passing to attenuating voltage is gradual as frequency increases. The high-frequency cut-off of a filter is the frequency at which voltages are attenuated by 3 dB, or about 30%. Low-pass settings on EOG amplifiers are typically adjustable in several steps from around 5 Hz up to 50 Hz. The setting is a tradeoff, because some useful information in the eye movement record has high frequencies like the noise. Cutting off these high frequencies will distort parts of the recording and prevent accurate measurement of rapid eye movements, particularly saccade velocities. Studies of the frequency content of eye movements show that little information is lost if frequencies above 100 Hz are filtered out, and that most information is below 50 Hz.[1] High-frequency cut-off should be set as high as possible, but as EOG is inherently noisy, settings are often limited to less than 50 Hz. A 30-Hz value will give acceptable recordings, and lower settings may be used when the chart record shows excessive noise, but velocity measurements will be artificially low. Ideally, all of the equipment used will be able to reproduce faithfully the rapid changes present in eye movements. Some chart recorders, however, cannot move the stylus fast enough to record the high-frequency signals, and the high-frequency cut-off will actually be limited by the mechanical characteristics of the recorder. Special consideration must be given to frequency response when the signals are digitized on a computer. The digitizing rate should be at least 100 Hz and preferably higher, and filters with a high-frequency cut-off of no more than half the sampling rate must be used before the signal is sent to the digitizer, in order to prevent a sampling artifact called aliasing.

Eye movement recordings contain times when the eyes are held steady and the corresponding EOG voltages should not change (such as during testing of lateral gaze). Drift artifacts are slowly changing voltages that mimic a slowly moving eye when it is actually still. Some EOG amplifiers have a high-pass filter to eliminate drift artifact. When this filter is used, only changing voltages pass through and constant voltages are allowed to fall to zero. The waveform of the voltage fall is exponential and has a time constant (usually specified in seconds) that indicates how long it takes for the voltage to drop to 37% of its original amplitude. High-pass settings, also called low-frequency cut-off, are often specified by a time constant that is inversely related to the lowest frequency that the filter will pass. The 3-dB point or "corner frequency" in Hz is equal to 0.16 divided by the time constant in seconds (0.16/Tc). This setting can only be used when the eyes are continually moving, as in caloric or optokinetic nystagmus. The slowly changing drift voltages are then allowed to fall to zero while the more rapidly changing eye movement voltages are passed on to the recorder, but information about the average eye position in the orbit is lost. When measuring any other eye movements, all low frequencies must be allowed down to zero low frequency, which is termed "direct current" and usually labeled "DC" on the low-frequency cut-off control. Amplifiers without this DC capability can handle only "alternating current" ("AC").

Some older ENG equipment has only AC coupling and is therefore limited to recording caloric nystagmus responses. Modern ENG laboratories should have DC recording equipment. Most nystagmus is affected by orbital position and loss of this information may be misleading, so all recordings should be made in the DC mode. Drift artifact is a nuisance, but can be minimized by proper attention to electrode resistance and by calibration checks.

Chart Recorders

After the EOG signals are appropriately amplified and filtered, they must be recorded in some fashion. The most common method is by chart recorder, where lines representing eye movements are drawn. Alternate methods include immediate digitization and storage on computer disk, or FM tape recording. All three methods may be used simultaneously. Detailed EOG recordings may have as many as eight channels of information: two horizontal and one vertical eye position channels, one channel for target position, and four additional channels for the velocity of each position signal. Recorders with fewer available channels require switching of input signals to document those of primary interest for each part of the ENG. Chart recorder paper is printed with a grid of fine lines, usually with 1-mm spacing, and paper speeds are adjustable over a range of millimeters per second. Timing marks, if available, are placed on the chart paper at 1-second intervals to document the recording speed. A heated stylus marking on thermal paper is a common method of recording signals and has the advantages of simplicity and cleanliness. Pen recorders using ink under pressure are typically more complex, require drying time for the ink, and are potentially messy, but the paper is usually easier to handle by folding, and the tracing line may be finer. Stylus motion from one edge of the recording strip to the other may inscribe a straight line or a rectilinear trace. If the recording point moves in an arc, the tracing is termed curvilinear and the paper should have a pattern of lines that are straight along the time axis and curved to match pen motion in the other direction. It may be difficult to measure curvilinear tracings and to calculate accurate slow-phase velocities due to the distortions in the waveform. Most modern recorders are rectilinear or nearly so, and measurement errors are small.

ELECTRODES AND PATIENT PREPARATION

Electrodes may be either the silver–silver chloride type or gold-cup type. For EOG recording a small size electrode is preferable for accurate placement near the eyes. The most popular electrodes consist of a small plastic cap containing a pellet of silver metal coated with silver chloride. Reproducibility and accuracy of eye movement records depend on maintaining a constant and symmetrical contact between the electrodes and skin. The patient should be inspected visually during electrode placement for skin lesions that would affect recording or comfort. Skin preparation can usually be limited to brisk cleaning of the skin with an alcohol wipe to clear off oils and makeup and assure good electrical and physical contact. Special skin preparation pastes are available. They are slightly gritty and are rubbed on the skin at the electrode location to mildly abrade the skin and produce better electrical contact. Deliberate skin abrasion is not usually necessary and is uncomfortable to the patient, and firm scrubbing with an alcohol pad should suffice. Commercial electrode preparation wipes containing a mild abrasive and cleanser combination are particularly convenient to use without being uncomfortable for the patient. The electrode design holds the silver pellet slightly away from the skin. This gap must be filled with a conducting gel that contacts both the metal surface of the electrode and the skin. Careful filling will prevent any air gaps and improve contact. Electrodes may be held on the skin with tape placed over the top or with double-sided sticky collars. Care must be taken to keep cleaning substances, gel, and tape out of the patient's eyes.

Placement of the electrodes on the skin is most important and is done by visual inspection so the electrodes line up with the movement to be recorded. Figure 4–3 is a photograph of a subject with electrodes placed for horizontal recording of each eye and a vertical channel for the right eye. A ground electrode, often larger, has been placed on the forehead, but grounds may also be placed on the earlobe. Note that the horizontal electrodes are in line with the

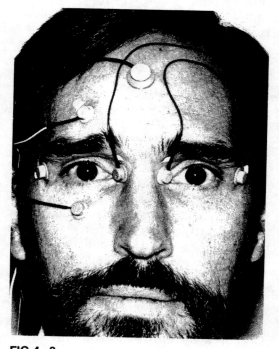

FIG 4–3.
Electrode placement for EOG recording. Silver–silver chloride electrodes are affixed to the patient's skin with adhesive collars. One larger ground electrode is placed on the forehead, and one pair is placed above and below the right eye to detect blinks and vertical eye movements. A pair of electrodes is placed just lateral to each eye, horizontally aligned with the pupil, to maximally sense horizontal movement and reject vertical movement.

pupils, so that horizontal movements are maximally recorded and vertical ones rejected. The electrode, gel, and skin combination can form a small battery and produce unwanted potentials that are maximal just after electrode placement and then decay. Allowing the electrodes to equilibrate on the patient for 15 minutes will lower impedance and reduce drift, and this period will also allow for a stable light adaptation to diminish variation from changing retinal metabolism. Both of these types of artifact will cause amplitude variation during recording, and electrode potentials will cause drift of the zero level. These effects require periodic recentering of the signal and recalibration of gain to maintain accuracy.

Electrodes tend to build up a charge when not in use, particularly if they are not cleaned well, creating more drift during recording. This effect can be minimized by careful cleaning after use, and if severe, by storing the electrodes in pairs in saline with their wires electrically connected. This keeps any possible electrode battery effect discharged. Poor electrical contact between electrode and skin, measured as high impedance, can create recording artifacts, particularly 60-Hz noise. Most commercial devices have an impedance checker built in, or separate ones are available and should be used to assure good electrode contact. Impedance is measured for each electrode after all are in place. Each impedance should be under 5,000 Ω, and faulty electrodes should be fixed or replaced. If impedance is measured in pairs, the reading should be under 10,000 Ω for each pair.

The first step in recording the ENG is to check the entire system with simple up, down, rightward, and leftward eye movements to ensure that all channels are working with the correct polarity. Assessment of the signal during fixation will determine if drift or noise levels are too high, requiring equipment or electrode adjustment. Initial calibration should always be done only with the eye being calibrated and viewing the stimuli while the other is covered. This will ensure that disconjugacy due to weakness or restriction will not be missed. If all of these procedures have worked correctly, eye movements of 1° should be visible and, with care, the sensitivity may be 0.5°. Amplification and analysis assume linearity of EOG voltages: the change in voltage should be the same for a 5° eye movement from center to 5° right as for a 5° movement from 20° right to 25° right. Deviations from linearity typically get larger as the eye moves farther from primary. The range of linearity is generally given as the region in which the nonlinearity error is no greater than the sensitivity. Each laboratory should check the sensitivity and linearity of their recording procedure to establish norms for interpretation of patient records. Movements of up to 30° are usually acceptably linear, and greater accuracy may be obtained by determining a plot of linearity for each patient and then applying the necessary correction to the eye movement records.

ELECTRO-OCULOGRAPHY ANALYSIS

As stated earlier, EOG records are usually ink or thermal traces on chart paper that can be reviewed during the testing and then analyzed in more detail at a later time. Eye movements that are digitized may be viewed on a computer monitor and simultaneously printed on a chart recorder, or first analyzed with computer assistance, after which only selected portions may be printed. Because digitized data can take up very large amounts of storage space on computer disks, digitization of the entire testing session may be impractical. Some laboratories save the entire session on FM tape that can be played back at a later time with signals digitized or written out on chart paper.

Any analysis of EOG records should begin with a verification of the calibration: known eye positions that were observed by the technician are correlated with the chart trace. Adjustment factors for gain and position must be calculated for application to measurements if there is not a simple relationship between distance on the chart in millimeters and degrees of eye movement. Time calibrations should also be noted, as chart speed settings may vary for specific tests. Ideally, blinks that were observed will have been marked on the chart at the beginning of the test session to assist in identifying them throughout the record. Blinks are usually easy to see in the vertical channel but also affect the horizontal channel as a result of "crosstalk," so portions of the trace with blink artifact should not be used for measurements. Slow-drift artifact and gain variation must be noted by comparing repeat calibrations during testing, and corrective calculations applied if necessary.

Initial tests usually concern fixation of calibration lights, and the trace of eye position during these fixations should be a straight line on the chart, parallel to paper motion, and on zero or in the center of the paper if fixation was in primary position. By convention, traces are viewed so time advances to the right, and rightward eye movements are plotted upward with positive values, whereas leftward movements are downward. High-frequency noise will show up as a thickening of the trace as the stylus oscillates. Small saccades away from fixation followed by a return saccade in a few hundred milliseconds constitute square wave jerks and should be noted. Rapid drift artifact will generate a sloped line and require continued readjustment of the offset control.

Rhythmic deviations from a straight line represent nystagmus if artifacts are not present. Vestibular nystagmus is usually a constant velocity drift of the eyes in one direction, with quick saccadic eye movements bringing the eyes back near the fixation position. The eye movement record of this jerk nystagmus has a sawtooth waveform, with an alternation of straight lines angled away from fixation (the slow phase) and lines nearly straight up or down, perpendicular to the paper motion, corresponding to the saccades (the fast phase). Figure 4–4 is a photograph of a sample recording including lateral gaze in both directions followed by a section of optokinetic nystagmus, similar in appearance to caloric nystagmus. Because eye motion is represented on the chart by distance up and down and time is represented by distance along the chart, the slope of a line determines the eye velocity during that period. Upward distance, measured in millimeters, can be converted to degrees of eye movement by multiplying the conversion factor (in degrees per millimeter) determined during calibration. Likewise, the time in seconds can be obtained by multiplying the distance along the paper in millimeters and the paper speed in seconds per millimeter. Paper speed is often selected in millimeters per second, so the inverse must be used for conversion. The two conversion factors may be combined to determine a single slope constant, which can then be multiplied by slope to obtain eye velocity as long as calibration and paper speed do not change. A calibration of 8°/10 mm (0.8°/mm), can be multiplied by a paper speed of 10 mm/sec to yield a constant of 8°/sec. A slow phase with 10 mm upward deviation and 5 mm along the time axis has a slope of 2.0, and if the example constant is applied, a rightward eye velocity of 16°/sec is calculated. A slope of −4.5 would correspond to a 36°/sec leftward eye movement. The traces of eye position are usually not exactly straight lines, and the slope is calculated from a best-visual-estimate straight line, often drawn on the paper. Slow-phase velocity should be averaged over several individual slow phases for a more robust measure, as there is some beat-to-beat variation.

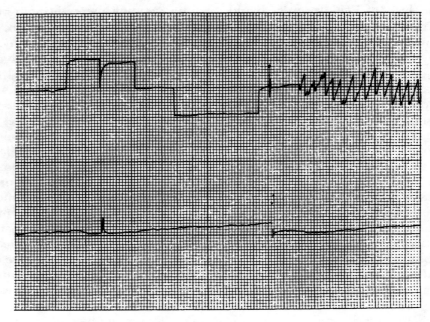

FIG 4–4.
Example EOG record of fixation and optokinetic nystagmus. This is a typical two-channel EOG tracing, with horizontal eye movement from bitemporal electrodes represented in the top channel and vertical movements in the bottom. The brief peaked waveforms seen in the lower channel are blinks and clearly affect the horizontal channel in this example. This tracing shows a rightward and then leftward fixation followed by left-beating optokinetic nystagmus generated by stripes moving to the subject's right.

Slope and eye velocity calculations are illustrated in Figure 4–5.

Nystagmus may also have a pendular waveform with the trace appearing almost sinusoidal, and exponential waveforms are found in some varieties of nystagmus where the slow-phase waveform is not a straight line. Saccades can generally be recognized by their high velocities of several hundred degrees per second. These high velocities cannot be measured by taking the slope of the trace during a saccade unless the paper speed is set very fast, and even then the accuracy is low because the eye velocity varies during the saccade. A velocity trace created by electronic differentiation is necessary to assess saccades and other high-velocity movements accurately and routinely.

The accuracy of measurements made from paper records depends on careful attention to detail, including calibration records, gain and offset adjustments, and noise levels. Most accuracy problems will affect both rightward and leftward eye movements, so EOG analysis of asymmetries may be adequate in spite of high noise levels or poor frequency band-pass characteristics. Assessment of higher resolution details such as saccade latency, saccade velocity, and small amplitude movements may be inaccurate, and the small movements may be missed entirely. Each laboratory must determine its own standards of normal and abnormal eye movements as determined by measurements from records, and "literature standard" values should not be accepted unless verified on the equipment.

Analysis of digitized records by computer depends largely on the capabilities and quality of the software programs. Most often the measurements are automated, saving considerable time, but these programs can be fooled by high noise levels, abnormal eye movements, and artifacts. Results of automated analysis should always be confirmed by at

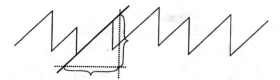

FIG 4–5.
Calculation of nystagmus slow-phase velocity. A schematic illustration of a left-beating nystagmus recording is shown. A straight edge, placed on the recording, may be used to draw a line, shown here as a *darker trace*, matching the slope of a slow phase and extending beyond the actual duration. *Dashed lines* indicate where measurements may be made for the duration *(horizontal direction)* and amplitude *(vertical direction)*. The slope is the ratio of the vertical to horizontal measurements, each in millimeters. The slow-phase velocity is the product of this slope and the slope constant determined from the calibration, as described in the text.

least a visual inspection of the record. Software analysis programs should allow the operator to display an eye movement record with computer-determined values visible so the record can be rejected from analysis if necessary or correct values inserted if appropriate.

SURVEY OF OTHER EYE MOVEMENT RECORDING METHODS

The EOG method of recording eye movements is still the workhorse of the clinical testing laboratory, but other techniques are gaining in popularity and some have great potential. Table 4–1 provides a brief survey of common techniques, noting the major advantages, disadvantages, and characteristics.[2,5,6] Electro-oculography has several advantages in clinical situations, including relatively low cost, good patient acceptance, and freedom to position the patient or perform provocative maneuvers. However, limitations in EOG sensitivity and linearity have virtually eliminated this technique from most research-oriented publications. Eye movement traces in newly published literature will primarily be recorded with magnetic search

coil or sometimes infrared reflection equipment. Computerized analysis of high-resolution video images is perhaps the most promising technique, with the possibility of recording all three dimensions of movement with high resolution and no patient contact. Careful clinical observation remains the important first step in any eye movement recording, to determine the appropriate methods to be used and understand their limitations. Complex waveforms are sometimes best appreciated by direct inspection, and observation of ocular fundus movements by ophthalmoscopy may detect tiny eye movements.[8] Frenzel goggles worn by the patient magnify the image of the eye for the observer and reduce visual supression of nystagmus by the patient.

Magnetic Search Coil

Magnetic search coil recording is the current research favorite. This technique requires the subject to wear a type of soft contact lens with an embedded coil of wire, and to be seated within a cage controlling a magnetic field. The current induced in the eye coil is proportional to the eye position in the magnetic field. This method can be used to measure horizontal, vertical, and torsional eye position with a sensitivity of $0.017°$ (one-sixtieth of a degree) or better in a research setting.[3] It is the only technique currently available for measuring torsional eye movements with accuracy. Head position in the magnetic field can be determined equally easily with a search coil affixed to the forehead or on a headband. Simultaneous head measurements are often desirable, as the technique actually measures eye position with respect to the magnetic fields, not with respect to the head, as do other methods. The major drawbacks of this method are the requirement to wear the contact lens, limitations due to testing in a magnetic field, and expense of equipment. Most patients can tolerate wearing the contact lens for about 30

TABLE 4–1.

Major Characteristics of Six Common Eye Movement Recording Techniques

Technique	Characteristics	Advantages	Disadvantages
Visual inspection	Full range; resolution to 10 minutes of arc with ophthalmoscope; vertical and torsional movements noted	No cost; brief exam allows easy comprehension of complex waveforms; may be able to correlate symptoms with eye movements	No permanent record produced; poor estimation of velocity or fine details of waveform
Electro-oculography	Range of ~40° with resolution of 1°; vertical movements recorded but not accurately; torsional movements not sensed; bandwidth of 35 Hz.	Inexpensive, noninvasive, well tolerated by children and noncooperative patients; vestibular stimulation in all planes possible; best general method for clinical setting	Low resolution and low bandwidth obscure fine details, particularly of saccades; baseline drift and artifacts may be problem; no torsional and poor vertical records
Infrared	Range limited to 20° with resolution of 0.1°; vertical recordings inaccurate; torsional movements not sensed; bandwidth >100 Hz	High resolution and non-contact	Moderately expensive (≥$5,000); horizontal record limited and poor vertical recording; difficult to use with vestibular stimulation; some limitation of field of view; eyes must be open
Magnetic search coil	Range of 40°, full with special equipment; resolution of 0.02°; records vertical and torsional movements accurately; bandwidth up to 1,000 Hz	Best method for high resolution of all types of eye movements, primarily for research	High cost (≥$20,000); contact; eye limit use in cooperative subjects of ~30 minutes
Photographic	Range limited to ~20° with accuracy of 1°, depending on sharpness of image; horizontal and torsional movements visible; bandwidth limited by frame rate with 16 ms between images common	Noncontact; may be used in unusual environments such as space	Very labor intensive; poor time resolution
Image analysis	Technology is developing; high resolution of horizontal, vertical, and torsional movements possible	Promise of resolution to match magnetic recordings without being invasive	Investigational; very expensive

minutes without discomfort. Figure 4–6 is a photograph of a magnetic search coil in a subject's eye.

Infrared Recording Devices

Infrared devices have to be worn as spectacle-like equipment. An infrared light is directed to shine on the eye, and photocells measure reflected light from the sclera. A typical infrared device is shown on a subject in Figure 4–7. The method depends on the different reflectance of the sclera and iris. The edge of the iris moves with the eye while the photocells remain stationary. The amount of reflected light sensed by the photocells is proportional to eye position. This tech-

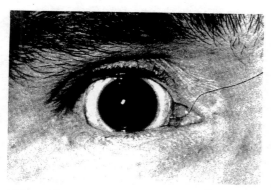

FIG 4–6.
Close-up photograph of a magnetic search coil in a subject's right eye. Note the annular shape of the contact lens, fitting just around the cornea, and the turns of fine wire embedded in the soft plastic. The pair of twisted wires is attached to the contact lens at the medial edge and is taped to the forehead before connecting with more substantial wire leads running to the amplifier.

nique does not touch the eye and is well tolerated by a cooperative subject. Linearity is better than EOG but in a narrower range, while vertical recording is difficult because of effects of the eyelid. Visual stimulation may be limited by the need to have the equipment placed in view of the subject. The relationship between the infrared photocells and the eye is critical for accuracy and stability of the signal, so vestibular stimulation or head motion that might cause the spectacles to slip are difficult to use with this method. Newer goggle versions of infrared record-

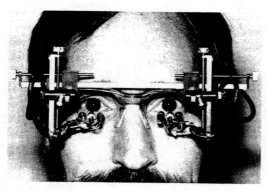

FIG 4–7.
Infrared recording equipment. Subject is shown wearing an adjustable frame hanging from lensless spectacles. Screws allow for three-dimensional adjustment of the two recording photocells and central illumination source just below each eye. Note the limitation of visual field from the equipment.

ers may be much easier to use, and maintain the sensitivity advantages while allowing some head motion.

Photographic and Video Recording Devices

Photographic techniques have been limited by the time resolution of the frames and the need to analyze each frame to extract eye position information. Newer video methods may improve time resolution significantly, and the intensive computerized image analysis becoming available may allow for a high-resolution signal for horizontal, vertical, and torsional movements to be generated on line without the need for any retrospective analysis by the operator. High cost is currently the significant disadvantage of this technique, but should eventually be in reach. Image processing methods are likely to become an important research tool in the future.

Videotaping of the eyes using a commercial portable home video camera is an easy and inexpensive way to document abnormal eye movements for teaching and comparison at future evaluations. No graphical record is produced, but resolution is good enough to see all but the smallest amplitude nystagmus. All types of ocular movements may be documented, including retraction nystagmus, pulsatile exophthalmos, and lid movements that will not show up using other methods. Combinations of horizontal, vertical, and torsional movements are much easier to appreciate by visual inspection than by reconstructions from separate graphical records. Video documentation is particularly valuable when the eye movements are associated with other signs of neurologic or vestibular dysfunction, and abnormalities of the examination can be permanently recorded.

Computer-Assisted Recording

Computerization of many aspects of stimulus generation and eye movement analysis has been a major advance in ENG testing over the past decade. Computer methods can be applied to the output signal of any of the recording methods as well as interact with the acquisition of data. Eye movement records can be stored in the computer memory and analyzed on the screen, with only relevant portions printed out. Numerical calculations are quickly and easily performed, encouraging qualitative comparisons. Computer-controlled visual displays can be altered in accordance with the recorded eye movement, allowing stabilized images or visual simulations of disease states to be generated. Digitization of data permits linearization techniques to be applied to greatly extend the range of any of the recording methods. While these computerized tools have great advantages, care must be taken to ensure that the eye movement input is not corrupted or incorrect, or only faulty computer analysis will be output. Quantitative computer analysis should always confirm, not replace, the visual assessment of the eye movements themselves and the eye movement record.

REFERENCES

1. Bahill TA, Kallman JS, Lieberman JE: Frequency limitations of the two-point central differentiation algorithm. *Biol Cybern* 1982; 45:1–4.

2. Carpenter RHS: *Movements of the Eyes*, ed. 2. London, Pion, 1988.

3. Collewijn J, Van Der Mark F, Jansen TC: Precise recording of human eye movements. *Vision Res* 1975; 15:447–450.

4. Kolder HE: Electo-oculography, in Heckenlively JR, Arden GB (eds): *Principles and Practice of Clinical Electrophysiology of Vision.* St Louis, CV Mosby, 1991, pp 301–313.

5. Leigh RJ, Zee DS: *The Neurology of Eye Movements*, ed 2. Philadelphia, FA Davis, 1991.

6. Young LR, Sheena D: Survey of eye movement recording methods. *Behav Res Methods Instrum* 1975; 7:397–429.

7. Yee RD, Schiller VL, Lim V, et al: Velocities of vertical saccades with different eye movement recording methods. *Invest Ophthalmol Vis Sci* 1985; 26:938–944.

8. Zee DS: Ophthalmoscopy in examination of patients with vestibular disorders. *Ann Neurol* 1978; 3:373–374.

CHAPTER 5

Background and Technique of Ocular Motility Testing

Timothy C. Hain, M.D.

There are four types of eye movements of particular interest in the evaluation of balance. *Saccades*, the fastest of eye movements, enable us to rapidly redirect our line of sight. *Pursuit* is the smooth following of moving objects in order to stabilize their image upon the fovea. *Optokinetic nystagmus* is the eye movement evoked by following of moving fields. *Fixation* is the eye movement associated with an effort to keep the eyes completely still. In most instances, these eye movements interact in a synergistic way to maintain clear vision of objects of interest.

In this chapter these types of eye movements are delineated, with the procedures or "paradigms" used to elicit and quantify them. We will present "minimal" procedures to elicit these responses as well as more sophisticated options. We will also discuss the technique of extracting parameters from recorded data, and indicate technical pitfalls unique to each type of eye movement.

SACCADES

The term "saccade" is derived from the French word *saquer*, which means "to pull." Saccades are rapid eye movements made to bring a point of regard onto the fovea. Saccades of all kinds begin abruptly and can be differentiated from other eye movements by their ex-

tremely high initial acceleration (up to 30,000°/sec^2 (Fig 5–1). They typically begin with about a 200-ms latency after the appearance of a target of interest. During the main portion of the saccade, which usually lasts 50 to 100 ms, the eye moves at a high velocity and vision is obscured. Saccades end as abruptly as they begin.

Saccades are produced and controlled by a number of central structures including occipitoparietal cortex, the frontal lobes, the basal ganglia, the superior colliculus, the cerebellum, and the brain stem.[12] Saccades can be separated into two varieties, based on their origin. "Reflexive saccades" are triggered by the appearance of a novel target. "Volitional saccades" are triggered by the intention of the subject. Reflexive saccades are initiated by neural structures close to visual input pathways, such as the superior colliculus, while volitional saccades are formulated in the frontal lobes. Both types of saccades share a final pathway in the brain stem.

Methods of Eliciting Saccades

Calibration Test

The "minimal" approach to assessing saccades is to observe them during calibration. The calibration procedure is the process of relating eye position to the electrical voltage produced by one's eye-movement recording device. The

20 Degree Saccade

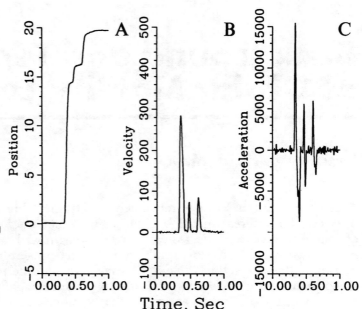

FIG 5–1.
Normal 20° saccade recorded using the scleral search coil (100-Hz bandwidth). **A,** position trace. Note that the saccade is hypometric, which is a normal pattern. **B,** velocity trace. **C,** acceleration/deceleration trace.

calibration procedure is not standardized, as it often must vary according to the recording method and geometry of the clinical laboratory. The calibration procedure is called the "calibration test" when saccades are to be assessed.

Most authors advocate a similar procedure for the calibration test.[2, 4, 7, 18] The test is performed with the subject seated upright and the head stabilized by a strap or chin rest. A light array, with four lights arranged in a cross (Fig 5–2) at 10° to 15° eccentricity, and a fifth light in the center, should be located between 1 and 2 m from the subject. A commercial device of this nature is currently available (Micromedical Technologies, Inc.; see Appendix). Marks on a screen can be substituted for lights, but lights are more convenient. Common red light–emitting diodes (LEDs) combined with current limiting resistors are the most suitable choice of target because of their long life, and because they can be turned on and off very rapidly. Note that in the electronystagmography (ENG) laboratory, two calibration arrays are the most convenient arrangement. One is used in the upright position for the gaze

test (which will be discussed subsequently) and for the recording of spontaneous nystamus. The other array is placed on the ceiling for the calibration test and to allow for a calibration procedure to be performed just prior to each caloric irrigation. The distances appropriate for placement of target lights can be calculated from the following formula:

$$\text{Eccentricity} = \text{distance} \times \text{tangent (desired } \angle) \qquad (5\text{–}1)$$

Thus, at a distance of 1 m, a 15° eccentricity can be achieved by placing the lights 27 cm from the center. The center of the cross should be at eye level. The subject is instructed to follow the light in the following sequence:

1. Gaze to the left (−15°) and back to center
2. Gaze to the right (+15°) and back to center
3. Gaze to the upper light (+15°) and back to center
4. Gaze to the lower light (−15°) and then back to center.

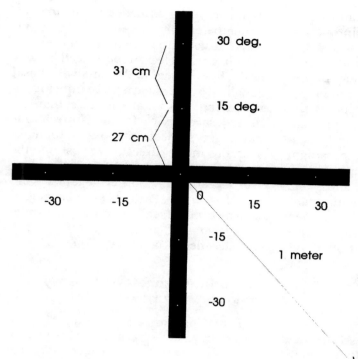

30 deg.

31 cm

15 deg.

27 cm

-30   -15   0   15   30

-15

1 meter

-15

-30

FIG 5–2.
A light array suitable for calibration and assessment of fixation. The lights at a 15° eccentricity are used for the calibration test, and the lights at 30° are used for the fixation test.

Each eye position is held for 3 seconds or more, to allow the subject enough time to get the eyes onto the target. While this paradigm includes only a single saccade size (15°), it is usually possible to evaluate saccadic accuracy and to detect gross disorders of velocity.

A chart recorder or appropriate computer software should be used that has two or more channels. One channel is used for horizontal eye position and the other for vertical eye position and blinks. If a chart recorder with more than two channels is available, a third channel allows one to make monocular recordings, which are particularly helpful if the eyes do not move together. A fourth channel can be used for target position or saccadic velocity. Saccadic velocity can be evaluated with a velocity coupler which allows a direct display of velocity on the pen recorder. For accurate measurements of velocity, it is important that the bandwidth of the entire recording system—including amplifier, velocity coupler, and chart recorder—extend to at least 40 Hz. More will be said about this later.

There are several obvious flaws in the calibration test. Because only a single saccade size is used, disorders that are more prominent in smaller or larger saccades may be missed. Because the position of the target is predictable, saccadic latencies are rarely useful.

A more sophisticated saccadic evaluation can be be obtained using computerized ENG laboratory equipment. Sources for computerized ENG equipment are listed in the Appendix. With the aid of computerized *saccade paradigms*, more data can be obtained about the site of central nervous system lesions. A major thrust of recently developed paradigms has been to distinguish between volitional saccades produced by cortical structures and reflexive saccades through brain stem structures.

Random Paradigm

There are four saccade paradigms suitable for use in computerized ENG equipment. In the *random paradigm*, saccades are elicited by a target whose location is not known to the subject until the time of presentation. A typical procedure consists of moving an LED or laser-galvanometer target from one position to the next position at 3- to 4-second intervals. The direction and time of target displacement are made unpredictable by varying them randomly. Baloh and associates[3] were one of the first groups to describe use of the random saccade paradigm to identify neurologic lesions. The random paradigm assesses the function of the afferent visual pathway, superior colliculus, and brain stem. Although not providing any information about volitional saccades, the approach is an improvement over the calibration test because it offers the possibility of obtaining latency information and also includes a larger selection of saccadic amplitudes.

Gap Paradigm

The *gap paradigm* can be used to elicit saccades of extremely short (between 90 and 130 ms) latency called "express saccades," which are a variety of reflexive saccades. In the gap paradigm, the target is briefly extinguished when stepping from one position to the next. Latency is measured from the time of target reappearance; therefore, forewarned by target extinguishing, some subjects can make saccades with shorter latency than when no warning is provided. These extremely short latency saccades were originally demonstrated in highly trained monkeys[8] and later also in humans.[9] Both the warning provided by the gap and a predictable target location facilitate their appearance. In monkeys, the ability to generate express saccades is abolished by lesions of the superior colliculus but not of the frontal lobes.[16]

Remembered Target and Anti-Saccade Paradigms

The *remembered target* and the *anti-saccade* paradigms are both aimed to elicit and evaluate volitional saccades, unlike the previous two paradigms, which were intended to elicit reflexive saccades. The remembered target paradigm provokes saccades to an unseen, remembered target. Saccades to remembered targets are formulated in the frontal lobes and released to proceed by way of the basal ganglia. Patients with basal ganglia disorders have more difficulty in producing volitional saccades than reflexive saccades.[11] In the anti-saccade paradigm subjects are asked to make saccades in the direction opposite to the target displacement. In this case, reflexive saccades are pitted against volitional saccades. Patients with basal ganglia disorders, schizophrenia, or frontal lobe lesions often make an inappropriate saccade to the visual target.

Saccadic Parameters: Latency, Velocity, Accuracy

Three parameters of saccadic eye movements are of clinical relevance in the quantification of saccades. Saccadic *latency* refers to the difference in time between the presentation of a target and the beginning of a saccade intended to acquire that target. Mean latencies of 200 ms are usual in normal subjects. A saccadic latency plot for a normal subject is shown in Figure 5–3.

Saccadic *velocity*, when not otherwise qualified, refers to the *peak* eye velocity obtained during the eye movement rather than the mean velocity. Saccades typically have peak velocities ranging from 50° to 700°/sec.[5] Peak velocity is a strong function of ocular displacement, and a plot of velocity versus displacement is called a "main sequence." Figure 5–3,B shows a main sequence for a healthy subject.

Saccadic *accuracy* refers to the prevalence of saccades that are larger than appropriate for the target displacement (hypermetric) or smaller than needed (hypometric). After making a saccade that is too large or too small, after a latency of about 100 to 200 ms, the subject then makes a corrective saccade to the target. The two types of saccadic inaccuracy, hypermetria and hypometria, are best seen in two different types of plots.

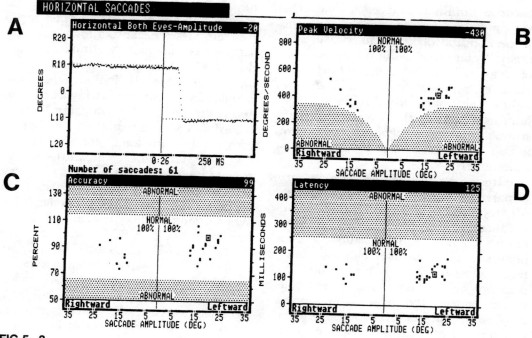

FIG 5–3.
Saccadic summary for a normal subject, made with an ICS MASTR ENG system. The recording method used was electro-oculography. **A,** normometric saccade. Target position is shown by the *dashed line* and eye position by the *solid line.* After a latency of about 200 ms, a normometric saccade is made to the target. **B,** saccadic velocity plot (main sequence). **C,** saccadic accuracy plot. This style of plot is appropriate for detecting hypometric saccades, which must be consistent and substantial to be abnormal. **D,** saccadic latency plot. *(Figure courtesy of ICS Medical Corporation, Schaumburg, Ill.)*

Saccadic hypometria must be reproducible and extreme to be abnormal, as normal subjects usually produce slightly hypometric saccades. It is best seen in a plot of the ratio of the amplitude of the first saccade to target amplitude, such as is found in Figure 5–3,C. Saccadic hypermetria, or "calibration overshoot," must also be reproducible to be significant. However, even a small amount of hypermetria is abnormal and may indicate the presence of a cerebellar lesion. Hypermetria is best judged from saccadic position plots, such as is shown in Figure 5–3,A. In such saccadic position plots, one looks for a second, corrective saccade directed oppositely to the initial saccade that was too large. Examples of hypermetric saccades will be given in Chapter 6.

Another type of saccadic inaccuracy occurs when saccades do not end crisply, but after decelerating abruptly, drift slowly onward or backward over approximately a half second. This is called "postsaccadic drift" or a "glissade." (Postsaccadic drift is an abnormal pattern and is illustrated in Chapter 6.) Finally, saccades may also be inaccurate in a more subtle way. An accurate vertical saccade might be made which had an unwanted horizontal component. The horizontal component would then require a horizontal corrective saccade to fixate the intended target. This is called "pulsion."

Technical Aspects of Recording Saccades

There are several methods of generating targets intended to elicit saccades. Marks on a wall, screen, or hand held calibration devices are the least expensive methods, and work well in subjects with good vision and attentional capabilities. An array of red LEDs controlled by switches or a computer is preferable because illuminated targets are easier to see and, more importantly, can be turned on and off so as to measure latency. A commercial "light bar" consists of an array of LEDs positioned behind a plate of material which diffuses the light. Light bars are discussed again later in regards to their use as a pursuit stimulator. A laser-galvanometer system is also a good method of producing saccade targets.

Filtering of the analog data is very important when measuring saccades. All amplifiers of biological signals incorporate a low-pass filter. In "AC" or alternating current coupled amplifiers, a high-pass filter is also included. Low-pass filters, are the only type of filtering included in "DC" or direct current coupled amplifiers, the effect of the filtering can be predicted from a parameter called the "time constant." High-pass filtering is intended to eliminate the effects of electrode drift, which can cause the pens to drift and "pin" against the recorder stops. It does this by responding slowly to constant, non-zero voltages, so as to gradually null them out. The difficulty with high-pass filtering is that the filter is unable to distinguish between constant non-zero voltage related to electrode drift, and a constantly held eye position. The larger the time constant of the high-pass filter, the less of a problem this presents. A value of 5 to 10 seconds is best, although many laboratories use a 3-second time constant.[6] Alternating current recordings are acceptable for registration of saccadic velocity and latency, but are not well suited to registration of postsaccadic drift because the electronic drift created by the filter may resemble ocular drift (for example, a glissade). Use of the DC recording technique is recommended as it avoids these difficulties.

Low-pass filters are used in both AC and DC recordings. Low-pass filtering affects both noise and saccadic velocity. For low-pass filters, the effect of the filtering can be predicted from a parameter called the "3 dB point" or the "cut-off." When low-pass filters are used for electro-oculography (EOG) recording a problem arises because a low-pass filter setting that adequately eliminates EOG noise also lowers measured saccadic velocity.[1] In general, it is desirable to use a low-pass filter cutoff setting as close to 100 Hz as possible. When using EOG to record saccades, the highest bandwidth compatible with adequate noise rejection is 40 Hz. Higher bandwidths are associated with random variation in peak velocity (due to "noise") and dispersion of points on the main sequence plot. When a methodology is available which has less noise than EOG (infrared or the scleral eye coil), saccades should be recorded with low-pass filter cutoff set to 100 Hz or more. Commercially available EOG amplifiers are generally not designed for saccadic testing and are often suboptimal because of low bandwidth.

Comparing saccades from each eye independently—monocular recording as opposed to the bitemporal technique in which EOG electrodes are placed across the temples—is also helpful. Monocular recording avoids pitfalls related to disconjugate eye motion which can occur due to convergence, ocular muscle paresis, and central disorders such as internuclear opthalmoplegia. These disorders are discussed in Chapter 6.

Use of a microprocessor system to present targets and correlate eye movements with target motion is desirable so that enough data on saccades can be processed to produce a result with reasonable statistical power. Ideally, one should present at least 40 target steps, including step sizes ranging from 5° to 30°. Data must be sampled at a rate at least twice the frequency cutoff of one's low-pass filter. This rate is called the "Nyquist frequency." A sampling rate of 100 Hz or more is appropriate for EOG recordings, which usually have amplifier bandwidths of 40 Hz or less. A 250-Hz sampling rate combined with an 100-Hz bandwidth is appropriate for infrared or scleral eye coil recordings.

SMOOTH PURSUIT

Pursuit eye movements consist of smooth following movements interspersed with "catch-up" saccades (Fig 5–4,A). Under natural conditions, pursuit can be elicited by visual, tactile, proprioceptive, and auditory targets.[13] In the oculomotor laboratory, pursuit is usually elicited either by a pendulum or a moving spot controlled by a computer.

Like saccades, pursuit is produced by several parallel central pathways. Pursuit can be separated into two components, which are called "predictive" and "random" pursuit. Predictive pursuit is probably produced mainly by way of the frontal cortex while pursuit of targets moving in an unpredictable fashion is generated by occipito-parietal-temporal cortex. Both pursuit pathways converge at the level of the brain stem.

Commonly used clinical pursuit paradigms provide information about a combination of random and predictive pursuit, the relative proportions of which are idiosyncratic to the individual being tested. As clinical oculomotor recording gains sophistication, one would expect eventual adoption of paradigms that can separate out predictive and random pursuit.

Predictable Waveforms

The "minimal" approach to registration of pursuit is called the "tracking test." Minor variants of the tracking test are advocated by most sources.[2, 4, 7, 18] A 2-m pendulum, such as illustrated in Figure 5–5, is positioned at a distance 1m from the subject, who is upright. On the end of the pendulum is a small, heavy, brightly colored object, such as a

SMOOTH PURSUIT AND OKN

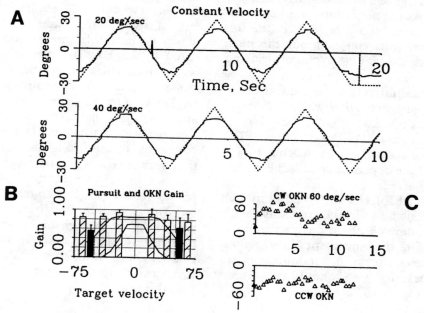

FIG 5–4.
Smooth pursuit and optokinetic (OKN) summary. Data were obtained from a normal subject by constant velocity stimuli. Recording method was infrared. **A,** two traces of smooth pursuit position versus time are shown. Horizontal eye position is indicated by the *solid line* and target position by the *dashed line.* **B,** mean eye velocity divided by target velocity (gain) is plotted against target velocity. The *hatched bars* indicate pursuit gain for 20°/sec and 40°/sec target velocities (constant velocity, triangular waveforms). The *filled bars* indicate optokinetic nystagmus gain for 60°/sec drum rotation. The *lines crossing the bars* indicate lower limits of normal pursuit gain for young *(upper line)* and elderly *(lower line)* subjects. **C,** optokinetic nystagmus. Each *triangle* indicates the mean velocity of a single slow phase.

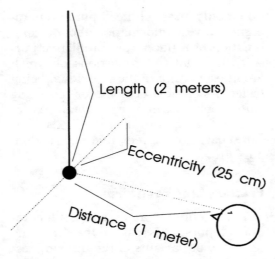

Length (2 meters)

Eccentricity (25 cm)

Distance (1 meter)

FIG 5–5.
A pendulum suitable for registration of sinusoidal pursuit.

colored golf ball, whose motion the patient is asked to follow. A pendulum that swings between ±25 cm eccentricity to either side of center provides a peak velocity of 31°/sec and frequency of 0.35 Hz. As the pendulum amplitude declines because of air resistance, the frequency remains constant but the peak velocity declines. Five cycles of tracking are recorded. Performance is usually judged qualitatively from the frequency and size of catch-up saccades.[6] Normal young individuals should be able to track perfectly at 40°/sec, 0.3 Hz. The subjective nature of the scoring procedure and the dependence of target velocity on the eccentricity with which the examiner displaces the pendulum bob are obvious flaws in the "tracking test."

The following equations can be used to calculate the placement of the pendulum. The period of a pendulum set up using these formulas should be verified with a stopwatch.

Amplitude = atan (eccentricity/distance)

Frequency = $1/(2\pi * sqrt(length/10))$

Peak velocity = amplitude * frequency * 2π

Period = 1/frequency   (5-2)

Where atan = arc tangent; sqrt = square root.

Note that frequency is related only to length. Shortening the pendulum causes a higher frequency and larger peak velocity for the same eccentricity. Frequencies greater than 0.5 Hz (1 m or less pendulum length) are not as useful as lower frequencies, as not all normal subjects can track well at frequencies this high.

More sophisticated pursuit paradigms can be produced by moving a target under computer control. The *sinusoidal paradigm* (Figs 5–6 and 5–7,A) is simply a computer-driven version of the pendulum test. The advantage of using the computer is that by presenting a pure sinusoidal motion of precisely known frequency and amplitude, sophisticated signal analysis techniques such as Fourier analysis can be substituted for the qualitative and subjective scoring method of the pendulum test.

In the *ramp* paradigm (Fig 5–7,B), targets are moved to and fro at constant velocity. A selection of velocities is chosen, typically 20°/sec and 40°/sec, with a sweep amplitude (such as 40°) which keeps the frequency less than or equal to 0.5 Hz. The major advantage of the triangular wave paradigm over the sinusoidal test is simplicity of analysis. Because both eye and target velocity are constants, gain can be calculated through simple division. The major disadvantage of the triangular paradigm is that because the target undergoes abrupt changes in velocity at the turn-around points, it is impossible to track "perfectly." The sinusoidal and triangular-wave paradigms both measure a mixture of predictive and nonpredictive pursuit, the relative proportions of each which are idiosyncratic to the individual being tested.

Nonpredictable Waveforms

The *Rashbass* and *sum-of-sines* paradigms are intended to measure nonpredictive pursuit. Both paradigms are mainly used by researchers and require a computer for stimulus presentation

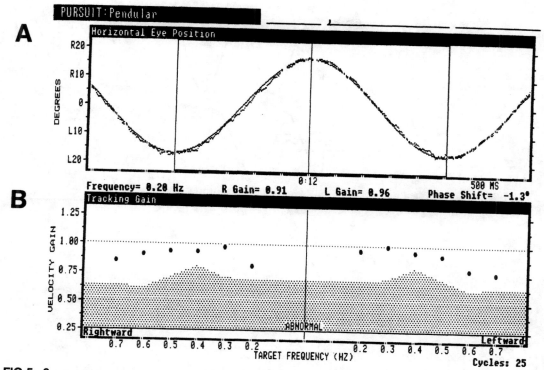

FIG 5–6.
Sinusoidal smooth pursuit summary (for discussion, see text). Recording method is EOG. *(Figure courtesy of ICS Medical Corporation, Schaumburg, Ill.)*

and analysis. In the Rashbass or "step-ramp" paradigm (Fig 5–7,C), the target is stepped away from the subject and then moved at constant velocity in the opposite direction.[15] Smooth tracking begins about 140 ms after the step, but visual feedback about how well the tracking is doing is not processed until about 220 ms after the step because of visual delays. Smooth eye motion between approximately 100 and 200 ms after the onset of target motion is attributed to nonpredictive pursuit. Generally the size of the step is adjusted so that the target crosses the fovea at approximately the time that tracking begins, making it unnecessary for the subject to produce an initial catch-up saccade. The direction, timing, and the velocity of the ramps are randomized.

The sum-of-sines or "SOS" paradigm (Fig 5–7,D) depends on mixing together of several sine waves of independent frequencies, with the premise that the overall waveform is unpredictable, and thus tracking performance indicates nonpredictive pursuit. The analysis of this sort of tracking can be easily accomplished with Fourier analysis.

Analysis of Pursuit Data

Regardless of the method by which the target is presented, analysis of pursuit translates into the problem of separating the smooth movements from the saccades, and correlation of the smooth following movement with target motion. Three parameters are commonly used to quantify smooth pursuit: gain, phase, and acceleration.

Pursuit *gain* refers to the ratio of eye velocity (during nonsaccadic portions) to target velocity. For situations where the target is moving at constant velocity, such as during the "step-ramp" paradigm, the pursuit gain is simply the average velocity (not including the sac-

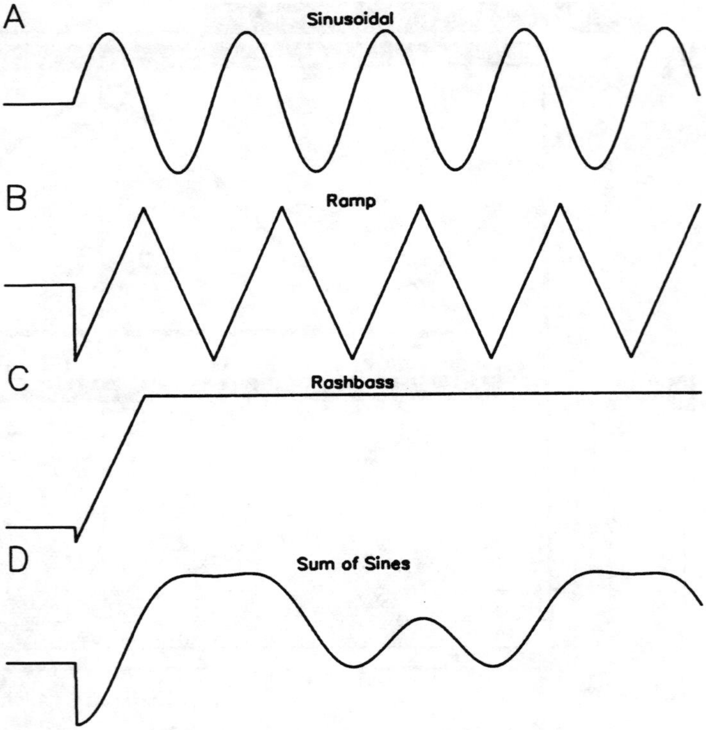

FIG 5–7.
Pursuit paradigms. **A,** sinusoidal paradigm. **B,** ramp paradigm (constant velocity). **C,** Rashbass (step-ramp) paradigm. **D,** sum of sines paradigm.

cades) or modal value of eye velocity divided by target velocity. When the target is moving sinusoidally, gain is calculated by dividing peak eye velocity, during nonsaccadic portions, by peak target velocity. In clinical testing, the pursuit stimulus is usually chosen so that gain in normal subjects is close to 1.0.

Pursuit *phase lag* refers to delay between the target and the tracking waveforms. Numerically, it is the difference in time between the waveforms, normalized to the period, and multiplied by 360°. As suggested earlier, for predictable waveforms of reasonable peak velocity, acceleration, and amplitude most normal subjects can track with zero phase lag, indicating that they can predict the target motion and produce the required waveform.[14]

Fourier analysis is a powerful engineering technique that can be used to extract gain and phase data produced by the sinusoidal and sum-of-sines paradigms. The ability to use Fourier analysis and to score pursuit objectively is the most compelling reason to use a computerized pursuit paradigm.

Pursuit *initial acceleration* refers to the rate of change of eye velocity within the first 100 ms after tracking is initiated. Initial acceleration is used instead of gain in an attempt to obtain a measure of pursuit that is not influenced by visual feedback, as at least 100 ms is required for pursuit to be initiated or modified by visual input. In theory, acceleration should be a relatively pure measure of one's capability to track unpredictably moving targets. Acceleration is a measurement more vulnerable to contamination by noise than is velocity, and accurate estimates of acceleration can only be obtained when using "clean" methods of measuring eye position such as the infrared or the scleral eye coil techniques. The Rashbass paradigm is usually used to present stimuli suitable for measurements of initial acceleration.

Technical Aspects of Recording Pursuit

There are three commonly used stimulators which can be used to elicit pursuit. The pendulum stimulator has already been discussed under the heading of the tracking test. *Light bars* are often supplied with commercial ENG equipment (for example, ICS, Micromedical, Nicolet; see Appendix). They consist of an array of red LEDs positioned behind a diffusor. By sequentially activating the LEDs, an illusion of a smooth continuous movement is created. Light bars are preferable to pendulums because of the ability to provide precise control of simulus speed and amplitude, and because the lighted targets are preferred to unlit targets, as they presumably produce tracking which is less sensitive to visual acuity. The quality of commercial light bars varies markedly among the sources listed in the Appendix, due to "granularity." Commercial bars have as few as 128 or as many as 512 LEDs in their arc. Light bars with fewer LEDs are unable to present as smooth target motion as those with larger numbers.

A mirror-galvanometer/laser system is the best method of producing a smooth-pursuit stimulus and is the method used by most oculomotor researchers. The laser spot is very bright, and brightness decreases the sensitivity of pursuit to visual acuity. The galvanometer can be moved smoothly, avoiding the issue of bar granularity. The parts needed to build a laser galvanometer system are available from General Scanning Inc. (see Appendix). Fully assembled systems can be purchased from several of the sources listed in the Appendix.

Filtering of the eye position analog data signal is not as significant a problem with pursuit as it was with saccades. While saccades contain power up to frequencies of 100 Hz, pursuit has little power above 1 Hz. However, a recording system with a 0 to 1-Hz bandwidth is not good enough, because saccades must be separated from pursuit. A bandwidth of at least 20 Hz is desirable. Alternating current coupling of EOG is acceptable for pursuit as long as the time constant is kept reasonably long (such as 10 seconds).

OPTOKINETIC NYSTAGMUS AND AFTERNYSTAGMUS

Optokinetic nystagmus (OKN) is the eye movement elicited by tracking of a *field*. This movement is produced in response to a moving full-field visual surrounding, such as is shown in Figure 5–8. The normal response, as shown in Figure 5–9,A, is a smooth following eye movement toward the direction of the moving pattern, interspersed by saccades which re-center the eye when its movement gets appreciably eccentric. The purpose of OKN is to stabilize an entire visual field, unlike pursuit, which has to do with maintaining the position of single target upon the fovea. When elicited in isolation, pursuit and OKN are often opposed. For example, when tracking a bird moving across a cloud-covered sky, one uses smooth pursuit; however, as one tracks the bird, the background moves in the opposite direction. Similarly, in the clinical laboratory, optokinetic nystagmus elicited by a drum is often opposed by an effort of the subject to fixate. On the other hand,

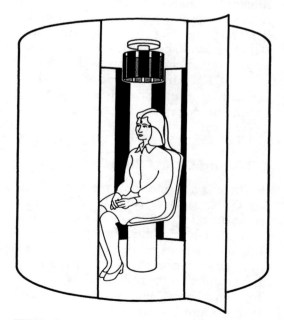

FIG 5–8.
Full-field visual stimulator suitable for elicitation of optokinetic nystagmus and afternystagmus. A small cage containing a light rotates and projects stripes upon the wall.

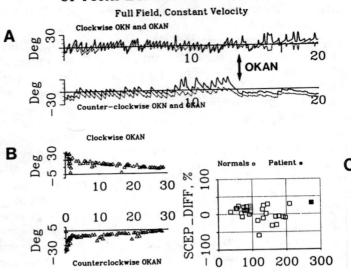

FIG 5–9.
Optokinetic afternystagmus
produced by a normal subject in
response to 60°/sec drum rotation.
Recording method is infrared. **A,**
position versus time traces of
optokinetic nystagmus. *Solid line*
indicates the right eye; *dashed line*
indicates the left eye. The drum is
illuminated through 12 seconds,
after which optokinetic
afternystagmus begins. **B,**
slow-phase velocity of optokinetic
afternystagmus. **C,** summary of
optokinetic afternystagmus with
patient's performance compared
with those of a group of healthy
subjects. SCEP = slow cumulative
eye position (see text).

during natural head movement, OKN
and pursuit are usually synergistic and
are produced by similar cortical and
brain stem structures.

After about 10 seconds of optokinetic
stimulation has been presented, if the
lights are extinguished, nystagmus continues for about 30 seconds. This is
called optokinetic afternystagmus
(OKAN) (see Fig 5–9). In humans,
OKAN is weak, but with averaging techniques it can be accurately measured.
Unlike OKN, OKAN is not produced by
cortical neuronal structures analogous
to pursuit, but rather is generated in the
brain stem.

OKN and OKAN Paradigms

There is no "minimal" method of testing OKN, as there is no technique adequate to elicit OKN other than a full-
field visual stimulus. In spite of this
difficulty, a variety of partial field devices are often used to produce an eye
movement that resembles OKN, including light bars and small motorized
drums. Light bar stimulators, in particular, are often supplied as standard
equipment by commercial vendors of
ENG equipment. Such stimulators produce an array of dots, which move to

the right or the left. The dots fill only a
small amount of the visual field, but in
normal subjects, this stimulus produces
a nystagmus which resembles the optokinetic nystagmus produced by a full-
field stimulus. Similar responses can be
obtained from hand-held drums. However, because only a small portion of the
visual field is stimulated, these devices
elicit pursuit rather than OKN, or in the
case of larger drums, a mixture of OKN
and pursuit. As such, a rationale is lacking for performing the OKN test at all
with this equipment, as pursuit can be
assessed in a more straightforward fashion during the tracking test.

Two paradigms are used to evoke
full-field optokinetic nystagmus. The
constant velocity OKN paradigm consists of presenting a horizontally moving
field to the subject for approximately 1
minute, followed by a 1-minute rest, after which the pattern is presented in the
opposite direction (see Fig. 5–10). "Field"
in this instance refers to a visual stimulus that fills 90% or more of the patient's
visual space. The subject should be positioned upright. Vertical and torsional
OKN can be produced by an appropriately designed stimulator, but are not
generally used in clinical laboratories.
The most practical device available to

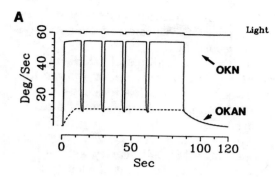

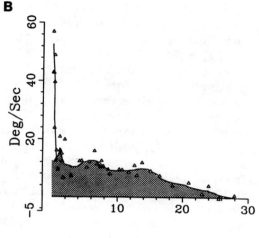

FIG 5–10.
Paradigm used to elicit optokinetic nystagmus and afternystagmus. **A,** an optokinetic surround is rotated at constant velocity, in this instance at 60°/sec. At approximately 15-second intervals, the lights are briefly extinguished to "sample" the initial portion of optokinetic afternystagmus. After stimulation of the subject for slightly more than a minute, the lights are extinguished for 2 minutes, and optokinetic afternystagmus is observed. The *solid line* indicates eye velocity. The *dashed line* indicates stored eye velocity, revealed as optokinetic afternystagmus after the lights are extinguished. **B,** example of OKAN from a normal subject. The area of the *shaded region* is the slow cumulative eye position of optokinetic afternystagmus.

produce a horizontally moving field is an optokinetic projector. Use of other devices is discussed later in the section dealing with technical considerations.

Data analysis is usually quite simple, as eye velocity becomes constant after about 10 seconds of stimulation. Typical velocities of stimulation are 30°, 40°, or 60° per second, as normal subjects can generally track these velocities very well. Because OKN and pursuit are pro-

duced by similar pathways in humans, it is helpful to use similar paradigms to elicit both OKN and pursuit (for example, sinusoidal paradigms or constant velocity paradigms) and to plot them together as shown in Figure 5–4,B.

The constant velocity OKN paradigm is well suited to elicitation of OKAN. One simply turns the lights off during the rest period, and continues recording. In this instance, it is important that the subject be upright, as head tilt with respect to gravity greatly influences OKAN. The entire OKAN decay curve should be shown graphically (see Fig 5–9) to assist the clinician in rejecting erroneous numerical results related to the variability and the low amplitude of human optokinetic nystagmus.

The *sinusoidal* OKN paradigm consists of presenting a selection of field frequencies/amplitudes as was done for the sinusoidal pursuit paradigm. The major disadvantage of the sinusoidal as opposed to the constant velocity OKN paradigm is that it cannot be used to produce OKAN. The advantage of sinusoidal OKN is that sinusoidal OKN can be directly compared with sinusoidal pursuit. Most ENG laboratories prefer constant velocity modes of stimulation.[6]

OKN Parameters: Gain and Phase

For the constant velocity OKN paradigm, gain consists of the ratio of eye velocity, excluding saccades, to field velocity. For a 60°/sec field velocity, normal subjects should track with a gain of at least 0.5, and gain should be symmetrical. For the sinusoidal OKN paradigm, gain is the ratio of peak eye velocity to peak field velocity. The OKN phase is relevant only to the sinusoidal paradigm, and is computed in the same way as was described for sinusoidal pursuit.

OKAN Parameters: Initial Velocity, Time Constant, and SCEP

For optokinetic afternystagmus, unlike the situation with pursuit and

OKN, the initial velocity parameter is preferred to gain. This is because OKAN velocity saturates with increasing velocity, causing gain to decrease with velocity although the amplitude of response remains constant. Initial velocity is calculated from the eye velocity in the 2nd second after the lights are extinguished. Data from the 1st second is not generally used because there are several transient processes that contaminate the initial "off" response. In humans, OKAN initial velocity for a 60°/sec field velocity is typically only about 10°/sec and is highly variable among normal subjects.[17]

For OKAN, the timing of the response is conventionally quantified by the time constant, which is the time required for the slow-phase velocity to decrease to 37% of the initial value. Like OKAN initial velocity, the time constant of OKAN is highly variable.[17] Another method of quantifying OKAN is to combine the response magnitude and duration information into a single number, called "slow-cumulative eye position" (SCEP). The SCEP is the integral of slow-phase eye velocity. Recent studies have suggested that the SCEP is more sensitive than either the initial velocity or time constant parameters to detection of vestibular lesions.[10]

Technical Considerations Important for Optokinetic Responses

The frequency content for OKN is similar to that of pursuit, and an EOG system with a bandwidth of 0 to 20 Hz, or an infrared system with a bandwidth of 0 to 100 Hz are appropriate. A DC coupled EOG is preferred to AC coupled EOG because of interactions between AC coupling and the beating field. The eyes normally deviate in the orbit in the direction of the fast phase during OKN. Accordingly, at least in theory, AC coupled EOG might cause artifactually larger slow-phase velocities because electronic drift might summate with the slow phase. Accordingly, as usual, DC coupled EOG is preferred over AC coupled recordings.

Infrared recordings of OKN are difficult to obtain because of interactions between eye deviation induced by OKN and the limited linear range of most infrared devices. The beating field may easily deviate average eye position beyond the ±15° of linearity available to most infrared recording devices. On the other hand, infrared is better suited to the recording of OKAN than is EOG because infrared does not drift and introduces very little noise.

There are two fundemental types of optokinetic stimulators. Full-field stimulators, such as cloth drums and optokinetic projectors, are the preferred alternative to light bar stimulators and small drums. They fill the entire visual fields with moving patterns. The most effective device is a large motorized cloth drum with alternating black and white stripes which surrounds the subject. The disadvantages of the cloth drum are unwieldiness and a higher cost than the partial field alternatives. The next most effective optokinetic stimulator is the projector, as shown in Figure 5–9. While the projector fills the entire visual field, it is less compelling than the cloth drum and for this reason may be associated with more erratic optokinetic responses. However, it is the most practical way to obtain a true optokinetic response.

The measurement of OKAN is fraught with formidable technical problems. OKAN is a weak and erratic response in humans.[17] The response is so weak that EOG electrode drift, electronic drift due to AC-coupled EOG amplifiers, and small amounts of spontaneous nystagmus are significant sources of error. Infrared and the scleral eye coils, however, are excellent methods of recording OKAN. Additionally, OKAN is easily suppressed by dim light. It is often difficult to obtain complete darkness in the ENG laboratory, and it is also difficult to determine how "complete" the darkness actually is. Enclosures that appear dark immediately after the lights are extinguished often turn out to be dimly illuminated after one sits in the dark for 5 minutes and dark becomes adapted.

FIXATION

Fixation is the eye movement associated with an effort to keep the eyes still with respect to the head. Fixation is an active process. For example, fixation might be used to diminish the intensity of a spontaneous nystagmus or to inhibit urges to make saccades. Fixation may be disturbed by saccadic intrusions, slow drifts and oscillations, or a combination of slow and fast movements such as vestibular and gaze-evoked nystagmus. Fixation paradigms attempt to detect three common types of disturbed fixation: gaze-evoked nystagmus, square wave jerks, and rebound nystagmus.

Paradigms to Assess Fixation

Similar procedures to evaluate fixation are advocated by most literature sources that consider it in any detail.[7, 18] Fixation is assessed in midposition and in eccentric gaze. In the ENG battery, the test is best performed immediately after the saccade test or pursuit test, and prior to the positional, caloric, optokinetic, and rotatory tests. Assessment of fixation in midposition is made in the following way. The subject's head is upright, as otherwise positional nystagmus might be superimposed. With the lights on, and with subject's eyes open and viewing a centered target at least 1 m away, eye position is recorded for 30 seconds. Next the eyes are closed, but the attempt to maintain center position is continued and eye position is recorded for another 30 seconds. Finally the lights are completely extinguished, the subject's eyes are opened, and eye position is recorded for another 30 seconds. If complete darkness is not available, one may substitute use of Frenzel's goggles.

The most common disturbance to fixation in primary position is small square wave jerks (Fig 5–11). Abnormal patterns of square wave jerks will be discussed in Chapter 6. In patients with vestibular disorders, nystagmus is a common finding, but because of its importance in the vestibular system evaluation it is discussed elsewhere in this volume.

After fixation is assessed in the primary position, it is assessed in eccentric gaze. The patient views an array of targets arranged in a cross (see Fig 5–2), in which the most eccentric points are 30° from the center. Note that the ±30° of the target array is not the same as the ±15° spacing of the calibration test and that a 30° or more spacing is required: smaller eccentricities are not effective. For a target array placed 1 m away, the eccentric targets should be placed 58 cm from the center target. For other distances, the formula of equation (5–1) can be used to calculate the eccentricities. The lights in the room are kept on. The patient looks from center to left and holds the left position for 10 seconds, and then returns gaze to center where gaze is again held for 10 seconds. The same procedure is followed for right, up, and down. It is important that eccentric gaze be held for at least 10 seconds so that an adequate sample of fixation can be obtained and also in order that the rebound nystagmus can be evaluated (see subsequent description). Because the assessment of fixation in eccentric gaze requires a visual fixation point, it cannot be performed with the subject's eyes closed or in conditions of total darkness. Similar procedures are advocated by most sources.[4, 7, 18]

An example of a normal gaze test, without nystagmus, is shown in Figure 5–12. The most common disturbance of fixation in eccentric gaze is gaze-evoked nystagmus, which will be discussed in Chapter 6. Spontaneous nystagmus may also disturb eccentric fixation, and its

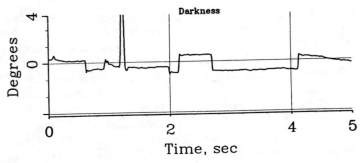

FIG 5-11.
Square wave jerks in a normal subject. Recording method is infrared (bandwidth is 50 Hz).

amplitude and direction may be modulated by gaze. This finding is discussed under the heading of "Alexander's law" in Chapter 6.

Rebound nystagmus is an abnormal nystagmus that occurs in patients with brain stem or cerebellar lesions.[19] It is a nystagmus that lasts about 5 seconds, beginning *after* the eyes are returned to the center. The slow phases are directed toward the point of previous lateral gaze. Rebound nystagmus does not occur in normal subjects when the procedures outlined earlier are used. Also, rebound does not occur after vertical gaze holding. An example of rebound nystagmus will be shown in Chapter 6.

Fixation Parameters

Inability to maintain steady gaze due to rhythmical slow eye movements or a combination of slow and saccadic eye movement is called "spontaneous nystagmus," while inability to maintain gaze purely due to saccadic eye move-

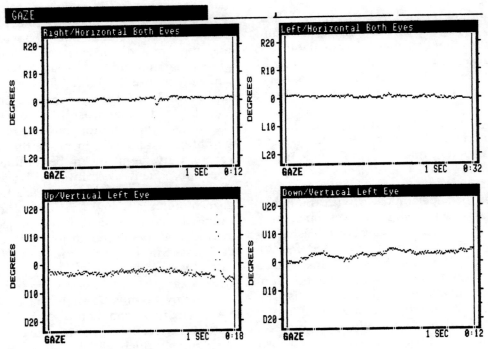

FIG 5-12.
Midposition and eccentric gaze test in a normal subject. Recording method is EOG. No nystagmus or drift is seen in right and left lateral gaze. *(Figure courtesy of ICS Medical Corporation, Schaumburg, Ill.)*

ments is called "fixation instability." If a nystagmus is recorded, then the variety of nystagmus should be identified and an attempt made to quantify the intensity. For example, for a typical vestibular nystagmus, the slow-phase velocity should be indicated. For a pendular (sinusoidal) nystagmus, which might be found in a patient with multiple sclerosis or with a congenital nystagmus, the frequency and amplitude should be noted. Also, in these situations, the *fixation index* should be calculated. The fixation index formula is as follows:

$$\text{Fixation index} = \frac{\text{SPd}}{\text{SPv}} \quad (5-3)$$

where SPd = slow phase velocity with eyes open; SPv = slow phase velocity while viewing target. If a condition in which the subject's eyes are open in darkness is not available for this study, then eyes open under Frenzel goggles or eyes closed conditions may be substituted. Low-fixation indices are found typically in patients with a nystagmus of a peripheral origin, while high-fixation indices are generally found in patients with central nervous system disorders. Any other source of impaired pursuit, such as sedating drugs or diminished visual acuity, may cause elevation of the fixation index.

Technical Considerations When Assessing Fixation

The major consideration in assessing fixation is one's method of preventing it. The eyes-open-in-darkness condition is generally agreed to be the best method of preventing fixation. The alternative of eye closure suffers from the major problem that the eyes tend to deviate in the orbit when they are closed (Bell's phenomenon), allowing for the possibility of contaminating midposition nystagmus with gaze-evoked nystagmus. Another problem with eye closure is that drowsy patients may fall asleep. While Frenzel's goggles can be used to reduce fixation, it is uncertain whether results obtained

with vision blurred by Frenzel's glasses can be legitemately compared with results obtained when light is completely occluded. Blackout goggles are another alternative that may be preferred.

Acknowledgments

Many of the figures in this chapter were made possible from data obtained from patients studied at the Johns Hopkins Hospital in collaboration with Drs. David S. Zee and Ronald J. Tusa.

REFERENCES

1. Bahill AT, Brockenbrough A, Troost BT: Variability and development of a normative data base for saccadic eye movements. *Invest Ophthalmol Vis Sci* 1981; 21:116–125.
2. Baloh RW, Honrubia V, Sills AW: Eye tracking and optokinetic nystagmus. *Ann Otol Rhinol Laryngol* 1977; 86:108–114.
3. Baloh RW, Konrad HR, Sills AW, et al: The saccade velocity test. *Neurology* 1975; 25:1071–1076.
4. Barber HO, Stockwell CW: Electronystagmography. St Louis, CV Mosby, 1976.
5. Becker W, Metrics in Wurtz RH, Goldberg ME (eds): *The Neurobiology of Saccadic Eye Movements.* Amsterdam, Elsevier, 1989, chap 2.
6. Brookler KH: Standardization of electronystagmography. *Am J Otol* 1991; 12:480–483.
7. Coats AC: ENG examination technique. *Ear Hear* 1986; 7:143–150.
8. Fischer B, Boch: Saccadic eye movements after extremely short reaction times in the monkey. *Brain Res* 1983; 260:21–26.
9. Fischer B, Ramsperger E: Human express saccades: Extremely short reaction times of goal directed eye movements. *Exp Brain Res* 1984; 57:191–195.
10. Hain, TC, Zee DS: Abolition of optokinetic afternystagmus by aminoglycoside ototoxicity. *Ann Otol Rhinol Laryngol* 1991; 100:580–583.
11. Lasker AG, Zee DS, Hain TC, et al: Saccades in Huntington's disease: Initiation defects and distractibility. *Neurology* 1987; 37:364–370.
12. Leigh RJ, Zee DS: *The Neurology of Eye Movement,* ed 2. Philadelphia, FA Davis, 1991.
13. Mather JA, Lackner JR: Multiple sensory and motor cues enhance the accuracy of pursuit movements. *Aviat Space Environ Med* 1980; 51:856–859.

14. McHugh ED, Bahill AT: Learning to track predictable target waveforms without a time delay. *Invest Ophthalmol Vis Sci* 1985; 26:932–937.

15. Rashbass C: The relationship between saccadic and smooth tracking eye movements. *J Physiol* 1961; 159:326–338.

16. Schiller PH, Sandell JH, Maunsell JHR: The effect of frontal eye field and superior colliculus lesions on saccadic latencies in the rhesus monkey. *J Neurophysiol* 1987; 57:1033–1049.

17. Tijssen M, Straathof C, Hain TC, et al: Optokinetic afternystagmus in humans: Normal values of amplitude, time constant and asymmetry. *Ann Otol Rhinol Laryngol* 1989; 98:741–746.

18. Uemura T, Suzuki J, Hozawa J, et al: *Neurotological Examination*. Baltimore, University Park Press, 1977.

19. Yamazaki A, Zee DS: Rebound nystagmus: EOG analysis of a case with a floccular tumor. *Br J Ophthalmol* 1979; 63:782–786.

Appendix: Sources for Oculomotor Testing Equipment

General Scanning, Inc.
500 Arsenal St.
Watertown, MA 02172

ICS Medical Corp.
2227 Hammond Dr.
Schaumburg, IL 60173

Micromedical Technologies
110 W. Walnut
Chatham, IL 62629

Neurokinetics, Inc.
130 Gamma Dr.
Pittsburgh, PA 15238

Nicolet Instruments Corporation
Biomedical Division
5225 Verona Rd.
P.O. Box 4451
Madison, WI 53711–0451

CHAPTER 6

Interpretation and Usefulness of Ocular Motility Testing

Timothy C. Hain, M.D.

There is much to be learned from the oculomotor test battery. The abnormalities that can be observed and their localization are summarized in Table 6–1. In the following text normal values for oculomotor testing are provided and common patterns of oculomotor abnormality receive comment. Most abnormalities will be illustrated, and can be compared with illustrations of normal oculomotor performance found in the preceding chapter. Unless otherwise noted, recordings of eye movements used for illustrations were made using an electro-oculography (EOG) system having a 0- to 40-Hz bandwidth.

SACCADES

Cerebellar disorders and degenerative disorders of the central nervous system can often be diagnosed through saccadic testing. The three saccadic parameters most relevant to clinicians are *peak velocity*, *latency*, and *accuracy*.

Disorders of Saccadic Velocity

Normal values for the velocity of 20° saccades are given in Table 6–2. Note that velocity is very sensitive to the method by which saccades are recorded. Normal saccadic velocity values obtained by infrared methods or scleral search coil recordings are usually higher than those obtained by means of EOG recordings.

Saccadic velocity is approximately proportional to saccadic amplitude for sizes between 5° and 20°. After amplitude reaches 20°, saccadic velocity undergoes a soft saturation with respect to further increases in amplitude. This pattern is seen on *main sequences*, which plot peak velocity against saccade size. The usual upper limit for saccadic velocity, no matter how big the saccade, is about 750°/sec. The author uses the function given in equation 6–1 for his limits of normal velocity. For the lower limit, the asymptote is set at 350°/sec. For the upper limit, the asymptote is 750°/sec. Saccade amplitude is designated by E and saccadic velocity, Ė. Saccadic velocity cannot be altered voluntarily and is not affected substantially by age or gender.

$$\dot{E} = \text{asymptote} * (1 - e^{-E/15})$$

There are several pitfalls to be aware of in measuring saccadic velocities. *Variability* is appreciable and one is advised to acquire about 40 saccades varying in size between 10° and 40° to develop a reasonable main sequence. Calibration error is another common problem. The calibration error may be related to subtle factors that are not evident when the oculomotor test is read. For example, patients with ocular motor palsies may be unable to get one or both eyes to the tar-

TABLE 6–1.

Summary of Abnormalities Observed in the Oculomotor Tests*

Abnormality	Significance
Saccade test	
Slowing	CNS or ocular disorder
Too fast saccades	CNS or ocular disorder
Asymmetrical velocity	CNS or ocular disorder
Prolonged latency	CNS or ocular disorder
Asymmetrical latency	CNS disorder
Dysmetria	CNS or ocular disorder
Pursuit test	
Low gain pursuit	Drug, CNS or visual disorder, inattention
Asymmetrical pursuit	CNS disorder
Reversed pursuit	Congenital nystagmus
OKN/OKAN test	
Low gain OKN	Pursuit disorder
Asymmetrical OKN	Pursuit disorder
Absent OKAN	Bilateral peripheral vestibular disorder
Asymmetrical OKAN	Peripheral vestibular disorder
Hyperactive OKAN	Mal de debarquement
Fixation	
Low fixation suppression	Pursuit disorder
Gaze-evoked nystagmus	CNS or ocular disorder
Rebound nystagmus	CNS disorder
Bizarre nystagmus	CNS disorder or congenital nystagmus
Square wave jerks	CNS disorder

*CNS, central nervous system; OKN, optokinetic; OKAN, optokinetic afternystagmus.

get. Patients with strabismus may alternate the eye that they view from, depending on the direction of gaze, and allow one eye to drift out away from the target. In these instances, measured saccadic velocities are wrong, because the calibration is inappropriate. Monocular record-ing and single-eye viewing are essential to avoid error in these sorts of patients. In patients without problems of ocular alignment, evidence that the calibration is stable over several trials must be available before diagnosing abnormalities of saccades.

Slow Saccades

There are three types of disorders of saccadic velocity. Saccades may be too slow, too fast, or have substantially different velocities in one eye or direction than the other. *Saccadic slowing* is diagnosed when mean saccadic velocity for a particular amplitude is less than the lower fifth percentile of normal. Causes of slow saccades are listed in Table 6–3.

When saccadic slowing is observed, drug ingestion should be the first consideration. Anticonvulsants, sedatives, and antidepressants are the most common culprits. Saccades can be slowed as much as 50% when subjects become drowsy. If the patient is wide awake and not taking a centrally acting medication, then the alternative diagnoses in Table 6–3 should be considered.

In some disorders, subtleties of the pattern of saccadic slowing will allow one to further narrow the list of diagnostic possibilities. One should try to judge whether the slowing involves all saccades, or just horizontal or vertical saccades. Metabolic conditions, such as drug ingestion and drowsiness, cause *global saccadic paresis*. Most degenerative conditions of the central nervous system that are accompanied by slow

TABLE 6–2.

Peak Velocity of 20° Saccades in Normal Subjects

Method	Velocity	Lower Limit
Infrared (300 Hz)*	657 ± 78	491
Eye coil (60 Hz)†	—	325
Electro-oculography (35 Hz)‡	410 ± 100	210
Electro-oculography (15 Hz)§	336 ± 42	252

*Bahill AT, Brockenbrough A, Troost BT: *Invest Ophthalmol Vis Sci* 1981; 21:116–125.
†Hain T: Unpublished data; seven normal subjects.
‡Baloh RW, Konrad HR, Sills AW; et al: *Neurology* 1975; 25:1071–1076.(estimated from Fig 6–7.)
§Henriksson NG, Pyykko I, Schalen L, et al: *Acta Otolaryngol* 1980; 89:504–512.

TABLE 6–3.

Causes of Slow Saccades

Drug ingestion
Drowsiness
Fatigue
Basal ganglia syndromes
   Huntington's chorea
   Progressive supranuclear palsy
   Wilson's disease
Cerebellar syndromes
   Olivopontocerebellar atrophy
   Ataxia telangiectasia
   Joseph's disease
Peripheral oculomotor nerve or muscle weakness
   Sixth cranial nerve palsy and third cranial nerve
     palsy
   Fisher syndrome
   Myasthenia gravis
   Progressive external ophthalmoplegia
   Mitochondrial myopathy
   Thyroid disorders
White matter diseases
   Adrenoleukodystrophy
   Internuclear ophthalmoplegia
Miscellaneous disorders
   Niemann-Pick disease
   Wernicke's ophthalmoplegia

saccades, such as cerebellar degenerations, Huntington's chorea, and the chronic progressive external ophthalmoplegias also cause a similar global pattern of slowing. Figure 6–1, A shows a graph of slow saccades in a patient with a mitochondrial myopathy, which is one of the causes of chronic progressive external ophthalmoplegia.

On the other hand, several disorders affect vertical saccades and horizontal saccades differentially. Disorders that affect vertical saccades to a greater extent than horizontal saccades include disorders of the midbrain, such as *progressive supranuclear palsy* (PSP), and the ocular muscle involvement typical of *thyroid disease*. Figure 6–1, B shows an example of a patient with PSP in which only the larger horizontal saccades are abnormally slowed. Another helpful point that may assist in identification of PSP and related disorders is *constriction of range*. For example, in Figure 6–1, B, while the target displacement was as large as 40°, this patient showed a paucity of saccades greater than 30°. Examples of disorders that af-

fect horizontal saccades to a greater extent than vertical saccades include focal lesions of the pons such as internuclear ophthalmoplegia, sixth nerve palsy, and disorders of the lateral and medial ocular muscles.

Ocular myasthenia may cause weakness of all ocular muscles, or be restricted to individual muscles. Thus, the

A

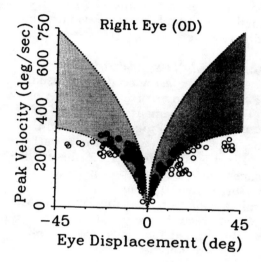

B

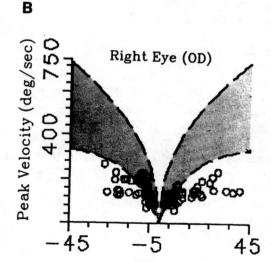

FIG 6–1.

Slow saccades. Peak eye velocity is plotted against eye displacement for the right eye. The region of normal velocity is shaded. **A,** slow saccades in a patient with a mitochondrial myopathy. **B,** slow saccades in a patient with progressive supranuclear palsy.

horizontal-vertical distinction does not help in the diagnosis. Rather, the diagnosis is usually made through observation of fluctuation of ocular alignment from minute to minute, restriction of eye movement to the central range, and postsaccadic drift (see the following section on postsaccadic drift for an example). Myasthenics may also develop a progressive slowing of saccades over time, due to fatigue. Ocular myasthenia is usually associated with ptosis, and ocular findings are usually affected by small amounts of intravenous edrophonium (the "tensilon" test).

Abnormally Fast Saccades

Abnormally fast saccades can usually be traced to an error in calibration or a noisy eye movement recording (Table 6–4). As an example of calibration error, consider the case when a patient makes a 5° saccade to a 15° target displacement. The calibration factor will be three times too large, and saccades will appear to be abnormally fast. "Noisy" recordings, resulting from a poorly applied EOG electrode or blink artifact are another cause of what appears to be inappropriately fast saccades. Because saccadic velocity is calculated from the peak velocity, velocity noise adds to the real peak velocity and results in incorrectly high velocities. This is particularly a problem with infrared recordings, which combine high bandwidth with susceptibility to blink artifact.

In rare instances, abnormally fast saccades may be real, and not due to a technical artifact. One cause is the *opsoclonus* syndrome or its relative, *ocular flutter*. In these conditions, patients make unintended saccades without intersaccadic interval, which may be ab-

normally fast for their size.[10] A rare cause of saccades that are too fast for their size are ocular disorders in which eye movement is *restricted*. A large saccade may be programmed centrally, but because the eye is brought up short by muscular restriction or rapid fatigue, a small saccade is made with the velocity appropriate to a bigger saccade. A clue here is that these patients never make saccades faster than the upper limit of normal for large saccades (about 750°/sec for recordings made with a 40-Hz bandwidth)

Asymmetrical Saccadic Velocity

Saccadic velocity, for a given amplitude, should be equal between eyes. Velocity should also be equal whether the eye is abducting or adducting. *Saccadic velocity asymmetry* then consists of significant inequality in velocity between eyes or directions. Of course, asymmetry between eyes can only be detected when monocular recordings are available. Unfortunately, the method by which velocity is measured can create an artifactual asymmetry. Studies done with EOG recordings suggest that adducting saccades are faster, while studies performed with infrared recordings suggest that abducting saccades are faster.[9] The difference between the peak velocities of abducting and adducting 20° saccades reported by Fricker and Sanders[13] in a population of 40 normal subjects ranged from −70° to 200°/sec (95% range, infrared method). We recommend establishing one's own fifth percentile lower limits of normal, for the method in use locally.

The most frequent causes of asymmetrical velocity are listed in Table 6–5. There are several potential asymmetry patterns, the most common of which is *normal abduction with slowed adduction*. This occurs mainly in internuclear ophthalmoplegia (INO) (Fig 6–2). Internuclear ophthalmoplegia is due to a lesion in the medial longitudinal fasciculus, which connects the paramedian pontine reticular formation and

TABLE 6–4.

Causes of Abnormally Fast Saccades

Calibration error
Opsoclonus/ocular flutter
Restriction syndromes

TABLE 6–5.

Causes of Asymmetrical Saccadic Velocity

Restriction syndromes
Ocular muscle palsies
Ocular nerve lesions
  Third nerve palsy
  Sixth nerve palsy
Nuclear lesions
Internuclear ophthalmoplegia
Conjugate gaze palsy
One-and-a-half syndrome

the oculomotor nucleus. The INO condition is most often found in patients with multiple sclerosis or cerebrovascular accidents involving the brain stem. The hallmark of INO is slowing of adducting saccades, accompanied by an overshoot of the abducting eye. The condition can be unilateral or bilateral. A reduction of adducting velocity into the abnormal range, accompanied by normal abducting velocity, for medium-size saccades

(about 20°), should cause one to consider INO. In this case, one should also examine the position traces of each eye, as shown in Figure 6–2. The combination of an overshoot of the abducting eye, with significant slowing of the adducting eye occurring simultaneously, confirms the diagnosis of INO.

Normal adduction with slowed abduction occurs most commonly in patients with palsies of the sixth cranial nerve. One should look for substantial slowing for a medium-size saccade. Note that calibration error is common in this situation, as the patient with a sixth nerve palsy will often be unable to fixate the target with both eyes when looking in the direction of paresis.

Several other patterns occur frequently in patients with cerebrovascular disease or demyelinating disease involving the brain stem. Preserved abduction in one eye, combined with slowing of all

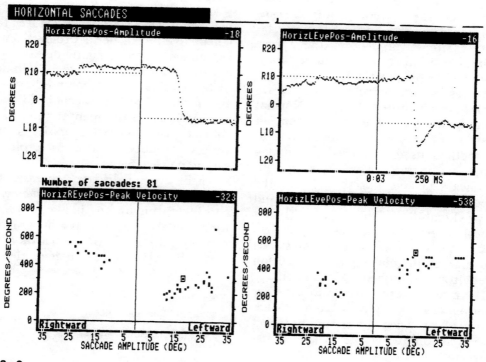

FIG 6–2.
Internuclear ophthalmoplegia. These data were recorded and plotted on the MASTR electronystagmography commercial system, (ICS Medical Corp., Schaumburg Ill). Position versus time plots for the right and left eyes are shown on the *upper left* and *upper right* plots, respectively. The "main sequence" plots are shown in the *bottom two plots.* In the saccade shown, the right eye is adducting, and the left eye is abducting. The adducting saccade is relatively slow, and the abducting eye shows a prominent overshoot.

other horizontal motion in both eyes, occurs in the one-and-a-half syndrome. Reduced speed of adduction in one eye combined with reduced abduction in the other eye occurs in conjugate gaze palsies. Slowing of all horizontal saccades, combined with normal vertical saccades occurs in bilateral pontine lesions which affect the burst cells, such as pontine hemorrhage. The interested reader can find more detail about these conditions in Leigh and Zee.[23]

Disorders of Saccadic Latency

Saccadic latencies are calculated from the difference in time between target displacement and the onset of the first saccade toward the new target position. In Chapter 5, several paradigms to elicit saccades were presented which differed mainly in their effects on saccadic latency. These included the *random, express saccade,* and *anti-saccade* paradigms. At this writing, only the random paradigm is being used clinically. In this simple procedure, the target changes position at unpredictable times, to unpredictable positions.

Representative normal values for latencies are given in Table 6–6. Normal saccadic latencies are independent of target amplitude and are insensitive to the method used to record eye movements, but vary according to target luminance, size, and contrast (whether the target is visual, auditory, or both) and the predictability of the target.[23] Thus it is best to establish normal values specific to one's own laboratory unless one is using commercial equipment within an environmentally controlled booth.

There are several pitfalls to consider when measuring latency. Latencies are relevant only when the timing of target motion is unpredictable. That is, patients may anticipate predictable targets, producing a latency that is impossibly short or even negative. Latency may also be reduced by input from nonvisual senses, such as noises associated with target displacement.[22] Saccadic latency is strongly affected by visual acu-

TABLE 6–6.

Normal Latencies of 20° Saccades*

229.8 ± 62.5 ms; *n* = 23 young subjects
275.2 ± 74.7 ms; *n* = 11 elderly subjects

*Data from Abel et al.[3]

ity, and delayed latencies are common in persons with cataracts or other disorders that reduce vision. Latency decreases about 15 ms per logarithmic unit of luminance above foveal threshold.[41] Thus a bright target is essential. A small laser produces an extremely bright target which is ideal for this purpose. If one is using a light-emitting diode based stimulator such as a light bar, it may be helpful to test in dim lighting to improve contrast and minimize effects of visual acuity.

Prolonged and Reduced Saccadic Latencies

A *general prolongation of saccadic latency* is an average latency greater than 400 ms. While general prolongation is associated with certain disease processes, as outlined in Table 6–7, in most instances this finding has no diagnostic significance because saccadic latencies are sensitive to the mental state of the subject. Uncooperative patients may simply produce erratic or prolonged saccadic movements.

There are no disease processes that cause a *general shortening of latency;* accordingly, this finding is always related to technical error, anticipation, or lack of cooperation. Lack of cooperation can cause the appearance of a general short-

TABLE 6–7.

Disorders of Saccadic Latency

General prolongation of latency
Inattention
Basal ganglia disorders
General shortening of latency
Anticipation
Extraneous saccades
Asymmetry in latency
Visual field cut
Hemi-inattention

ening of latency if one is testing a subject who makes large numbers of extraneous saccades, because latency is calculated from the time between target displacement and eye movement. When many extraneous movements are being made, if one occurs by chance just after target displacement, an abnormally short latency may be registered.

Asymmetrical Saccadic Latencies

On the other hand, *asymmetry in latency* between saccades into one or the other hemifield is useful clinically, as it may indicate the presence of a lesion involving parietal or occipital cortex. Figure 6–3 shows an example of such a patient. What is helpful in this instance is that saccades in one direction provide a control for saccades in the opposite direction. This pattern is frequent in patients who have had cerebrovascular accidents. Patients with occipital lesions may not see targets in the blind parts of their fields and may produce a "staircase" of searching saccades, the first of which has a prolonged latency.[37] Patients with parietal lobe lesions have inattention to the side of their lesion, and may produce no saccade at all or make saccades with prolonged latency to that side.[25]

Disorders of Saccadic Accuracy

Causes of the four most common patterns of saccadic inaccuracy—overshoot dysmetria, undershoot dysmetria, glissades, and pulsion—are listed in Table 6–8. These disorders are caused both by ocular disorders and central nervous system disorders.

There are several pitfalls to be aware of when considering the diagnosis of dysmetria. *Blink artifact* is the most troublesome because many subjects blink with every saccade, unless otherwise instructed. Blink artifact can be easily seen in Figures 6–4 and 6–6 where there are brief deflections in the vertical trace, lasting about 200 ms, accompanied by synchronous deflections in the horizontal traces. Blinks contribute a technical arti-

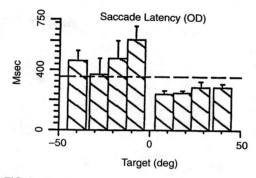

FIG 6–3.
Asymmetrical saccadic latency. Average saccadic latencies for each target amplitude are plotted. Data are from a patient with a large, left-sided occipitoparietal tumor.

fact due to interactions with the EOG and infrared methods of measuring eye movements. Only the magnetic scleral eye coil technique of measuring eye movements is immune to blink artifact. EOG recordings are mainly affected in the vertical lead, but in infrared recordings, both the horizontal and vertical components are affected. When EOG recordings are used, it is quite common for the direction of blink artifact to differ between each eye, or for blink artifact to be strong in one eye and absent in the other. These problems are usually related to errors in electrode placement. Blinks are also accompanied by a small eye movement,[29] and also may interact centrally with saccades causing overshoot.[16] Blink artifact is best avoided

TABLE 6–8.
Disorders of Saccadic Accuracy

Overshoot dysmetria
  Cerebellar disturbances
  Ocular muscle or nerve weakness
  Internuclear ophthalmoplegia
  Visual field deficits
Undershoot dysmetria
  Cerebellar disturbances
  Basal ganglia disorders
    Parkinsonism
    Progressive supranuclear palsy
  Visual field deficits
Glissades
  Cerebellar disturbances
  Ocular muscle or nerve weakness
Pulsion
  Posterior inferior cerebellar artery syndrome
  Superior cerebellar artery syndrome

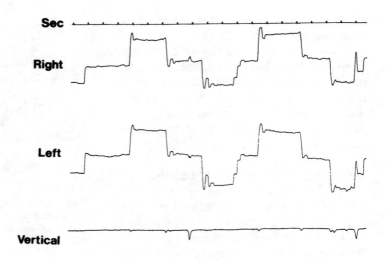

Sec

Right

Left

Vertical

FIG 6-4.
Overshoot dysmetria. This record demonstrates consistent and permanent saccadic overshoot resulting from a midline cerebellar vermis lesion.

Target

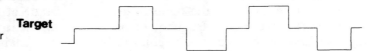

by having a vertical lead recording available, which allows one to ignore saccades with superimposed blinks, and by instructing the patient to avoid blinking during the testing. When a vertical lead is not available, such as in Figures 6-2 and 6-7, it is quite difficult to be sure that a saccade of unusual configuration is truly aberrant, and one may have to fall back on direct visual inspection of the patient.

A more subtle pitfall relates to calibration error. Certain commercial electronystagmography systems calculate metrics by comparing the actual saccade displacement to the target displacement. In this situation, an incorrect calibration can cause a numerical dysmetria, which is an artifact of the calibration error. This mistake can easily be detected by inspecting the eye position traces, as true dysmetria is always accompanied by corrective saccades.

Overshoot Dysmetria

In *overshoot dysmetria*, the initial horizontal saccade is too large and the corrective saccade occurs in the opposite direction to the target displacement.

Figure 6-4 shows recordings of overshoot dysmetria in a patient with a cerebellar lesion.

Overshoot dysmetria is not always abnormal. In normal subjects, transient overshoot dysmetria is common in saccades directed toward a primary position, in saccades less than about 10° in size, and saccades made to a stimulus appearing in a novel location. Normal subjects will, however, readjust their saccades to a predictable target location and, after several refixations to the same place, stop producing overshoots. Overshoot dysmetria is abnormal when it is frequent (at least 50% of the time), of significant size (greater than 2°), and when it occurs in centrifugal saccades larger than 20°. While numerical criteria for overshoot are available,[40] we do not feel these are necessary, as the diagnosis is usually obvious from inspection. Enduring overshoot dysmetria is a classic sign of a cerebellar lesion.[30,32] It also can occur in the abducting eye in internuclear ophthalmoplegia, in patients with visual field disturbances, and in the stronger eye of a habitual pareticeye fixator.

Undershoot Dysmetria

In *undershoot dysmetria*, the initial saccade is too small and the corrective saccade continues onward toward the target. Undershoot dysmetria does not carry the same pathologic connotation as does overshoot dysmetria, as undershoot is common in normal subjects. Normal subjects will show about 1° to 2° of undershoot for 20° and larger target displacements.[24] Constant and significant (first saccade < 50% of target displacement) undershooting is suggestive of a basal ganglia disorder such as Parkinson's disease or PSP. Figure 6–5 is a graph of hypometric saccades produced by a patient with PSP. Patients with visual field deficits may also produce inaccurate saccades, but overshooting is the more common pattern, as in this way a hemianoptic patient can put the target into his or her seeing field. Patients with poor vision, such as those with cataract, may simply be guessing as to new target location, and can produce undershoot or overshoot patterns.

Pulsion

The term *"pulsion"* is applied to vertical saccades that are pulled to the right or left, requiring a horizontal corrective saccade to fixate the target. Both upward and downward saccades are pulled in the same horizontal direction. Pulsion towards the side of lesion, or "ipsipulsion," occurs after infarcts in the distribution of the posterior inferior cerebellar artery.[26] Pulsion away from the side of lesion, or "contrapulsion," may occur after infarcts in the distribution of the superior cerebellar artery.[28] Most clinical laboratories do not attempt to record pulsion.

Glissades

The term *"glissade"* designates a saccade that does not end crisply, but rather glides to its end point. "Onward glissades" occur when the eye continues to glide in the same direction as the faster part of the saccade; "backward" glissades occur when the eye drifts in the opposite direction to the main saccadic movement. Figure 6–6 illustrates backward glissades in a patient with myasthenia gravis. Glissades occur in conditions in which the brain stem miscalculates the "pulse" of oculomotor activity needed to get the eye to new position or the "step" of innervation needed to hold the eye in place against elastic restoring forces. Thus, glissades are often said to be due to a "pulse-step mismatch." Patients having rapid changes in oculomotor function, such as ocular myasthenics, are particularly prone to developing a glissadic pattern, because the amount of neural firing required to obtain a given eye position and to hold

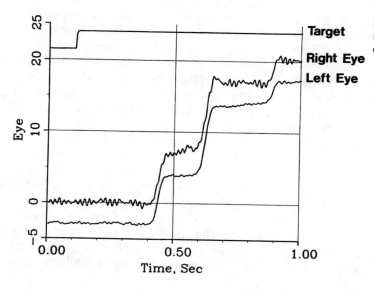

FIG 6–5.
Undershoot dysmetria in a patient with progressive supranuclear palsy.

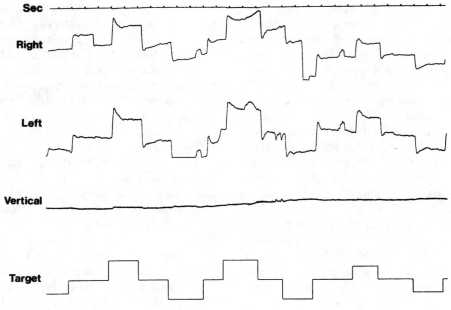

FIG 6−6.
Glissades in a patient with a cerebellar disorder.

it there against elastic restoring forces is constantly varying. Myasthenics also may demonstrate a briefer drift called *"quiver,"*[39] an example of which is shown in Figure 6−7. Patients with cerebellar lesions may produce glissades because they are unable to adjust their pulse-step ratio. Patients with internuclear ophthalmoplegia show onward prolonged glissades in the adducting eye, and briefer backward glissades in the abducting eye (see Fig 6−2).

The main pitfall to consider when trying to decide if a patient has glissades is the adequacy of head stabilization. If the head is free to move and does so during a saccade, the eye component of a combined head-eye saccade may resemble a glissade. Infrared recordings also have a special problem as they may show a glissade-like artifact related to changes in eyelid position that accompany saccades.

PURSUIT

Both the sinusoidal and the triangular wave pursuit stimuli are used for clinical testing. Sinusoidal stimuli are appropriate for detecting symmetrical disturbances of pursuit, and triangular wave stimuli are used to detect pursuit which is better in one direction than the other. Pursuit gain, which is the ratio of eye velocity to target velocity, is affected by target velocity, acceleration, and frequency. For the sinusoidal pursuit stimulus, these three stimulus parameters are mutually interdependent, as discussed in Chapter 5. For the triangular wave pursuit stimulus, velocity is constant, and acceleration appears as periodic pulses. Accordingly, frequency and velocity can be varied independently of acceleration. Unfortunately, perfect tracking of the triangular wave stimulus is impossible because of the abrupt accelerations at turn-around time.

Registration of smooth pursuit is of minor diagnostic utility, because disturbances of pursuit are usually nonspecific. Pursuit performance is strongly affected by attention, and inattentive or uncooperative subjects can perform poorly without having any significant central lesion. Another source of difficulty is that the lack of a standard pursuit paradigm asso-

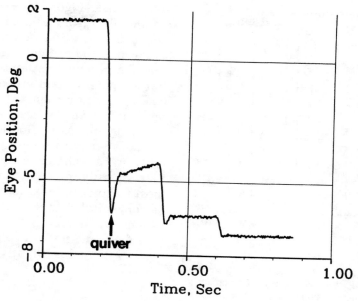

FIG 6–7.
Quiver in a patient with myasthenia gravis. These data were obtained with the scleral eye coil, after injection of edrophonium (Tensilon).

ciated with a well-defined normal data set. Simple sinusoidal pursuit paradigms can be characterized by pairs of three variables (frequency, amplitude, and peak velocity), and pursuit tracking performance is a function of all three variables. Most laboratories have used idiosyncratic combinations of paradigm variables, which has resulted in the generation of many small normal data sets that cannot be compared to others. There is considerable variability even when the paradigm variables are similar. This variability may be related to factors that are difficult to quantify, such as the degree of alertness present in subjects or the visibility of the pursuit target. Pursuit is easily disrupted by common centrally acting medications such as anticonvulsants, minor tranquilizers, and preparations used for sleep. Finally, it is also clear that pursuit performance declines with age.[42]

Normal Limits for Smooth Pursuit

Figure 6–8 summarizes the lower limits of normal sinusoidal pursuit gain from a commonly used commercial elect-

ronystagmography system. Note the strong effects of frequency, age, and gender. These normal values may not apply to data obtained from other equipment, or even if the same vendor's equipment is used in different lighting conditions. Similar normal data for pursuit according to age are not available for triangular wave testing.

Symmetrical Disturbances of Pursuit

Symmetrical reduction of smooth pursuit is encountered frequently. Table 6–9 lists the most common causes of reduced pursuit gain. For the reasons advanced earlier, one should be conservative when diagnosing abnormalities of pursuit. Clinically, it is adequate to classify patients with symmetrical pursuit into those with perfect pursuit, those with moderately impaired pursuit, and those with no pursuit at all. This classification can usually be done by eye from the position trace, when one uses a reasonable sinusoidal stimulus (for example, 0.5 Hz, ± 20° amplitude).

Those with perfect or near perfect

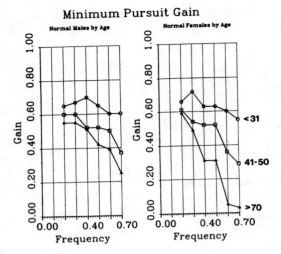

Minimum Pursuit Gain

Normal Males by Age   Normal Females by Age

FIG 6–8.
Minimum pursuit gain for normal subjects. These data were obtained using ICS Medical Corporation's MASTR ENG system,[21] and indicate the lower limit of normal for sinusoidal pursuit, using a stimulus amplitude of 17°. *Circles* are used to indicate data from patients less than 31 years old, *squares* for persons between 41 and 50 years of age, and *triangles* for persons over 70 years of age.

pursuit, as judged from the lack of catch-up saccades, or from pursuit gains greater than 0.8, are considered normal. Persons with some, but not perfect pursuit are in a grey zone. Typically they have pursuit gains greater than 0.2 but less than 0.8. Such moderately impaired pursuit tracking might be related to inattention or to medication, to an underlying central nervous system disorder, or to advanced age.

Persons with no pursuit at all, operationally defined as pursuit gain less than 0.2, are the most important patients to be identified, because they will nearly always have a central nervous system

TABLE 6–9.
Disorders of Smooth Pursuit

Advanced age
Brain stem disorders
Cerebellar disorders
Cerebral cortical disturbances
Congenital nystagmus
Drug ingestion
Inattention
Visual disorders

disturbance. Figure 6–9 shows an example taken from a patient with a cerebellar degeneration. A staircase of saccades must be present, which indicates that the patient is attempting to track. Rarely, pursuit gain greater than 1.0 is noted. This is recognized by the occurrence of "backup" saccades (saccades directed against target motion). If backup saccades are not present, one will inevitably find a technical error. Pursuit gain that is truly greater than 1.0 occurs most frequently in patients with a form of congenital nystagmus called "latent nystagmus," during triangular wave pursuit. Some normal subjects can also track with gains slightly greater than 1.0.

Asymmetrical Pursuit

Pursuit which is significantly worse in one direction than another is termed asymmetrical. While rare, asymmetrical pursuit is more often of clinical utility than is symmetrically reduced pursuit, because it is a specific indicator for a central nervous system disorder. One can easily detect pursuit asymmetry if a plot is available in which there is an indication of mean gain and the standard

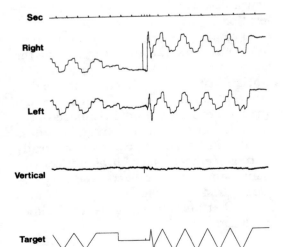

FIG 6–9.
Reduced gain pursuit and staircase of saccades indicating that patient is attempting to follow target. This patient had a vermal cerebellar degeneration.

deviation in each direction. One must use a pursuit stimulus in which velocity is constant, such as the triangular wave paradigm, in order to be able to compare rightward and leftward gain.

There are several causes of asymmetrical pursuit (Table 6–10). Patients with *acute parietal or frontal lesions* may transiently exhibit better pursuit directed contralateral to their lesion. Pursuit asymmetry resulting from a cortical injury typically persists for only several weeks.

Unidirectional spontaneous nystagmus may be superimposed on pursuit and cause asymmetry. Spontaneous nystagmus due to peripheral vestibular lesions, when weak, may not affect pursuit at all, but when it is strong (for example, 20°/sec in the dark), it may overwhelm the pursuit system. Spontaneous nystagmus resulting from *central lesions* may go uncorrected by the pursuit system and result in a pronounced asymmetry pattern. These patients present with a spontaneous nystagmus that is poorly suppressed by fixation, reduced and asymmetrical pursuit, and gaze-evoked nystagmus. An example is shown in Figure 6–10. In these instances it is helpful to measure pursuit gain only around regions where the eye is crossing primary position, as in this way the effects of gaze can be eliminated.

In patients with a form of congenital nystagmus called *latent nystagmus*, a pursuit asymmetry can be recorded which alternates direction according to the viewing eye. These patients usually have a history of amblyopia. As no pursuit asymmetry or nystagmus may be seen with both eyes viewing, this condition can cause confusion if the patient alternates fixation during the oculomotor battery.

TABLE 6–10.

Causes of Asymmetrical Pursuit

Acute parietal lobe disorder
Acute frontal lobe disorder
Superimposed nystagmus

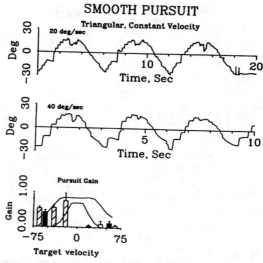

FIG 6–10.
Asymmetrical pursuit. This recording is from a patient after removal of a posterior fossa meningioma. A complex pattern of nystagmus is shown which is related to the combination of spontaneous nystagmus, gaze-evoked nystagmus, and diminished pursuit tracking. On the *bottom* plot, *hatched bars* indicate pursuit gain for triangular wave tracking, and *filled bars* indicate gain of optokinetic nystagmus (60°/sec constant velocity). Eye movements were recorded with the infrared technique.

Reversed Pursuit

In certain patients with congenital nystagmus, the eyes will make saccades in the direction of target motion and slow, smooth movements against target motion. Some authors prefer to avoid using the term "reversed pursuit" under these circumstances because eye velocity is not proportional to target velocity in these patients.[1]

Miscellaneous Pursuit Abnormalities

In patients with *poor peripheral vision*, such as those with retinal pigmentary degenerations, from time to time the eyes may "get lost" during tracking, showing a characteristic pattern of searching saccades. However, because the patient can find the target intermittently, numerical figures for tracking may be normal. Figure 6–11 shows an example of such a case. The term "*disor-*

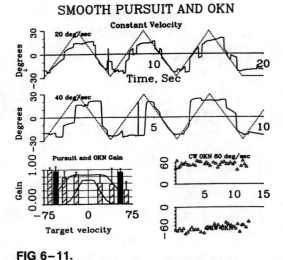

FIG 6–11.
Disorganized pursuit. This patient has poor peripheral vision resulting from a hereditary retinal degeneration. The patient intermittently finds the target with his fovea and tracks it quite well, but also gets quite far from the target from time to time. The *bottom plot* is organized as described in Figure 6–10, except that optokinetic nystagmus is also plotted at the bottom right. Eye movements were recorded with the infrared technique.

ganized pursuit" is sometimes applied to severely abnormal pursuit falling into one of the categories mentioned earlier. *Disconjugate eye movements* may occur rarely during pursuit. In most cases it is not necessary to scrutinize the pursuit trace, because the same underlying disorders that cause disconjugate pursuit, also cause disconjugate saccades.

OPTOKINETIC NYSTAGMUS AND OPTOKINETIC AFTERNYSTAGMUS

Disorders of Optokinetic Nystagmus

Optokinetic nystagmus (OKN), like pursuit, has only minor diagnostic utility. Although OKN is more specific than pursuit, as it is not as affected by inattention and medication as is pursuit; it is also less sensitive. Presumably the relative lack of sensitivity of OKN to ocular and central disorders occurs because OKN is the *sum* of two tracking mecha-

nisms, namely, the smooth pursuit system, which uses foveal vision, and a separate tracking system, which uses both foveal and extrafoveal vision.

Normal values for OKN gain are similar to those given for pursuit gain, or slightly greater, but OKN gain is less strongly reduced at high frequencies.[27] While normal values are available for OKN phase, it is uncertain whether or not phase is affected by disease. Practically, OKN is best evaluated by comparing it to smooth pursuit, using the normal values developed for pursuit.

There are several *pitfalls* unique to optokinetic testing. While less sensitive to attention than pursuit, because OKN is disturbing to some patients, there may be an active attempt made to suppress OKN by fixating on a nonmoving object in the room. This pattern is easily recognized because these persons are generally otherwise healthy individuals, and because their initial responses are robust. Also, as discussed in Chapter 5, many commercial "optokinetic simulators" are actually devices which elicit smooth pursuit. If one is using such a device, the diagnostic points listed later, which depend on noticing differences between pursuit and optokinetic responses, do not apply.

Symmetrically Reduced OKN Gain

Table 6–11 lists causes of OKN abnormalities. There are three specific patterns of abnormal OKN, the first of which is *symmetrically reduced OKN gain*. Reduced OKN occurs in visual disorders, in pursuit system disorders, and in disorders of fast phases. While smooth pursuit is most affected by visual acuity, which represents foveal vision, OKN is pro-

TABLE 6–11.
Causes of Abnormal Optokinetic Nystagmus

Visual disorders
Pursuit system disorder
Fast-phase disorder
Superimposed nystagmus
Congenital nystagmus

duced both by foveal and extrafoveal vision, and thus may persist even when visual acuity is poor. In disorders which selectively affect foveal vision, a slow buildup of OKN may occur to a constant velocity stimulus.[7] In disorders which spare foveal vision but abolish peripheral vision, such as extremely severe retinal pigmentary degenerations, no buildup of OKN is seen. Another context in which pursuit is normal but OKN is symmetrically reduced are patients with fast-phase disorders. The most common clinical disorder of this type is PSP, a degenerative disorder of the brain stem, in which saccades are slowed and difficult to initiate. Accordingly, patients with PSP may have normal pursuit to a sinusoid or triangular wave target, but poor OKN to a drum moving at constant velocity because their OKN "hangs up" in the orbit (Fig 6-12). In other words, the eyes deviate out to the orbital edge and just stay there, instead of undergoing periodic resetting quick phases which bring the eye back to the center. These patients show a similar disorder of vestibular fast phases, and get "hung-up" when rotated at constant velocity. In the later stages of PSP, both pursuit and OKN are lost.

Asymmetrical OKN Gain

Asymmetrical OKN is not as helpful for diagnosis of central nervous system disorders as asymmetrical pursuit, mainly because it occurs so infrequently. Presumably asymmetrical OKN is uncommon because it requires lesions in two tracking systems: foveal and extrafoveal. Only a minor asymmetry of OKN appears following complete unilateral peripheral vestibular lesions. Asymmetrical OKN also appears briefly following unilateral parietooccipital lesions.

Reversed Optokinetic Nystagmus

Reversed or inverted OKN occurs in patients with congenital nystagmus, which is discussed under the heading of fixation. In these patients, the nystagmus beats in the direction of stripe movement. However, the slow-phase velocity of the nystagmus does not scale with the stimulus speed.[1]

Disorders of Optokinetic Afternystagmus

Optokinetic afternystagmus (OKAN) is the nystagmus that follows a constant velocity optokinetic stimulation, after the lights have been turned off. It is a weak response in humans, generally decaying from an initial value of about 10°/second to zero, over about 15 seconds. A good normal data base of normal subjects exists for the study of OKAN.[36] OKAN is characterized by three parameters; *initial velocity*, the *time constant of decay*, and the *slow-cumulative eye position* (SCEP). The most useful of these parameters is the SCEP. The lower limit of normal for SCEP used in the author's laboratory is 40°.

The major *pitfall* to be aware of when attempting to use OKAN for clinical diagnosis is that OKAN varies substantially in the same individual from trial to trial.[36] Averaging can be used to overcome this problem.

Conditions that may result in abnormal OKAN are listed in Table 6-12.

Symmetrical Reduction of OKAN

There are three abnormal patterns to OKAN: complete loss, significant asymmetry, and hyperactive OKAN. *Complete*

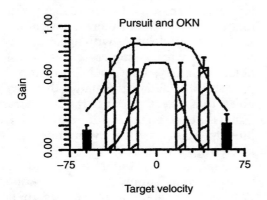

FIG 6-12.
Reduced optokinetic nystagmus *(filled bars)* with normal pursuit function *(hatched bars)* for a patient with progressive supranuclear palsy.

TABLE 6–12.

Causes of Abnormal Optokinetic Afternystagmus

Optokinetic nystagmus disorders
Peripheral vestibular lesions
Central vestibular lesions
Mal de debarquement syndrome

loss of OKAN, or bilateral reduction of the SCEP to less than 40°, occurs very commonly in patients with bilateral vestibular loss.[15,44] Figure 6–13 shows an example from a patient with antibiotic induced ototoxicity. Optokinetic afternystagmus can also be lost in central lesions that affect vestibular connections.[8]

Asymmetrical Reduction of OKAN

Asymmetry of OKAN occurs in patients with unilateral vestibular loss (Fig 6–14). A stronger response is found for drum rotation toward the side of lesion. Asymmetrical OKAN also occurs in many subjects who otherwise test as normal, for uncertain reasons. Because of this normal variability, a significant directional preponderance in OKAN occurs in only about half of patients with complete unilateral vestibular loss.

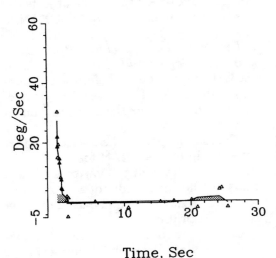

FIG 6–13.
Reduced optokinetic afternystagmus (OKAN) in a patient with bilateral loss of vestibular function resulting from antibiotic ototoxicity. The *cross-hatched area* indicates remaining OKAN.

Hyperactive OKAN

Abnormally increased OKAN may be found in patients with "mal de debarquement," a condition in which the vestibular system is overactive, and causes a prolonged "land sickness."[11]

FIXATION

The utility of the fixation test is related to identification of central disorders. Five abnormalities of fixation will be discussed, namely impaired fixation suppression, gaze-evoked nystagmus, rebound nystagmus, congenital nystagmus, and square wave jerks.

Impaired Fixation Suppression

The diagnosis of *impaired fixation suppression* is made by observing the effect upon an ongoing nystagmus of asking the subject to fix his or her eyes on a clearly visible target, upon any ongoing nystagmus. The *fixation index* is the ratio of nystagmus peak slow-phase velocity with fixation to nystagmus intensity with fixation removed (for example, complete darkness or subject's eyes closed).

For nystagmus induced by caloric input, Takemori and Cohen[35] found the normal mean fixation index to be 48 ± 10%. However, it is questionable whether this value is an appropriate normal value for several reasons. It seems likely that fixation index should increase with age, as the pursuit declines with age, but fixation data by age of subject are not available. Similarly, fixation suppression is probably affected by the many other variables that affect pursuit. It also seems likely that the efficiency of fixation is related to the intensity of nystagmus one is attempting to suppress.

Peripheral vestibular nystagmus is usually well suppressed by fixation. Congenital nystagmus, which is to be discussed later, and many varieties of central nystagmus are unaffected by or even increased by fixation. Nystagmus

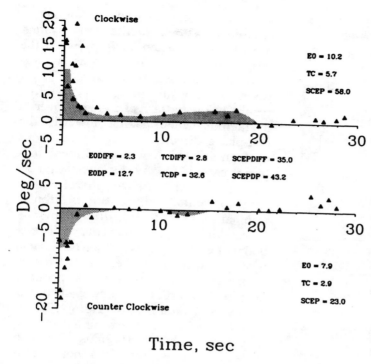

EO = 10.2

TC = 5.7

SCEP = 58.0

EODIFF = 2.3   TCDIFF = 2.8   SCEPDIFF = 35.0

EODP = 12.7   TCDP = 32.6   SCEPDP = 43.2

EO = 7.9

TC = 2.9

SCEP = 23.0

FIG 6–14.
Asymmetrical optokinetic afternystagmus in a patient with unilateral loss of vestibular function (right side) due to resection of an acoustic neurinoma. The *shaded regions* indicate the area underneath the velocity trace used to calculate the slow-cumulative eye position. The initial velocity *(E0)*, time constant *(TC)*, and slow-cumulative eye position *(SCEP)*, are all greater for stimulation towards the right (clockwise). This asymmetry is also reflected in the difference and preponderance figures, listed in the space between the two velocity traces.

which is increased by fixation is called "fixation nystagmus."

Gaze-Evoked Nystagmus

A second point of information to be gained from the fixation test is the *adequacy of gaze holding,* as impaired gaze holding may indicate the presence of a central lesion. *Gaze-evoked nystagmus* is a drift of the eye which is only present for certain directions of gaze. When EOG recordings are used, any persistent nystagmus for ocular displacements of 30° or less are considered abnormal. When using infrared recordings, small amounts of weak (0.5°/sec to 3.0°/sec) gaze-evoked nystagmus may be recorded in normal subjects.[2]

Causes of gaze-evoked nystagmus are listed in Table 6–13. Several distinct patterns of gaze-evoked nystagmus can be identified by scrutiny of the eye position trace. The most common variety consists of a drift towards the center of the orbit, interspersed by corrective outgoing saccades attempting to acquire a target which has drifted off the fovea

(Fig 6–15). In this situation, the initial rate at which the eye drifts is directly proportional to how far the eye is from center, because elastic restoring forces are proportional to displacement. Accordingly, as the eye approaches center, the rate of drift decreases, accounting for the characteristic *decreasing exponential trajectory of ocular drift.* The decreasing exponential pattern may be difficult to appreciate if the patient makes frequent saccades to the target, and one must look for a slow phase in which the patient allowed his or her eye to drift close to the center. Gaze-evoked nystagmus on lateral gaze and upward gaze is common, whereas gaze-evoked nystagmus on downward gaze is infrequent. Certain patients with congenital nystag-

TABLE 6–13.

Causes of Gaze-Evoked Nystagmus

Medication
Brain stem or cerebellar disorder
Normal variant
Ocular muscle fatigue
Congenital nystagmus

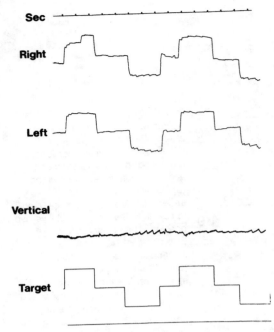

Sec

Right

Left

Vertical

Target

FIG 6–15.
Gaze-evoked nystagmus in a patient with a cerebellar degeneration. This patient also had a downbeat nystagmus (see *vertical lead*), which increased on left gaze.

mus or with acquired central nystagmus varieties have *increasing exponential* velocity patterns. More will be said about this shortly under the heading "Congenital Nystagmus."

Two factors may contribute to the *amount* of gaze-evoked nystagmus found in individual patients. The first relates to the patterns of neural firing associated with maintenance of eye position against elastic restoring forces. Central disorders, particularly those involving the cerebellum, can disrupt the neural "step" of firing, which holds the eye in place against elastic forces, and cause centripetal drift. A second consideration relates to how proficiently the patient can use visual tracking mechanisms such as pursuit or optokinetic responses to offset and eliminate drift, even though it is self-generated.

Gaze-evoked nystagmus which is greater when the subject is looking in one direction than in the other occurs in several situations. In vestibular disor-

ders, when gaze-evoked nystagmus is combined with a spontaneous nystagmus, they add when gazing toward the fast phase of the spontaneous nystagmus and subtract when the gaze is toward the opposite direction. This often results in the pattern of a greater overall nystagmus when gazing towards the fast-phase direction of the spontaneous nystagmus. This common clinical pattern is called "*Alexander's law,*"[31] and occurs in patients with peripheral and in some patients with central vestibular imbalance (Fig 6–16). *Brun's nystagmus,* which occurs in patients with cerebellar lesions, refers to asymmetrical nystagmus in which there is little or no spontaneous nystagmus in a primary position, but an asymmetry exists at the extremes of lateral gaze (Fig 6–17). Patients with INO often exhibit a disconjugate gaze-evoked nystagmus in which the abducting eye exhibits a more prominent nystagmus than the adducting eye (see Fig 6–2).

Rebound Nystagmus

Rebound nystagmus is a primary position nystagmus that is provoked by prolonged eccentric gaze holding. It appears after the eyes are returned to primary position. An example is shown in Figure 6–18. An abnormal amount of rebound consists of at least three beats of clear nystagmus, with the slow-phases directed toward the previous position of gaze. Rebound after gaze holding for periods more prolonged than 30 seconds, or for eccentricities larger than about 45° is of uncertain significance, as healthy subjects may exhibit rebound under such circumstances.[14] Vertical rebound nystagmus is rare.

Rebound nystagmus is always pathologic and is related to brain stem or cerebellar disease. Accordingly, if an unusually large gaze-evoked nystagmus is observed, one should automatically look for rebound nystagmus. On the other hand, gaze-evoked nystagmus without

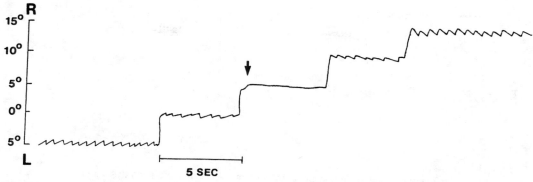

FIG 6–16.
Asymmetrical gaze-evoked nystagmus. The record of this patient, with a brain stem infarct, also demonstrates Alexander's law. In primary position (zero degrees), a spontaneous nystagmus is seen, which is nulled at 5°, more intense at 5° left, and reversed beyond 5° right. Eye movements are recorded with the infrared method. *(Courtesy of Glen Krol, Illinois Eye and Ear Infirmary, Chicago.)*

rebound is usually of little significance. Rebound is always associated with poor pursuit.

Congenital Nystagmus

Congenital nystagmus is a term applied to a diverse group of abnormal eye movements that are noted at birth or shortly thereafter. Congenital nystagmus is included under the category of disorders of fixation because it can frequently present as a severe gaze-evoked nystagmus, and because it is often increased by attempts at fixation. Figure 6–19 shows an example of congenital nystagmus in a patient with albinism, showing rounding of slow phases, with convexity in the direction of gaze. Such "increasing exponential velocity profiles" are typical of congenital nystagmus. No special procedure is required to elicit congenital nystagmus other than that described for registration of gaze-evoked nystagmus.

There are several types of acquired nystagmus that appear similar to congenital nystagmus. *Nystagmus of the blind* is a constantly present nystagmus that may undergo periodic changes in direction. *Spasmus nutans* consists of a pendular, dysconjugate nystagmus accompanied by head-nodding, which occurs in children. Similar acquired pen-

dular nystagmus in adults can be caused by multiple sclerosis, and follow brain stem infarctions. Occasional central nystagmus patterns, such as those related to *Wernicke's encephalopathy*, may have increasing exponential velocity profiles similar to those seen in some forms of congenital nystagmus.

One must be cautious when using infrared oculography for registration of congenital nystagmus and gaze-evoked nystagmus, because artifact due to transducer nonlinearity can cause an or-

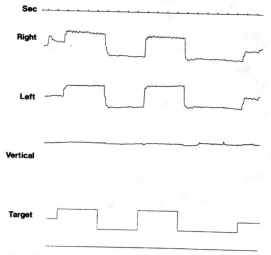

FIG 6–17.
Brun's nystagmus. This patient with a cerebellar lesion had much more nystagmus on right gaze than on left gaze. The nystagmus is also disjunctive, as it is much stronger in the right eye than in the left eye.

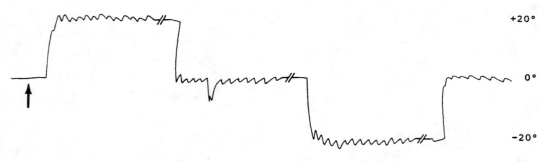

FIG 6–18.
Rebound nystagmus. Patient with an Arnold-Chiari malformation. Initially there is no nystagmus in primary position. On gaze holding at 20° right, a right-beating nystagmus appears. On return to central position a left-beating nystagmus appears, which gradually dies away. On left gaze, a left-beating appears, and a right-beating nystagmus appears after return to primary position. Eye movements were recorded with the infrared method. (*Courtesy of Dr. A. Kumar, Illinois Eye and Ear Infirmary, Chicago.*)

dinary gaze-evoked nystagmus to resemble the increasing exponential pattern described earlier. Also, care must be taken that an unusually intense gaze-evoked nystagmus is not mistaken for congenital nystagmus.

Square Wave Jerks

The last point of information to be derived from the fixation test relates to *square wave jerks*. These are inappropriate saccades that take the eye off the target, followed by a nearly normal intersaccadic interval (approximately 200

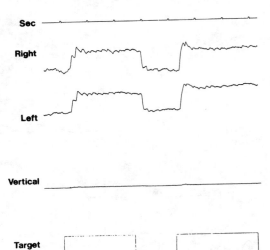

FIG 6–19.
Congenital nystagmus in a patient with albinism.

ms), and then a corrective saccade that brings the eye back to the target.[23] Square wave jerks are illustrated in Figure 6–20. Multiple sources have been suggested as generators for square wave jerks including the cerebral hemisphere,[34] the cerebellum,[4,12,43] and superior colliculus.[20] Table 6–14 shows the commonly reported clinical associations.

As square wave jerks are universally found in normal subjects, the main criteria for abnormality is frequency. There are two factors that can affect frequency: age and fixation. Increasing age is associated with increasing frequency. Herishanu and Sharpe[19] reported a mean frequency of 4.7 occurrences per minute in young subjects and 27 per minute in the elderly. Another factor influencing frequency is the state of fixation. Shallo-Hoffmann and associates[33] reported that, for normal young subjects, the mean frequency was 4.4 per minute when recorded in light with visual fixation, 8.5 per minute when re-

TABLE 6–14.

Causes of Square Wave Jerks

Cerebral lesions
Cerebellar disorders
Basal ganglia disorders
Catecholamine depletion
Strabismus
Normal aging

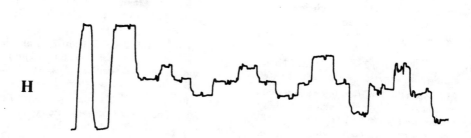

H

V

FIG 6–20.
Square wave jerks in a patient with progressive supranuclear palsy. Frequent small square waves are seen superimposed upon a saccade sequence. The initial large horizontal movements are between ±20°.

corded in dark without visual fixation, and 5.4 per minute when recorded with the subject's eyes closed.

The clinical utility of square wave jerks is to point toward the possibility of a central disorder. In young normal persons, square wave jerks occur infrequently. Accordingly, when they are found frequently in a young patient (more than 1 per second), the possibility of a cerebellar disorder should be considered. In the elderly, square wave jerks are common and are rarely of significance. However, in certain conditions such as progressive supranuclear palsy (see Fig 6–20), the diagnosis cannot be made without finding frequent square wave jerks.[38]

REFERENCES

1. Abadi RV, Dickinson CM: The influence of preexisting oscillations on the binocular optokinetic responses. *Ann Neurol* 1985; 17:578–586.

2. Abel LA, Parker L, Daroff RB, et al: End-point nystagmus. *Invest Ophthalmol Vis Sci* 1978; 17:539–544.

3. Abel L, Troost T, Dell'Osso L: The effects of age on normal saccadic characteristics and their variability. 1983; V is Res 23:33–37.

4. Alpert JN, Coats AC, Perusquia E: "Saccadic nystagmus" in cortical cerebellar atrophy. *Neurology* 1975; 25:276–280.

5. Bahill AT, Brockenbrough A, Troost BT: Variability and development of a normative data base for saccadic eye movements. *Invest Ophthalmol Vis Sci* 1981; 21:116–125.

6. Baloh RW, Konrad HR, Sills AW, et al: The saccade velocity test. *Neurology* 1975; 25:1071–1076.

7. Baloh RW, Yee RD, Honrubia V: Optokinetic asymmetry in patients with maldeveloped foveas. *Brain Res* 1980; 186:211–216.

8. Baloh RW, Beykirch K, Tauchi P, et al: Ultra-low vestibulo-ocular reflex time constants. *Ann Neurol* 1988; 23:32–37.

9. Becker W: Metrics, in Wurtz RH, Goldberg ME (eds): *The Neurobiology of Saccadic Eye Movements.* Amsterdam, Elsevier, 1989, vol 8, chap 2.

10. Bergenius J: Saccadic abnormalities in patients with ocular flutter. *Acta Otol* (Stockh) 1986; 102:228–233.

11. Brown JJ, Baloh RW: Persistent mal de debarquement syndrome: A motion-induced subjective disorder of balance. *Am J Otol* 1987; :218–222.

12. Dale RT, Kirby AW, Jampel RS: Square wave jerks in Friedreich's ataxia. *Am J Ophthalmol* 1978; 85:400–406.

13. Fricker SJ, Sanders JJ: Internuclear ophthalmoplegia and associated abnormalities in eye motion timing (differential delays). *Neurology* 1975; 25:281–285.

14. Gordon SE, Hain TC, Zee, DS, et al: Rebound nystagmus. *Soc Neurosci Abstr* 1986; 12:1091.

15. Hain TC, Zee DS: Abolition of optokinetic afternystagmus by aminoglycoside ototoxicity. *Ann Otol Rhinol Laryngol* 1991; 100:580–583.

16. Hain TC, Zee DS, Mordes M: Blink-induced saccadic oscillations. *Ann Neurol* 1986; 19:299–301.

17. Henriksson NG, Pyykko I, Schalen L, et al: Velocity patterns of rapid eye movements. *Acta Otolaryngol* 1980; 89:504–512.

18. Hershey LA, Whicker L, Abel LA, et al: Saccadic latency measurements in dementia. *Arch Neurol* 1983; 40:592–594.

19. Herishanu YO, Sharpe JA: Normal square wave jerks. *Invest Ophthalmol Vis Sci* 1981; 20:268–272.

20. Hikosaka O, Wurtz RH: Effects on eye movements of a GABA agonist and antagonist injected into monkey superior colliculus. *Brain Res* 1983; 272:368–372.

21. ICS Medical Corporation: Pursuit testing with computers—a status report. ENG Report. Schaumburg, Ill, ICS Medical Corporation, February 1988.

22. Konrad HR, Rea C, Olin B, et al: Simultaneous auditory stimuli shorten saccade latencies. *Laryngoscope* 1989; 99:1230–1232.

23. Leigh RJ, Zee DS: *The Neurology of Eye Movement*, ed 2. Philadelphia, FA Davis, 1991.

24. Lemij HG, Collewijn H: Differences in accuracy of human saccades between stationary and jumping targets. *Vision Res* 1989; 29:1737–1748.

25. Meienberg O, Zangemeister WH, Rosenberg M, et al: Saccadic eye movement strategies in patients with homonymous hemianopia. *Ann Neurol* 1981; 9:537–544.

26. Meyer KT, Baloh RW, Krohel GB, et al: Ocular lateropulsion: a sign of lateral medullary disease. *Arch Ophthalmol* 1980; 98:1614–1616.

27. Peterka RJ, Black FO, Schoenhoff MB: Age-related changes in human vestibulo-ocular and optokinetic reflexes: Pseudorandom rotation tests. *J Vestibular Res* 1990; 1:61–71.

28. Ranalli PJ, Sharpe JA: Contrapulsion of saccades and ipsilateral ataxia: A unilateral disorder of the rostral cerebellum. *Ann Neurol* 1986; 20:311–316.

29. Riggs LA, Kelly JP, Manning KA, et al: Blink-related eye movements. *Invest Ophthalmol Vis Sci* 1987; 28:334–342.

30. Ritchie L: Effects of cerebellar lesions on saccadic eye movements. *J Neurosci* 1976; 39:1246–1256.

31. Robinson DA, Zee DS, Hain T, et al: Alexander's law—its behavior and origin in the human vestibulo-ocular reflex. *Ann Neurol* 1984; 16:714–722.

32. Selhorst JB, Stark L, Ochs AL, et al: Disorders in cerebellar ocular motor control. II: Macrosaccadic oscillation. An oculographic, control system and clinico-anatomical analysis. *Brain* 1976; 99:509–522.

33. Shallo-Hoffmann J, Petersen J, Muhlendyck H: How normal are "normal" square wave jerks. *Invest Ophthalmol Vis Sci* 1989; 30:1009–1011.

34. Sharpe JA, Herishanu YO, White OB: Cerebral square wave jerks. *Neurology* 1982; 32:57–62.

35. Takemori S, Cohen B: Loss of visual suppression of vestibular nystagmus after flocculus lesions. *Brain Res* 1974; 72:213.

36. Tijssen MA, Straathof CS, Hain TC, et al: Optokinetic afternystagmus in humans: Normal values of amplitude, time constant, and asymmetry. *Ann Otol Rhinol Laryngol* 1989; 98:741–746.

37. Troost BT, Weber RB, Daroff RB: Hemispheric control of eye movements. 1: Quantitative analysis of refixation saccades in a hemispherectomy patient. *Arch Neurol* 1972; 27:441.

38. Troost BT, Daroff RB: The ocular motor defects in progressive supranuclear palsy. *Ann Neurol* 1977; 2:397–403.

39. Yee RD, Cogan DG, Zee DS, et al: Rapid eye movements in myasthenia gravis. II: Electrooculographic analysis. *Arch Ophthalmol* 1976; 94:1465–1472.

40. Weber RB, Daroff RB: The metrics of horizontal saccadic eye movements in normal humans. *Vision Res* 1971; 11:921–928.

41. Wheeless LL, Cohen GH, Boynton RM: Luminance as a parameter of the eye-movement control system. *J Opt Soc Am* 1967; 57:394–400.

42. Zackon DH, Sharpe JA: Smooth pursuit in senescence. Effects of target acceleration and velocity. *Acta Otol* 1987; 104:290–297.

43. Zee DS, Yee RD, Cogan DG, et al: Ocular motor abnormalities in hereditary cerebellar ataxia. *Brain* 1976; 99:207–234.

44. Zee DS, Yee RD, Robinson DA: Optokinetic responses in labyrinthine-defective human beings. *Brain Res* 1976; 113:423–428.

CHAPTER 7

Background, Technique, Interpretation, and Usefulness of Positional and Positioning Testing

Thomas Brandt, M.D.

TESTS FOR POSITIONAL AND POSITIONING NYSTAGMUS: AN INTRODUCTION*

When the head or head and body move from one position to another, the semicircular end organ receptors and central vestibular pathways are stimulated in such a way that a compensatory eye movement occurs, helping to maintain fixation on a target during the movement. When the movement is completed, the cupulae should once again be at rest, and no imbalance in the resting afferent activity should occur. In this situation no nystagmus occurs after the head has—or head and body have—moved from point "A" to point "B." However, if for some reason an imbalance occurs following the movement, nystagmus will result. If the nystagmus occurs as a result of the *active* motion of the head or head and body, the nystagmus is said to be *positioning* in origin. If the nystagmus occurs as a result of the new *static* body position, the nystagmus is said to be *positional* in origin. One must be aware of the precedence of

*Introduction prepared by Gary P. Jacobson, Ph.D., and Craig W. Newman, Ph.D.

spontaneous nystagmus when performing this subtest of the electronystagmography (ENG) test battery. That is, if a patient demonstrates a coarse left-beating nystagmus on the test for spontaneous nystagmus (for example, sitting with eyes closed and alerted), it is expected that this nystagmus will contaminate the rest of the positional and positioning tests. Therefore for this patient if a left-beating nystagmus is observed during positional and positioning testing it is most likely spontaneous nystagmus and not positional/positioning nystagmus.

The positional/positioning test battery described by Barber and Stockwell[2] included the following tests: Hallpike maneuver (head-hanging right, head-hanging left), and the following positional test positions: head and body left lateral, head and body right lateral, supine, sitting (spontaneous test), and supine with head hanging in the center position. These positions are illustrated in Fig 7–1. All of these positional test positions were conducted for at least

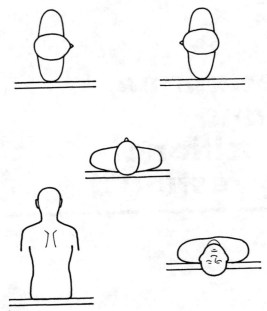

FIG 7–1.
Diagram of standard positions used in positional test battery. *Top left;* right lateral; *top right;* left lateral; *middle;* supine; *Bottom left;* sitting (also referred to spontaneous nystagmus test); *bottom right,* supine, head-hanging.

20 seconds with the patient's eyes open and then the same amount of time with the patient's eyes closed and undergoing alerting exercises (in this manner, if nystagmus was noted with eyes closed but not with the eyes open, a judgment could be made as to whether the patient could visually suppress the nystagmus). A number of investigators have noted that a significant number of clinically normal individuals will generate a low-velocity nystagmus during positional testing. For instance, Barber and Wright[3] reported that 92 (82%) of 112 healthy subjects demonstrated a position-induced nystagmus in at least one of the positions with eyes closed. This nystagmus could be either direction-fixed (nystagmus beating in one direction regardless of the body position) or direction-changing (the nystagmus was right-beating when the patient was turned to the right, and left-beating when the patient was turned to the left). Given their experience, Barber and Wright empirically defined the presence of positional nystagmus as being a sign

of abnormality only if (1) the direction of the nystagmus changed within a single head or head and body position, (2) the nystagmus was present and greater than 3°/sec in at least the majority of positions, or (3) if the slow-phase velocity of the nystagmus exceeded 6°/sec in a single head or head and body position.[3] Using these criteria the authors found that 95% of their healthy subjects would have been classified as being normal.

It is significant to note that Aschan[1] has described a classification system for positioning/positional nystagmus. This system describes positioning and positional nystagmus in terms of its duration. Type I is persistent and direction-changing. Thus, in the left lateral position the patient may demonstrate a left-beating nystagmus, and in the right lateral position the patient may demonstrate a right-beating nystagmus. Type II is direction-fixed nystagmus (nystagmus beating in the same direction regardless of the position). Both types I and II may be observed in both peripheral and central vestibular system disorders. Type III is nystagmus that stops during the time the patient is in the critical head position. The most common form of type III positional/positioning nystagmus—benign paroxysmal positioning (BPPV)—is discussed in detail later in this chapter. It has been reported that it is unusual for nystagmus that accompanies BPPV to have a down-beating component, or for the nystagmus not to be paroxysmal in onset. These characteristics may point to a central vestibular system origin of this nystagmus.

As discussed, with few exceptions the clinical significance of positional nystagmus is unclear. It would appear that with the exception of a nystagmus that changes direction within a single position (such as direction-changing nystagmus within a single head or head and body position), positional nystagmus that persists at equivalent slow-phase velocity with the subject's eyes closed or open (both of which are usually seen in central vestibular system disease) and

BPPV that is accompanied by a nystagmus with a strong downbeating component, most types of positional nystagmus can be observed in both peripheral and central vestibular system disease.* Because one purpose of conducting the ENG examination is to obtain semiobjective support for a patient's complaint, our current recommendation is to perform the positional test examination as described by Barber* and Brandt (later in this chapter). If a significant positional nystagmus exists (defined by the criteria of Barber and Brandt), and the clinical importance of the finding is obscure (for example, it is not possible to differentiate the origin as being peripheral or central, or to determine whether the left or right side peripheral vestibular system is abnormal) this finding simply is presented to the referral source as semiobjective support for the patient's complaint of vertigo that occurs during a change in head or head and body position.

Chapter 7, by Dr. Thomas Brandt, reflects the changing view of the importance of positional/positioning testing. The author describes a testing protocol that is quite different from that described by Barber and Stockwell.[2] Brandt has included only those examinations that provide information that is *clinically useful.* For instance, the reader is asked to note that the test protocol described by Brandt eliminates the right lateral, left lateral, supine, and head-hanging positions. The author prefers to use only three different maneuvers for both positioning and positional testing. This protocol is consistent with the modifications in the conventional positional and positioning test that have been advocated by Barber.* With eyes open and using Fenzel's lenses, the patient is moved briskly from a sitting position to a supine, head-hanging position with the head either straight, turned left, or turned right. Brandt indicates that both positional- and position-

ing-induced nystagmus can be detected using these same maneuvers. That is, if a particular head position is maintained long enough in a single position, the positioning response ends within a few seconds and the positional response (if present) will persist for as long as the critical head position is maintained. The author reports that this method is clinically efficient in that it is not necessary to perform different maneuvers in order to elicit both positional and positioning responses.

Positional and positioning vertigo and nystagmus syndromes can be attributed to either peripheral or central vestibular dysfunction[21] (Table 7–1). Positional and positioning testing are an integral part of the examination of balance function even if the patients do not complain about symptoms associated with head motion. Simple observation of positional and positioning nystagmus by use of Frenzel's lenses often allows one to establish the diagnosis. ENG recording of the eye movements evoked by these tests provides reliable documentation but does not contribute substantially to the success rate of diagnosis.

POSITIONAL AND POSITIONING TESTING

Careful history-taking is the key to diagnosis and is still much more important than electro-oculography or modern brain imaging techniques in the evaluation of vestibular system disease. The examiner should attempt to elicit from the patient a report of head motion intolerance or of vertigo (for example, positioning vertigo), oscillopsia, and nausea associated with changes in head position (for example, positional vertigo).

Positional/Positioning Test Technique

A distinction should be made between a positioni*ng* response and a positio*nal* response. Positioning nystagmus

*Barber HO: Positional nystagmus. *ENG Report*, Oct 1983.

TABLE 7–1.

Vertigo and/or Nystagmus Associated With Head Motion or Changes in Head Position Relative to the Gravitational Vector

Central vestibular (pontomedullary brain stem or vestibulocerebellum)
    Positional downbeat nystagmus
    Downbeat nystagmus/vertigo
    Upbeat nystagmus/vertigo
    Central positional nystagmus without major vertigo
    Central positional vertigo with nystagmus
    Basilar insufficiency
Vestibular nerve
    Neurovascular compression ("disabling positional vertigo")
Peripheral labyrinth
    Benign paroxysmal positioning vertigo
    Cupula/endolymph gravity differential (buoyancy mechanism)
        Positional alcohol vertigo/nystagmus
        Positional "heavy water" nystagmus
        Positional glycerol nystagmus
        Positional nystagmus with macroglobulinaemia
    Perilymphatic fistula
    Meniere's disease
    Vestibular atelectasis
    Physiological "head extension vertigo" or "bending over vertigo"
Vestibular head motion intolerance (oscillopsia and unsteadiness of gait)
    Bilateral vestibulopathy
    Ocular motor disorders (defective vestibulo-ocular reflex)
    Neurovascular cross-compression ("vestibular paroxysmia")
    Vestibulocerebellar ataxia
    Perilymphatic fistula
    Post-traumatic otolith vertigo
    Vestibulocerebellar intoxication (e.g., alcohol, phenytoin)

and vertigo are precipitated by rapid head extension or lateral head tilt which evokes an enhanced postrotatory response. This may be contrasted with positional nystagmus and vertigo, which are due to the position of the head relative to the plane of gravity rather than the velocity of head movement.

Positioning and positional testing may be detected with the same maneuvers. The test protocol is summarized in Table 7–2. The most provocative positioning test is to briskly tilt the patient as a unit from a sitting to a supine, head-hanging position with the head straight or turned to the left or to the right. An alternative procedure is to tilt the sitting patient laterally by grasping the head bitemporally (Fig 7–2). If the examiner observes the eye movements long enough following the head tilt, then he or she will be able to recognize both *positioning responses* (which cease

after a period of time that may last from a few seconds to a maximum of 1 minute) and *positional responses* (which persist as long as the head position is maintained). Eye movements should be observed in each position for at least 20 seconds (if no nystagmus occurs) or up to several minutes (if nystagmus occurs). In this way, it is possible to differentiate between paroxysmal positioning nystagmus and central vestibular positional nystagmus (positional nystagmus that does not attenuate with visual fixation). Positioning maneuvers, if provocative of nystagmus or vertigo, are repeated several times in both directions (right ear down, upright, left ear down) in order to evaluate carefully the position-induced response in terms of latency, duration, reversal, and fatigability of the nystagmus. Eye movements (in primary position and or lateral gaze) are observed both in the offending head

TABLE 7–2.

Protocol for Positional/Positioning Test

1. The patient is placed in the sitting position wearing Frenzel's lenses with his/her eyes open. The patient's head is grasped bitemporally, and the patient is tilted laterally (e.g., right ear down, back to upright, and then left ear down) with the head turned 45° in order to detect disorders of the posterior semicircular canal,* or,
   The sitting patient is briskly tilted as a unit to a supine head-hanging position with the head straight, or turned to the left, or turned to the right.*
2. The patient is placed in the recumbent position (supine) and rolled rapidly about the longitudinal axis to the right and to the left in order to detect the rare case of horizontal canal benign paroxysmal positioning vertigo.*
3. Eye movements are observed (either visually, or both visually and with electronystagmographic recordings) for at least 20 seconds if no nystagmus occurs. Eye movements should be observed for up to several minutes if nystagmus occurs to differentiate between paroxysmal positioning nystagmus and central vestibular positional nystagmus.

   *All of these maneuvers can be used to detect position*al* as well as position*ing* nystagmus and vertigo. The thinking is that if the particular head position is maintained long enough the positioning nystagmus will cease and the positional nystagmus will remain as long as the head position is maintained.

   Thus, for the conventional testing it is not necessary to perform different maneuvers for positional and positioning responses. All disorders described in this chapter can be identified by these simple three maneuvers. Several variants in these procedures have been described elsewhere which, to our experience, do not enhance the diagnostic sensitivity or specificity of the positional/positioning test.

position and after return of the patient into the primary sitting position.

Spontaneous Nystagmus

The spontaneous nystagmus test protocol is shown in Table 7–3. The patient's eyes are first inspected with his/her head stationary at a normal upright position and with fixation on a target straight ahead. Spontaneous vestibular nystagmus and other ocular oscillations that are present when the patient is in the static, sitting position are often confusing to clinicians because these results contaminate positional and positioning testing. Spontaneous vestibular nystagmus of peripheral origin is exaggerated or becomes overt when fixation is removed. Therefore, with the patient in

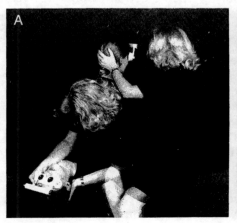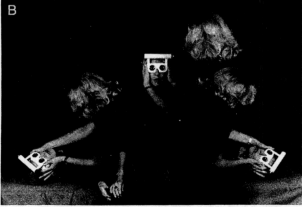

FIG 7–2.
Positioning and positional tests are performed by a brisk tilt of the patient en bloc from a sitting to a supine, head-hanging position **(A)** or by a lateral tilt with the patient's head slightly turned to the left or to the right **(B).** Eye movements are observed by the examiner; the patient is wearing Frenzel's lenses, which largely suppress voluntary fixation.

TABLE 7–3.

Protocol for Spontaneous Nystagmus Test

1. The patient is instructed to sit with the eyes open.
2. Eye movements are observed with the patient wearing Frenzel's lenses and given alerting exercises to perform.
3. Eye movements are observed during visual fixation of a stationary target straight ahead (central gaze) and during lateral gaze to the right, to the left, up, and down.
4. A first-degree nystagmus is said to exist if nystagmus is present only with the patient's gaze directed toward the fast phase. A second-degree nystagmus is said to exist if nystagmus beating toward the fast phase is also present with central gaze. A third-degree nystagmus is said to exist if the nystagmus is present in all gaze positions.
5. Vigorous head shaking is useful to transiently enhance spontaneous vestibular nystagmus, particularly in patients with weak first-degree or second-degree nystagmus where partial central compensation for the unilateral peripheral vestibular imbalance has occurred.

the same static position, Frenzel's lenses are used for evaluation of involuntary ocular oscillations in the absence of fixation.

Evaluation of the positional response may be difficult in all patients suffering from additional spontaneous nystagmus or other ocular oscillations that override fixation. Normal vestibular end organs generate resting firing frequency that is the same bilaterally. This continuous excitation is transmitted to the vestibular nuclei by way of vestibular nerves. Pathologic processes affecting an end organ or the vestibular nerve alter its firing frequency, thereby creating a tone imbalance. The imbalance causes nystagmus and vertigo. Therefore, spontaneous nystagmus denotes the presence of a tonic imbalance in the peripheral vestibular system.

Head-Shaking Nystagmus (High-Frequency Testing)

The well-known clinical method of provoking spontaneous nystagmus by passive head shaking of a patient wearing Frenzel's lenses[77, 78] reveals a unilateral labyrinthine loss even if it is appar-

ently centrally compensated. The patient is asked to vigorously shake his or her head side-to-side (horizontal yaw plane; vertical pitch plane) for 10 seconds before the eyes are observed for transient nystagmus. Hain et al.[60] were able to show that horizontal head shaking in the yaw plane elicits horizontal nystagmus with slow phases that are initially directed toward the side of the lesion and upward. They assume that "head-shaking nystagmus is generated by the combination of a central velocity-storage mechanism, which perseverates peripheral vestibular signals and Ewald's second law which states that high-velocity vestibular excitatory inputs are more effective than inhibitory inputs."[60]

Using a simple vestibulo-ocular reflex (VOR) bedside test (Fig 7–3), Halmagyi and Curthoys[61] observed that there is no central compensation of the directional asymmetry (for example, unilateral abnormality) of high-frequency canal function. When the head is rotated rapidly toward the side of the lesion, patients with unilateral vestibular loss make clinically evident, oppositely directed, compensatory refixation saccades. This indicates a unilateral high-frequency deficiency of the VOR, produced by functional asymmetry of the remaining labyrinth. This simple bedside test is also useful for the detection of bilateral vestibular loss.[12]

If the head is passively turned quickly (say faster than 1 Hz and 100°/s^2 peak acceleration[61] then the compensatory eye movement to maintain gaze in space is mediated by the vestibular system rather than the optokinetic pursuit reflex or cervico-ocular reflex. With bilateral vestibulopathy, despite attempted fixation on a stationary target, the gaze shifts with the head (because compensatory eye movements are inappropriate). Gaze in space is corrected after the head movement by a compensatory saccade toward the fixation target (see Fig 7–3), which can be easily detected by the observer. These tests do not exclude the possibility that parts of the vestibular

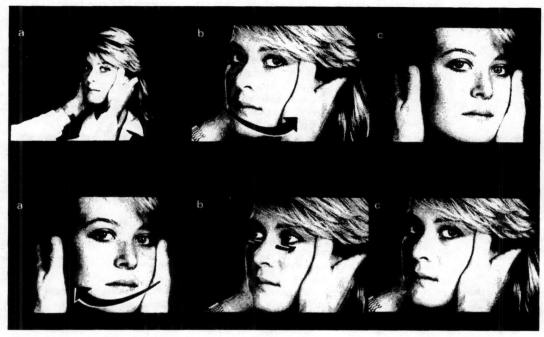

FIG 7–3.
Vestibulo-ocular reflex bedside test. *Top,* normal gaze fixation during rapid head turn toward intact side. In *a* and *b,* with the face turned a little to the right and the eyes fixed on a distant target, the subject (professional model) waits for her head to be moved rapidly to left by examiner; *c* after leftward head movement, gaze is still fixed on target so that no refixation saccades are required. *Bottom,* clinical signs of right semicircular canal paresis. Abnormal gaze fixation during rapid head turn toward lesioned side. In *a,* with the face turned a little to the left and with the eyes fixed on a distant target, the subject waits for head to be moved rapidly to right. Position *b* follows rightward head turn with head to right; *c* leftward or compensatory saccade is now required to refix gaze. *(From Halmagyi GM, Curthoys IS: Arch Neurol 1988; 45:737–739. Used by permission.)*

labyrinth may still function, especially the vertical semicircular canals or the otoliths.

CLINICAL ENTITIES: POSITIONING TESTING

Benign Paroxysmal Positioning Vertigo

In benign paroxysmal positioning vertigo (BPPV), initially described by Barany in 1921,[16] brief attacks of (mostly rotational) vertigo and concomitant positioning rotatory-linear nystagmus are precipitated by rapid head extension as well as by lateral head tilt toward the affected ear. It is the most common cause of vertigo in the elderly and is due to cupulolithiasis of the posterior semicircular canal[114, 116] or by canalolithia-

sis. In these patients there is a frequent history of spontaneous recovery, and, there exists the possibility of a most effective mechanical therapy by performing positioning maneuvers.[20]

Definitive diagnostic criteria for BPPV (Table 7–4) are based on the time history of the burst of rotational vertigo and sometimes nausea associated with the typical positioning nystagmus. Both symptoms are induced by rapid head and body movements from the sitting to the head-hanging right or left position. Other criteria include:

1. *Latency.* Vertigo and nystagmus begin 1 or more seconds after the head is tilted toward the affected ear, and increase in severity to a maximum.

2. *Duration less than 1 minute.* Nystagmus reduces gradually after 10 to 40

TABLE 7–4.

Diagnostic Criteria for Benign Paroxysmal Positioning Vertigo

Clinical syndrome	Brief attacks of rotational vertigo and rotatory-linear nystagmus precipitated by rapid head tilt toward the affected ear or by head extension
	Typical rotatory nystagmus that beats toward the undermost ear, has a latency of 1 to 3 sec, a duration less than 1 min, a reversal on righting, and fatigues with repetitive provocation
	Direction of fall is toward the affected ear and forward
Incidence/age/sex	Idiopathic forms (50%): Most common cause of vertigo in the elderly (6th and 7th decades); female:male ratio = 2:1
	Symptomatic forms (50%) (e.g. post-traumatic, postviral neurolabyrinthitis): adolescence to old age; female:male ratio = 1:1.
Pathomechanism	"Cupulolithiasis or canalolithiasis": dislodged otoconia (degeneration, trauma) settle in the posterior semicircular canal and cause gravity-dependent cupula deflection
Course/prognosis	Mostly benign with spontaneous recovery within weeks or months (70%), but persistent (when untreated) in about 20% to 30%, or shows recurrence at variable periods for years
Management	Most effective physical therapy by positioning maneuvers on a serial basis; in rare intractable cases, plugging of the posterior semicircular canal
Differential diagnosis	Central positional nystagmus/vertigo, perilymphatic fistulas, drug- or alcohol intoxication, Meniere's disease, neurovascular cross-compression, Waldenström's disease, psychogenic vertigo

seconds and ultimately abate even with maintenance of the precipitating head position.

3. *Linear-rotatory nystagmus.* The nystagmus is best seen when the patient is wearing Frenzel's lenses (for example, 20 diopter lenses), which prevent suppression by fixation. The nystagmus is linear-rotatory, with the fast phase beating toward the undermost ear or upward when the patient's gaze is directed toward the uppermost ear (Fig 7–4).

4. *Reversal.* When the patient returns to the seated position, the vertigo and the nystagmus may reoccur less violently in the opposite direction.

5. *Fatigability.* Constant repetition of this maneuver will result in ever lessening symptoms.

During the initial course of the disease, when patients are standing in the normal head-upright position they may complain of other symptoms of otolithic vertigo. These include the sensation of feeling as if they are walking on pillows. This sensation probably arises from the unequal excess loading of the two utri-cular otoliths. Central mechanisms provide compensation within one to three weeks.[21, 22]

Mechanisms Underlying BPPV: Cupulolithiasis

The early assumption by Barany[116] and Dix and Hallpike[40] that the underlying lesion must be situated in the vestibular end organ and must involve the otoliths was later supported by Schuknecht[113, 115] and Schuknecht and Ruby.[116] Schuknecht and his co-workers postulated a mechanical pathogenesis termed "cupulolithiasis." They found basophilic deposits on the cupula in the posterior semicircular canals in patients who manifested unilateral BPPV prior to death from unrelated disease. These deposits exceeded the size of those found in more than 30% of temporal bones in a control population. They argued that inorganic particles, detached from the otoconial layer by spontaneous degeneration or head trauma, gravitate to and become settled on the cupula of the posterior semicircular canal, which is situated directly inferior to the utricle when

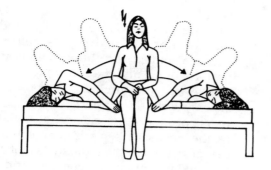

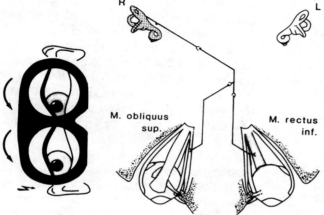

M. obliquus sup.

M. rectus inf.

FIG 7–4.
Benign paroxysmal positional vertigo and nystagmus are precipitated by rapid lateral head tilt toward the affected ear or by head extension **(top)**. The typical nystagmus (best seen with Frenzel's lenses) beats toward the undermost ear, rotating counterclockwise with right ear lesions *(bottom left)*, and clockwise with left ear lesions. The rotatory-linear nystagmus reflects ampullofugal stimulation of the posterior semicircular canal with activation of ipsilateral superior oblique and contralateral inferior rectus eye muscles *(bottom right)*.

the head is upright (Fig 7–5). The posterior semicircular canal thus serves as a receptacle for the detached sediment. In fact, otoconia are easily dislodged by linear accelerations or centrifuging in animals.[66, 72] Otoconial debris become displaced in old age,[76] and lodge either in the posterior semicircular canals[126] or in the cochlea in cochleosaccular degeneration.[58]

The cupula normally has the same specific gravity as the endolymph and is a transducer of angular accelerations only. When heavily loaded, it should theoretically become sensitive to changes in head position relative to the vertically oriented earth gravitational field (gravitational vector: see "the buoyancy hypothesis" later in this chapter). The common view is that BPPV simply reflects transformation of the affected cupula from a transducer of angular acceleration to one of linear acceleration, secondary to the

acquired specific gravity differential ("heavy otoconial debris acting on cupula") between the cupula and endolymph.[49, 103, 114] This view cannot be correct for several reasons: BPPV is a positioning rather than a positional vertigo/nystagmus because it is induced only by rapid changes in head position, and the paroxysmal nystagmus is compatible with the cupulogram of an ampullofugal stimulation of the posterior semicircular canal rather than with ampullopetal positional effects as expected. Schmidt[112] was able to reverse the direction of paroxysmal positioning nystagmus by making his patients bend rapidly forward. On the bases of utriculo-cupula interaction as described by Fluur,[46] he argued that BPPV is the consequence of a disinhibited angular reaction of the posterior canal arising from disturbed utricular function. We believe, however, that either cupulolithiasis or canalolithiasis are

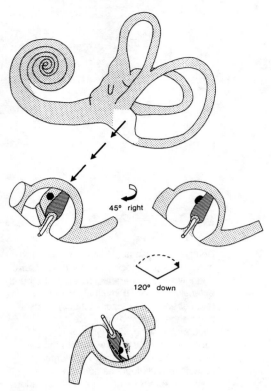

FIG 7–5.
Mechanism of cupulolithiasis, as a possible cause of benign paroxysmal positioning vertigo. Inorganic "heavy" particles detached from the otoconial layer (by degeneration or head trauma) gravitate to and become settled on the cupula of posterior semicircular canal. The "heavy" material causes a specific gravity differential between cupula and endolymph with postrotatory overexcitability. After rapid head tilt towards the affected ear or after head extension, when the posterior semicircular canal is moved in the specific plane of stimulation, an ampullofugal deflection of the cupula occurs with rotational vertigo and concomitant nystagmus.

causative, in that the "heavy cupula" creates an overexcitability of the posterior canal to angular accelerations[21, 22] or a free-floating clot of inorganic particles (heavier than endolymph) gravitates and produces push or pull forces on the cupula.

The intensity of positional nystagmus depends on the velocity of the positioning maneuver, and BPPV attacks can be avoided if the challenging position is assumed very slowly (longer than 6 seconds).

The suggestion that the posterior semi-circular canal plays the critical role in BPPV is in accordance with the finding that an ampullofugal cupula deflection causes a contraction of the ipsilateral superior oblique and the contralateral inferior rectus eye muscles.[120] It is also consistent with the pattern of eye movements produced by selective stimulation of the posterior semicircular canal, as demonstrated in the monkey by Cohen et al.[32] and in man by Morgenstern and Farrenkopf.[96] It is further supported by Gacek,[49] who cured patients with chronic unilateral BPPV by selective dissection of the ipsilateral posterior ampullary nerve. The presence of cupulolithiasis and canalolithiasis has been shown histologically, and it could provide an explanation of fatigability. The detached particles could disperse from the cupula into the endolymphatic space, and this would account for the diminution of the symptoms.

Etiologic Condition

In the early stages, BPPV is usually experienced on awakening in the morning rather than on first lying down. Studies in large series of patients[11, 80] supports the common clinical finding that the following conditions figure in the etiology of BPPV: head (labyrinthine) trauma, viral neurolabyrinthitis, vertebrobasilar ischemia (anterior inferior cerebellar artery), postsurgery (ear and general), prolonged bedrest due to unrelated diseases, and most often idiopathic causes (aging).

In the series of 240 patients described by Baloh et al.,[11] the origin of BPPV was idiopathic in about half of the cases. In the remainder the most commonly identified causes were head trauma (17%) and viral neurolabyrinthitis (15%). We found that out of a total of 104 patients with unilateral BPPV, 12% had suffered from vestibular neuritis days to years previously.[29] The age at onset of BPPV ranges from adolescence to old age, and in the idiopathic group exhibits a peak incidence in the 6th and 7th decades. In contrast, onset tends to be earlier on average in symptomatic forms of BPPV. There is a striking female preponderance exceeding a ratio of two women to one man in the idiopathic group,[11, 79] whereas sexes are about equally distributed in the post-traumatic and postviral neurolabyrinthitis forms.

When patients present with post-traumatic BPPV[14, 51] it is sometimes difficult to determine retrospectively whether the trauma really caused the vertigo or vice versa. In about 10% of the cases, observed BPPV is bilateral (mostly asymmetrical) and is particularly associated with post-traumatic forms.[87] The relatively frequent coincidence of BPPV following vestibular neuritis was first explained on the basis of ischaemia of the anterior vestibular artery[84]; however, it is more likely to be due to viral inflammation of the vestibular nerve, and in some cases promotes the concept that vestibular neuritis results in a partial rather than complete unilateral vestibular paresis.[29] This may occur because BPPV requires preserved function of the posterior canal. The natural history of BPPV is considered benign because of its spontaneous recovery within weeks or months, but in about 20% to 30% of the patients the condition persists (when untreated) or reoccurs after variable periods for years.

Nystagmus

Visually observed paroxysmal positioning nystagmus (best seen with the eyes behind Frenzel's lenses) is similar in direction in all cases, and is beating toward the undermost and affected ear, with a rotatory component clockwise (when following leftward movement) or counterclockwise (when following rightward movement), as seen by the investigator. As indicated earlier, these patterns of eye movements and the characteristics of a short latency, limited duration, reversal on return of the patient to the upright position, and fatigability on repetitive provocation are sufficient to establish the diagnosis.

A closer look however, in particular at the gaze-dependent differential effects on the direction and the conjugation of induced eye movements, reveals much more complexity and explains some of the seemingly contradictory descriptions in the literature. What Harbert[62] rediscovered in 1970 was already part of the original description by Barany[15] in 1921. This was that positioning nystagmus is mainly rotatory and beats toward the undermost ear when gaze is directed toward the undermost ear, but beats mainly in a linear-oblique direction toward the forehead when the gaze is directed toward the uppermost ear.

The neuronal network mediating the VOR of the vertical canals is based on sensory convergence within a three-neuron reflex arc. It links a set of extraocular muscles with their primary action aligned to the particular spatial plane of either the anterior or posterior canal. Sensorimotor transformation from canal planes to the planes of eye movements has been demonstrated at the level of second-order neurons within the vestibular nuclei. These neurons projecting to oculomotor neuron pools always contact their two respective principal eye muscles in the excitatory as well as in the inhibitory (push-pull operational mode) vestibulo-ocular motor link.[52, 53]

Ampullofugal stimulation of the posterior semicircular canal causes excitation of the ipsilateral superior oblique and the contralateral inferior rectus muscles.[32, 53] This causes both eyes to move downward with the slow phases and to move upward with the quick phases of the nystagmus (see Fig 7–4). Monocular ENG recordings of horizontal and vertical components demonstrated a larger horizontal component in the ipsilateral eye and a larger vertical component in the contralateral eye, both of which can be explained by the different angle of insertion of the oblique and rectus muscles.[13] Furthermore, the amplitude of the horizontal component in each eye depends on the direction of gaze relative to the head, and ENG recordings sometimes appear inconsistent with visual observation, such that reversals of the horizontal component with changes in gaze position and dissociated eye movements as well as downbeating nystagmus were reported.[11, 81]

Vertigo and Postural Imbalance

The occurrence of BPPV with the patient supine is very discomforting and makes patients afraid of falling backward, an almost unique complaint. In the upright body position vertiginous attacks produced by changes in head position are incapacitating and can be dangerous, such as when a patient is looking up at the ceiling while standing on a ladder. In this situation, BPPV can cause a catastrophic fall. Although the nystagmus pattern in BPPV attacks has been well described, less information is available on the direction and magnitude of postural destabilization.

Posturographic measurements have been made in patients with BPPV in whom attacks were elicited by head tilt while they were standing on a posturographic platform. These measurements revealed a characteristic pattern of postural instability[27]: after a short latency, patients exhibit large sway amplitudes, predominantly forward-and-backward (Fig 7–6), with a mean sway frequency range below 3 Hz. The amount of instability decreases gradually within 30 seconds in parallel to the diminution of the sensation of vertigo and of the nystagmus. When subjects close their eyes, the tendency to fall can hardly be compensated for by interference of corrective somatosensory input.

Patients standing on a force-measuring platform show a shift of the mean position of the center of gravity forward and toward the direction of the head tilt (see Fig 7–6), with a concurrent increase in sway amplitude. Mean sway amplitudes increase by a factor of 4 in the forward-backward plane and a factor of 3 in the lateral plane. Some patients exhibit a superimposed 3 Hz for-

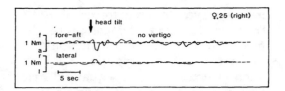

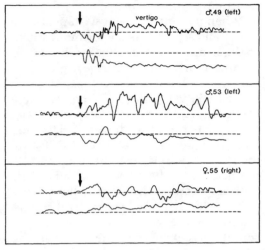

FIG 7–6.
Original recordings of forward-backward *(fore-aft)* and lateral body sway of four patients suffering from BPPV. When vertigo is elicited (patients 2, 3, and 4), a destabilization occurs mainly in the forward-backward direction with simultaneous increase in amplitude of sway and shift of the center of gravity forward and laterally, with the lateral shift always occurring toward the affected ear. If no vertigo is evoked, postural instability is minimal and only reflects the slight shift of body mass due to head tilt (patient 1).

ward-backward sway, an oscillator-like tremor of body posture as described in chronic alcoholics with paleocerebellar atrophy.[39]

The measurable shift of the center of gravity in the forward direction, and ipsilateral to the tilted head, can be interpreted as the motor compensation for the initial subjective vertigo in the opposite direction, the diagonal plane being identical to the spatial plane and working range of the ipsilateral posterior canal.[28] Thus, compensation for the initial perceived (subjective) fall caused by the lesion occurs in such a way that a measurable (objective) fall results in the opposite direction. Posturographic data are consistent with the hypothesis that the posterior canal is responsible for the generation of paroxysmal peripheral positioning vertigo.

Posturographic measurements performed by Black and Nashner[17] were unable to distinguish three groups of patients: those with unilateral or bilateral loss of peripheral vestibular function, those with BPPV without peripheral vestibular deficit, and those with the combination of both BPPV and peripheral vestibular deficit. Patients were exposed to either a stable or a moving foot support, and to variable visual surroundings. The authors concluded from their results that the BPPV patients principally use visual information to compensate for the postural destabilization induced by a vestibular irritation, whereas a peripheral vestibular deficit causes a disturbed adaptive reorganization of visual and postural references for orientation in space. Vestibulospinal compensation results, therefore, from either suppression of vestibular inputs or from simultaneous selection of an alternative reference for orientation: vision or support. Clinicians are well aware that patients in the acute phase of BPPV also complain of unsteadiness in gait and postural balance, which they describe as "walking on pillows." These symptoms can be classified as otolithic vertigo, and can be attributed to the suddenly unequal weights on the maculae of the two utricles which generate a vestibular tone imbalance. Impairment of control of posture and gait usually shows a gradual improvement in the following days or weeks, which reflects either central compensation or peripheral restitution of the equal weights.

It is not easy to examine utricular function in isolation in human subjects, but one possible source of information is dynamic ocular counterrolling, a reflex that appears to depend on the utricular otolith organs. Markham et al.[88] described abnormal ocular counterrolling in 16 of 18 patients with BPPV tested by rotating the body about two axes with the head fixed in relation to the body. The two axes were the naso-occipital

and the submental-vertex (barbecue rotation), which provided a more sensitive indicator of utricular dysfunction than the naso-occipital. The most common dysfunctions were disconjugate eye movements and hypoactivity. Further, subjects were more sensitive to ipsilateral tilt than to contralateral. This agrees with our own experience in patients with acute BPPV, who show significant deviations of the subjective visual vertical when they adjust a test bar to perceived vertical.

Management

Based on the mechanical hypothesis of cupulolithiasis we constructed an effective physical therapy for these patients in order to promote the loosening and ultimate dispersion of the degenerated otolithic material from the cupula of the posterior canal.[23] Specifically, patients are instructed to provoke systematically vertigo attacks by repeatedly tilting their upper trunk and head in the challenging position, with the lateral aspects of their occiput resting on the bed. This ensures proper plane-specific stimulation of the posterior semicircular canal. They remain in this position until the evoked vertigo subsides, or for at least 30 seconds and then by a 180° assuming the opposite head-down position for a further 30 seconds. The sequence of positioning is repeated about five times during each session. The maneuvers are carried out by the patients themselves every 3 hours while awake, and are terminated after 2 consecutive vertigo-free days. In extreme cases, when patients are subject to nausea, or in particularly anxious patients, vestibular sedative drugs such as dimenhydrinate or scopolamine are given during the first 1 to 3 days of the physical therapy.

This simple physical approach has lead to relief in the majority of cases[23, 67] within 1 to 4 weeks (Fig 7–7), even if the vertigo had lasted for months before the initiation of the therapy. In post-traumatic forms a slight but minimally distressing BPPV may persist

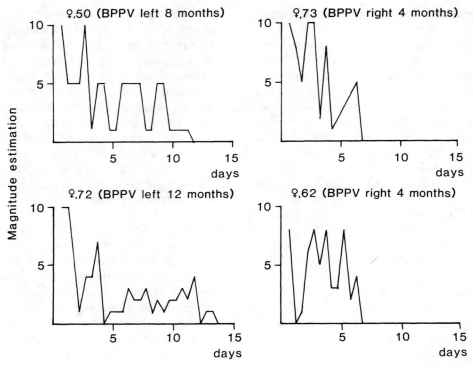

FIG 7–7.
Time course of individual recovery during the course of physical therapy in four patients with BPPV. Daily subjective estimates of vertigo reflect the irregular time course of recovery, which is different for each patient and independent of the duration of the disease prior to therapy onset. The abrupt relief of symptoms followed by equally abrupt worsening is seen in the *patients at the right* supports a purely physical mechanism rather than central compensation by habituation: after 7 days possibly the cupula became free of heavy otoconia and thus no more vertiginous attacks were elicited by positioning maneuvers (From Brandt T: *Vertigo: Its Multisensory Syndromes.* London, Springer, 1991. Used by permission.)

which is unresponsive to physical training. The time course of individual recovery, undulating and with abrupt remissions, supports a purely physical mechanism rather than central compensation by habituation (see Fig 7–7).

In the rare patients not responding even to prolonged physical therapy, surgical transection of the posterior ampullary nerve by a middle ear approach can be considered.[48, 49] This operation provides relief of vertigo; it is, however, not easy to locate the posterior ampullary nerve surgically, and sensorineural hearing loss is one of several possible postsurgical complications.[41, 49] In our experience with hundreds of BPPV patients there are only a few individuals who did not respond well to physical therapy and who ultimately required selective surgi-

cal transection of the posterior ampullary nerve. Recently, an alternative surgical procedure of transmastoid posterior semicircular canal occlusion has been described for intractable BPPV.[102] Drug therapy with anti–motion sickness medications reduces nausea but has not been proved to be a particularly efficacious treatment of BPPV.

Horizontal Semicircular Canal BPPV?

McClure[86] described paroxysmal nystagmus in some patients which possibly originated from stimulation of the horizontal semicircular canal. This was supported by Katsarkas,[79] who reported a small number of patients with unusual paroxysmal positioning nystagmus (for example, it may be purely horizontal or rotatory-linear, with the fast phases in the opposite direction to that usually observed). This is possibly compatible with excitation of the posterior or horizontal semicircular canal of the lowermost ear, or with excitation of the superior canal of the uppermost ear. In four of five patients with suspected horizontal canal BPPV sinusoidal rotational tests revealed a reduced phase shift of eye velocity relative to head velocity at 0.04 Hz compared with normal subjects.[90] This change was attributed to either reduced elasticity of the cupula or increased viscous friction of the canal fluid.

Bending-Over Vertigo

A combination of mechanisms similar to that described for head-extension vertigo (discussed later in this chapter) would be applicable in explaining the common symptom of vertigo upon bending over at the waist.[24] An added consideration is the transient increase in intracranial pressure (secondary to increased cephalic venous pressure) being transmitted to the perilymphatic space surrounding the endolymphatic membrane.

CLINICAL ENTITIES: POSITIONAL TESTING

Spontaneous Nystagmus: Peripheral Vestibular System Disease

Spontaneous vestibular nystagmus is mostly horizontal-rotatory (clockwise, left beating; or counterclockwise, right beating). The nystagmus is typically reduced in amplitude by fixation (fixation suppression) and enhanced by eye closure or use of Frenzel's (high plus diopter) lenses. According to Alexander's law, spontaneous nystagmus is increased with gaze shifts toward the fast phase, and decreased with gaze shifts toward the slow phase of the nystag-

mus. This may mimic gaze-evoked nystagmus in a patient with moderate spontaneous nystagmus which is completely suppressed by fixation straight ahead but still present with the gaze directed toward the fast phase. Positional testing may unspecifically facilitate spontaneous nystagmus.

In the acute stage of peripheral (labyrinth, vestibular nerve) vestibular system disease (for example, vestibular neuritis, herpes zoster oticus), horizontal spontaneous nystagmus beats toward the unaffected ear. After recovery, spontaneous nystagmus in some patients transiently reverses its direction *(Erholungsnystagmus or recovery nystagmus)* when the centrally compensated lesion regains function. The direction of spontaneous nystagmus is less conclusive in other labyrinthine disorders such as Meniere's disease or perilymph fistulas.

Spontaneous Nystagmus: Central Nervous Systems Disease

A spontaneous nystagmus that is *purely* horizontal (for example, as opposed to horizontal rotary) in direction and not attenuated by fixation is caused by a central lesion. More often central spontaneous nystagmus is mixed linear-rotary or purely rotary or vertical. It is evoked by acute lesions adjacent to the vestibular nuclei, such as in pontomedullary infarction (Wallenberg's syndrome).

Periodic Alternating Nystagmus

This occurs with a variety of cerebellar conditions and is a spontaneous horizontal nystagmus that reverses its direction approximately every 2 minutes.

Acquired Pendular Nystagmus

This type of nystagmus is usually a small-amplitude, vertical (torsional) oscillation at a frequency of 2 to 7 Hz, sometimes disconjugate or purely monocular. Multiple sclerosis is the most common cause.

Downbeat Nystagmus

When downbeat nystagmus occurs in the primary position of gaze, or more particularly on lateral gaze, it is often accompanied by oscillopsia and postural instability. It is due to a lesional tone imbalance of the vertical VOR in the pitch plane and is almost specific to structural lesions of the paramedian craniocervical junction (25% of patients with Arnold-Chiari malformation).

Upbeat Nystagmus

This type of nystagmus in the primary position of gaze with concomitant oscillopsia and postural instability is a pendent of downbeat nystagmus and most probably reflects an imbalance of vertical VOR in the pitch plane. Static head tilt to the prone and supine positions modifies the characteristics of upbeat nystagmus in most cases[45]; it may be enhanced but is mostly suppressed (Fig 7–8). Two separate brain stem lesions in the pontomesencephalic junction and in the medulla near the perihypoglossal nuclei are likely to be responsible for this syndrome.

Congenital Nystagmus

Congenital nystagmus is usually horizontal, with abnormal wave forms. It is activated by fixation, modulated by gaze direction, and diminished by convergence. Some patients exhibit additional head oscillations or a head turn; changes in head position relative to the gravitational field are ineffective. An inverted optokinetic nystagmus (as tested by an hand-held rotatory optokinetic drum) is almost pathognomonic. History taking is most important, as the condition is usually diagnosed during infancy.

Spontaneous Nystagmus: Influence of Drugs/Medications

The list of drugs that may have adverse effects on eye movements and balance is impressive (Tables 7–5 and 7–6). The administration of these drugs in therapeutic doses may result in spontaneous nystagmus.

Positional Nystagmus/Vertigo With Specific Gravity Differential Between Cupula and Endolymph: The Buoyancy Hypothesis

Transient positional nystagmus has been repeatedly described following the ingestion of water-soluble molecules with differing specific gravities, such as alcohol or heavy water. The semicircu-

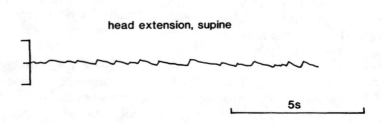

FIG 7–8.
Original ENG recording of vertical eye movements in a patient with upbeat nystagmus. The nystagmus is damped by static head tilt to the supine position *(bottom)*.

TABLE 7–5.

Toxic Oculomotor Disturbances*

Oculomotor Sign	Toxic Agent
Gaze-evoked nystagmus or saccadic pursuit	Phenytoin, carbamazepine, barbiturates, alcohol, benzodiazepines, methadone, chloral hydrate, marijuana
Slow saccades	Barbiturates, alcohol, benzodiazepines, fentanyl, vestibular sedatives (dimenhydrinate, scopolamine)
Impaired vestibulo-ocular reflex (VOR)	Vestibular sedatives (dimenhydrinate, scopolamine), barbiturates, alcohol, benzodiazepines
Exaggerated VOR	Industrial solvents (xylene, styrene, trichloroethylene, methylchloroform)
Internuclear ophthalmoplegia	Phenytoin, barbiturates, tricyclic antidepressants, bromides, hepatic coma
External ophthalmoplegia	Phenytoin, barbiturates, tricyclic antidepressants (imipramine, doxepin, amitriptyline)
Vertical gaze palsy	Barbiturates/primidone
Skew deviation	Lithium, hepatic coma
Downbeat nystagmus/vertigo	Phenytoin, barbiturates, lithium, alcohol, magnesium depletion, vitamin B_{12} deficiency
Upbeat nystagmus/vertigo	Antiepileptics, tobacco
Periodic alternating nystagmus	Phenytoin
Central positional nystagmus	Barbiturates, mercury compounds, industrial solvents (xylene, styrene, trichloroethylene, methylchloroform)
Labyrinthine positional nystagmus	Alcohol, glycerol, "heavy" water
Opsoclonus	Amitriptyline, haloperidol, lithium, thallium, chlordecone, DDT

*From Brandt T: *Vertigo: Its Multisensory Syndromes*. London, Springer, 1991. Used by permission.

lar canals selectively transduce angular velocity and acceleration, and under normal circumstances are insensitive to gravitational orientation and linear acceleration. A major reason for the lack of sensitivity is that the cupula and endolymph have the same specific gravity (the sensory hair cells are embedded in the cupula, which is housed in the ampulla of the canals). The neutral buoyancy of the cupula in the endolymph prevents any out-of-balance forces when linear accelerations are applied. If a considerable specific gravity differential occurs between cupula and endolymph, then the semicircular canals should become sensitive to changes in head position within the gravitational field (see Fig 7–9), resulting in positional rotatory vertigo and nystagmus. The direction of nystagmus and vertigo should be dependent on the particular head position (according to the different planes of the horizontal and vertical semicircular canals) and on whether the specific gravity of the cupula is greater or less than that of the endolymph. Thus, nystagmus should be direction-changing with either head position right lateral or left lateral, beating toward the undermost ear, with the cupula heavier than endolymph.

This hypothesis, known as *the buoyancy hypothesis*, requires that ingested compounds of different specific gravity diffuse at different speeds into the cupula and endolymph, thus causing the transient density gradient. Experiments were prompted with ethanol,[94] deuterium oxide,[95] and glycerol,[103] which all induced positional nystagmus consistent with the hypothesis.

Several questions are raised when considering the pathophysiologic concept of a gravity differential between cupula and endolymph which causes either a positional (alcohol, glycerol, heavy water, macroglobulinemia) or a positioning vertigo/nystagmus (cupulolithiasis). Why is positional alcohol nystagmus (see Fig 7–9) maintained over minutes and hours in the precipi-

TABLE 7–6.

Oculomotor Abnormalities Caused by Toxic Agents*

Drugs and toxic agents	Oculomotor abnormalities
Phenytoin	Gaze-evoked nystagmus, saccadic pursuit, external ophthalmoplegia, internuclear ophthalmoplegia. Rare: periodic alternating nystagmus, downbeat nystagmus/vertigo
Carbamazepine	Gaze-evoked nystagmus, saccadic pursuit, impairment of optokinetic nystagmus, external ophthalmoplegia, downbeat nystagmus/vertigo, oculogyric crises
Barbiturates/primidone	Gaze-evoked nystagmus, saccadic pursuit, impairment of optokinetic nystagmus, slow saccades, vertical gaze palsy, external ophthalmoplegia, impairment of vestibulo-ocular reflex (VOR), internuclear ophthalmoplegia, central positional nystagmus, impaired vergence, decreased accommodative convergence/accommodation ratio
Alcohol	Labyrinthine positional vertigo, saccadic pursuit, slow saccades, downbeat nystagmus/vertigo
Benzodiazepines	Saccadic pursuit, slow saccades, impairment of VOR, impairment of gaze-holding
Tricyclic antidepressants	Internuclear ophthalmoplegia, external ophthalmoplegia, opsoclonus
Tricyclic antidepressants and L-tryptophan	Ocular oscillations and myoclonus
Bromides	Internuclear ophthalmoplegia
Vestibular sedatives	Impairment of VOR, slow saccades
Lithium	Alternating skew deviation, opsoclonus, downbeat nystagmus/vertigo
Thallium	Opsoclonus
Phenothiazines	Internuclear ophthalmoplegia, oculogyric crises
Methadone	Saccadic pursuit, saccadic hypometria
Haloperidol	Opsoclonus
Marijuana	Gaze-evoked nystagmus, saccadic pursuit
Amphetamine	Increased accommodative convergence/accommodation ratio
Mercury	Spontaneous and/or positional nystagmus, impairment of optokinetic nystagmus
Chemotherapeutic anticancer agents	Vestibular/hearing loss
Loop diuretics (ethacrynic acid, frusemide)	Transient vestibular/hearing loss, impaired VOR
Aminoglycoside antibiotics (gentamicin, streptomycin)	Permanent vestibular hearing loss
Acetylsalicylic acid	Transient vestibulocochlear impairment
Industrial solvents (xylene, trichloroethylene)	Central positional nystagmus, exaggerated VOR, impaired fixation suppression of VOR

*From Brandt T: *Vertigo: Its Multisensory Syndrome.* London, Springer, 1991. Used by permission.

tating head position? Is it because the gravity-dependent deflection force is greater than the physiologic restoring force? This phenomenon would be consistent with a constant deflection of the cupula, providing constant stimulation to the hair cells. In this model, the gravitational force would be balanced by the elastic restoring force of the cupula tissue at some deflected position. The nor-

mal time constant (7 seconds time constant of the cupula) seems to be the result of the endolymph viscosity opposing the elastic restoring force intrinsic to the cupula when the stimulus is removed. What is perhaps mysterious, however, is the apparent lack of adaptation of the hair cells implied by this long-duration response.

On the other hand, if the concept of

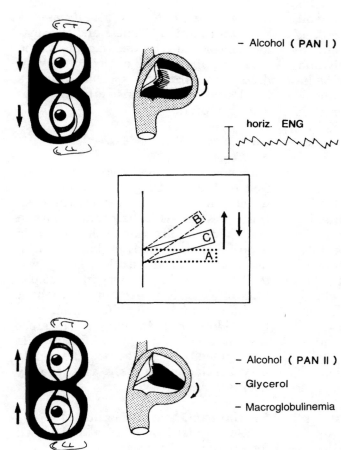

- Alcohol (PAN I)

horiz. ENG

- Alcohol (PAN II)
- Glycerol
- Macroglobulinemia

horiz. ENG

FIG 7–9.
Ingestion of water-soluble molecules with differing specific weights such as alcohol, heavy water, or glycerol causes the specific gravity differential between cupula and endolymph (buoyancy hypothesis) with positional nystagmus and vertigo. During the resorption phase of alcohol, nystagmus beats toward the undermost ear (*PAN I*, with the cupula relatively lighter than endolymph). Positional nystagmus beats toward the uppermost ear during alcohol-reduction phase (*PAN II*) as well as in glycerol-, heavy water-, and macroglobulinemia-induced positional nystagmus (with the cupula relatively heavier than endolymph). The gravity-dependent deflection force on the cupula (*B in insert*) must be greater than the physiologic restoring force (*C in insert*) in order for the positional nystagmus to last as long as the precipitating head position is maintained.

cupulolithiasis ("heavy cupula") is valid, then it remains unclear why patients with BPPV do not suffer from additional positional vertigo/nystagmus. Similarly, compounds with differing specific weights such as alcohol or heavy water should be able to induce not only positional but also positioning nystagmus with rapid changes in head position. In the case of alcohol this positioning nystagmus [positional alcohol vertigo/nystagmus (PAN)] should beat toward the same direction as positional nystagmus during the resorption phase (PAN I, when the cupula is relatively lighter) and toward the opposite direction during the reduction phase (PAN II, when the cupula is relatively heavier). Further experiments are needed in order to clarify these discrepancies between theory and clinical manifestation.

Positional Alcohol Vertigo/ Nystagmus

Barany[15] described the direction-changing characteristics of PAN in humans with changes in head position (beating toward the undermost ear), which was later proved in animals.[36, 50, 106] Walter[127] reported that the direction of PAN reverses (beating toward the uppermost ear) hours after alcohol intake. This phenomenon was later termed PAN II by Aschan et al.[8, 9] and Money et al.[94, 95] Peripheral labyrinthine origin of PAN was suggested by observations that it does not occur after loss of labyrinthine function in humans[64] and in animals.[100] This argument, however, is not convincing because central positional nystagmus is also dependent on peripheral graviceptive input.

Alcohol is lighter than endolymph, and when blood levels approach 40 mg/dL, alcohol diffuses into the cupula, rendering it lighter than endolymph, thereby transforming the semicircular canals into gravity-sensitive receptors.[95] Nystagmus and vertigo then occur when the subject lies down. In phase I of PAN, the nystagmus beats toward the undermost ear (Fig 7–9; Table 7–7). With time, blood alcohol diffuses into the endolymph, equalizing its specific gravity to that of the cupula. There is then a "silent (intermediate) period", beginning between 3.5 and 5 hours after cessation of alcohol ingestion, when positional vertigo is absent. Alcohol selectively diffuses out of the cupula before it leaves the endolymph. This causes the cupula to be transiently denser than the endolymph, thus initiating phase II of PAN, which begins between 5 and 10 hours after cessation of drinking when there is a falling blood level at about 20 mg/dL. In PAN II, nystagmus beats to the uppermost ear.

Positional vertigo may persist until all alcohol eventually leaves the endolymph (equalizing the specific gravities of the endolymph and the cupula), but this may not transpire until many hours after the blood alcohol level has

reached zero. PAN II is usually associated with motion sickness and is a major concomitant of the hangover. The "morning after" drink of alcohol may indeed reequalize the specific gravities and lessen, at least transiently, the untoward symptoms.[24]

Positional "Heavy Water" Nystagmus

Money and Myles[95] described ingestion of 100 to 200 g deuterium oxide, which caused a vigorous lateral positional nystagmus lasting some hours in man, with a directional characteristic opposite to that of postural alcohol nystagmus. Deuterium oxide ("heavy water") has a molecular weight of 20.030 (that of water is 18.016), and is thought to diffuse earlier into the cupula than the endolymph. As long as a great enough specific gravity deferential is maintained between the two, the cupula may act inappropriately as a gravity transducer.

Positional Glycerol Nystagmus

The standard doses of glycerol used for obtaining diagnostic audiograms in patients with suspected Meniere's disease can cause transient positional nystagmus. This was first observed in a sin-

TABLE 7–7.

Positional Alcohol Nystagmus (PAN)

Phase	Nystagmus	Time	Mechanism
PAN I (resorption phase)	Direction changing rotational vertigo and *nystagmus* with head right or left, beating toward the *undermost ear*	30 min after oral administration; duration, 3 to 4 hr	With blood levels of 25 to 40 mg/100 mL, diffusion into the cupula makes alcohol lighter than endolymph, and sensitive to gravity changes
"Silent (intermediate) period"	No positional vertigo/nystagmus	3 to 5 hr after alcohol ingestion	Alcohol diffuses also into the endolymph: equal specific gravity of cupula and endolymph
PAN II (reduction phase)	"Hangover vertigo" with direction changing positional *nystagmus* with head right or left, toward the *uppermost ear*	5 to 10 hr after alcohol ingestion	Alcohol stays longer in the endolymph, causing a specific gravity differential with the cupula being "heavier"

gle case by Angelborg et al.[7] and later studied more systematically by Rietz et al.[103] In their study, five of six subjects exhibited a positional nystagmus that was maximal 120 minutes after glycerol ingestion, shortly after peak serum levels were achieved. From their data, Rietz et al.[103] inferred that different transport velocities of the compound result in a postural nystagmus toward the uppermost ear. This concept is supported by animal studies in guinea pigs in which Yoshida et al.[131] found that endolymphatic pressure dropped 15 minutes after intravenous administration of glycerol (when glycerol enters the cupula?) lasting for at least another 25 minutes, at which point glycerol entering the endolymph (re)balances the osmotic gradient. The duration of postural glycerol nystagmus, most pronounced between 90 and 240 minutes after oral ingestion,[103] indicates that glycerol does not enter the endolymph for at least 2 hours after oral administration.

Positional Nystagmus With Macroglobulinemia (Waldenström's Disease)

Malignant lymphoproliferative Waldenström's disease with macroglobulinemia can have auditory and vestibular manifestations in as many as 10% to 20% of those afflicted.[42, 85] Various explanations of these manifestations have been proposed: increased blood viscosity with obstruction in the venules,[6] stagnation or sudden release of clotting factors,[104, 107] associated neurologic dysfunction,[19] or hemorrhage.[4] Vascular vertigo in the hyperviscosity syndrome is most likely due to obstruction of the venules and capillaries with peripheral vestibular hypoxia.[6] This mechanism does not explain positional vertigo in Waldenström's disease.

Keim and Sachs[83] reported on 5 patients, 3 of whom gave a history of periodic dizziness with postural changes. They were able to record a direction-changing positional nystagmus with a latent period and fatigue in 1 patient, who simultaneously reported rotatory vertigo with nausea and visual disturbance. The 2 others, symptom-free at the time of otoneurologic investigation, did not exhibit positional nystagmus. Because molecular weights in macroglobulinemia of over one million are possible, as opposed to normal gamma globulin values with a molecular weight of approximately 150,000, Keim and Sachs[83] stress the increased specific gravity of the cupula as the causative factor, which varies with concentration of the circulating protein and the diffusion characteristics.

Central Positional Vertigo

When the position of the head is brought to an off-vertical, lateral, or head-hanging position a change in graviceptive (otolithic) input occurs. This change is the precipitating factor for central positional vertigo. The most probable explanation for this response is a vestibular tone imbalance with directional positional nystagmus and rotational/linear vertigo caused by disinhibition of the vestibular responses on perception, eye-, head-, and body position.[21] Thus, it is not (as one might speculate) the head position–dependent dislocation of the mass and intracerebral structures which causes the manifestations.

There are a variety of central positional vertigo syndromes resulting as a consequence of a mass (tumor, hematoma) near the fourth ventricle and the vestibular nuclei (Fig 7–10). These are characterized by rotational vertigo, nystagmus, and postural imbalance, which may be abrupt and more violent than in peripheral labyrinthine dysfunctions. This severe form of central positional vertigo, which initially immobilizes the patient, gradually improves within days to weeks. The central vestibular pathways involved are not yet known. It is known, however, that the typical site of the lesion is dorsolateral to the fourth ventricle.

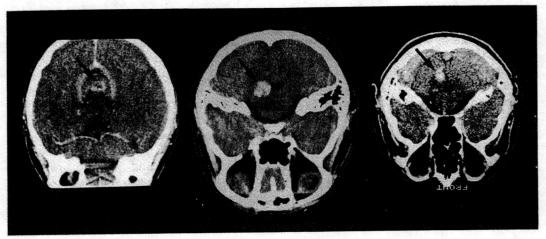

FIG 7–10.
Severe central positional vertigo is usually induced by infratentorial lesions *(arrows)* dorsolateral of the fourth ventricle (computed tomographic scans *left* and *center,* in patient with cerebellar hemorrhages) or the vestibulocerebellum (cystic vermis tumor, scan at *right*).

Positional nystagmus without concomitant vertigo is always central; however, the direction of the nystagmus varies. It may beat diagonally or toward the undermost or uppermost ear. Frequently it is bilateral and direction changing when the head is tilted toward the right or left, respectively.

The frequency of central positional nystagmus is usually low and constant, which distinguishes it from BPPV. Differentiation between central positional nystagmus and BPPV is based not only on the direction of the nystagmus but also on the lack of a latency period after movement to the provoking position. In addition, there is a lack of fatigability and habituation on repetitive stimulation.

Central positional nystagmus is indicative of a posterior fossa lesion. The probable locations are the caudal brain stem and the vestibulocerebellum; however, the condition does not allow for a more precise localization. Computed tomography and magnetic resonance imaging are also insufficient in determining the location of the lesion. The possible causes are similar to those of positional downbeating nystagmus, and we have also seen it with rapidly developing hydrocephalus if it involves the

fourth ventricle. It is our experience that central positional nystagmus occurs frequently in the elderly (lacunar ischemia?) and often recovers spontaneously (central compensation?).

There is some evidence, from experiments in animals, that posterior cerebellar vermis lesions may cause positional nystagmus which mimics BPPV.[5] The clinical relevance of this central "pseudo-BPPV has been repeatedly stressed[56, 109, 128]; however, it should not be overestimated because of its rarity. Other reports that *Borrelia* infections are a possible causative factor for both peripheral and central positional nystagmus[105] still need to be proved and analyzed more thoroughly.

Positional Downbeating Nystagmus

Positional downbeating nystagmus, with only slight vertigo with the patient in the head-hanging position, is indicative of a vestibulocerebellar nodular lesion. It may be related to the downbeat nystagmus syndrome, which also shows activation on head extension. Experimental extirpation of the nodulus in the cat causes postural downbeat nystagmus.[43] This has also been confirmed by clinical experience.[65, 82] Physiologically, the nodulus may have an inhibitory influence on the gain of the VOR.[44] Lesional postural downbeat nystagmus can be abolished by additional bilateral labyrinthectomy.[5] Thus, without labyrinthine graviceptive input there is no positional nystagmus.

Positional downbeating nystagmus, with or without slight positional vertigo in the head-hanging position, is a frequent and often the only clinical sign in neurologic patients. It may spontaneously recover or persist. It may be caused by multiple sclerosis, ischemia, intoxication, craniocervical malformation, or cerebellar degeneration; however, sometimes there is no identifiable cause in elderly patients. Brain imaging techniques in most cases do not show a vestibulocerebellar lesion.

"Basilar Insufficiency"

Nystagmus, vertigo, and postural imbalance induced with the head maximally rotated and/or extended while standing and terminated abruptly by returning the head to a neutral upright position are frequently reported experiences. Clinicians usually attribute these symptoms to intermittent basilar insufficiency caused by a functional compression of the vertebral artery, particularly in elderly patients with atheromas or with cervical spondylosis and osteophytes narrowing the transverse foramina.[37, 118, 130]

Transient attacks of vertigo of central origin are the most common early symptom of basilar insufficiency because of the steep pressure gradient from the aorta to the terminal pontine arteries, which are long, tenuous, circumferential arteries and therefore provide a most vulnerable blood supply for the vestibular nuclei.[130] The possibility cannot be excluded that transient ischemia of the labyrinths may also contribute, as blood supply originates from the same source. Experimental studies on blood flow in cadavers reveal that extreme head positions may reduce flow through one or another of the vertebral or carotid vessels.[124] Thus, vestibular vertigo and ataxia and drop attacks can be undoubtedly precipitated by extreme extension or rotation of the neck, at least when a partial obstruction of the arteries combines with a sudden fall of systemic blood pressure, for example, in a patient rising from a chair and looking up. An association of dysfunctions that convinces the clinician in the diagnosis is that of vertigo with visual illusions, field defects, diplopia, dysphagia, dysarthria, drop attacks, or motor symptoms.

Head-Extension Vertigo

Apart from basilar insufficiency, however, symptoms of to-and-fro vertigo and postural imbalance occur frequently in healthy people, such as that elicited by overhead work while standing on an unstable wobbling ladder or in situations in which visual cues conflict with proprioceptive input (looking up at moving clouds).

Vertigo and postural imbalance terminate abruptly when the head is flexed to a neutral position. The symptoms are also often attributed to intermittent vertebral artery occlusions caused by the head posture, particularly in the elderly. The symptoms, however, occur frequently in young people, and a physiologic explanation is presented based on an unusual combination of multisensory inputs from the stabilizing systems.[24, 26] The "normal" instability related to this head position can be determined by attempting to balance on one foot with the eyes closed and head extended as compared with the neutral head position.

The otoliths are beyond their optimal functioning range in the offending head-extended position.[26] When the body is supine, the otoliths are in the same position relative to the plane of gravity but are not, in this situation, involved in postural control. The otoliths are also out of optimal range with head flexion, but vertigo is not induced. Flexion, however, is a common position.

Repetitive challenges are required for

central adjustments of motor responses to the patterns of multisensory inputs to develop. Infrequently occurring stimulation patterns would not be associated with appropriately calibrated engrams.

Visual cues, correcting for the postural imbalance, would be less effective with one's head extended because of the change in egocentric spatial coordinates (with respect to retinal shift up-and-down becomes forward-and-backward). Moreover, the direction of compensatory body sway must be corrected to reflect the change in coordinates. In situations in which visual cues are absent (eyes closed or in darkness) or conflicting (looking up at moving clouds), the postural imbalance is greatly worsened. When somatosensory input is varied (for example, when the person is standing on a piece of foam rubber, as in patients with sensory polyneuropathy), the symptoms of instability also increase.

OTHER POSITIONAL/ POSITIONING ENTITIES

Head Motion Intolerance With Bilateral Vestibulopathy

The characteristics and origins of bilateral vestibulopathy are summarized in Table 7–8. Bilateral vestibular loss causes unsteadiness of gait and oscillopsia associated with head movements or when walking. This is due to an inappropriate VOR, and excessive motion of images on the retina was measured in these patients while walking.[57] The condition can be identified by a simple bedside test of the VOR (see Fig 7–2) as well as by the decreased ocular motor responses to thermic irrigation and angular acceleration.

Some ototoxic drugs (for example, streptomycin, gentamicin) are known to damage the peripheral vestibular sensory cells in advance of those in cochlea (hair cell damage of the inner ear). Kanamycin, tobramycin, and neomycin preferentially damage the auditory sensory cells,[115] whereas more recent ami-

TABLE 7–8.

Profile of Bilateral Vestibulopathy*

Clinical syndrome
  Symptoms
    Unsteadiness of gait (particularly in dark)
    Oscillopsia with head movements (e.g., when walking)
  Signs
    Oculomotor hyporesponsiveness to thermic irrigation and angular rotation
    Pathologic vestibulo-ocular reflex bedside test
Etiology
  Ototoxic drugs
  Meningitis, labyrinthine infections
  Bilateral sequential vestibular neuritis
  Tumors (neurofibromatosis)
  Endolymphatic hydrops (delayed endolymphatic hydrops)
  Polyneuropathy
  Autoimmune inner ear disease
  Otosclerosis
  Paget's disease
  Congenital malformation
  Familial vestibular areflexia
  Vertebrobasilar ischaemia (?)
  Vestibular atelectasis (?)
  Vestibular aging (?)
  Idiopathic bilateral vestibulopathy(?)
Management
  Controlled physical exercise consisting of voluntary head movements about different axes when fixating a target, and balance training (recruitment of compensatory nonvestibular control capacities, somatosensory and visual)

*From Brandt T: *Vertigo: Its Multisensory Syndromes.* London, Springer, 1991. Used by permission.

noglycosides such as dibekacin or ribostamycin are less ototoxic.[110] Hair cells and cochlear neurons may be transiently (reversibly) damaged by diuretics (ethacrynic acid; furosemide) or high-dose salicylate therapy.[99, 115] Combined use of loop-inhibiting diuretics and aminoglycoside antibiotics can cause permanent hearing loss.[10] Permanent loss of hair cells sometimes occurs with alkylating anticancer chemotherapeutics.[115]

Independent of those produced by ototoxins, single cases of "progressive vestibular degeneration" of unknown cause have been described with the following factors in common: repeated episodes of dizziness relatively early in life, bilateral loss of vestibular function with retention of hearing, and freedom from other neurologic disturbances.[38, 55, 59]

Bilateral vestibulopathy may occur for other more common reasons such as meningitis, labyrinthine infection, bilateral tumors (Fig 7–11), endolymphatic hydrops, inner ear autoimmune disease, or congenital malformation.[31, 119] Autoimmune disease of the inner ear can produce both vestibular and auditory loss.[69] Permanent bilateral loss of vestibular function has also been described for bilateral sequential vestibular neuritis.[117] There are, however, a considerable proportion of patients presenting with seemingly idiopathic bilateral vestibulopathy.[12] There is reason to assume that these patients reflect a heterogenous group of causes, some of which may be vascular.

Management

Controlled physical exercises, including voluntary head movements about all three axes and balance training, can improve the condition in patients with permanent bilateral vestibulopathy. This will recruit nonvestibular sensory capacities such as the cervico-ocular reflex or proprioceptive (somatosensory) control of stance and gait. The latter process of multisensory compensation is indirectly demonstrated by the significantly higher gain of cervico-ocular reflexes and arthrokinetic nystagmus in labyrinthine-defective subjects.[18]

Clinical Evidence for Cervical Vertigo?

The frequency and intensity of cervical vertigo should not be overestimated. Pain arising from the cervical spine with tenderness and limitation of movement of the neck, if associated with rotational vertigo and nystagmus, should not be called cervical vertigo. The characteristic symptom of cervical vertigo (Table 7–9) is more likely to be a sensa-

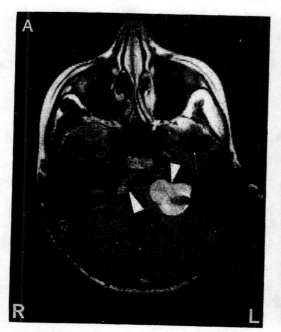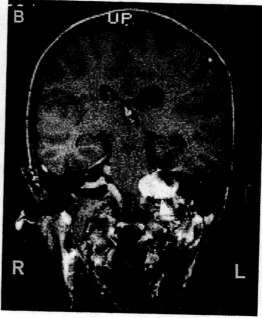

FIG 7–11.
Magnetic resonance images of a patient suffering from neurofibromatosis. Axial **(A)** and frontal **(B)** orientation after application of intravenous gadolinium-DTPA as a contrast agent [echo delay time (TE), 17 ms; pulse sequence repetition time (TR), 500 ms]. Multiple neuromas involve cranial nerves bilaterally. **A**, there is an intracanalicular acoustic neuroma *(arrow)* as well as hypoglossal neuroma. **B**, 3 years after surgical removal of an acoustic neuroma, an extracanalicular neuroma has reoccurred *(arrows)* pressing on and dislodging the pontine brain stem. (Courtesy of Dr. Vogl, Department of Radiology, University of Munich.)

TABLE 7-9.

Profile of Cervical Vertigo*

Experimental cervical vertigo (unilateral suboccipital anaesthesia)
    Rabbit, cat, monkey
        Ataxia with ipsilateral deviation of gait
        Positional nystagmus
        (contraversive horizontal nystagmus)
    Humans
        Sensation of floating and unsteadiness of gait
        Ataxia with increased ipsilateral and decreased
            contralateral extensor muscle tone
        Ipsiversive tendency to fall, and deviation of gait
        Ipsiversive past-pointing
        No spontaneous or positional nystagmus
Clinical cervical vertigo
    Ataxia and unsteadiness of gait associated with
        some neck pain or limitation of neck movement
    Mechanism
        Tone imbalance of upper two cervical root
            inputs?
    Incidence
        Unknown, no pathognomonic diagnostic test

*From Brandt T: *Vertigo: Its Multisensory Syndromes.* London, Springer, 1991. Used by permission.

tion of numbness or floating with ataxia of stance and gait, as can be inferred from the experimental vertigo induced by unilateral suboccipital local anaesthesia.[35] It is not known how traumatic, degenerative, inflammatory, or rheumatic disease affect neck sensory input.

This explains the various hypotheses, for example regarding cervical vertigo following whiplash injury. Suggested causes are the neuromuscular mechanism,[54] the neurovascular mechanism,[71, 129] or mechanical vascular obstruction of the vertebral artery.[33] The incidental observation of an improvement of post-traumatic vertigo and ataxia by use of a neck collar[68] was made earlier by Longet[86] in 1845. But head trauma and whiplash injury do not affect only neck structures. The otoliths are obviously more vulnerable to acceleration; damage causes otolith vertigo with a similar benign course to that of neck pain.[22] Furthermore, whiplash injuries frequently damage the brain,[101, 125] which makes interpretation of an abnormal vestibulo-ocular test difficult.[108, 123] Postural testing with head

extension as proposed by DeJong and Bles,[34] or nystagmus induced by passive head rotations[70, 98, 111] cannot clearly differentiate between healthy and diseased subjects.

Vertigo and/or Tinnitus Associated With Neurovascular Compression ("Disabling Positional Vertigo," "Vestibular Paroxysmia")

Neurovascular cross-compression of the root entry zone of the cranial nerves V, VII, and IX can cause local demyelination and axonal hyperactivity (for example, by transversely spreading ephaptic activation), accompanied by the distressing symptoms of trigeminal neuralgia, hemifacial spasm, and glossopharyngeal neuralgia. Compressing vessels which had made indentations on the relevant nerve or nerve root entry zone have been found surgically, and the efficacy of microvascular decompression as a successful treatment of these symptoms is well established.[74] These findings suggest that it is reasonable to search for a group of patients presenting with typical paroxysmal vestibular and/or cochlear symptoms, analogously caused by neurovascular compression of the eighth cranial nerve.

If vertigo is the major complaint, vascular compression must be causing abnormal impulse activity of the vestibular portion of the eighth cranial nerve. If vertigo and tinnitus are present, then both vestibular and cochlear portions of the eight nerve are compressed by one or more vessels, either the anterior inferior cerebellar artery (AICA), the posterior inferior cerebellar artery (PICA), or a vein. Compression may be due to vascular malformation of the posterior fossa,[30] arterial ectasia,[132] or simply to arterial aging with elongation and looping. It is well established that pulsatile compression of the caudal cranial nerves is more likely to be symptomatic when the central (oligodendroglia) myelin rather than the peripheral myelin is involved.

For the eighth cranial nerve this means that the entire intracranial portion from brain stem to the internal auditory canal (1 to 1.5 cm) may be particularly vulnerable. This syndrome was first described by Jannetta et al.[73] and later termed "disabling positional vertigo" by the same authors,[75, 93] a description for a most heterogeneous collection of signs and symptoms, and far from a reliable diagnosable disease entity. The lack of a well-defined syndrome, and of a diagnostic test, make it difficult for the nonsurgical clinician to "believe in" this interesting disease. However, it is possible that it plays an important role in the group of vertigo patients who do not respond to other treatment.

Hesitation in the diagnosis of this disorder is highly justifiable because retromastoid craniotomy and microvascular decompression of the eighth cranial nerve is the recommended procedure once the diagnosis has been established. This surgical procedure is still associated with a mortality of about 1% and a considerable morbidity of about 10%,[47, 97] even though others report lower mortality/morbidity rates. Selection criteria for the operation that have been proposed are insufficient, because they do not reliably exclude causes of vertigo other than neurovascular compression. Too many patients will be incorrectly selected for an unnecessary and risky operation. The surprisingly high improvement rate (16 of 21 patients became symptom free after operation[93]) is not significant proof of the diagnosis, since other common vertigo syndromes such as "phobic postural vertigo" can be treated rapidly and successfully by psychiatric methods. Furthermore, it is necessary to remember that decades passed before it was demonstrated that the success of "endolymphatic sac shunt operations" in the management of Meniere's disease was a result of a placebo effect.[122] This is the reason why the following description of the so called "disabling positional vertigo" should be accepted with critical reserve.

In their original paper Jannetta et al.[75] reported on 9 patients, all of whom showed vascular compression of the superior or inferior vestibular nerve (or both) at the brain stem, and 8 of whom experienced total relief of symptoms after microvascular decompression:

"We have found a certain kind of balance disorder that does not fulfill the criteria of the established syndromes just discussed (Meniere's disease, benign paroxysmal positional vertigo, vestibular-neuritis) and that does not respond to medical treatment. Patients with this disorder experience a constant positional vertigo or disequilibrium so severe that they are disabled and constantly nauseated; thus, the vertigo cannot be called benign."[75]

A more recent description of the syndrome in another 21 patients[93] is even less specific and more ambiguous. To complicate matters and further stretch the clinical spectrum of neurovascular compression syndromes, Møller[92] reports on 10 patients, all of whom had classical symptoms of Meniere's disease, but who, in addition, had audiologic signs indicating involvement of the auditory nerve. Because vertigo on its own does not allow identification of the site of the lesion, results of audiovestibular tests and brain stem auditory evoked potentials (BAEP) served as the basis for deciding which was most probably the affected side and the side that would eventually be subjected to surgical exploration. Those BAEP recordings with unilaterally increased latencies between the waves I and III were reported to be the most helpful. These patterns are similar to those seen in acoustic neuromas and indicate functionally significant lesions of the proximal cochlear portion (waves II) of the eighth cranial nerve.

First reports from other clinical centers do not clarify the muddle of signs and symptoms seemingly characteristic for this mysterious disease. Of 10 patients diagnosed as having neurovascular compression of the eighth cranial nerve, all were middle-aged and hypertensive, and most complained of paroxysmal vertigo lasting from hours to days, which was aggravated by changing head position (movement). Also, patients had persistent tinnitus and progressive unilateral hearing loss.[121] In contrast to the findings of Jannetta et al.[75] and Møller et al.,[93] there was no positional vertigo, and wave I of BAEP was prolonged in 6 cases, whereas the interpeak latency of waves I to III was normal in 5 cases.

In conclusion there is some evidence that neurovascular compression of the eighth cranial nerve can cause paroxysmal attacks and a persistent disabling vertigo/ataxia syndrome (mostly with tinnitus and some hearing loss) and that this can be successful treated by microvascular decompression procedures.

The proposed name of the disease, "disabling positional vertigo," is misleading. "Vestibular paroxysmia" might be a more appropriate term.[25] It is not only the position of the head but the movement (change in position) that seems to aggravate vertigo and postural imbalance in many patients. Neither the regular surgical finding of close vessel-nerve contact at the brain stem, nor the surprisingly high improvement rate following microvascular decompression unequivocally confirm the proposed diagnosis.

There is no pathognomonic sign for vestibular paroxysmia, and many elderly patients will exhibit some unilateral or bilateral deficit of cranial nerve function which may easily persuade the uncritical clinician to undertake an unnecessary posterior fossa craniotomy. Antivertigo drugs have been reported to be ineffective in these patients, but there is no evidence that antiepileptic drugs, such as carbamazepine, have been thoroughly tested. Carbamazepine, the drug of first choice for trigeminal neuralgia, was indeed effective in a few vertigo patients in whom we suspected a neurovascular compression syndrome of the eighth cranial nerve. Further information is required if the clinical picture presented by the eighth cranial nerve neurovascular compression syndrome is to be accurately defined.

CONCLUSIONS

Benign paroxysmal positioning vertigo due to cupulolithiasis or canalolithiasis is the most important disorder described in this chapter because it is the most common cause of vertigo in the elderly. Brief attacks of rotational vertigo and concomitant positioning-induced rotatory-linear nystagmus are precipitated by rapid extension of the head or by lateral head tilt toward the affected ear. Definitive diagnostic nystagmus criteria are latency of 1 to several seconds, beating direction rotating toward the undermost ear, duration of less than 1 minute, reversal of nystagmus direction with return of the patient to the upright position, and fatigability with repetition of the maneuver. Spontaneous recovery is common, but there is a highly effective form of mechanical therapy that involves the use of positioning maneuvers.

Positional alcohol (vertigo) nystagmus, when elicited by lateral head position, beats toward the undermost ear during the resorption phase of alcohol (PAN I) and toward the uppermost ear during the reduction phase (PAN II). It can be explained by the buoyancy hypothesis: A specific gravity differential between cupula and endolymph occurs when alcohol (which is lighter than endolymph) diffuses into the cupula, thereby transforming the semicircular canals into gravity-sensitive receptors.

Until recently there are no reliable clinical tests available by which to establish the diagnosis of cervical vertigo following whiplash injury, or neurovascular cross-compression ("vestibular paroxysmia"). Most cases of transient post-traumatic vertigo that manifests with head motion intolerance and unsteadiness of gait may be otolith vertigo. Central compensation (rearrangement) would account for the gradual recovery within days to weeks, supporting the view that exercise is the best therapy.

Central positional vertigo and/or nystagmus are disorders of intraaxial posterior fossa structures, particularly when involving vestibular nuclei and their connecting pathways to the vestibulocerebellum. These disorders are often associated with other oculomotor abnormalities such as saccadic smooth pursuit, gaze-evoked nystagmus, and upbeat or downbeat nystagmus. Positional nystagmus without vertigo is always central of origin. But lesions dorsolateral of the vestibular nuclei may cause a severe form of positioning/positional vertigo that includes nausea and vomiting. A lesional or toxic (drugs) disinhibition of (inhibitory) vestibulocerebellar Purkinje cell input onto vestibulo-ocular reflexes may be causative.

Positional and positioning tests may be contaminated by spontaneous vestibular nystagmus secondary to a peripheral (vestibular neuritis, Meniere's attack) or central (AICA or PICA infarction; Wallenberg's syndrome) vestibular tone imbalance. Spontaneous vestibular nystagmus is typically suppressed by fixation. Involuntary ocular oscillations which override fixation, such as congenital nystagmus or downbeat nystagmus or upbeat nystagmus, may mimic positional nystagmus in that they are modified in intensity by gaze direction (congenital nystagmus) or by static head tilt to the prone or supine position (downbeat/upbeat nystagmus).

REFERENCES

1. Aschan G: The pathogenesis of positional nystagmus. *Acta Otolaryngol [Suppl]* 1961; 159:90–93.

2. Barber HO, Stockwell CW: *Manual of Electronystagmography*. St Louis, Mosby–Year Book, 1976; pp 142–152.

3. Barber HO, Wright G: Positional nystagmus in normals. *Adv Otorhinolaryngol* 1973; 19:276.

4. Afifi AM, Tawfeek S: Deafness due to Waldenström macroglobulinaemia. *J Laryngol Otol* 1971; 85:275.

5. Allen G, Fernandez C: Experimental observations in postural nystagmus: Extensive lesions in posterior vermis of the cerebellum. *Acta Otolaryngol* 1960; 51:2–14.

6. Andrews JC, Hoover LA, Lee RS, et al: Vertigo in the hyperviscosity syndrome. *Otolaryngol Head Neck Surg* 1988; 98:144–149.

7. Angelborg C, Klockhoff I, Stahle J: The caloric response in Menière's disease during spontaneous and glycerin-induced changes of the hearing loss. *Acta Otolaryngol* 1971; 71:462–468.

8. Aschan G: Different types of alcohol nystagmus. *Acta Otolaryngol* 1958; 140:69–78.

9. Aschan G, Bergstedt M, Goldberg L, et al: Positional nystagmus in man during and after alcohol intoxication. *J Stud Alcohol* 1956; 17:381–405.

10. Baloh RW: *Dizziness, Hearing Loss, and Tinnitus: The Essentials of Neurootology*. Philadelphia, FA Davis, 1984.

11. Baloh RW, Honrubia V, Jacobson K: Benign positional vertigo. *Neurology* 1987; 37:371–378.

12. Baloh RW, Jacobson K, Honrubia V: Idiopathic bilateral vestibulopathy. *Neurology* 1989; 39:272–275.

13. Baloh RW, Sakala SM, Honrubia V: Benign paroxysmal positional nystagmus. *Am J Otolaryngol* 1979; 1:1–5.

14. Barber HO: Positional nystagmus especially after head injury. *Laryngoscope* 1964; 73:891–944.

15. Barany R: Experimentelle Alkoholintoxikation. *Monatsschr Ohrenheilkd* 1911; 45:959–962.

16. Barany R: Diagnose von Krankheitserscheinungen im Bereiche des Otolithenapparates. *Acta Otolaryngol* 1921; 2:434–437.

17. Black FO, Nashner LM: Vestibulo-spinal control differs in patients with reduced versus distorted vestibular function. *Acta Otolaryngol [Suppl]* 1984; 406:110–114.

18. Bles W, Klören T, Büchele W, et al: Somatosensory nystagmus: Physiological and clinical aspects. *Adv Otorhinolaryngol* 1983; 30:30–33.

19. Bolch KJ, Maki DG: Hyperviscosity syndrome associated with immunoglobulin abnormalities. *Semin Hematol* 1973; 10:113–124.

20. Brandt T: Vertigo and dizziness, in Asbury AK, McKhann GM, McDonald I (eds): *Diseases of the Nervous System*. Philadelphia, WB Saunders, 1986, pp 561–576.

21. Brandt T: Positional and positioning vertigo and nystagmus. *J Neurol Sci* 1990; 95:3–28.

22. Brandt T: *Vertigo, Its Multisensory Syndromes.* London, Springer-Verlag, 1991.

23. Brandt T, Daroff RB: Physical therapy for benign paroxysmal positional vertigo. *Arch Otolaryngol* 1980; 106:484–485.

24. Brandt T, Daroff RB: The multisensory physiological and pathological vertigo syndromes. *Ann Neurol* 1980; 7:195–203.

25. Brandt T, Dieterich M: Vertigo due to neurovascular compression, vestibular paroxysmia? *Nervenarzt* 1990; 61:376–378.

26. Brandt T, Krafczyk S, Malsbenden I: Postural imbalance with head extension: Improvement by training as a model for ataxia therapy. *Ann NY Acad Sci* 1981; 374:636–649.

27. Büchele W, Brandt T: Vestibulo-spinal ataxia in benign paroxysmal positional vertigo. *Aggressologie* 1979; 20:221–222.

28. Büchele W, Brandt T: Benign paroxysmal positional vertigo and posture, in Bles W, Brandt T, (eds): *Disorders of Posture and Gait.* Amsterdam, Elsevier, 1986, pp 141–156.

29. Büchele W, Brandt T: Vestibular neuritis—a horizontal semicircular canal paresis? *Adv Otorhinolaryngol* 1988; 42:157–161.

30. Büttner U, Stöhr M, Koletzki E: Brainstem auditory-evoked potential abnormalities in vascular malformation of the posterior fossa. *J Neurol* 1983; 229:247–254.

31. Chambers BR, Mai M, Barber HO: Bilateral vestibular loss, oscillopsia, and the cervico-ocular reflex. *Otolaryngol Head Neck Surg* 1985; 93:403–407.

32. Cohen B, Tokumasu K, Goto K: Semicircular canal nerve, eye and head movements: The effect of changes in initial eye and head position on the plane of the induced movement. *Arch Ophthalmol* 1966; 76:523–531.

33. Compere WE: Elektronystagmographic findings in patients with "whiplash injuries." *Laryngoscope* 1968; 78:1226–1233.

34. DeJong JMBV, Bles W: Cervical dizziness and ataxia, in Bles W, Brandt Th (eds): *Disorders of Posture and Gait.* Amsterdam, Elsevier, 1986, pp 185–206.

35. DeJong PTVM, DeJong JMBV, Cohen B, et al: Ataxia and nystagmus induced by injection of local anesthetics in the neck. *Ann Neurol* 1977; 1:240–246.

36. DeKleyn A, Versteegh C: Untersuchungen über den sogenannten Lagenystagmus während akuter Alkoholvergiftung beim Kaninchen. *Acta Otolaryngol* 1930; 14:356–377.

37. Denny-Brown D: Recurrent cerebrovascular episodes. *Arch Neurol* 1960; 2:194–209.

38. Diamant H: Sound localization and its determination in connection with some cases of severely impaired function of vestibular labyrinth, but with normal hearing. *Acta Otolaryngol* 1946; 34:576–586.

39. Dichgans J, Mauritz KH, Allum JHJ, et al: Postural sway in normals and atactic patients: Analysis of the stabilizing and destabilizing effects of vision. *Aggressologie* 1975; 17C:15–24.

40. Dix R, Hallpike CS: The pathology, symptomatology and diagnosis of certain common disorders of the vestibular system. *Ann Otol Rhinol Laryngol* 1952; 6:987–1016.

41. Epley JM: New dimensions of benign paroxysmal positional vertigo. *Otolaryngol Head Neck Surg* 1980; 88:599–605.

42. Fahey JL, Barth WF, Solomon A: Serum hyperviscosity syndrome. *JAMA* 1965; 192:464–467.

43. Fernandez C, Alzate R, Lindsay JR: Experimental observation on postural nystagmus. II: Lesions of the nodulus. *Ann Otol Rhinol Laryngol* 1960; 69:94–114.

44. Fernandez C, Fredrickson JM: Experimental cerebellar lesions and their effect on vestibular function. *Acta Otolaryngol* 1964; 192:52–62.

45. Fisher A, Gresty M, Chambers B, et al: Primary position upbeating nystagmus: A variety of central positional nystagmus. *Brain* 1983; 106:949–964.

46. Fluur E: Positional and positioning nystagmus as a result of utriculo-cupular integration. *Acta Otolaryngol* 1974; 78:19–27.

47. Friedman W, Kaplan B, Gravenstein D, et al: Intraoperative brainstem auditory-evoked potentials during posterior fossa microvascular decompression. *J Neurosurg* 1985; 62:552–557.

48. Gacek RR: Further observations on posterior ampullary nerve transection for positional vertigo. *Ann Otol Rhinol Laryngol* 1978; 87:300–306.

49. Gacek RR: Cupulolithiasis and posterior ampullary nerve transection. *Ann Otol Rhinol Laryngol [Suppl 112]* 1984; 93:25–29.

50. Goldberg L, Störtebecker TP: Criteria of alcohol intoxication in animals in relation to blood alcohol. *Acta Physiol Scand* 1941; 3:71–81.

51. Gordon N: Post-traumatic vertigo, with special reference to positional nystagmus. *Lancet* 1954; 1:1216–1218.

52. Graf W, Ezure K: Morphology of vertical canal related second order vestibular neu-

rons in the cat. *Exp Brain Res* 1986; 63: 35–48.

53. Graf W, McCrea RA, Baker R: Morphology of posterior canal-related secondary vestibular neurons in rabbit and cat. *Exp Brain Res* 1983; 52:125–138.

54. Gray LP: Extra-labyrinthine vertigo due to cervical muscle lesions. *J Laryngol Otol* 1956; 70:352–361.

55. Graybiel A, Smith CR, Guedry FE, et al: Idiopathic progressive vestibular degeneration. *Ann Otol Rhinol Laryngol* 1972; 81:165–179.

56. Gregorius FK, Grandall PH, Baloh RW: Positional vertigo with cerebellar astrocytoma. *Surg Neurol* 1976; 6:283–286.

57. Grossmann GE, Leigh RJ: Instability of gaze during locomotion in patients with deficient vestibular function. *Ann Neurol* 1990; 27:528–532.

58. Gussen R: Saccule otoconia displacement into cochlea in cochleosaccular degeneration. *Arch Otolaryngol* 1980; 106:161–166.

59. Guttich H, Stark R: Doppelseitiger, praktisch vollkommener, wahrscheinlich angeborener Vestibularisausfall. *HNO* 1965; 13:177–180.

60. Hain TC, Fetter M, Zee DS: Head-shaking nystagmus in patients with unilateral peripheral vestibular lesions. *Am J Otolaryngol* 1987; 8:36–47.

61. Halmagyi GM, Curthoys IS: A clinical sign of canal paresis. *Arch Neurol* 1988; 45:737–739.

62. Harbert F: Benign paroxysmal positional nystagmus. *Arch Ophthalmol* 1970; 84:298–302.

63. Hardy DG, Rhoton AL: Microsurgical relationship of the superior cerebellar artery and the trigeminal nerve. *J Neurosurg* 1978; 49:669–678.

64. Harris CS, Guedry FE, Graybiel A: *Positional Alcohol Nystagmus in Relation to Labyrinthine Function. NSAM 839*, NASA R-47. Pensacola, Fla, Naval School of Aviation Medicine, 1962.

65. Harrison MS, Ozsahinoglu C: Positional vertigo. *Arch Otolaryngol* 1975; 101:675.

66. Hasegawa T: Die Veränderung der labyrinthären Reflexe bei zentrifugierten Meerschweinchen. *Pflügers Arch* 1933; 232:454–465.

67. Herdman SJ: Treatment of benign paroxysmal positional vertigo. *Phys Ther* 1990; 70:381–388.

68. Hinoki M, Terayama K: Physiological role of neck muscles in the occurrence of optic eye nystagmus. *Acta Otolaryngol* 1966; 62:157–170.

69. Hughes GB, Kinney SE, Barna BP, et al: Practical versus theoretical management of autoimmune inner ear disease. *Laryngoscope* 1984; 94:758–767.

70. Hülse M: *Die zervikalen Gleichgewichtsstörungen*. Berlin, Springer-Verlag, 1963.

71. Hyslop G: Intra-cranial circulatory complication of injuries of the neck. *Bull NY Acad Med* 1952; 28:729–733.

72. Igarashi M, Nagaba M: Vestibular end-organ damage in squirrel monkeys after exposure to intensive linear acceleration, in *Third Symposium on the Role of the Vestibular Organs in Space Exploration*. NASA SP-152. 1968, pp 63–61.

73. Jannetta PJ: Neurovascular cross-compression in patients with hyperactive dysfunction symptoms of the eighth cranial nerve. *Surg Forum* 1975; 26:467–468.

74. Jannetta PJ: Treatment of trigeminal neuralgia by microoperative decompression, in Youmans J (ed): *Neurological Surgery*, vol 6, WB Saunders, Philadelphia, 1982, pp 3589–3603.

75. Jannetta PJ, Møller MD, Møller AR: Disabling positional vertigo. *N Engl J Med* 1984; 310:1700–1705.

76. Johnson LG, Hawkins JE: Sensory and neural degeneration with aging, as seen in microdissections of the human inner ear. *Ann Otol* 1972; 81:179–193.

77. Jung R: Nystagmographie. Zur Physiologie und Pathologie des optisch-vestibulären Systems beim Menschen, in von Bergmann G, Frey W, Schwieck H (eds): *Handbuch der Inneren Medizin*, ed 4, vol 51. Berlin, Springer-Verlag, 1953, pp 1325–1379.

78. Kamei T: Der biphasisch auftretende Kopfschüttelnystagmus. *Arch Otolaryngol* 1975; 209:59–67.

79. Katsarkas A: Nystagmus of paroxysmal positional vertigo: Some new insights. *Ann Otol Rhinol Laryngol* 1987; 96:305–308.

80. Katsarkas A, Kirkham T: Paroxysmal positional vertigo. A study of 255 cases. *J Otolaryngol* 1978; 7:320–330.

81. Katsarkas A, Outerbridge JS: Nystagmus of paroxysmal positional vertigo. *Ann Otol Rhinol Laryngol* 1983; 92:146–150.

82. Kattah JC, Kolsky MP, Luessenhof AJ: Positional vertigo and the cerebellar vermis. *Neurology* 1984; 34:527–529.

83. Keim RJ, Sachs GB: Positional nystagmus in association with macroglobulinaemia. *Ann Otol* 1975; 84:223–227.

84. Lindsay JR, Hemenway WG: Postural vertigo due to unilateral sudden partial loss of vestibular function. *Ann Otol Rhinol Laryngol* 1956; 65:692–708.

85. Logothetis J, Silverstein P, Coe J: Neurological aspects of Waldenström's macroglobulinaemia. *Arch Neurol* 1960; 3:564–573.

86. Longet FA: Mémoroises sur les troubles qui surviennent dans l'équilibration, la station et al locomotion des animaux après la section des parties molles de la nuque. *Gaz Med Paris* 1845; 13:565–567.

87. Longridge NS, Barber HO: Bilateral paroxysmal positioning nystagmus. *Can J Otol* 1978; 7:395–400.

88. Markham CH, Diamond SG, Juichi I: Utricular dysfunction in benign paroxysmal positional vertigo, in Graham MD, Kemink L (eds): *The Vestibular System: Neurophysiologic and Clinical Research*, New York, Raven Press, 1987, pp 275–283.

89. McClure JA: Horizontal canal BPV. *J Otolaryngol* 1985; 14:30–35.

90. McClure JA: Functional basis for horizontal canal BPV, in Barber HO, Sharpe JA (eds): *Vestibular Disorders*. Chicago, Year Book, 1988, pp 233–238.

91. Merchant SN, Schuknecht HF: Vestibular atelectasis. *Ann Otol Rhinol Laryngol* 1988; 97:565–576.

92. Møller MD: Controversy in Meniere's disease: Results of microvascular decompression of the eighth nerve. *Ann J Otol* 1988; 9:60–63.

93. Møller MD, Møller AR, Jannetta PJ, et al: Diagnosis and surgical treatment of disabling positional vertigo. *J Neurosurg* 1986; 84:21–28.

94. Money KE, Johnson WH, Cerlett BMA: Role of semicircular canals in positional alcohol nystagmus. *Am J Physiol* 1965; 208:1065–1070.

95. Money KE, Myles WS: Heavy water nystagmus and effects of alcohol. *Nature* 1974; 247:404–405.

96. Morgenstern C, Farrenkopf J: Die Funktion des hinteren vertikalen Bogenganges beim Menschen. *Arch Otorhinolaryng* 1980; 227:482.

97. Morley TP: Case against microvascular decompression in the treatment of trigeminal neuralgia. *Arch Neurol* 1985; 42:801–802.

98. Moser M: Zervikalnystagmus und seine diagnostische Bedeutung. *HNO* 1974; 22:350–355.

99. Myers E, Bernstein J, Fostiropolous G: Salicylate ototoxicity: A clinical study. *N Engl J Med* 1965; 273:587.

100. Nito Y, Johnson WH, Money KE, et al: The nonauditory labyrinth and positional alcohol nystagmus. *Acta Otolaryngol* 58:65.

101. Ommaya AK, Faas F, Yarnell P: Whiplash injury and brain damage. *JAMA* 1968; 204:285–289.

102. Parnes LS, McClure JA: Posterior semicircular occlusion for intractable benign paroxysmal positional vertigo. *Ann Otol Rhinol Laryngol* 1990; 99:330–334.

103. Rietz R, Troia BW, Yonkers AJ, et al: Glycerol-induced positional nystagmus in human beings. *Otolaryngol Head Neck Surg* 1987; 97:282–287.

104. Ronis ML, Rojer CL, Ronis BJ: Otologic manifestations of Waldenström's macroglobulinaemia. *Laryngoscope* 1966; 76:513–523.

105. Rosenhall U, Hanner P, Kaijser B: Borrelia infection and vertigo. *Acta Otolaryngol* 1988; 106:111–116.

106. Rothfeld J: Über den Einfluß akuter und chronischer Alkoholvergiftung auf die Funktion des Vestibularapparates. *Monatsschr Ohrenheilkd* 1913; 47:1392–1393.

107. Ruben JR, Distenfeld A, Berg P: Sudden sequential deafness as the presenting symptom of macroglobulinaemia. *JAMA* 1969; 209:1364–1365.

108. Rubin W: Whiplash with vestibular involvement. *Arch Otolaryngol* 1973; 97:85–87.

109. Sakata E, Ohtsu K, Shimura H, et al: Positional nystagmus of benign paroxysmal type (BPPV) due to cerebellar vermis lesions. Pseudo-BPPV. *Auris Nasus Larynx* 1987; 14:17–21.

110. Sato K: Histopathological study on the vestibular toxicity of six aminoglycoside antibiotics. *Drugs Exp Clin Res* 1982; 8:259.

111. Scherer H: Halsbedingter Schwindel. *Arch Otorhinolaryngol* [suppl II] 1985; 2:107–124.

112. Schmidt CL: Zur Pathophysiologie des peripheren, paroxysmalen, benignen Lagerungsschwindel (BPPV). *Laryngol Rhinol Otol* 1985; 64:146–155.

113. Schuknecht HF: Positional vertigo. Clinical and experimental observations. *Trans Am Acad Ophthalmol Otolaryngol* 1962; 66:319–331.

114. Schuknecht HF: Cupulolithiasis. *Arch Otolaryngol* 1969; 90:765–778.

115. Schuknecht HF: *Pathology of the Ear*. Cambridge, Mass, Harvard University Press, 1974.

116. Schuknecht HF, Ruby RRF: Cupulolithiasis. *Adv Otorhinolaryngol* 1973; 22:434–443.

117. Schuknecht HF, Witt RL: Acute bilateral sequential vestibular neuritis. *Am J Otolaryngol* 1985; 6:255–257.

118. Sheehan S, Bauer RB, Meyer JS: Vertebral artery compression in cervical spondylosis. *Neurology* 1960; 10:968–986.

119. Simmons FB: Patients with bilateral loss of caloric response. *Ann Otol Rhinol Laryngol* 1973; 82:175–178.

120. Szentágothai I: The elementary vestibulo ocular reflex arc. *J Neurophysiol* 1950; 13:395–407.

121. Ter Bruggen JP, Keunen RWM, Tijssen CC, et al: Octavus nerve neurovascular compression syndrome. *Eur Neurol* 1987; 27:82–87.

122. Thomson J, Bretlau P, Tos M, et al: Placebo effect in surgery for Meniere's disease. *Arch Otolaryngol* 1981; 107:271–277.

123. Toglia JU: Acute flexion-extension injury of the neck. *Neurology* 1976; 26:808–814.

124. Toole JF, Tucker SH: Influence of head position upon cerebral circulation. *Arch Neurol* 1960; 2:616–623.

125. Torres F, Shapiro SK: Electroencephalograms in whiplash injuries. *Arch Neurol* 1961; 5:28–35.

126. Vyslonzil E: Über eine umschriebene Ansammlung von Otokonien in hinteren häutigen Bogengängen. *Monatsschr Ohrenheilkd* 1963; 97:63.

127. Walter HW: Alkoholmißbrauch und Alkoholnystagmus. *Dtsch Z Ges Gerichtl Med* 1954; 43:232–241.

128. Watson P, Barber HO, Peck J, et al: Positional vertigo and nystagmus of central origin. *Can J Neurol Sci* 1981; 8:133–137.

129. Weeks V, Travelli J: Postural vertigo due to trigger areas in sterno-cleidomastoid muscle. *J Pediatr* 1955; 47:315–327.

130. Williams D, Wilson TG: The diagnosis of the major and minor syndromes of basilar insufficiency. *Brain* 1962; 85:741–747.

131. Yoshida M, Lowry LD, Liu JJC: Effects of hyperosmotic solutions on endolymphatic pressure. *Am J Otolaryngol* 1985; 6:297–301.

132. Yu Y, Moseley I, Pullicino P, et al: The clinical picture of ectasia of the intracerebral arteries. *J Neurol Neurosurg Psychiatry* 1982; 45:29–36.

CHAPTER 8

Background and Technique of Caloric Testing

Gary P. Jacobson, Ph.D.
Craig W. Newman, Ph.D

The caloric examination is usually the most informative subtest of the electronystagmography (ENG) test battery because caloric test results can be used to validate a tentative diagnosis of asymmetric function in the peripheral vestibular system.

The principle advantage of the caloric test lies in the ability of an investigator to evaluate selectively the physiologic integrity of a patient's left or right horizontal semicircular canal. By irrigating the external ear canal with cool or warm water it is possible to affect changes in the movement of endolymph of the ipsilateral horizontal semicircular canal, and thereby alter the level of afferent neural activity emanating from the ipsilateral vestibular end organ. From the background material presented by Drs. Honrubia and Hoffman in Chapter 2 we know that the caloric stimulus is nonphysiologic in that normal everyday movements of the head and of the head and body are accompanied by simultaneous movements of the motion transducers (the otoliths and cupula) of *both* the left and right end organ systems.

There are three primary disadvantages of caloric testing. First, although we are infusing the external ear canal with warm or cool water (with reference to body temperature) or air that is con-

trolled thermostatically, the actual level of stimulation at the end organ level may vary greatly depending on the heat-transferring capacities of the surrounding bone and air in the middle ear space. Second, like the auditory system, the vestibular system responds to natural head (or head and body) movements that cover a wide frequency range (for example, from approximately 0.01 to 8 Hz).[37, 51, 88, 99] Caloric stimulation is analogous to head rotation at a frequency of 0.003 Hz.[42] Thus, conducting a caloric examination in isolation without rotational testing is analogous to conducting pure-tone threshold audiometry at 125 Hz and inferring from these data the hearing sensitivity over the rest of the frequency range of hearing (and the integrity of the entire auditory end organ). Third, in caloric testing we have adopted the misleading practice of making inferences about the physiologic health of the entire membranous labyrinth (three semicircular canals, utricle, and saccule) based on testing that is capable only of evaluating the horizontal semicircular canal over an extremely narrow portion of its operating range. This can be a dangerous and inaccurate assumption.

The importance of the caloric test as an integral component of the site of lesion vestibular test battery makes the accurate performance of this test essential. The purposes of the present chapter are: (1) to present the historical development of caloric test procedures; (2) to describe conventional methodologies and unconventional permutations of the alternating binaural bithermal (ABB) caloric test, and to describe conventional measurement techniques; (3) to describe methods of calibrating caloric systems; and (4) to discuss those variables that may affect the caloric response.

It is interesting that since the ABB caloric test was first described in 1942 by Fitzgerald and Hallpike,[33] the original methodology has remained unchanged with few exceptions over the subsequent 50 years. These exceptions have included the following:

1. Addition of electro-oculographic instrumentation (also called electronystagmography, or ENG), and photoelectric nystagmographic recording techniques (PENG), which have permitted the examiner a method of quantifying accurately vestibular system function;
2. Inclusion of fixation suppression testing;
3. Appreciation of the effects of certain variables on the caloric response; and
4. The recent advent of computerized data collection and analysis techniques.

The clinical significance of various types of caloric test results will be discussed in Chapter 9.

HISTORICAL PERSPECTIVE

Background

Caloric testing began in 1868 when Schmiederkam observed that nystagmus could be elicited by irrigating the ears with water.[79(p 209)] However, it was not until 1906 that Barany developed the caloric test.[8] Jung and Mittermaer[52] were the first to develop the use of the EOG as a means of providing a permanent record of nystagmus. Finally, Henriksson[45] and Stahle[80] were the first to comment that caloric nystagmus became reduced or absent in the presence of visual fixation. Prior to this time caloric testing was conducted routinely with the subject's eyes opened and fixated on a stationary point.

It was Robert Barany who formulated the hypothesis that thermal convection currents set up within the membranous labyrinth were the origin of caloric nystagmus.[8, 9] Barany observed that when water cooler than body temperature was infused into the ear canal of a patient sitting upright, a nystagmus was elicited, with a fast phase directed toward the opposite ear. Alternatively, when water warmer than body temperature was infused into the ear canal a nystagmus was elicited with a fast phase directed toward the same side. Additionally, the nystagmus could be made to reverse direction if the patient's head was directed downward such that the crown of the head was pointed toward the floor.

The method of caloric transduction described by Barany is illustrated in Figure 8–1. When warm water is infused in the external auditory meatus the skin of the ear canal is heated, resulting in a temperature change which is transmitted to the horizontal semicircular canal. Additionally, heat transfer is conducted to the vestibule through the air in the middle ear space.[44] The endolymph closest to the canal wall is heated, causing it to become relatively less dense than the surrounding endolymph. Because less dense fluids rise, and more dense fluids fall, the heated endolymph rises and is replaced by more dense endolymph, which is in turn heated and in turn rises. The fluid movement that results from the heating of the endolymph is called a "convection current." Warm water irrigations for the

Utriculopetal movement of cupula

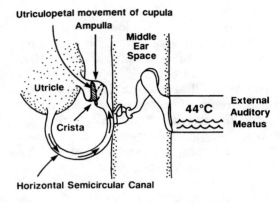

Utriculofugal movement of cupula

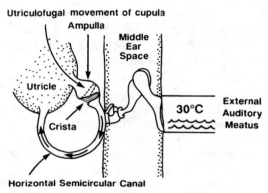

FIG 8–1.
Schematic diagram illustrating how thermal convection currents set up in membranous labyrinth lead to utriculopetal movement of cupula for warm caloric stimulation and utriculofugal movement of cupula for cool caloric stimulation. (Adapted from Baloh RW, Honrubia V: *Clinical Neurophysiology of the Vestibular System*, ed 2. Philadelphia, FA Davis, 1990.)

horizontal semicircular canal result in utriculopetal movement (toward the utricle) of the horizontal semicircular canal cupula. Utriculopetal movement of the right cupula is analogous to the movement induced in the right horizontal semicircular canal by a rightward head turn. The resulting effect in the right cristae is a depolarization of the dendrites at the base of the hair cells. This creates a net increase in electrical activity over the resting spontaneous activity. The activity routed through the medial longitudinal fasciculus results in a slow deviation of the eye to the opposite direction (leftward in the present example) and a fast correcting saccade toward the same side as the caloric infu-

sion (toward the right in the present example).

It has been demonstrated that the convection current associated with a massive 10°C change in endolymphatic temperature results in only a 1.5- to 2.6-μm cupular deflection.[43] The nystagmus direction (determined by the direction of the fast phase of the nystagmus beat) reverses if the patient's head is inverted. This is illustrated in Figure 8–2. In the current example, if the head position is reversed such that the face is pointing downward (subject prone), the irrigation of the ear canal with warm water results in a deflection of the cupula away from the utricle, resulting in a hyperpolarization of the end organ, which creates a decrease in the resting discharge rate. This is analogous to what occurs in the right semicircular canal following a head turn toward the left. The result is a slow deviation of the eye toward the right and a fast correcting saccade toward the left. Under normal testing conditions, cool water irrigations result in slow-phase eye movements toward the ear stimulated and fast-phase eye movements away from the stimulated ear. Alternately, warm water irrigations result in slow-phase eye movements away from the ear stimulated and fast phases toward the stimulated ear (the mnemonic is "COWS": cold opposite, warm same). This phenomenon is depicted in Figure 8–3. Barany received the Nobel Prize in 1914 for his observations of thermal stimulation of the vestibular system.

It is now believed that thermal convection currents are the primary but not the sole mode of transduction within the horizontal semicircular canal system during caloric testing. Recent experiments conducted under weightless conditions aboard the Spacelab scientific space laboratory have demonstrated that caloric nystagmus can be elicited in the absence of the gravitational field that is required for convection currents to exist. (See "Controversies in Caloric Testing" at the end of this chapter.)

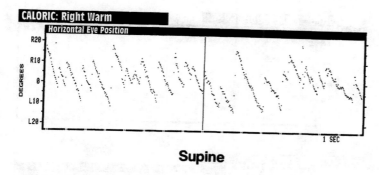

Supine

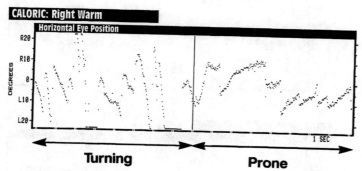

Turning   **Prone**

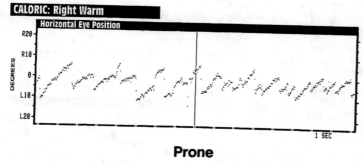

Prone

FIG 8–2.
Caloric nystagmus elicited following irrigation of the right ear with warm water. Notice that the nystagmus reverses direction when the subject is moved from the supine (face-up) position to the prone (face-down) position. Changing the subject's body position also changes the direction of endolymph flow from utriculopetal to utriculofugal. (See text for discussion.)

Attempts to Evaluate Vestibular System Function Through Caloric Testing

Minimal, Maximal, and Directional Preponderance Tests

A number of caloric examinations were developed in the beginning of the twentieth century. Most of these examinations were developed in Germany and are referred to as minimal, maximal, or directional preponderance tests. The *minimal tests*, for example, those of Demetriades-Mayer, Veits-German, and Töröck,[32(pp 137-138)] employed small amounts (5–10 mL) of cold water as a stimulus to the labyrinth obviating the discomfort associated with caloric testing using larger volumes of water (thus, the term

"minimal test" is used). The patient's head was placed in a "neutral" position (not optimal for stimulation of the labyrinth), and the ear was irrigated with the water over a period of 5 to 10 seconds. Following the interval of 30 to 60 seconds required for the heat transfer to take place, the patient's head would be placed in an optimal position for labyrinthine stimulation and the patient would be instructed to open his or her eyes. The latency, duration, and/or frequency of the nystagmus was measured and compared following stimulation of each ear. The minimal tests were used to determine the physiologic threshold for a response from the labyrinth. The *maximal tests*, for example, those of Barany,[32(p137)] employed larger volumes of water (50 to 250 mL)

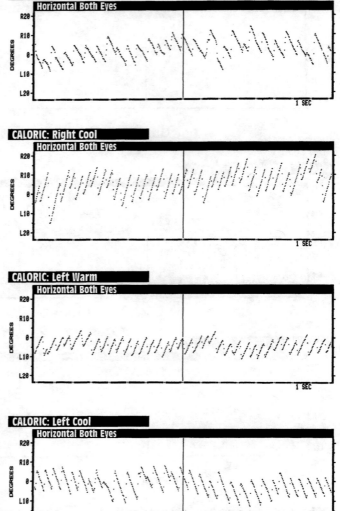

FIG 8–3.
Nystagmus responses extracted from examination of a healthy subject (*UW* = unilateral weakness value; *DP* = directional preponderance value). Notice that nystagmus responses elicited by irrigating the ear with cool water result in fast phases that beat toward the opposite ear. Alternatively, nystagmus elicited by irrigating the ear with warm water results in fast phases that beat toward the same ear ("COWS": cold-opposite, warm-same).

UW = 6% on the left   **DP = 12% to the left**

delivered over longer time periods (20 to 40 seconds). These tests were used to investigate the function of patients (1) who had little or no response to minimal stimulation, (2) who had a preexisting spontaneous nystagmus that contaminated the minimal tests, or (3) who had a preexisting gaze nystagmus of central nervous system origin. The *directional preponderance* tests include the cold-warm contrast test[32(p140)] and the ABB test.[33] These examinations were used to detect the phenomenon of the propensity for the eyes to demonstrate a nystagmus fast phase that beat stronger in one direction rather than the other following cool and warm water irrigations. This phenomenon, observed with the subject's eyes open, was first reported by Fitzgerald and Hallpike[33] in patients with temporal lobe disease. This observation might be referred in present-day vernacular as directional preponderance of fixation suppression ability (see Chapter 9).

Alternate Binaural Bithermal Caloric Test

In 1942, Fitzgerald and Hallpike[33] reported the use of a bithermal water caloric test. For this test the patient was placed in a supine position with the head elevated 30°. Tanks of water were placed on raised shelves above the patient's head. One tank contained water heated to 44° C (110° F) and a second tank contained water heated to 30° C (87° F). Because these temperatures were 7° C above and below body temperature, they were referred to as warm and cool caloric stimuli, respectively. A hose from the cool tank was placed in the patient's ear, and the gravitational pull created by the weight of the water caused the water to flow out of the tube. The ear was irrigated with 250 mL of cool water over a period of 40 seconds. The patient's eyes remained open during this test, and the magnitude of the induced caloric nystagmus was quantified according to its duration. Following this phase of the test, a time interval was provided in which the temperature of the ear canal, middle ear, and surrounding bone was allowed to normalize. Then the three other irrigations were conducted. In conjunction with Barany's observation the warm water irrigation produced a nystagmus with a fast phase directed toward the stimulated ear, whereas the cool water irrigation produced a nystagmus with a fast phase directed toward the unstimulated ear.

INSTRUMENTATION FOR CALORIC TESTING

A number of different caloric irrigators are now available for use. They share in their ability to deliver a precise volume of stimulus to the ear drum. They differ in the type of media that is controlled by the irrigator. The two major types of irrigators deliver either air or water stimuli (air and water caloric irrigators). The third type delivers a water caloric stimulus through an expandable rubber receptacle that is placed in the patient's ear canal. This device was designed by Kenneth Brookler and Guenter Grams[21] and is called the Brookler-Grams "closed-loop" system. These caloric stimulators circulate the cool or warm water continuously throughout the system so that the temperature is maintained at a preset level at any particular instant. This is to be compared with those water caloric systems that must be "purged" prior to irrigation to bring the water temperature up to the proper level. (See Appendix.)

Air Irrigator

An air irrigator system consists of an air flow regulator, a heater, and thermostat. The air is delivered either through a hose or a speculum (Fig. 8–4,A). Air is supplied to the air caloric irrigator from either an external air pump or air supplied from the wall sources that are located in most hospitals. The air is heated with a Peltier thermoelectric device. This device heats air in proportion to the amount of current flowing through a feedback circuit. This feedback circuit includes a thermistor which measures the temperature of the air (Fig 8–4,B). The thermistor is located at the tip of the delivery system because air is a poor conductor of heat. Thus, the placement of the thermistor at the tip of the irrigator makes it possible to measure the temperature of the air at the last possible moment prior to when the air leaves the delivery system.

The advantage of the latter delivery system is that the tympanic membrane can be visualized during the irrigation. The chief advantage of the air caloric system is that of convenience. There is no water to recover as it runs out of the ear canal, and an ear with a tympanic membrane perforation can be irrigated without concern of infection from the use of nonsterile water.

A

B

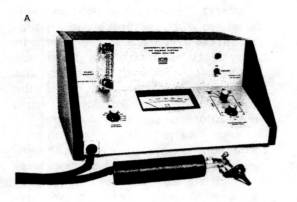

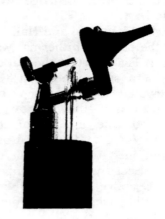

FIG 8–4.
A, photograph of air caloric irrigator. Note controls on the front panel that permit flow rate, irrigation time, and irrigation temperature to be regulated by the examiner. **B,** close-up photograph of delivery head of air caloric irrigator. Note the thermistor at tip of irrigator. The thermistor transmits information about the temperature at the irrigation tip. This feedback circuit permits air temperature to be kept at a constant temperature. *(Photographs courtesy of ICS Medical; Schaumberg, Ill.)*

Conventional Water Irrigator

The water irrigator is the conventional caloric irrigation system. The stimulator consists of two "baths" containing 30° C and 44° C water, respectively (Fig. 8–5). A temperature-sensing device submerged in each bath is connected to a thermostat that will heat the water when the water temperature decreases beyond a preset level. This level is normally slightly greater than 30° or 44° C due to the decrease in temperature that occurs as the water travels from the baths to the irrigation tip (see Appendix). A highly sensitive thermostat is important for the maintenance of cor-

rect water temperature. An inordinate amount of time will be required to bring the bath back to the correct temperature if the water temperature must decrease too far before the thermostat recognizes the change. Thus, it is important for the thermostat to be capable of detecting small variations in water temperature and to cause corrections for these deviations to occur quickly.

There is usually a foot pedal connected to the irrigator that opens and closes a solenoid switch that gates the flow of water. An internal timer is used to establish the duration of the water flow (usually 30 to 40 seconds). The solenoid switch controls when the flow of

FIG 8–5.
Photograph of conventional water caloric irrigator *(Photograph courtesy of ICS Medical, Schaumberg, Ill.)*

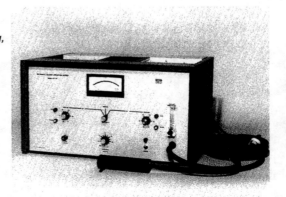

water stops. The volume of water per unit time (flow rate) may be controlled by one of two methods. First, a control may be present that regulates the water pump. When the control is increased the water pump will push water more quickly through the delivery tube. Second, the flow rate may be controlled by varying systematically the internal diameter of the delivery tip. For this method the internal diameter of the delivery tip is designed to be small at the point of exit of the water and large at the base of the base of the tip. To increase water flow the plastic tip is shortened until an internal diameter is reached that permits the appropriate volume of water to be delivered over a 40-second period (for example, 250 mL).

There are variations in the design of the water irrigators. These differences usually involve how water is delivered to the ear. It is preferable that the hoses be insulated so that the decrease in water temperature is limited as the water flows from the bath to the irrigation tip. Also (as noted earlier), there are irrigators that circulate precisely heated water through the entire tube continuously, so that no purging needs to be performed prior to initiation of irrigation. Also, the design of the irrigation tip differs from manufacturer to manufacturer. Some delivery tips are simply "tips," while others consist of large handles that have a delivery tip projecting out of them.

Two final issues deserve mentioning with respect to water caloric irrigators. Most clinical centers use tap water for caloric irrigations. The alternative is to use distilled water. The advantage of distilled water is that, unlike tap water, it does not contain organic material, and thus, will not contain sediment or promote the growth of algae. All water irrigators require routine maintenance. This routine maintenance includes calibration but also includes cleaning of the holding tanks and tubing.

Finally, electrical safety must be as-

sured for all patients tested in the ENG laboratory. During the caloric irrigation there is a direct connection between the patient and the irrigator and ENG recorder. Therefore, if the ENG recorder, the caloric irrigator, or the patient are not properly grounded it is possible for current to pass from one machine to the other with the patient as the bridge between the two. The result can be a dangerous electrical shock. Therefore, as is required in all medical centers the electrical safety of ENG equipment (such as, current leakage and grounding) should be evaluated on a regular basis.

Closed-Loop Water Irrigation System

The inconveniences associated with the need to purge the water caloric system as well as with recovery of the water media have been eliminated with the advent of the "closed-loop" irrigation system.[21] This system consists of the two standard bithermal baths and thermostatic control of temperature (Fig 8–6). However, water flow through the system is constant (to obviate the need for purging the system), and a silicone balloon is connected to the tip of the

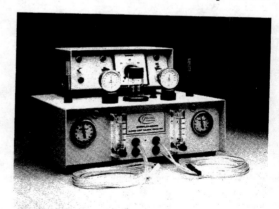

FIG 8–6.
Photograph of Brookler-Grams closed-loop water caloric irrigator. Note separate delivery tubes for cool and warm water. Also note that within each irrigator tube (for example, for warm and cool irrigations) is a delivery and removal tube. This permits the continuous circulation of water when the system is not being used *(Photograph courtesy of Life-Tech, Inc., Austin, Texas.).*

water delivery system so that no water is dispensed into the ear canal (hence the term "closed-loop"). The thin-walled silicone rubber balloon is placed in the patient's ear. Water fills the balloon, causing it to expand and fill the ear canal when the irrigation is initiated. Because the water flow is continuous through the tube and back to the tank, the water temperature is correct when irrigation commences. Inflation and deflation of the balloon as well as the timing of the duration of the irrigation are controlled by the irrigation unit.

METHOD FOR CONDUCTING CALORIC TESTS (AIR AND WATER)

Alternating Binaural Bithermal Test

Figures 8–7,A–D, illustrate the sequence of activities involved in performing the alternate binaural bithermal caloric test. Prior to the beginning of each caloric irrigation, a set of 10° saccadic recalibrations should be conducted to ensure that 10 mm of paper movement represents 10° of eye movement (Fig. 8–7,C). The caloric test is usually administered with the patient in the supine (face-up) position with the head elevated slightly to a 30° angle. Alternatively, the patient may have the examination performed while seated with the head flexed backward 60°. Both maneuvers are designed to bring the horizontal semicircular canal cupula into a near vertical position where the forces of the convection current can deflect it optimally. It has been our experience that the test is best tolerated when the patient is supine. This is a more comfortable, natural position for the patient to be in for the somewhat long duration of this test (generally 30 to 45 minutes).

The ears should be inspected visually with an otoscope prior to the caloric irrigation. In particular, the ear canal should be examined for the presence of large amounts of cerumen that could impede the flow of water or air to the eardrum. Also important to note is the condition of the eardrum. This may be done during the otoscopic evaluation (Fig 8–7,B) but may also be done through tympanometric testing (Fig 8–7,A) prior to the caloric irrigations. If there are signs that the eardrum is perforated, measures should be taken to avoid passing water into the middle ear cavity.* There may be occasions when it is necessary to conduct a caloric test in the presence of unilateral or bilateral tympanic membrane perforations. In these situations, calculations of symmetry of vestibular system responsiveness will be impossible because the heat-transmitting properties of the middle ear space will be different for the ear or ears with tympanic perforation. The diagnostic question in these situations is usually whether peripheral vestibular system function exists at all.

Following the visual inspection of the ear canal a catch basin is placed under the patient's ear (Fig 8–7,D). We have found it useful to place towels beneath the basin so that the basin is placed directly beneath the auricle. This produces two benefits. First, there is little possibility that water will leak out from the space beneath the ear and the basin and saturate the patient. Second, this leaves both hands of the examiner free to open the ear canal and insert the irrigation tip properly. Then, the water irrigation system is purged. If one were to begin irrigating directly from the water tank, the first 10 to 15 seconds of the irrigation (roughly 25% to 50% of the irrigation duration) would consist of water that had been cooling in the irrigation hose. Therefore, it has become the practice of clinicians to purge the water in the hose prior to the irrigation. From a practical standpoint, purging consists of

---

*An alternative to water caloric testing is to conduct the examination using an air caloric stimulator. In the absence of an air caloric irrigator, a finger cot may be placed deeply in the ear canal, and water may be infused into the finger cot.

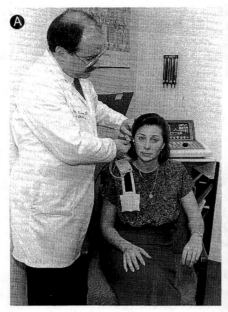

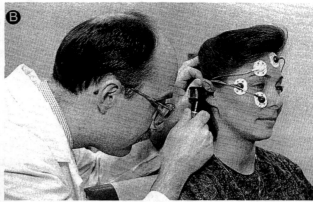

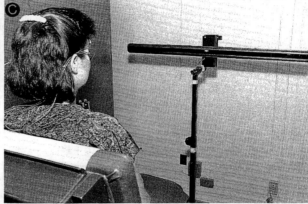

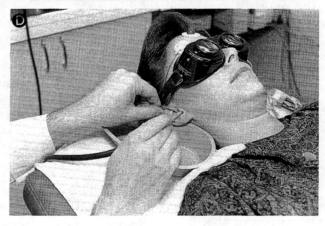

FIG 8–7.
A–D, sequence of events leading to the alternate binaural bithermal caloric test. The integrity of the patient's tympanic membrane is assessed either using tympanometry **(A)** or otoscopy **(B). C,** recalibration of eye movements is performed. **D,** the patient is supine with head elevated 30°. A catch basin is placed beneath the subject's ear, and the delivery tip is inserted. The test is being conducted in semidarkness with the patient's eyes opened and with the patient wearing Frenzel's lenses.

running one full irrigation cycle into a sink or receptacle. When the cycle is completed and the water flow is terminated, the water at the irrigation tip should be close to the calibrated temperature. It is important to begin irrigating immediately following this procedure.

It is critically important that the caloric examination be discussed with the patient in detail prior to the initiation of the test. In particular, telling the patient that they will, or may, become "dizzy" or "nauseous," or that "they may vomit" will gain one little and in general will "program" the patient to expect these unpleasant reactions. The patient should be told that they will be feeling cool (or warm) water in the ear and that it will be present for 40 seconds. The water will feel cold (or hot) initially and will gradually feel only cool (or warm). Further, they should be instructed that after approximately 30 seconds they may feel as though they are "turning," that this is a normal sensation, and that this sensation will disappear after about 1 to 2 minutes. For the more sophisticated patients it often helps to explain the mechanism that is responsible for the caloric response. The patient should be instructed that they will be asked to talk with the examiner during the test and that this conversation is necessary to ensure the accuracy of the test. Where applicable, during this instruction period (depending on the type of irrigation system one is using) the examiner should be purging the delivery system so that following the instructions, the delivery tip can be placed in the patient's ear canal and the first irrigation can commence. Measures should be taken to eliminate visual fixation (for example, through closing of the patient's eyes, darkening, or semi-darkening of the room, or by placing Frenzel goggles over the patient's eyes), and the first irrigation should be performed.

The first caloric irrigation tends to elicit the largest response. This may be due to the extra alerting that occurs when the patient does not know what to expect. It is important to engage the patient in a conversation that will distract his or her attention from the caloric irrigation and/or the sensation that ensues. These activities have been referred to as "alerting exercises" or "mental tasking." The practical significance of alerting maneuvers is that nystagmus may be intermittent or absent in an unalerted patient. These observations could be inadvertently interpreted as lack of function on the side of the absent caloric response. Additionally, certain central nervous system disorders may manifest themselves in dysrhythmic caloric induced nystagmus. Figure 8–8 shows the caloric response from two normal subjects during periods of time when they were not adequately alerted. The neuro-

physiology of alerting is not completely understood. It is clear, however, that the cortex exerts some control over the brain stem vestibular centers. When the cortex is occupied with cognitive tasks this control is potentiated and the brain stem reflex is unimpeded. Alerting tasks have traditionally involved serial additions or subtractions. However, these tasks are not particularly interesting and only serve to make the examination more difficult for some patients to tolerate (especially those who are poor at arithmetic).

There is good evidence in fact that simple conversation is more effective than serial arithmetic for releasing induced nystagmus.[57] One final observation is that many patients will have a combination of vestibular and auditory system disease. These patients will have great difficulty engaging in conversation when their better ear (if they have a better ear) is being irrigated. For these circumstances it is best to establish a signal (such as a pat on the shoulder) that can be administered when the patient should begin the alerting exercises. On this rare occasion it may be necessary to have patients do some repetitive task. These tasks can be made interesting without being prohibitively difficult. Examples of these tasks include the serial naming of states that begin with the letters of the alphabet (beginning with "A" and progressing through "W"), or describing rooms in their home.

Occasionally, one caloric irrigation will be substantially smaller than the other three. When this occurs it is the responsibility of the examiner to determine why this unlikely event has occurred. In most instances the sources of a single small response are poor irrigation technique or inadequate alerting of the patient. Therefore, in all instances this irrigation must be repeated. Also, as stated earlier, it is essential that eye movement calibration be conducted prior to each caloric irrigation. Proctor et al.[70] found that corneoretinal potentials showed a systematic change over

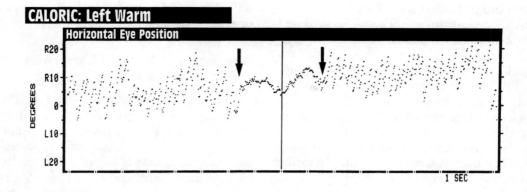

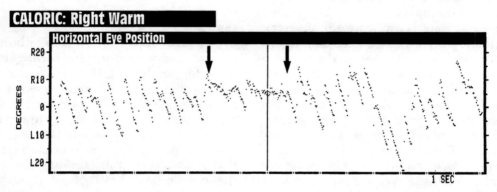

FIG 8–8.
Caloric nystagmus records elicited from two normal patients (top and bottom, respectively) during periods of time when patients were not adequately alerted *(areas between arrows)*.

time in normal subjects. Specifically, the potential decreased approximately 7% over a period of time required to conduct eight caloric irrigations. The lack of light over this time period was responsible for this change (corneoretinal potential is greatest in light). Based on these findings it might be expected that the maximum nystagmus to the four caloric irrigations might show a continuous (albeit small) decline if recalibrations are not performed. Also, for these reasons it is recommended that ambient light be kept constant for the period of caloric testing (do not turn on room lights and then turn them off prior to each irrigation).

Technique for Fixation Suppression Testing

Following the caloric irrigation, and in the midst of the alerting tasks, the nystagmus response will appear to reach a peak (evaluated visually by the steepness of the slopes of the slow component of the nystagmus response). It is at this point that the fixation suppression (FS) test should be administered. It cannot be overemphasized that it is important to evaluate patients for FS at the peak of the caloric response when the eye velocity is greatest. This will make the determination of FS unambiguous. Also, Kato et al.[55] have demonstrated that FS measures derived from a strong stimulus are more informative than those derived from a weak stimulus.

The patient is instructed to open his/her eyes and fixate his/her vision on a stationary target placed at central gaze at least 1 m from the head. This target may be a light-emitting diode that is mounted on the ceiling or the examiner's finger held at least 1 m from the patient at central gaze (Fig 8–9). Within 1 to 2 seconds (to permit the patient to fix their gaze on the point source) the caloric nystagmus should attenuate markedly. This phenomenon is known as "fixation suppression" or as "vestibuloocular reflex cancellation." The absence of this reduction of nystagmus following fixation has been referred to as paradoxical caloric response,[62] ocular fixation reversal phenomenon,[94] and failure of FS,[26] which is the term that will be used within this text. Calculations of FS will be described later in this chapter.

It should be noted that Bell's phenomenon may complicate the determination of FS ability (discussed later). Bell's phenomenon refers to the averting (rolling up) and adducting (moving toward midline) of the eyes that occurs upon eye closure. There is tremendous intersubject variability in the magnitude of Bell's phenomenon. Thus, for some patients it is possible for caloric nystagmus to be absent or periodically suppressed if the eyes are rolling behind closed lids. Hood and Korres[49] reported that the entire caloric response could be suppressed by Bell's phenomenon. Therefore, a patient with a particularly strong Bell's phenomenon may show what appears to be a complete absence of caloric response with eyes closed but will show a response with eyes opened.[49]

Alternating Binaural Bithermal Air Caloric Testing

The air caloric stimulator has the advantage of being able to be used in the presence of tympanic membrane perforations. It has also been reported that the technique is better tolerated by pediatric and adult patients than is water caloric testing. Last, the use of the air stimulator obviates the need to contend with the retrieval and disposal of water following water caloric irrigations.

The procedures for conducting binaural air caloric testing are identical to those for conducting binaural water caloric testing. The difference has to do with the care that one must take in the placement of the irrigating tip in the external auditory ear canal. The optimal delivery system for air caloric stimulation is a delivery tube running through the handle and head of an otoscope. With this system the tympanic membrane may be visualized throughout the irrigation (Fig 8–10). Because air is a poor conductor of heat it is critical that the delivery port be placed as deeply as possible in the ear canal. The air stream should be directed toward the tympanic membrane. The patient should be pre-

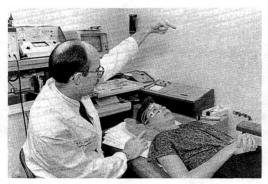

FIG 8–9.
Examiner conducting fixation suppression test. The patient is being asked to fixate her gaze on the examiner's finger. This test is being performed just following the peak of the caloric response.

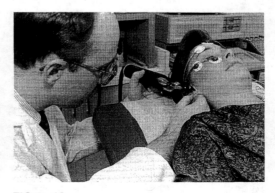

FIG 8–10.
Air caloric irrigation. The speculum is inserted in the patient's ear, and attempts are made to visualize the tympanic membrane during the irrigation.

pared by the examiner for the noise associated with the air caloric stimulus.

The effectiveness of air as a caloric medium has been a subject of discussion over the past 17 years. Capps et al.[23] introduced the air caloric stimulator as a substitute for the conventional water caloric stimulator. The investigators demonstrated that the irrigation of an ear with 0° C water (5 mL) or air (60 seconds) yielded the same magnitude of nystagmus slow-phase eye velocity, amplitude, and frequency. The water media resulted in a longer response duration than the air stimulus. The investigators observed that 24° C and 50° C air temperature (air flow, 8 L/min) resulted in nystagmus velocities that were identical to those obtained following water irrigation using 30° C and 44° C water for cool and warm irrigations, respectively.

Some investigators have demonstrated a lesser nystagmus intensity and larger intersubject variability for air caloric stimulation when water stimulation was used as a "gold standard."[28, 30] Coats et al.[28] demonstrated that when the air irrigation tip was moved from an optimal depth outward 7 mm toward the external auditory meatus the nystagmus slow-phase velocity (SPV) decreased 40% and 20% for the warm and cool irrigations, respectively. For these reasons and in an attempt to decrease the intrasubject variability the investigators recommended that the temperatures of 27.5° C and 45.5° C be used for cool and warm air caloric irrigations. Additionally, the authors recommended that an irrigation duration of 100 seconds be used and that the flow rate be increased 13 L/min.

Benitez et al.[17] reported that the maximum nystagmus SPV to cool and warm air caloric stimulation (27.4° C and 45° C, respectively, 6 L/min, 60 seconds) was 33% and 20% of that following conventional bithermal water caloric stimulation. Greven et al.[40] also demonstrated that the nystagmus

evoked by air caloric stimulation was less intense than that elicited by water caloric stimulation. However, Ford and Stockwell[35] demonstrated equivalent nystagmus velocity when comparing air and water caloric stimulation (24° C 50° C for cool and warm air caloric irrigations, 8 L/min, 60 seconds). The equivalency of air and water caloric stimuli have been reported by other investigators (for example, Tole[87]). Equivalent responses from air and water stimulation in clinical populations was observed by Suter et al.[83] Most investigators have observed that nystagmus duration is increased for water compared with air stimulation techniques.

In the hands of a meticulous, experienced clinician it is possible to obtain equivalent responses following air and water caloric stimulation. Factors of depth of insertion of the delivery tip and the orientation of the delivery tip in the ear canal are important in the ensuring of this equivalency.[17, 28, 36] It is clear that air caloric testing is more technically demanding than water caloric testing, and for these reasons the present authors continue to favor water caloric stimulation techniques over air techniques in the absence of tympanic perforations. (See "Problems, Pitfalls, and Artifacts" for caloric inversions following air caloric irrigations in the presence of medium or large tympanic perforations.)

Simultaneous Binaural Bithermal Test

Although Riesco-MacClure[73] described a simultaneous binaural bithermal caloric test in 1964 (using 15° C or 48° C water), it was Brookler[19, 20, 47] who is credited with popularizing this test in recent years. Brookler described a standardized method for conducting a bithermal caloric examination that has been referred to as the simultaneous bithermal test (SBT). For this examination, instead of alternately irrigating each ear with cool and then warm caloric stimuli, the ears are simultaneously irrigated first with cool water, then following a 5-minute interval they are irrigated simultaneously with warm water. The water is delivered through a "Y" tube to both ears. The total water flow is 250 mL, and the temperatures are the same as required for the ABB test (30° C and 44° C). Conventional ENG instrumentation is used to record the induced nystagmus. There are no quantitative measurements for this test. Only the presence or absence of nystagmus is observed as well as the direction of the induced nystagmus following each of the caloric irrigations. The SBT test was offered not as a replacement but as an adjunct to the ABB test.

Monothermal Caloric Tests

For these examinations only two warm caloric irrigations or two cool caloric irrigations are conducted. Percent differences in the magnitude of the responses obtained from each ear are calculated. For the most part, these examinations are used as screening tests (if the ENG examination up to the caloric test is normal) or are considered adjunctive tests (the Torok Monothermal Differential Caloric Test).

Monothermal Warm

Several investigators have attempted to decrease the amount of time required to conduct the ABB caloric test by conducting the examination at one temperature (monothermal caloric testing). Both monothermal cool and monothermal warm caloric screening tests have been proposed, although the monothermal warm caloric test has been the most popular of the two. The technique of the monothermal test is to administer only two of the four caloric irrigations that are used in the bithermal test. The average SPV obtained following the two irrigations is placed in a symmetry formula:

$$\frac{(LW - RW)}{(LW + RW)} \times 100$$

where LW = left warm and RW = right warm.

If the percent difference between the sides exceeds a critical value (which varies from published report-to-report but usually is between 25% and 29%), the monothermal test is called abnormal. It is important to understand that some investigators have suggested that the monothermal warm test be used as a replacement for the alternate binaural bithermal caloric test. Other investigators (including the present authors) suggest that the monothermal warm test be used as a "screening" test [hence the name monothermal warm screening test (MWST)]. It is understood that the MWST can be performed only if no abnormalities have been identified during the ENG up to the caloric test part of the ENG test battery. Also, the MWST calculations can be performed only if the SPV derived from each of the two warm irrigations exceeds 11°/sec. It should be understood that the ABB caloric test must be performed if the difference between sides exceeds the critical upper limit. The reason for this is if the critical value is exceeded it will not be possible to determine whether a patient is demonstrating a unilateral weakness or a directional preponderance based on two warm irrigations. Finally, the FS test is conducted during each of the warm irrigations. The MWST is described in greater detail in Chapter 9.

It is noteworthy that attempts have been made to develop a monothermal cool screening test (for example, see Becker[14]); however, cool stimuli have been associated with a larger number of false-negative predictions than warm stimuli. The reason monothermal warm caloric testing is associated with a smaller number of false-negative results than monothermal cool testing is unclear. It may be that the identification of abnormality in a pathologic vestibular system is associated with attempts at challenging the system to operate at levels above its resting discharge rate, rather than by evaluating the system with stimuli that are designed to decrease the spontaneous activity of the peripheral system close to its lower limit of function.

Monothermal Differential Caloric Test

This examination as described originally by Torok[93, 95] is a two-part test designed to identify the presence of vestibular recruitment and vestibular decruitment. Vestibular recruitment refers to the unusually rapid growth in the responsiveness of the vestibular system to increases in the intensity of the (caloric) stimulus. Vestibular decruitment refers to the observation of no increase or a decrease in the responsiveness of the vestibular system to increases in stimulus intensity. The stimulus is made more intense by increasing the volume of the caloric stimulus (from 10 mL to 100 mL of water). It has been the contention of the authors that vestibular recruitment (like loudness recruitment in the auditory system) is observed in the presence of peripheral vestibular system disease, such as end organ disease,[58] whereas decruitment phenomena are observed in the presence of central vestibular system disease (eighth cranial nerve and central vestibular pathways).[59, 95]

In the first part of the test the patient's ear is infused with 10 mL of 20° C water over a 5-second period. The patient is initially seated upright with the head pitched forward 30°. This position is designed to take the horizontal semicircular canal out of the plane of maximal stimulation (the cupula is oriented approximately parallel to the ground). After 1 minute, when the thermal changes are uniform, the patient's head is brought back 90° from the original position (60° degrees backward from verti-

cal). This position is designed to bring the horizontal canal into a plane of maximal stimulation (the cupula is vertical). The PENG recording techniques developed by Torok et al.[96] are utilized to record the induced nystagmus.

The second (more intense) irrigation is conducted using 100 mL of water at the same temperature (20°/C). The irrigation is performed with the patient's head tipped back 60° from vertical (optimal position for horizontal canal stimulation). The irrigation occurs over a 20-second period. The variable used to quantify nystagmus intensity is called culmination frequency. (See the section "Measurement of Caloric Data" for a description of culmination frequency.)

Indications and Technique for Ice Water Caloric Testing

In the absence of caloric responses to standard bithermal stimuli it is important to conduct ice water irrigations to verify the absence of any residual function. The ice water test is conducted with very cold water (10° C) either obtained from a drinking fountain or by filling a cup with water and ice. The patient turns the head so that the test ear faces upward (Fig 8–11,A). Two milliliters of water are drawn up into a syringe and infused into the ear canal. The patient maintains this head position for 20 seconds with the water in place, at which time the head is turned so that the water can run out of the ear canal. The patient's head is brought into the optimal position for caloric testing (30° up from supine, as illustrated in Fig 8–11,B), and the nystagmus is recorded. Some have stated that because of the discomfort of the test, the ice water irrigation may "release" a latent spontaneous nystagmus. A latent spontaneous nystagmus can be differentiated from caloric nystagmus by placing the patient in the prone position after the nystagmus has been observed in the supine position. The probability of latent spon-

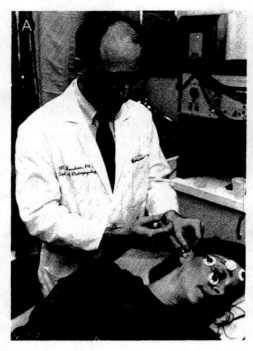
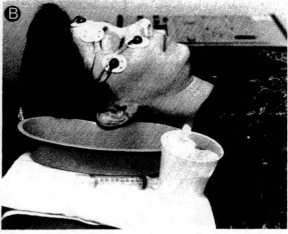

FIG 8–11.
A, patient in correct position for ice water test. **B,** patient's head is brought into position for optimal stimulation of the horizontal semicircular canal.

taneous nystagmus is good if the nystagmus direction does not reverse when the patient is inverted from the supine to the prone position.

MEASUREMENT OF CALORIC DATA

There are a number of different measurement issues in caloric testing. First it is important to find a measurement variable that shows a small coefficient of variation (that is, small variation within a group of subjects). Additionally, it is important to develop methods for using this variable or these variables to differentiate normal from abnormal vestibular systems.

Measurement Variables

A number of measurement variables have been used to quantify caloric-induced nystagmus. These have included duration, latency, amplitude, frequency, and velocity (Figs 8–12 and 8–13).

Duration

Nystagmus duration (see Fig 8–12) was the measurement variable used in the bithermal technique of Fitzgerald and Hallpike.[33] A stopwatch was started at the beginning of the irrigation, and timing was terminated at the point that nystagmus was no longer visible to the examiner. A time chart was made to depict graphically the asymmetries in the duration of the response. However, the duration of nystagmus is influenced by a number of factors unrelated to the responsiveness of the inner ear. The duration of the response is directly proportional to the amount of time required for the endolymph to reach its ambient temperature. That is, the endolymph in the horizontal semicircular canal is influenced by physiologic properties of the middle ear and temporal bone, which vary from person to person.

Latency

Following the development of electronystagmographic instrumentation it was possible to quantify nystagmus in greater detail. Nystagmus latency (see

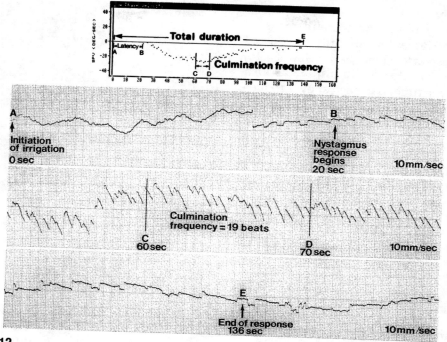

FIG 8–12.
Measurement parameters of latency, culmination frequency, and total duration are depicted graphically in a nystagmus velocity profile *(graph at top of figure)* and in the actual data *(bottom three nystagmus traces)* that have been abstracted from a caloric test.

Fig 8–12) refers to the interval from the initiation of the caloric irrigation to when the nystagmus response begins. Many factors, however, determine the latency of caloric nystagmus, including the heat-transmitting properties of the temporal bone and middle ear space (as noted earlier), and the alertness of the patient.

Amplitude

The amplitude of the nystagmus refers to the magnitude (measured in degrees) of the nystagmus measured from

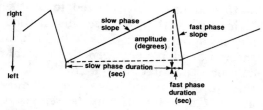

FIG 8–13.
Schematic diagram illustrating variables of slow and fast phase durations and slopes.

the base of the nystagmus "beat" to its peak (see Fig 8–13). Thus, amplitude describes the distance the eye travels (measured in degrees) during a slow phase of a nystagmus beat. This measurement variable in isolation fails to provide useful information, as both low- and high-amplitude nystagmus may have the same velocity.

Frequency

Nystagmus frequency refers to the number of nystagmus beats that occur within a given time period. The time period may be (1) 5 or 10 seconds, or (2) the duration of the entire caloric response. The "culmination frequency" is a term that refers to the total number of nystagmus beats that occur within a 10-second period at the peak of the caloric response (see Fig 8–12).[58, 89] Torok[91] stated that culmination frequency has a smaller standard deviation than the more popular measurement of slow-phase eye velocity.

Velocity

Velocity is the most useful measurement variable for quantifying the caloric response (Figs 8–14 and 8–15). Nystagmus velocity (amplitude as measured over time) has been shown to have the lowest coefficient of variation, reported by Henriksson[45] as 38%, and the greatest sensitivity to the presence of asymmetries in peripheral vestibular system function.[45]

Nystagmus SPV incorporates both amplitude and duration information and is quantified as the number of degrees of eye excursion over a 1-second period (°/sec). The SPV has been quantified by the highest velocity of a single nystagmus beat. More typically, SPV is quantified as an average of either of the following:

1. The three nystagmus beats with the greatest SPV at the peak of the caloric response;
2. All nystagmus beats in a 5-second period
3. All nystagmus beats in a 10-second period at the peak of the caloric response; or
4. Ten beats at the peak of the caloric response regardless of the sampling interval.

It has been our preference to calculate nystagmus velocity based on the average SPV of ten consecutive nystagmus beats at the peak of the caloric response. The choice of the average SPV of ten consecutive beats is an attempt to control for the sampling error that occurs when a fixed time of measurement is used. For example, for one ear, three beats of nystagmus might occur in a 5-second period, whereas five beats of nystagmus might occur for the other ear within the same period of time.

There are two methods for hand-measuring nystagmus velocity. These methods are illustrated in Figures 8–14 and 8–15,A–G. In the first method a line is drawn through the slow phase of a beat of nystagmus (see Fig 8–14). The line is

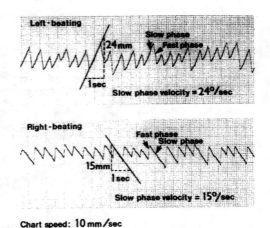

Chart speed: 10 mm/sec
Calibration: 1 mm = 1 deg of eye movement

FIG 8–14.
Illustration of common method for hand-measuring nystagmus slow-phase velocity for two pieces of nystagmus data *(top and bottom traces)*.

extended above and below the limits of this beat so that it reaches the margins of the paper. One then counts 10 mm horizontally, as the paper speed is normally 10 mm/sec and SPV is specified in the degrees (that is, amplitude) per second (time) as a unit of measure. The last step is to create a right triangle by connecting the 10-mm time mark to the diagonal line running through the nystagmus beat. The number of millimeters that constitute this vertical line up to the intersection are the number of degrees per second for that nystagmus beat (since eye movements are calibrated so that 1 mm of vertical pen excursion equals 1° of eye movement). The SPV of a number of nystagmus beats are calculated and averaged.

A second method that may be used to average the velocities of a number of nystagmus beats is illustrated in Figures 8–15 and has been referred to as the "gridding" method. To use this method one need only have an 8½ × 11-inch sheet of blank paper, a pencil, and a calculator. The first step is to block-off three (or five, or ten) beats of nystagmus at what appears visually to represent the peak of the nystagmus response. The bottom corner of the vertical side of the paper is placed next to the base of the

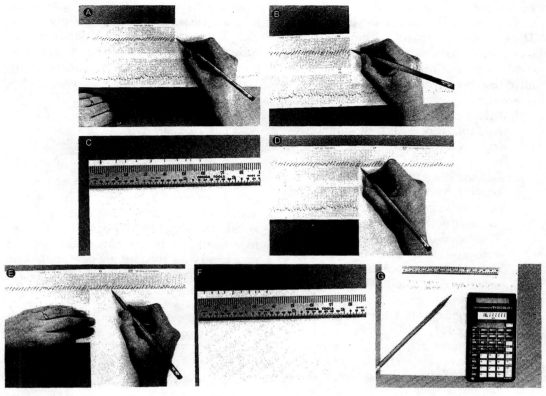

FIG 8–15.
A–G, Photographs depicting "gridding" method of hand-measuring caloric nystagmus slow-phase velocity. **A–C,** the "height" (amplitude) of ten consecutive nystagmus beats are stacked on a sheet of paper. The height is then measured in millimeters. **D–F,** the "width" (duration) of ten consecutive nystagmus beats are stacked on a sheet of paper. The duration is then measured in millimeters. **G,** the values are placed in a velocity formula (amplitude/time × 10.). The result is the average slow-phase velocity for ten consecutive nystagmus beats.

first beat of nystagmus. A tick is placed on the paper at a position representing the height of the peak of the first nystagmus beat (see Fig 8–15,A). This pencil tick becomes the reference base for the second beat of nystagmus. A second tick is placed over the first one, representing the height of the second nystagmus beat, and so on until the desired number of nystagmus beats have been sampled (see Fig 8–15,B). The horizontal part of the paper is used to "grid" the duration of each of the sampled nystagmus beats. The corner edge of the paper is placed next to the base of the first nystagmus beat. A pencil tick is placed on the paper at a point representing the time from the base to the peak of the nystagmus beat (Fig 8–15,D). This pencil tick becomes the point of reference for the

measurement of the second beat of nystagmus. The second beat of nystagmus is measured the same way, and so on (Fig 8–15,E). Finally, the height (in millimeters) is measured on the vertical axis (nystagmus amplitude, see Fig 8–15,C) and this value is divided by the total ticks (in millimeters) on the horizontal axis (nystagmus time; see Fig 8–15,F). This value is then multiplied by a factor of 10 and the result represents the average velocity in degrees per second (amplitude/time) for the total number of nystagmus beats (see Fig 8–15,G).

Calculation of Parameters

The caloric test is used to determine if the level of function of one peripheral vestibular system differs in a statistically significant manner from the other. Thus, there are three primary and one secondary measurement techniques used to determine normalcy of the caloric response. These methods are:

1. Interaural (left ear versus right ear) differences in nystagmus SPV (referred to as unilateral weakness);
2. Differences in the SPV of right-beating as compared with left-beating caloric responses (referred to as directional preponderance);
3. The capability of the central nervous system to exert control over the vestibular nuclei and thereby attenuate caloric nystagmus when the eyes are opened and gaze is fixed on a point (referred to as FS); and
4. The overall hyper- or hypoexcitability of the peripheral vestibular systems (referred to as hyperactive responses and bilateral caloric weakness).

   What constitutes clinical significance in these calculations and the diagnostic implications of these findings will be discussed in detail in Chapter 9.

Formula for Determining Symmetry of Function

The calculation in equation (8-2) is designed to compare the responses obtained from the left ear with those obtained from the right ear. Data are provided on symmetry of function, which also allow determination of unilateral weakness to be computed. The formula used to calculate these differences is as follows:

$$\frac{(LC + LW) - (RC + RW)}{(LC + LW + RC + RW)} \times 100$$

where the LC, LW, RC and RW refer to the average SPV values for the left cool, left warm, right cool, and right warm

caloric irrigations. LC + LW give total left-side responses; RC + RW give total right-side responses. The denominator contains the total of all responses. The result of this equation is multiplied by 100 to yield a percent difference between the left and right sides.

Formula for Calculating Directional Preponderance

Fitzgerald and Hallpike[33] originally described the phenomenon of directional preponderance in their historic article that described the alternate binaural bithermal caloric test. The following formula enables calculation of the propensity for nystagmus beating in one direction to be greater than the nystagmus beating in the opposite direction (directional preponderance).

$$\frac{(LC + RW) - (RC + LW)}{(LC + LW + RC + RW)} \times 100$$

where LC (left cool) + RW (right warm) = total of right-beating caloric responses, and RC (right cool) + LW (left warm) = total of left-beating responses, and the denominator is expressed as in the preceding formula. The practical significance of the observation of directional preponderance will be described in Chapter 9.

Formula for Assessment of Fixation Index

The fixation index (FI) is used to assess the intactness of connections between the vestibular nuclei and the midline cerebellar structures. Fixation index is calculated by using a modification of the FI formula developed by Demanez and Ledoux.[31]

$$FI = \frac{SPV\ (EO)}{SPV\ (EC)}$$

where SPV (EO) represents the average slow-phase nystagmus eye velocity that occurs for 5 seconds after the eyes are opened and fixated (allowing up to 2 seconds for visual fixation to occur) and SPV (EC) represents the average slow-phase nystagmus eye velocity that occurs for 5 seconds before the eyes are opened at the point of greatest nystagmus velocity.

Other Issues: Display of Data

Once caloric data have been collected and analyzed the data must be presented to the referral source in the form of a report or summary. Several types of reports have been developed over the years. Some reports consist of little more than a sheet of paper having check-marked boxes and a table of numbers representing the slow-phase velocities for each of the caloric irrigations and the percent directional preponderance and unilateral weakness. Other report forms consist of these summaries with the addition of illustrative raw data. This raw data may consist of extracted ENG strips that have been pasted on paper. Similarly, the newer commercially available ENG systems permit illustrative raw data to be printed on standard 8½ × 11-inch computer printer paper. The requirement of any report is that the data should be displayed in a clear and understandable manner.

Several types of pictorial formats have been offered for illustrating the results of the caloric test. If a pictorial format is used, there should be no ambiguity as to the meaning of the illustration. The following are examples of display types that permit a rapid visual appraisal of the intensity of the caloric response.

Fitzgerald and Hallpike Method.— The earliest technique for illustrating postcaloric intensity was developed by Fitzgerald and Hallpike.[33] The measurement variable was the duration of the caloric response. The investigators created a scale that consisted of an abscissa below which were placed numbers representing time measured in seconds (Fig 8–16). An arrowhead was used to de-

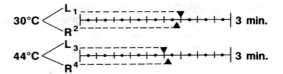

FIG 8–16.
Data representation technique used by Fitzgerald and Hallpike[33] to illustrate nystagmus duration.

note the time value representing the duration of a given caloric response. There were four of these scales for each caloric examination, representing the results of the two warm and two cold caloric tests. This display technique permitted the reader a clear representation of asymmetries in the caloric response.

Butterfly Chart.—Claussen and von Schlachta[25] developed another visual display method for plotting the intensity of caloric-induced nystagmus. The measurement variable for this technique is nystagmus frequency. Warm and cool responses for the right and left ears are plotted in a rectangular coordinate system that produces a butterfly-shaped graph (Fig 8–17). Responses on the "butterfly" chart are plotted by marking the maximum frequency on the four vertical scales (right warm, right cool, left warm, and left cool) and then connecting the four marks with the 0 point located in the center of the graph.

Pods.—The MASTR (ICS Medical) computerized ENG system permits the display of a nystagmus velocity "envelope" following each caloric irrigation. This envelope is actually a graph with time (in seconds) on the abscissa (as in the Fitzgerald and Hallpike report technique) and nystagmus velocity (measured in degrees/per second) represented on the ordinate. A computer algorithm is used to measure the velocity of each caloric nystagmus beat. The result of each measurement is a "dot" that is placed on the graph. The normal caloric response begins with low-velocity nystagmus. The nystagmus builds to a crescendo and then gradually declines. The

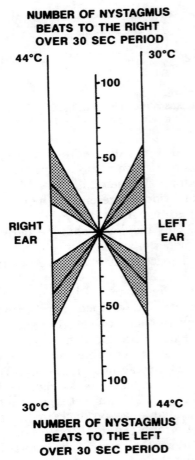

FIG 8–17.
Data representation technique used by Claussen[25] to illustrate nystagmus frequency.

scatter plot of these data from a healthy individual looks like a normal bell-shaped curve. The left ear caloric responses are represented on separate sides of the graph, and the velocity scatter plots are placed one above the other. The velocity profiles following warm and cool caloric stimulation are opposite in direction. Therefore, if the velocity profiles for left ear cool and warm caloric responses for a healthy individual are placed directly over each other the result is a picture that resembles a pea pod (hence the term "pods"). Figure 8–18 illustrates responses obtained from a normal subject. Cool and warm caloric data for the right and left ears are shown on the right and left sides of the figure, respectively. In this example,

responses begin approximately 25 seconds after the onset of the irrigation, reaching a maximum slow-phase velocity between 60 and 80 seconds, followed by a decline in response intensity. In healthy subjects, responses to cool and warm irrigations are almost mirror images of each other (that is, warm caloric irrigations tend to elicit slightly stronger mean nystagmus velocities). Further, response strength is essentially equivalent between the right and left ear.

It is the recommendation of the present authors that a signed cover letter summarizing the findings of the entire ENG examination, together with a summary sheet giving numeric data and raw traces illustrating abnormalities, should be forwarded to the referral source. This will permit the referral physician who is less sophisticated in ENG examination the option of reading a summary letter, whereas the physician who is more sophisticated will have the opportunity to evaluate the numeric data.

STIMULUS-RELATED AND SUBJECT-RELATED VARIABLES KNOWN TO AFFECT THE CALORIC RESPONSE

Stimulus-Related Variables

Water Temperature

A number of investigators have examined the relationship between warm and cool temperature effects and caloric responses.[4, 35, 45, 63] Higher intensities with shorter response times have been associated with warm water in comparison to cool water stimuli.[78] In this connection, Baertschi et al.[3] indicated that warm water irrigations result in increased blood flow through the skin and bone, resulting in increased thermal conduction of heat to the horizontal canals, and producing a strong caloric response; however, the caloric response declines rapidly because the warm irrigation acts to equalize temperature dif-

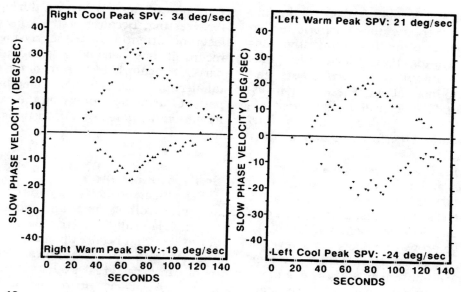

FIG 8–18.
Data representation technique (Pods) used by ICS Medical Corporation to represent nystagmus velocity over time.

ferences faster than cool irrigations. Therefore, warm irrigations have shorter response times. In contrast, cool water irrigation gives rise to less intense responses with longer durations. The arterioles in the external meatus and temporal bone constrict, causing a reduction in heat transmission to the horizontal canals. Further, the decay time of the resultant temperature difference is increased, causing a longer response time. Sills et al.[78] indicated that from a clinical standpoint, temperature effects must be taken into account particularly when evaluating a directional preponderance in a patient having only one ear tested or in the case of a unilateral weakness.

Finally, it is critical that the calibration of the water stimulus be as accurate as possible. The warm and cool caloric temperatures are only 7° C above and below normal body temperature. This means that a 1° variation away from the ideal 30° C or 44° C will result in a 14% difference in the magnitude of the stimulus. It is unclear what effect this degree of deviation from the ideal temperature will have on the caloric response.

Habituation

Repeated irrigation of the same ear with the same caloric stimulus will result in a gradual decrement in the caloric response.[34] This phenomenon has been termed vestibular habituation. Fluur and Mendel[34] examined 24 subjects, half of whom received repeated warm water irrigations and half of whom received repeated cool water irrigations. The caloric response was allowed to end before the next irrigation began. Each subject received between 8 and 12 caloric irrigations for each temperature. The examiners found for warm water irrigations that there was a regular decrement in the duration of the caloric response but that the response never did disappear. The authors were able to completely extinguish the caloric response following cool water irrigations.

Subject-Related Variables

Subject Attention, Arousal, and Vigilance

It is a common occurrence that during caloric irrigation little nystagmus may be observed until the patient is asked to perform some type of alerting exercise. This practice of conducting alerting exercises during caloric testing grew out of a number of investigations demonstrating that caloric nystagmus may be inhibited by drowsiness and boredom in a patient. These same investigations demonstrated that brisk caloric nystagmus may be elicited by having a patient perform mental alerting exercises.

Collins et al.[29] observed a caloric nystagmus of longer duration when their subjects were performing serial arithmetic tasks. The investigators also noted that the electronystagmograms of relaxed or drowsy subjects often revealed the presence of slow sinusoidal (pendular) eye movements. These eye movements were described by Barber and Wright[12] under similar conditions. Sokolovski[79] evaluated the effects of three conditions of mental alertness and visual fixation on caloric nystagmus: (1) visual fixation without mental activity; (2) visual fixation with mental activity; and (3) no visual fixation with mental activity. These authors found that the velocity, duration, frequency, and amplitude of the caloric nystagmus were superior in the third alerted condition. Torok[92] found that subjects were as likely to have consistent caloric responses if they were asked to remain relaxed and keep their eyes open in darkness as if they were forced to complete arithmetic calculations under the same fixation conditions. Torok argued for a flexible approach to tasks for maintaining the ENG record, which could be tailored to each subject. Barber and Wright[12] developed a standardized taped list of questions (difficulty of questions ranging from 30 months' mental age to sophisticated mathematic calculations) for patients undergoing caloric testing. The authors commented on the presence of nystagmus suppression and dysrhythmia (beat-to-beat fluctuation in the amplitude and frequency of nystagmus that has been attributed to the presence of central vestibular system disease) occurring in patients who were not adequately alerted during caloric testing. Because of the known effects of attention on the nystagmus record it has become a standardized part of the caloric test protocol for mental alerting tasks to be performed by the patient during and following the caloric irrigation (as noted earlier in this chapter).

Bell's Phenomenon

Bell's phenomenon refers to the reflex averting (rolling up) and adducting (moving laterally toward one another) of the eyes that occurs upon eye closure. The magnitude of the upward movement can be as great as 151°.[39] Indeed, as stated earlier, Hood and Korres[49] demonstrated that the caloric response could be completely suppressed by Bell's phenomenon.

Attempts have been made to quantify Bell's phenomenon. Goebel et al.[39] reported a mean upward deviation of 151° upon eye closure in 20 normal subjects. The authors reported that 89% of their sample demonstrated a decreased nystagmus regularity during voluntary eye elevation. This nystagmus dysrhythmia decreased once the eyes returned to baseline. The investigators demonstrated further that the effects of the Bell's phenomenon could be offset by approximately 47° by initiation of mental exercises by the subject. The authors also reported that 53% of their sample demonstrated bursts of nystagmus inhibition that correlated with the involuntary vertical eye movements (see Figure 4, page 1130, in reference 39).

The experience of the present authors is somewhat different from that of Goeble and associates. In our investigation of seven healthy young neurologically intact subjects, in which electro-oculographic instrumentation and monocular recording techniques were used, we found a mean upward deviation of 40° (±12°) and a mean lateral deviation of 9° (± 8°) following bilateral eye closure. The magnitude of the vertical eye deviation is reasonably close to the 55° vertical movement following eye closure reported previously by Takemori et al.[86]

Subject Age

A number of investigations have been conducted since the late 1930s that have served to describe the effect of age on caloric nystagmus. These investigations have been published in international journals without the benefit of English language translation or abstracts. The interested reader is directed to reviews of these early studies found in Mulch and Petermann[64] and Oosterveld.[65] In general, these studies have demonstrated that decrements in vestibular responsiveness occur with age regardless of the measurement parameter that is chosen to quantify the magnitude of the caloric response. For instance, we have observed a weak but statistically significant negative correlation between total cool SPV and subject age and, total SPV (the grand total SPV from all four caloric irrigations), and subject age (see Table 9–6).

In an early study, Arslan (2) evaluated 50 healthy subjects between the ages of 49 and 84 years. The investigator reported that, in general, middle-aged subjects showed hypoactive responses and subjects aged 70 years and older showed hyperactive responses. Almost 20 years later, van der Laan and Oosterveld[98] reported their observations from a group of 334 normal subjects. The authors reported a lower nystagmus frequency and greater nystagmus amplitude in younger subjects (up through the 3rd decade of life) compared with older subjects. The nystagmus frequency increased and amplitude decreased in the older age groups. The investigators suggested that these findings in the older age groups (subjects over 50 years of age) could be explained by decreased blood supply (due to atherosclerosis) reaching the vestibular end organ.

Bruner and Norris[22] reported their observations culled from examinations of 293 caloric examinations from indi-viduals with negative findings on vestibular system testing. The authors quantified nystagmus latency, amplitude, frequency, average maximum SPV, and duration. The only statistically significant parameters to show age-dependent changes were nystagmus frequency for cool caloric stimuli, maximum SPV, frequency for warm caloric stimulation, and total (combined warm and cool) caloric stimulation. In general, the authors found these nystagmus parameters to peak in the 60- to 70-year-old age group and to decline thereafter.

In a much-quoted study, Mulch and Petermann[64] evaluated caloric responses in 102 subjects aged 11 to 70 years. The authors quantified the total number of beats of nystagmus, maximum SPV, frequency, and amplitude over a 10-second period. Like Bruner and Norris,[22] Mulch and Petermann reported significant age-dependent increases in the total number of beats, maximum frequency, amplitude, and SPV up to about 60 years of age, after which decrements in function occurred.

Karlsen et al.[54] reported their results following conventional bithermal caloric testing in 75 subjects aged 18 to 81 years. The authors quantified nystagmus amplitude, latency, duration, frequency, and SPV following irrigations. All parameters showed an age-related decrement. The suggestion from this investigation was that there is a decline in vestibular system responsiveness beginning around age 65 to 70, which is in general agreement with previous studies.

Ghosh[38] reported the results of serial vestibulometry on 78 subjects that were divided into seven age groups spanning 10 to 71+ years. In serial vestibulometry, the ear was irrigated with water at 45° C, 33° C, 29° C, 25° C, 21° C, and 17° C. The maximum SPV following each irrigation was the measurement parameter. The author reported that there were greater age-related differences in the caloric nystagmus SPV at the extremes of irrigation temperatures. Age had a general effect of decreasing SPV. The mean performance of subjects above the age of 51 years fell outside normal limits. No parametric analyses were reported, although the general finding of reduced caloric SPV as a function of age is consistent with the findings of previous research.

Drugs

The ingestion of certain drugs may affect the physiological control of eye movements and/or the patient's level of arousal. Both of these factors may invalidate and/or complicate the interpretation of ENG findings.

It is well known that ocular motility studies may be affected by therapeutic and toxic doses of various drugs[5, 61] Smooth pursuit is known to be impaired by phenytoin,[18] phenobarbital and other barbiturates,[72 75] and alcohol.[7] Gaze-evoked nystagmus is produced by ingestion of phenytoin,[46, 60, 74] carbamazepine,[97] and barbiturates.[71] Downbeat nystagmus has been reported in two epileptic patients taking phenytoin, which disappeared when the dosage was reduced.[1] Similarly, Wheeler and his co-workers[100] documented a reversible downbeat nystagmus produced by ingestion of carbamazepine in an epileptic patient with no evidence of structural abnormality on computed tomographic scanning. Saccadic system abnormalities including reduced peak velocity,[56] increased latency,[56] and hypometria[7] have been attributed to alcohol intoxication. Thus, abnormal eye movements caused by a number of drugs should not be misinterpreted as pathologic nystagmus associated with central nervous system disease.

Although the ocular motility subtests of the ENG battery are particularly susceptible to various drugs, as indicated, the caloric examination also may be influenced by certain agents. Haciska[41] evaluated caloric responses obtained from eight young adults, 1 hour after ingestion of a barbiturate (200 mg of sodium amylobaritone-amytal sodium). It was observed that when the subject's eyes were closed, the nystagmus was either absent or weak. However, when the eyes were open and fixation was attempted, regular strong beats of nystagmus appeared. Haciska concluded that barbiturates depress function in the reticular formation, the site of origin for the fast phase of nystagmus. In contrast, physiology within the medial longitudinal fasciculus is unaffected. This makes it possible for the conjugate slow phase of nystagmus to occur. Thus, during barbiturate intoxication the eyes deviate in the direction of the slow phase and remain in a lateral position during eye closure. However, following eye opening the gaze system brings the eyes to midline. The force of the slow component generated by the medial longitudinal fasciculus deviates the eyes laterally, and this is followed by a refixation saccade. This may be misinterpreted as failure of fixation suppression. In addition to barbiturates, Barber and Stockwell[11] have indicated that failure of fixation suppression for caloric nystagmus may result from antiepileptic drug (AED) intoxication as well. The latter authors also attributed this phenomenon to drug interference with reticular formation activity.

The mild sedative effects of barbiturates, antihistamines, and tranquilizers may result in a lowering of the patient's level of alertness,[11, 82] which in turn, may suppress caloric-induced nystagmus. Although alerting exercises may be used assiduously, it might be difficult or even impossible for the examiner to maintain an adequate level of arousal necessary for conducting the caloric examination. In this situation, it is important for the clinician to be aware of this potential source of error and not inadvertently interpret the obtained responses (or lack thereof) as reduced or absent vestibular function.

From the foregoing discussion it is apparent that the ingestion of certain drugs may (1) cause impaired smooth pursuit, gaze-evoked nystagmus, or saccadic system deficits to occur that are normally associated with the presence of central nervous system disease; (2) abolish or impair fixation suppression ability; and/or (3) suppress caloric nystagmus. It is recommended that patients should be instructed to discontinue medications and to eliminate the intake of alcohol for 48 hours prior to the ENG examination. Prior to testing, the examiner should confirm compliance with instruction. Exceptions to these instructions include those patients who are taking antiepilepsy medications, and psychiatric patients who are taking behavior-mediating medications (for example, antipsychotic medications). If there are any questions whether a patient referred for ENG testing can be told to discontinue taking their medications for a 48-hour period, the responsible clinician should consult the referring physician. We have found that (for the most part) referring physicians are unaware of the effects that medications have on the vestibulo-ocular reflex or on ocular motility. Likewise, most referring physicians are agreeable, when possible, to having their patients not take these medications for the period of time necessary to obtain an interpretable test. It is incumbent on the clinician to note any medications or drugs ingested by the patient and to interpret the ENG findings accordingly, or, more preferably, to reschedule the examination.

Recording Variables

Illumination and Visual Fixation

A number of studies have analyzed the effects of different types of visual fixation on the caloric response. The initial study conducted by Fitzgerald and Hallpike[33] was conducted before the advent of electro-oculographic (electronystagmographic) techniques, and thus nystagmus could not be observed behind closed eyelids. Therefore, patients were evaluated with their eyes open and fixating their gaze on a distant point, much the same way that fixation sup-

pression testing is conducted today. After electronystagmography became available, studies were conducted with the purpose of examining the effects of different types of ocular fixation and room illumination on caloric nystagmus. The ultimate purpose of these studies was to determine optimal data recording conditions for conducting the caloric examination.

The caloric test is usually conducted under one of three conditions: (1) with the patient's eyes open in a completely dark room; (2) with the patient's eyes closed in a semi-darkened room, and (3) with the patient's eyes open and wearing Frenzel's lenses in a semi-darkened room. It is extremely difficult to create a light-proofed environment that is required to eliminate visual fixation during the caloric test. However, conducting the examination with eyes opened in darkness eliminates the effect of Bell's phenomenon on the caloric response. Most clinicians conduct the examination with the patient's eyes closed in a semi-darkened room. Baloh et al.[6] examined these testing conditions and determined that the coefficient of variation of the caloric response was lowest with the patient's eyes opened in a dark room. The next best recording technique was with the patient's eyes opened and wearing Frenzel's lenses. The authors noted that nystagmus was periodically suppressed and there was slowing of the fast component when the examination was conducted with the patient's eyes closed.

Like Baloh et al.,[6] Karlsen et al.[53] examined visual fixation during caloric testing. These authors observed that nystagmus SPV was equivalent in both the "eyes open in darkness" and "eyes closed in darkness" conditions. Further, in contrast to the findings of Baloh and co-workers, the coefficient of variation was found to be largest for the conditions where Frenzel's lenses were used (such as eyes opened and lighted lenses, eyes opened with unlighted lenses, eyes opened with lighted lenses and strobe lighting). In fact, the authors reported that caloric nystagmus was suppressed in the lighted lenses conditions (presumably because of the subject's ability to fixate their gaze on objects within the glasses).

The clinician should be aware that the visual conditions under which the caloric test is performed are not trivial considerations. The present authors recognize the practical limitations that must be dealt with in a hospital or outpatient clinic. We recommend that caloric testing be conducted with eyes opened in darkness, or with eyes closed in a semi-darkened room. The importance of effective alerting exercises is critical if the latter technique is used.

Head/Body Position

Coats and Smith[27] conducted a meticulous study of the caloric response as subject body position (12 subjects) was varied over 360°. Data from this study (see Figures 5 and 6 from reference)[27] illustrated that the maximum caloric response occurred when the head (and body) was positioned between 0° and 60° upward from the supine position for both warm and cool caloric irrigations. From their data it appears that small deviations in the position of the head from the ideal 30° vertical (with the subject in the supine position) probably have little effect on the magnitude of the caloric response.

Variables Affecting Fixation Suppression Ability

Caloric Temperature

It is surprising that little is known about the effect that specific stimulus variables have on FS. For instance, it is generally accepted that warm water (44° C) caloric stimuli elicit stronger slow-phase nystagmus velocities (SPV) than cool caloric (30° C) stimuli.[24, 69] It is also known that the pursuit system can follow smoothly moving targets with a gain of 1.0 for targets that move from 30° to 60° per second. As this upper limit is exceeded the target slips off of the retina and the smooth eye movements are replaced by catch-up saccades. It would follow that if the pursuit system plays a role in cancellation of vestibulo-ocular reflex that caloric stimuli associated with greater SPVs would be associated with lesser amounts of vestibulo-ocular reflex cancellation. An investigation conducted by Jacobson and Henry[50] demonstrated temperature-dependant changes in FS ability. It was shown that warm caloric stimulations were associated with poorer FS ability. It is interesting to note that these differences were small (mean difference in FS ability = 0.12) and they were associated with relatively small differences in the mean maximum SPV for the cool and warm caloric irrigations (20.31°/sec and 29.59°/sec, respectively).

Effects of Age on Fixation Suppression Ability

The same investigation by Jacobson and Henry[50] showed a relationship between FS ability and subject age but only for the warm caloric stimulus. The authors explained this finding based on the assumptions that (1) warm caloric stimuli yield larger SPV's than cool caloric stimuli, and (2) that FS is mediated by the pursuit pathway. It is known that the upper limit for normal pursuit gain (a gain of 1.0) for healthy subjects is 30°/sec for target excursions of ± 10° from primary gaze.[77] A pursuit gain of 1.0 for elderly subjects is not seen for target velocities greater than 5°/sec.[77] The mean age of the subjects in the study conducted by Sharpe and Sylvester[77] was 72 years. The mean age of the subjects who participated in the study conducted by Jacobson and Henry[50] was 57 years. In fact, 61% of the subject population was 60 years of age or older. Thus, it is likely that FS ability differed in the older subjects because the warm caloric irrigations resulted in a nystagmus SPV that exceeded the age-related limits of the pursuit subsystem.

Practice Effects

Takemori[84] has reported that fixation suppression ability in normals improved with repeated testing.

PROBLEMS, PITFALLS, AND ARTIFACTS ASSOCIATED WITH CALORIC TESTING

Perverted Nystagmus

In a patient with normal anatomy, there is no circumstance where stimulating the horizontal semicircular canal can result in a vertical nystagmus or a vertical component to a primarily horizontal nystagmus. The observation of vertical nystagmus during caloric testing has been referred to as "perverted" nystagmus.[4, 10] This type of nystagmus occurs rarely and denotes disease affecting the vestibular nuclei. The vestibular nuclei process afferent activity from the peripheral system. The outflow from the vestibular nuclei is then routed through the oculomotor system.

It is important to be aware that other sources may account for the presence of a vertical component during caloric testing. During calibration it is important to determine whether the vertical channel shows pen movement during horizontal eye movements. It is possible for the vertical electrodes to record a small potential difference during horizontal eye movements. If this phenomenon can be detected during calibration and during oculomotor subsystem testing, contamination of the vertical channel by horizontal nystagmus may be expected during caloric testing.

Eye Blink Artifact in the Horizontal Channel

Eye blink activity can be observed in the horizontal channel of the two-channel nystagmus record (Fig 8–19). However, the biphasic eye movement generated by eye blinking is usually sharply peaked without a definite slow or fast phase. It is helpful in these instances to attempt to correlate in time the eye blinking in the vertical channel with the

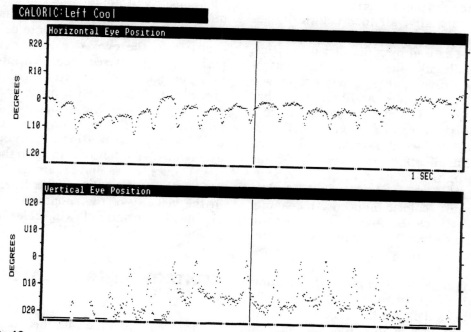

FIG 8–19.
Example of eye blink artifact. Note the synchronization of peaks in the horizontal channel *(top)* with the eye blinks in the vertical channel *(bottom)*.

questionable nystagmus in the horizontal channel. If the two are correlated in time it is probable that the horizontal nystagmus is eye blinking artifact.

Weak or Absent Responses

As discussed earlier, one of the four caloric irrigations may yield a minimal response. This may occur in the presence of both a unilateral weakness on the ipsilateral side and a directional preponderance for nystagmus beating toward the opposite ear. Alternatively, this may occur because the irrigation was less than optimal or because the patient was not properly alerted. It has been suggested[11] that the sign of an adequate water irrigation is the presence of a drop of water on the eardrum. It is always wise to visualize the eardrum prior to the caloric irrigation. This accomplishes two purposes. First, otoscopy will identify the presence of large amounts of cerumen that could obstruct the flow of water or air. Second, visualizing the eardrum provides information about what direction to orient the delivery tube during the irrigation.

Occasionally, all four caloric irrigations will not yield nystagmus. This may be caused by a number of reasons. It has already been stated that inattentive or drowsy subjects may not show a caloric nystagmus. Additionally, it has been noted that many medications that act on the central nervous system will affect the vestibulocular reflex arc. These medications may have a profound effect on the intensity of caloric nystagmus. Also, those patients who fail to generate caloric-induced nystagmus with eyes closed may have a saccadic system deficit. These patients are often unable to generate saccades during saccadic system testing. During caloric testing only the slow phase (the vestibular phase) of the nystagmus occurs. The eyes behind closed lids become tonically deviated in the direction of the slow phase. This phenomenon may only be observed when the patient's eyes are open. Thus, when an absent caloric response occurs it is important to observe the position of the patient's eyes during fixation suppression testing as soon as the eyes are opened. The finding of saccadic system abnormality of this type implicates the pontine brain stem reticular activating system. Finally, it has been noted by ourselves and others that some subjects who do not demonstrate caloric responses will demonstrate normal responses to rotational testing. It is known that water or air caloric stimulation is analogous to a rotational stimulus at around 0.003 Hz. Rotational testing usually begins at or about 0.01 Hz. Thus, it is possible that these patients have reduced peripheral vestibular system function at the lower end of its operating range.

Spontaneous or Congenital Nystagmus Superimposed on Caloric Response

Spontaneous nystagmus can complicate the interpretation of the gaze, optokinetic, positional, and positioning tests. Spontaneous nystagmus can also complicate the caloric test. Spontaneous nystagmus algebraically adds to or subtracts from the evoked caloric nystagmus. Thus, a 30°/sec right-beating caloric response will be attenuated by a preexisting 15°/sec, left-beating spontaneous nystagmus. The same caloric response will be eliminated by a preexisting 30°/sec, left-beating spontaneous nystagmus. It often occurs that the responsiveness of an end organ can be assessed only by calculating the difference in the velocity of the spontaneous nystagmus before and following caloric irrigation.

CONTROVERSIES IN CALORIC TESTING

In recent years a number of published reports have been critical of Barany's theory of caloric transduction.[48, 66–68, 76, 81, 101] These papers were published for the most part following the voyage of Spacelab I in November 1983.[13] During this mission, caloric stimulations were conducted on two subjects. The caloric medium was air, and both ears were irrigated simultaneously with air at 15° C for one ear and 44° C for the other ear. The intent was to create as intense a stimulus as possible. If the thermal convection theory was the only method for transduction, no nystagmus should have resulted from the caloric stimulation in microgravity, because the relative differences in the density of endolymphatic fluids would not exist. However, nystagmus (albeit weak) was elicited by the air stimulus (5°/sec for one subject and 19°/sec for the second subject). These observations were supported during investigations of nystagmus following caloric stimulation in parabolic flight under microgravity conditions by Oosterveld et al.[66] Paige[67] plugged the horizontal semicircular canal of squirrel monkeys and subjected them to ice water caloric irrigations. The inactivation of the semicircular canal did not result in the absence of caloric nystagmus. Finally, Coats and Smith,[27] after the experiments of Behrman,[15, 16] investigated the effects of body position on the presence of caloric nystagmus. The investigators conducted caloric stimulations with their subjects fixed on a table that could be rotated about the binaural axis. The nystagmus was measured every 30° of movement of the table through the full 360° degrees rotation. The authors demonstrated that the evoked nystagmus intensity was clearly greater in subjects in the face-up than in the face-down condition. The thermal convection theory would have predicted an equal and opposite direction and intensity of nystagmus when the table was inverted. Taken together these findings have caused investigators to search for alternative or adjunctive explanations for the presence of caloric nystagmus.

It is now believed that there are at least two additional routes of thermal stimulation in the vestibular system. These are (1) through direct thermal stimulation of the vestibular end organ and/or neural elements, and (2) through volume expansion of endolymph and the resulting mechanical transduction of the end organ.

Direct Thermal Stimulation of the Vestibular End Organ and/or Neural Elements

From data obtained by Coats and Smith[27] as reinterpreted by Hood,[48] it was illustrated that caloric responses of subjects in the face-up position were stronger than in the face-down position irrespective of irrigation temperature. It was hypothesized that the caloric stimulus directly heated or cooled the end organ independent of convection. Heating neural elements tends to increase their level of firing over the spontaneous level, and cooling tends to decrease the firing level. According to this theory warm stimulation would result in an excitatory response that was a combination of convective and direct thermal forces. When the subject was inverted (face-down), the convective effect would reverse (and result in a nystagmus beating in the opposing direction), but the direct thermal effect would not reverse and would subtract from the convective response. The same mechanism would occur for cool caloric stimulation. The convective and direct thermal forces would act to reduce activity on the ipsilateral side and result in a nystagmus beating to the opposite direction. Inverting the position of the subject would reverse the convective flow of endolymph and reverse the nystagmus but would not reverse the direct thermal effect on the affected end organ. Therefore, the evoked nystagmus would result from an admixture of excitatory and inhibitory influences. The net result would be a nystagmus intensity that was of lesser degree with the subject in the face-down position. Hood[48] reported from his recalculations of Coats and Smith's data that the direct thermal effect contributed 42% and 34%, respectively, to the total nystagmus responses of warm and cool stimulation with the subject in the position of maximum response.

Direct Volume Expansion From Thermal Stimulation

A second explanation for the results reported by Coats and Smith[27] has been offered by Wit et al.[101] According to this theory, the heat transfer following caloric stimulation results in an overall expansion of the fluid. In a closed system like the membranous labyrinth of the horizontal semicircular canal, warm caloric stimulation results in uniformly distributed pressure being exerted on the cupula. Thus, a warm stimulation would be expected to increase and cool stimulation would be expected to decrease the volume of endolymph and the resulting endolymphatic pressure on the cupula. This increase or decrease of pressure would result in an increase (depolarization) or decrease (hyperpolarization) of spontaneous activity on the affected side.

REFERENCES

1. Alpert JN: Downbeat nystagmus due to anticonvulsant toxicity. *Ann Neurol* 1978; 4:471–473.
2. Arslan M: The senescence of the vestibular apparatus. *Pract Otol Rhinol Laryngol* 1957; 19:475–483.
3. Baertschi AJ, Johnson RN, Hanna GR: A theoretical and experimental determination of vestibular dynamics in caloric stimulation. *Biol Cybern* 1975; 20:175–186.
4. Baloh RW, Honrubia V: *Clinical Neurophysiology of the Vestibular System.* Philadephia, FA Davis, 1979.
5. Baloh RW, Honrubia V: (1990). *Clinical Neurophysiology of the Vestibular System,* ed 2. Philadelphia, FA Davis, 1990.
6. Baloh RW, Sills AW, Solingen L, et al: Caloric testing: Effect of different conditions of ocular fixation. *Ann Otol Rhinol Laryngol* [Suppl] 1977; 43:1–6.
7. Baloh RW, Sharma S, Moskowitz H, et al: Effect of alcohol and marijuana on eye movements. *Aviat Space Environ Med* 1979; 50:18–23.
8. Barany R: Untersuchungen uber den vom vestibularapparat des ohres reflectorisch ausgelosten rhytmischen nystagmus und seine begleiterscheinungen. *Monatschr Ohrenheilk* 1906; 40:193–297.
9. Barany R, Witmaack K: Funktionelle prufung des vestibularapparates verhandl. *Dtsch Otolog Gesellsch* 1911; 20:37–184.
10. Barber HO, Stockwell C: *Manual of Electronystagmography.* St Louis, CV Mosby, 1976.
11. Barber HO, Stockwell CW: *Manual of Electronystagmography.* St Louis, CV Mosby, 1980.
12. Barber H, Wright G: Release of nystagmus suppression in clinical electronystagmography. *Laryngoscope* 1967; 77:1016–1027.
13. Baumgarten R, von Benson A, Brand U, et al: Effects of rectilinear acceleration and optokinetic and caloric stimulations in space. *Science* 1984; 225:208–224.
14. Becker GD: The screening value of monothermal caloric tests. *Laryngoscope* 1979; 89:311–314.
15. Behrman W: Uber indifferenlagen und nystagmusgebiete. *Acta Otolaryngol* [Suppl.] 1940; 40:1–61.
16. Behrman W: Uber indifferenlagen und nystagmusgebiete. Versuche mit horizontal liegenden, nach einseitiger kalorischer reizung um ihre landsachse rotierten personen. *Acta Otolaryngol* 1942; 30:298–310.
17. Benitez JT, Bouchard KR, Choe YK: Air calorics: A technique and results. *Ann Otol Rhinol Laryngol* 1978; 87:216–223.
18. Bittencourt PRM, Gresty MA, Richens A: Quantitative assessment of smooth-pursuit eye movements in healthy and epileptic subjects. *J Neurol Neurosurg Psychiatry* 1980; 43:1119–1124.
19. Brookler KH: Simultaneous bilateral bithermal caloric stimulation in electronystagmography. *Laryngoscope* 1971; 81:1014–1019.
20. Brookler KH: The simultaneous binaural bithermal: A caloric test utilizing electronystagmography. *Laryngoscope* 1976; 86:1241–1250.
21. Brookler KH, Baker AH, Grams G: Closed loop water irrigation system. *Otolaryngol Head Neck Surg* 1979; 87:364–365.
22. Bruner A, Norris TW: Age related changes in caloric nystagmus. *Acta Otolaryngol* [Suppl] 1979; 282:1–17.
23. Capps MJ, Preciado MC, Paparella MM, et al: Evaluation of the air caloric test as a

routine examination procedure. *Laryngoscope* 1973; 83:1013–1021.

24. Chambers BR, Gresty MA: The relationship between disordered pursuit and vestibulo-ocular reflex suppression. *J Neurol Neurosurg Psychiatry* 1983; 46:61–66.

25. Claussen CF, von Schlachta I: Butterfly chart for caloric nystagmus evaluation. *Arch Otolaryngol* 1972; 96:371–375.

26. Coats AC: Central electronystagmographic abnormalities. *Arch Otolaryngol* 1970; 92:43–53.

27. Coats AC, Smith SY: Body position and the intensity of caloric nystagmus. *Acta Otolaryngol* 1967; 63:515–532.

28. Coats AC, Herbert F, Atwood, GR: The air caloric test. *Arch Otolaryngol* 1976; 102:343–354.

29. Collins W, Guedry F, Posner J: Control of caloric nystagmus by manipulating arousal level and visual fixation distance. *Ann Otol Rhinol Laryngol* 1962; 71:187–202.

30. Cooper JC, Mason RL: Variability of air calorics vs water: statistical implications. *Arch Otolaryngol* 1979; 105:113–115.

31. Demanez JP, Ledoux A: Automatic fixation mechanisms and vestibular stimulation. Their study in central pathology with ocular fixation index during caloric tests. *Adv Otorhinolaryngol* 1970; 17:90–98.

32. Fischer JJ: *Labyrinth: Physiology and Functional Tests*. New York; Grune & Stratton, 1956.

33. Fitzgerald G, Hallpike CS: Studies in human vestibular function. I: Observations on the directional preponderance ("nystagmusbereitschaft") of caloric nystagmus resulting from cerebral lesions. *Brain* 1942; 62(part 2):115–137.

34. Fluur E, Mendel L: Habituation, efference and vestibular interplay. *Acta Otolaryngol* 1962; 55:65–80.

35. Ford CR, Stockwell CW: Reliabilities of air and water caloric responses. *Arch Otolaryngol* 1978; 104:380–382.

36. Gao Y-Z, Sze Y-Y, Shen L: The air caloric test and its normal values. *Adv Otorhinolaryngol* 1983; 31:191–197.

37. Gauthier GM, Piron JP, Roll JP, et al: High frequency vestibulo-ocular reflex activation through forced head rotation in man. *Avia Space Environ Med* 1984; 55:1–7.

38. Ghosh P: Aging and auditory vestibular response. *Ear Nose Throat J* 1985; 64:264–266.

39. Goebel JA, Stroud MH, Levine LA, et al: Vertical eye deviation and nystagmus inhibi-

tion during mental tasking. *Laryngoscope* 1983; 93:1127–1132.

40. Greven AJ, Oosterveld WJ, Rademakers WJAC, et al: Caloric vestibular test with the use of air. *Ann Otol Rhinol Laryngol* 1979; 88:31–35.

41. Haciska DT: The influence of drugs on caloric-induced nystagmus. *Acta Otolaryngol* 1973; 75:477–484.

42. Hamid MA, Hughes GB, Kinney SE: Criteria for diagnosing bilateral vestibular dysfunction, in Graham MD, Kemink JL (eds): *The Vestibular System: Neurophysiologic and Clinical Research*. New York, Raven Press, 1987, pp 115–118.

43. Harada Y, Ariki T: A new theory for thermal influences on endolymphatic flow. *Arch Otorhinolaryngol* 1985; 242:13–17.

44. Harrington JW: Caloric stimulation of the labyrinth experimental observations. *Laryngoscope* 1969; 79:777–793.

45. Henriksson NG: Speed of slow component and duration in caloric nystagmus. *Acta Otolaryngol* 1956; 46(Suppl 125):1–29.

46. Herishanu Y, Osimand A, Louzoun Z: Unidirectional gaze paretic nystagmus induced by phenytoin intoxication. *Am J Ophthalmol* 1982; 94:122–123.

47. Hoffman RA, Brookler KH, Baker AH: The accuracy of the simultaneous binaural bithermal test in the diagnosis of acoustic neuroma. *Laryngoscope* 1979; 89:1046–1052.

48. Hood JD: Evidence of direct thermal action upon vestibular receptors in the caloric test. *Acta Otolaryngol* 1989; 107:161–165.

49. Hood JD, Korres S: Vestibular suppression in peripheral and central vestibular disorders. *Brain* 1979; 102:785–804.

50. Jacobson GP, Henry KG: Effect of temperature on fixation suppression ability in normal subjects: The need for temperature and age-dependent values. *Ann Otol Rhinol Laryngol* 1989; 98:369–372.

51. Jell RM, Stockwell CW, Hixon WC: The vestibulo-ocular reflex in man during voluntary head oscillation under three visual conditions. *Aviat Space Environ Med* 1982; 53:541–548.

52. Jung R. Mittermaier R: Zur objektiven registrierung und analyse verschiedener nystagmusformen: Vestibulaer, optokinetischer und spontaner nystagmus in ihren wechselbeziehunger. *Arch Ohren Nasen Kehlkopfh* 1939; 146:410–439.

53. Karlsen EA, Goetzinger CP, Hassanein R: Effects of six conditions of ocular fixation on caloric nystagmus. *Arch Otolaryngol* 1980; 106:474–476.

54. Karlsen EA, Hassanein RM, Goetzinger CP: The effects of age, sex, hearing loss and water temperature on caloric nystagmus. *Laryngoscope* 1981; 91:620–627.

55. Kato I, Kimura Y, Aoyagi M, et al: Visual suppression of caloric nystagmus in normal individuals. *Acta Otolaryngol* 1977; 83:245–251.

56. Katoh Z: Slowing effects of alcohol on voluntary eye movements. *Aviat Space Environ Med* 1988; 59:606–610.

57. Kileny P, McCabe BF, Ryu JH: Effects of attention-requiring tasks on vestibular nystagmus. *Ann Otol Rhinol Laryngol* 1980; 89:9–12.

58. Kumar A: Diagnostic advantages of the Torok monothermal differential caloric test. *Laryngoscope* 1981a; 91:1679–1694.

59. Kumar A: Reliability of central vestibular signs in identification of posterior fossa pathology. *Adv Neurol* 1981b; 30:291–299.

60. Kutt H, Winters W, Kokenge R, et al: Diphenylhydantoin metabolism, blood levels, and toxicity. *Arch Neurol* 1964; 11:642–648.

61. Leigh RJ, Zee DS: *The Neurology of Eye Movements*, ed 2. Philadelphia, FA Davis, 1991.

62. Maccario M, Backman JR, Korein J: Paradoxical caloric response in altered states of consciousness. Clinical and EEG correlations in toxic metabolic encephalopathies. *Neurology* 1972; 22:781–788.

63. Mehra YN: Electronystagmography: A study of caloric tests in normal subjects. *J Laryngol Otol* 1964; 78:520–529.

64. Mulch G, Petermann W: Influence of age on results of vestibular function tests. *Ann Otol Rhinol Laryngol* 1979; 56:1–17.

65. Oosterveld WJ: Changes in vestibular function with increasing age, in Hinchcliffe R (ed): *Hearing and Balance in the Elderly*. New York, Churchill Livingstone, 1983; pp 354–372.

66. Oosterveld WJ, Greven AJ, Gursel AO, et al: Caloric vestibular test in the weightless phase of parabolic flight. *Acta Otolaryngol* 1985; 99:571–576.

67. Paige GD: Caloric responses after horizontal canal inactivation. *Acta Otolaryngol* 1985; 100:321–327.

68. Pau HW, Limberg W: Fluid kinetics of endolymph during calorization. *Acta Otolaryngol* 1990; 109:331–336.

69. Proctor L, Glackin R: Factors contributing to variability of caloric test scores. *Acta Otolaryngol* 1985; 100:161–171.

70. Proctor L, Hansen D, Rentea R: Corneoretinal potential variations. Significance in electronystagmography. *Arch Otolaryngol* 1980; 106:262–265.

71. Rashbass C: Barbiturate nystagmus and mechanics of visual fixation. *Nature* 1959; 183:897–898.

72. Rashbass C, Russell GFM: Action of a barbiturate drug (amylobarbitone sodium) on the vestibulo-ocular reflex. *Brain* 1961; 84:329–335.

73. Riesco-MacClure JS: Caloric tests: Methods and interpretation. *Ann Otol Rhinol Laryngol* 1964; 73:829–837.

74. Riker WK, Downes H, Olsen GD, et al: Conjugate lateral gaze nystagmus and free phenytoin concentrations in plasma: Lack of correlation. *Epilepsia* 1978; 19:93–98.

75. Schalen L, Pyykko I, Korttila K, et al: Effects of intravenously given barbiturate and diazepam on eye motor performance in man. *Adv Otorhinolaryngol* 1988; 42:260–264.

76. Scherer H, Clarke AH: The caloric vestibular reaction in space. *Acta Otolaryngol* 1985; 100:328–336.

77. Sharpe JA, Sylvester TO: Effect of aging on horizontal smooth pursuit. *Invest Ophthalmol Vis Sci* 1978; 17:465–468.

78. Sills AW, Baloh RW, Honrubia V: Caloric testing: Results in normal subjects. *Ann Otol Rhinol Laryngol* [Suppl] 1977; 43:7–23.

79. Sokolovski, A: The influence of mental activity and visual fixation upon caloric-induced nystagmus in normal subjects. *Acta Otolaryngol* 1966; 61:209–220.

80. Stahle J. Electro-nystagmography in the caloric and rotary tests. *Acta Otolaryngol* [Suppl] 1958; 137:5–83.

81. Stahle J: Controversies on the caloric response. *Acta Otolaryngol* 1990; 109:162–167.

82. Steenerson R, Van De Water S, Systma W, et al: Central vestibular findings on electronystagmography. *Ear Hear* 1986; 7:176–181.

83. Suter CM, Blanchard CL, Cook-Manokey BE: Nystagmus responses to water and air caloric stimulation in clinical populations. *Laryngoscope* 1977; 87:1074–1078.

84. Takemori S: Visual suppression test. *Ann Otol Rhinol Laryngol* 1977; 86:80–85.

85. Takemori S, Suzuki M: Cerebellar contribution to oculomotor function. *J Oto Rhinol Laryngol* 1977; 39:209–217.

86. Takemori S, Ono M, Maeda T: Cerebral contribution to the visual suppression of vestibular nystagmus. *Arch Otolaryngol* 1979; 105:579–581.

87. Tole JR: A protocol for the air caloric test and a comparison with a standard water ca-

loric test. *Arch Otolaryngol* 1979; 105:314–319.

88. Tomlinson RD, Saunders GE, Schwartz DWF: Analysis of human vestibulo-ocular reflex during active head movements. *Acta Otolaryngol* 1980; 90:184–190.

89. Torok N: Significance of the frequency in caloric nystagmus. *Acta Otolaryngol* 1948; 36:38–50.

90. Torok N: Some observations on culmination and directional preponderance of the post-stimulatory nystagmus. *Laryngoscope* 1962; 72:79–103.

91. Torok N: Nystagmus frequency versus slow phase velocity in rotatory and caloric nystagmus. *Ann Otol Rhinol Laryngol* 1969; 78:625–639.

92. Torok N: The effects of arousal upon vestibular nystagmus. *Adv Oto rhinolaryngol* 1970; 17:76–89.

93. Torok N: Standard evaluation of the reactive nystagmus. *Arch Otolaryngol* 1972; 96:448–452.

94. Torok N: Differential diagnosis of the caloric nystagmus. *Equilibrium Res* 1973; 3:70–79.

95. Torok N: Vestibular decruitment in central nervous system disease. *Ann Otol Rhinol Laryngol* 1976; 85:131–135.

96. Torok N, Guillemin V, Barnothy JM. Photoelectricnystagmography. *Ann Otol Rhinol Laryngol* 1951; 60:917–927.

97. Umeda Y, Sakata E: Equilibrium disorder in carbamazepine toxicity. *Ann Otol Rhinol Laryngol* 1977; 86:318–322.

98. van der Laan FL, Oosterveld WJ: Age and vestibular function. *Aerospace Med* 1974; 45:540–547.

99. Vercher J-L, Gauthier GM, Marchetti E, et al: Origin of eye movements induced by high frequency rotation of the head. *Aviat Space Environ Med* 1984; 55:1046–1050.

100. Wheeler SD, Ramsay E, Weiss J: Drug-induced downbeat nystagmus. *Ann Neurol* 1982; 12:227–228.

101. Wit HP, Spoelstra AA, Segenhout JM: Barany's theory is right but incomplete. *Acta Otolaryngol* 1990; 110:1–6.

Appendix: Calibration of Water Caloric Irrigators

The stimulus for water caloric testing is either 30° C or 44° C water presented to the ear over a 30-second period for a total volume of 250 mL (8.3 mL/sec). The temperature, flow rate, and duration of caloric irrigations must be precisely controlled. The instruments needed to calibrate the water caloric stimuli consist of a stopwatch, a graduate that will hold at a minimum 250 mL of water, and a laboratory-grade thermometer that measures temperature in degrees centigrade. The objective is to deliver 250 mL of water over a 40-second interval. This water should be 30° C for the cool caloric irrigations and 44° C for the warm caloric irrigations.

Duration of the irrigation can be measured with the stopwatch. This is done by simultaneously starting the stopwatch while initiating irrigation by pressing on the footswitch. When the timer on the irrigator interrupts the irrigation, the stopwatch is stopped and the time is noted. There is an adjustment on the water caloric irrigators that permits the duration of the irrigation to be varied. If duration of the irrigation is less or more than 40 seconds an adjustment is made on the timer and the irrigation is measured again with the stopwatch.

The total flow (for example, 250 mL) is evaluated by running the water into a graduate during the irrigation. At the end of 40 seconds the total volume of water is measured. If the total volume is less than 250 mL, one of two methods may be used to increase the total volume depending on the brand of irrigator that is purchased: (1) the pump can be adjusted to force more water through the delivery system during the 40 seconds, or (2) the delivery tip can be systematically shortened, thereby increasing the internal diameter of the tip and allowing more water to flow in the 40-second period. If the total water volume is more than 250 mL during the 40-second period, the pump can be adjusted to produce less water flow, or a new tip can be put on the delivery hose and the process of shortening the tip to produce the desired total volume can be started again.

The method of determining water temperature is a bit more complicated. The incorrect method of measuring water temperature is by placing the laboratory thermometer directly into the water bath. It is important to remember that although water is a good temperature-conducting medium there is still some heat loss as the water passes from the bath to the irrigating tip. Therefore, measurements of water temperature are made at the irrigation tip as the water exits. It is important to purge the system (if the irrigation system is not a "closed-loop" system) before temperature measurements are made. If the temperature is greater or less than the desired temperature, an adjustment can be made to the thermostat on each bath to increase or decrease the temperature. If an adjustment is made to increase the temperature of the bath, the warming light will illuminate and will terminate when the feedback circuit within the bath verifies that the water has reached the chosen temperature. The measurement should be made again with the thermometer, and adjustments should be made until the water is 30° or 44° C. Be aware that 5 to 10 minutes may elapse, once an adjustment has been made, before the water reaches the desired temperature.

CHAPTER 9

Interpretation and Usefulness of Caloric Testing

Gary P. Jacobson, Ph.D.
Craig W. Newman, Ph.D.
Edward L. Peterson, Ph.D.

Chapter 8 presented in detail the methodologies and techniques used to conduct the caloric examination. The current chapter is an extension of the preceding discussion and focuses on the clinical significance and underlying neurophysiologic bases of abnormal results of the caloric test. More specifically, the purposes of the present chapter are (1) to present strategies for developing laboratory normal upper limits based on statistical techniques, (2) to define caloric abnormalities, and (3) to present clinicopathologic correlates of data obtained from conventional and unconventional caloric techniques.

ESTABLISHING LABORATORY UPPER LIMITS FOR CALORIC TEST RESULTS

Reference ranges are used commonly in medicine to alert physicians when patients demonstrate test values unlikely to occur relative to the entire population of patients. Values that fall outside a reference range do not necessarily imply that the subject is ill or abnormal.

Reference ranges are constructed by taking a sample of observations from normal individuals. These data values are used in statistical techniques designed to find those points between which a certain percentage of the values from the population are expected to fall. Those extreme values not included in the reference range still have originated from normal subjects. They represent *unlikely* values in the *normal* population and not, necessarily, *likely* values from the abnormal or ill population.

There are a large number of statistical approaches to the construction of reference ranges.[102, 107] Two approaches are considered in this chapter: one parametric, and one nonparametric.

Parametric Approach

If data are sampled from a set of values known to be distributed with a Gaussian (normal) distribution, the distributional properties of the sample are well known. Relevant to the construction of a reference range, the percent of data likely to fall between k standard deviations on each side of the mean is known for all k. Hence, a reference region is defined as:

$$\overline{X} \pm ks$$

where $\overline{X}$ and s are the sample mean and standard deviation respectively, and k is chosen to include a specified percentage of the distribution of values. For any choice of percent coverage, $100(1 - \alpha)\%$, k is chosen to equal the $100(1 - \alpha/2)$ centile of the standard normal distribution. This is available in any standard set of statistical tables.[25]

As example, a 95% reference range would exclude the top and bottom 2.5% of the set of normal values. This corresponds to an interval ranging ± 1.96 standard deviations around the mean. The traditional ± 2 standard deviations corresponds to a 95.5% reference range.

If this approach is to be used, then it is important to verify that the data satisfy the distributional assumption of normality. This can be checked either subjectively by examining a histogram of the data to see if it appears as a bell-shaped curve, or examining the empirical distribution function graphed on normal probability paper. Objective tests for normality are available.[109] Figure 9–1 shows a frequency histogram of the directional preponderance obtained from a group of normal subjects. Note that the shape of this distribution appears to approximate a bell-shaped curve (Gaussian distribution).

If the data are not normally distributed then it may be possible to consider transforming the data to make it normally distributed. Figure 9–1 illustrates data that are not normally distributed. This is a distribution of total cool caloric slow-phase velocity (SPV) values

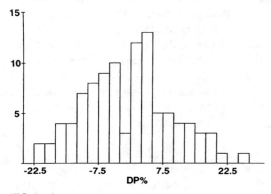

FIG 9–1.
Frequency histogram of percent directional preponderance obtained from 100 healthy subjects. The distribution approximates a bell-shaped curve.

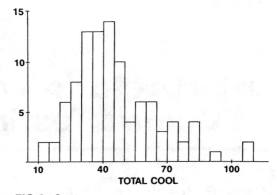

FIG 9–2.
Frequency histogram of total cool caloric slow-phase velocity (SPV) (left cool maximum SPV + right cool maximum SPV) obtained from 100 healthy subjects. Notice that this distribution has observations extending far into the righthand tail and is not normal.

(left cool SPV plus right cool SPV) obtained from a sample of normal subjects. It can be seen in this figure that there are scores extending far to the right of the peak in the distribution.

A common distribution encountered in the laboratory is the loginormal distribution. This distribution is skewed toward zero, and the outcomes are always positive. Applying a logarithmic transformation to data of this type will result in the transformed data following a normal distribution. If the data are not normally distributed and no suitable transformation can be found then this parametric approach should not be used. In these cases the nonparametric procedure outlined in the following section should be used.

The data must also be examined for outliers. These are points whose values are very much different from the rest of the data. Outliers can be seen in Figure 9–2 to the far right of the distribution. When using the parametric approach in the construction of a reference range the effect of an outlier can be quite dramatic. It shifts the mean and inflates the estimated standard deviation, both of which are used to compute the reference range.

There are formal statistical tests available to detect outliers,[113] but we feel that the statistical significance of an apparent outlier is unimportant. We would not recommend exclusion of an extreme point based solely on any statistical criteria. A scientific rationale must be available before excluding a point. It may be that extreme points reflect the true underlying mechanism.

Nonparametric Approach

In nonparametric statistics the underlying distributional form of the data are not assumed to be known. Estimation and testing in nonparametric procedures are based on the relative order, or ranks, of the data.

The construction of the reference ranges consists of ordering the data from smallest to largest and choosing the appropriate ranked data points corresponding to the percentiles chosen. To compute a $100 (1-\alpha)$ % reference range, excluding $100 (\alpha/2)$% of the high and low data, the lth smallest and the lth largest observations are chosen. The number l is defined as $(\alpha/2) (N + 1)$.

As example, consider construction of the 90% reference range from a set of 99 observations from the smallest, $X_{(1)}$ to the largest, $X_{(99)}$. For a 90% confidence interval, $\alpha = 0.10$, which implies that the reference ranges excludes the highest 5% and the lowest 5% of the observations. For this example $l = (0.1/2) (100) = 5$, so we would choose the fifth lowest and the fifth highest observations. The reference range would be $X_{(5)}$ and $X_{(95)}$ (Note: the fifth largest value is equal to $(99 + 1) - 5 = 95$).

For most values of n, l will not be a whole number. In these cases the reference range points are computed by interpolating between the two ordered sample values whose ranks are nearest to each side of l. As example, consider a 90% reference range where the sample size is $n = 100$. In this case $l = (0.1/2) (100 + 1) = 5.05$. The 5.05th smallest observation would lie between $X_{(5)}$ and $X_{(6)}$, the fifth and sixth smallest observations. Using linear interpolation the reference range lower point would equal $X_{(5)} + 0.05$ $[X_{(6)} - X_{(5)}]$, or 5% of the distance between the fifth and sixth smallest observations added to the fifth smallest observation.

The 5.05th largest observation would lie between the fifth and sixth largest observations, $X_{(96)}$ and $X_{(95)}$, respectively. It would be the 96th largest observation minus 5% of the difference between the 95th and 96th largest observations $(X_{(96)} - 0.05 [X_{(96)} - X_{(95)}])$.

Summary

The estimation of the reference range by the parametric approach requires that the data, or suitable transformation of the data, be normally distributed. We believe that in many cases this assumption is not correct. Additionally, when the data are normally distributed, the nonparametric approach does almost as well. This argues that the nonparametric approach is preferable. Another strength of the nonparametric approach is that it is robust to outliers. Tables 9-1 and 9-2 show upper limits of normal and reference ranges computed for a sample of caloric test variable scores obtained from normal subjects. Note that some of the data are normally distributed (that is, these variables are associated with nonsignificant "*p*" values obtained in the test for normality), whereas other data for other variables are not normally distributed. Upper limits, or reference ranges for these variables, may be computed from percentile data.

It is important to reiterate a limitation of a reference range constructed solely on the basis of data indicating ranges of normal populations. Typically, a reference range is set up to identify people with unusual values. For this information to be of clinical use the value must imply that the person is ill or abnormal. To assess this, the distribution of values for individuals having abnormalities must also be estimated. As example, if all values are equally likely to occur from a normal or abnormal indi-

TABLE 9–1.

Reference Ranges for Other Caloric Variables*

Variable	p-Value for Normality	Normal Theory 90% Low	Normal Theory 90% High	Normal Theory 95% Low	Normal Theory 95% High	Percentile 90% Low	Percentile 90% High	Percentile 95% Low	Percentile 95% High
Monothermal warm‡	0.155	—	24.5	—	28.7	—	24.3	—	26.3
Monothermal cool‡	0.898	—	25.1	—	29.7	—	26.8	—	29.9
Total warm	0.001[†]	17.0	117.7	7.4	127.3	26.2	122.4	18.7	146.4
Total cool	0.001[†]	14.5	77.5	8.4	83.5	20.7	84.0	15.6	97.8
Total response	0.001[†]	36.5	190.2	21.8	204.9	51.6	206.4	37.6	220.9

*Please note that both total warm, total cool, and total response data are not normally distributed. Therefore, it is suggested that values obtained from percentile measurements be used to establish critical upper limits.
[†]These data did not demonstrate a Gaussian distribution.
‡High upper limits are 95% and 97.5%, respectively.

TABLE 9–2.

Directional Preponderance (DP) and Unilateral Weakness (UW) Data Obtained From a Subsample of Otologically Normal Subjects (n = 100)*

		Upper Limits of Normal			
		Normal Theory		Percentile	
Variable	p-Value for Normality	95%	97.5%	95%	97.5%
DP	0.363	17.5	20.7	16.9	19.3
UW	0.001	17.3	20.3	16.3	18.0

*Please note that the UW data are not normally distributed. Therefore, data collected from this particular sample suggests that it may be more appropriate to use percentile values (refer to text).

vidual, then a reference range is of little utility. On the other hand, if all abnormal individuals have high values relative to normal individuals, then the reference range is of high clinical utility. These points must be kept in mind when constructing a reference range, and, further, when interpreting the meaning of numerical values that fall in or out of that range.

SIGNIFICANT FINDINGS AND CLINICAL CORRELATES

Alternate Binaural Bithermal Caloric Test

Unilateral Weakness

A clinically significant unilateral weakness is defined as an interaural (for example, ear versus ear) difference in mean maximum SPV of 20% or greater. An example of data demonstrating uni-

lateral weakness is shown in Figure 9–3). Note that the velocity of the nystagmus slow phases is steeper for the left cool and left warm responses, compared with the right cool and right warm responses. These differences resulted in a significant 100% caloric reduction on the right side. The significance of this finding is fairly straightforward. In a unilateral weakness, there is an asymmetry in the magnitude of information entering the brain stem to drive the vestibulo-ocular reflex (VOR) arc (for example, to generate nystagmus slow phases). Thus, the interpretation of this finding is that the patient is demonstrating evidence of a significant peripheral vestibular system deficit. Unfortunately, the definition of the word "peripheral" is different for caloric testing than it is for testing the auditory system. In this instance, the word "peripheral" refers to any point distal to the second-order neuron in the

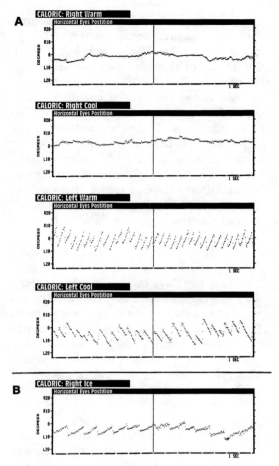

UW = 100% on the right   DP = 8% to the left

FIG 9-3.
Example of right unilateral weakness denoting a right peripheral vestibular system deficit (for example, ipsilateral end organ, eighth cranial nerve, or root entry zone of eighth cranial nerve). There was no caloric response following irrigation of the right ear with cool or warm water. Robust responses were obtained following irrigations of the left ear (100% unilateral weakness). A response to ice water irrigation could be obtained from the right ear. Therefore, there was evidence of residual function (albeit with an abnormally increased threshold) on the right side.

VOR arc (that is, originating at the level of the vestibular nucleus). Thus, a unilateral weakness can be caused by damage occurring within the vestibular end organ (the semicircular canal system), the vestibular portion of the eighth cranial nerve, or the root entry zone of the eighth cranial nerve. Thus, the finding of a significantly reduced caloric response on one side provides lateralizing

information (the disorder is usually ipsilateral to the side demonstrating the reduction) but does not provide localizing information (end organ, or nerve, or root entry zone). Extremely useful adjunctive localizing information may be derived from results of audiometric and evoked potential examinations.

Review of Available Data and Unilateral Weakness

End Organ Origin.—The most common cause of the unilateral weakness is end organ disease. The most common ear disease that causes a unilateral weakness is Meniere's disease. In a large series of patients with Meniere's disease it was reported that unilateral weakness occurs in 60% to 74% of the cases.[64, 117, 125] Indeed, some investigators[64, 125] believe that the finding of a significant unilateral weakness is as important for the diagnosis of Meniere's disease as the finding of fluctuant hearing loss, tinnitus, and episodic vertigo. It is interesting that in contrast with tumors of the eighth cranial nerve and meningiomas (Belal and Linthicum;[19] discussed later), the finding of an absent caloric response is a relatively rare occurrence in Meniere's disease.[64] Also, there has been some dispute about the relationship between the duration of the disease and the degree of caloric reduction. Stahle and Bergman[117] reported that there did not appear to be any systematic relationship between the duration of the disease and the degree of caloric reduction on the affected side.[117] However, Hulshof and Baarsma[64] reported that the degree of unilateral weakness was found to increase with the duration of symptoms.

Unilateral weakness of peripheral origin also may be caused by bacterial destruction of the membranous labyrinth that occurs in congenital, secondary, and tertiary stage syphilis and in bacterial meningitis that leads to labyrinthitis. Additionally, unilateral weakness of vascular origin may occur in migraine and in cerebrovascular disease affecting the posterior circulation. Belal and Linthicum[19] reported that syphilitic otitis results in osteitic changes in the otic capsule, ruptures in the membranous labyrinth, and degeneration of sensorineural structures. The effects of the disease are greatest in congenital syphilis. Wilson and Zoller[136] have reported that 64% of the ears of their subjects with congenital syphilis demonstrated significant caloric reductions, as opposed to 0% and 6% of subjects with secondary and tertiary syphilis.

A number of investigators have reported that it is not unusual to observe significantly reduced caloric responses in patients with common migraine headache, basilar artery migraine, or vertebrobasilar insufficiency. Kuritzky et al.[82] reported that 22% of 40 ears of subjects with common and classic migraine demonstrated reduced caloric responses. In a similar study, Toglia and his co-workers[126] reported that 44% of patients with common migraine demonstrated a significant unilateral weakness on caloric testing. Eviatar[47] evaluated children with basilar artery migraine and discovered that 44% of her subjects demonstrated a unilateral weakness on caloric testing. It is believed that the migraine may result from prolonged vasoconstriction and poor perfusion of the labyrinth. This would result in an ischemic injury to the vestibular labyrinth. Finally, Grad and Baloh[57] evaluated 84 patients with evidence of vertigo caused by cerebrovascular disease and reported that 42% of their subjects demonstrated a unilateral weakness on caloric testing.

Neural Origin.—The most common neural origins of the unilaterally reduced caloric response are the acoustic neuroma (and other tumors of the cerebellopontine angle) and vestibular neuronitis. Less common neural origins of unilateral weakness are demyelinating diseases, for example, multiple sclerosis (MS), and benign intracranial hypertension. A number of investigators (for example, references 9, 20, 61, 83, and 97) have reported caloric examination results for patients with acoustic neuromas and meningiomas of the cerebellopontine angle. The general trend of the results of these studies has been that between 30% and 60% of patients with tumors compressing the eighth cranial nerve demonstrate a total lack of caloric responsiveness. The other patients usually demonstrate unilateral weakness values of 30% to 35%.[9, 83] Interestingly, Laird et al.[83] found that it was not possible to differentiate patients with acoustic neuromas from patients with meningiomas on the basis of caloric test results.

Vestibular neuronitis is a disease typified by a single attack of vertigo that may last for days or weeks. The patient does not complain of hearing loss or tinnitus or other neurologic symptoms. The caloric examinations of these patients show a total absence of response (58% of the sample reported by Begenius and Borg[21]) or a marked unilateral weakness.[21, 37, 134] In fact, an ipsilateral unilateral weakness has been reported to occur in 97% to 100% of the cases.[21, 37, 134] It is interesting that patients with vestibular neuronitis may expect to recover some function with time. Begenius and Borg[21] reported that 95% of their subjects regained some function over a period of 1 year after an attack of vestibular neuronitis.

Central Origins.—Demyelinating diseases can affect the eighth cranial nerve or the vestibular nuclei at the pontomeduallary junction. The effect of the disease is to slow conduction through the nerve or brain stem, and in its severest form to block neural conduction completely. Grenman et al.[58] reported that 18% of their sample of patients with definite MS demonstrated unilateral weakness on caloric testing. Additionally, Johnsen et al.[69] reported 49 patients with MS who demonstrated abnormalities on balance function testing. Of this sample 13 patients (16%) demonstrated a unilateral weakness. The majority of these patients were classified as probably having MS. Thus, it appears that patients with MS who demonstrate remitting and exacerbating symptoms may demonstrate abnormalities on caloric testing. It may be possible through magnetic resonance imaging to determine whether the site of damage is at the level of the nerve or brain stem.

Finally, both Wennmo and Hindfelt[133] and Parker and Weiss[98] have reported the results of caloric testing for patients with brain stem disease. The types of brain stem diseases have included infarctions, demyelinating disorders (for example, MS) and degenerative disorders (for example, progressive supranuclear palsy) and tumors (for example, of the fourth ventricle). Both investigators reported that unilateral weakness occurred in 60% of their samples. These findings have supported the observations by Cohen and Uemura,[36] who created electrolytic lesions at the level of the root entry zone of the eighth cranial nerve at the level of the vestibular nuclei and found that these lesions resulted in the equivalent of a unilateral weakness and a decruiting response (see the section on differential monothermal testing, later in this chapter) in these animals.

A summary listing of the causes of unilateral weakness is shown in Table 9–3.

Directional Preponderance

In contrast to a unilateral weakness, which indicates an asymmetry in response to caloric stimulation of the left and right *ears*, a directional preponderance exists when the nystagmus response is greater in one *direction* than in the other. In our laboratory a clinically

TABLE 9–3.

Listing of Caloric Findings* Reported in the World Literature for Various Diseases

Disease	UW	DP	FFS	BW	PCR	HYP	PERV	DYS	REC	DEC
Amyotropic lateral sclerosis		X	X	X				X		
Aqueductal stenosis		X								
Arnold-Chiari malformation		X								
Ataxia										
Charlevoix-Saguenay			X							
Friedreich's	X	X	X	X	X			X		
Atrophy										
Brain stem										
Cerebellar (pure)									X	
Cerebral						X			X	
Olivopontocerebellar		X				X	X			
Parenchymal cerebellar	X				X					
Progressive muscular		X	X	X				X		
Basilar impression			X							
Benign intracranial hypertension	X	X		X		X				
Cerebral hemispherectomy	X									
Chronic alcoholism										
Cerebrovascular accident										
Brain stem	X				X	X				
Basilar artery aneurysm										
Cerebellar		X								X
Cerebral (unspecified)				X			X			X
Frontoparietal lobe				X						X
Parietal lobe				X						X
Subdural hematoma						X				X
Superior saggital sinus thrombosis				X						X
Temporal lobe hematoma		X								

(Continued.)

TABLE 9–3   (cont.).

Disease	UW	DP	FFS	BW	PCR	HYP	PERV	DYS	REC	DEC
Vertebrobasilar insufficiency		X	X			X				X
Diabetes										X
Disease										
Acute progressive demyelinating				X						
Lyme		X		X		X		X		
Meniere's										
Parkinson's			X				X			
Wilson's			X							
Epilepsy						X				X
Head trauma		X			X				X	
Hemangiomata (head and neck)						X				
Herpes zoster oticus									X	
Hydrocarbon exposure	X									
Hydrocephalus										X
Hypothyroidism										X
Infection										
Inflammatory brain stem disease			X							
Inflammatory cerebellar disease			X							
Otitis media				X						
Vestibular neuronitis	X	X				X				X
Viral encephalitis			X		X					
Labyrinthitis		X								
Meningitis	X									
Lupus			X							
Mega cisterna magna										X
Migraine										
Basilar artery	X									
Classic	X									
Common	X	X								
Multiple sclerosis	X		X			X	X	X		X
Organic mercurial intoxication			X							
Otosclerosis		X				X				
Ototocity				X						
Palsy										
Bell's										X
Progressive supranuclear	X		X	X						
Primary lateral sclerosis			X							
Psychosomatic disorder						X				
Spinocerebellar degeneration			X							
Syndrome										
MLF			X							
Cogan's			X							
Millard-Gubler		X								
Wallenburg's		X		X						
Wernicke-Korsakoff		X		X						
Syphilis (lues)	X	X		X						
Syphilis (neuro)										X
Syringomyelia			X							
Tumor										
Arachnoid cyst										X

(Continued.)

TABLE 9-3 (cont.).

Listing of Caloric Findings* Reported in the World Literature for Various Diseases

Disease	UW	DP	FFS	BW	PCR	HYP	PERV	DYS	REC	DEC
Bilateral acoustic neuroma			X							
Cerebellar hemisphere										
Cerebellar (unspecified)					X					
Cerebellar vermis	X								X	
Cerebral (unspecified)						X				
Corpus collosum			X							
Extra-axial brain stem (CP angle) (cranial nerve VIII, meningioma, epidermoid)	X	X	X						X	
Fourth ventricle	X		X				X			
Frontal lobe	X	X								
Frontoparietal lobe		X								
Intra-axial brain stem tumors (astrocytoma, medullablastoma, ependymoma, glioma)			X					X		X
Medullary										X
Parietal lobe			X							
Parieto-occipital										
Pinealoma			X							
Pseudotumor cerebri				X						
Spenoid wing		X								
Temporal lobe		X		X						
Temporaparietal lobe			X							

*UW, unilateral weakness; DP, directional preponderance; FFS, failure of fixation suppression (failure of vestibulo-ocular reflex cancellation); BW, bilateral weakness; PCR, premature caloric reversal; HYP, hyperactive caloric response; PERV, perversion; DYS, dysrhythmia; REC, recruiting response (e.g., Torok); DEC, decruiting response (e.g. Torok); MLF, medial longitudinal fasciculus.

significant directional preponderance is defined as a 27% or greater difference in intensity of the maximum SPV between the two right-beating responses (right warm and left cool) and the two left-beating responses (left warm and right cool). See Chapter 8 for the formula for calculating directional preponderance. An example of data illustrating a clinically significant directional preponderance toward the left is illustrated in Figure 9-4. It is apparent that the SPV of the left warm and right cool responses (left-beating) are stronger in comparison to the responses obtained from left cool and right warm (right-beating) irrigations. These findings illustrate an imbalance in resting vestibular system activity which results in greater left-beating caloric nystagmus.

The clinical significance of directional preponderance has been a source of controversy and has been debated for over 50 years. A directional preponderance is most often seen in patients who have a strong spontaneous nystagmus. In this instance it is not surprising that these patients demonstrate caloric responses that are stronger for irrigations that result in nystagmus beating toward the direction of the spontaneous nystagmus. Alternatively, these patients demonstrate weaker responses when the caloric nystagmus is beating against the direction of the spontaneous nystagmus. It is important to be aware that directional preponderance has been observed in otherwise healthy normal subjects. Because of this some believe[33, 70] that a directional preponderance may not always represent evidence of a vestibular system disease. However, others feel that the directional preponderance is evidence of disease in either the periph-

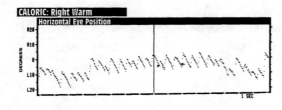

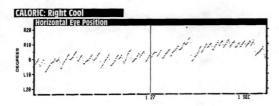

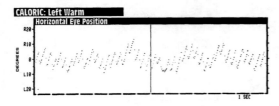

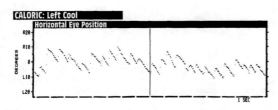

UW = 19% on the right   DP = 30% to the left

FIG 9–4.
Example of statistically significant directional preponderance. Left-beating nystagmus (from right cool, left warm caloric irrigations) attained higher peak velocities than right-beating nystagmus (from left cool, right warm caloric irrigations).

TABLE 9–4.

Direction of Nystagmus (Determined by Fast Phase) for a Directional Preponderance Based on Site of Lesion

Site	Directional Preponderance	
	Away From Involved Side	Toward Involved Side
Labyrinth	X	
Cranial nerve VIII	X	
Brain stem (vestibular nuclei to oculomotor nuclei)	X	X*
Cortex		X

*Most common.

Review of Available Data on Directional Preponderance

The phenomenon of directional preponderance was first described in 1923 by Dusser de Barenne and de Kleyn (see Fitzgerald and Hallpike[49]) in experimental studies using rabbits. de Barenne and de Kleyn observed that removal of one cerebral hemisphere led to a directional preponderance with the fast phase beating toward the ablated hemisphere. The early clinical studies reporting directional preponderance focused on patients with cortical lesions. It is noteworthy that response duration was the measurement variable used to quantify caloric-induced nystagmus. Thus, the patient's eyes remained open during the examination in order to allow the investigator direct observation of the caloric response. Therefore, in addition to evaluating the symmetry of end organ function (for example, measuring nystagmus duration), these early investigators may have been indirectly measuring the symmetry of fixation suppression ability (see Review of Available Data later in this chapter). In Fitzgerald and Hallpike's landmark study,[49] they reported their observations of directional preponderance in 20 patients with cortical lesions, based on clinical, operative, or postmortem findings. A directional preponderance of caloric nystagmus to the side of the lesion was demonstrated in 10 patients with disease localized within or involv-

eral or central vestibular system. In fact, directional preponderance has been observed in disorders restricted to the vestibular end organ, vestibular branch of the eighth cranial nerve, brain stem, and cerebral cortex. In addition, direction of the directional preponderance may vary according to these anatomic sites (Table 9–4). Thus, a significant directional preponderance has no localizing value. Diseases that have been associated with a directional preponderance on caloric testing are discussed here and are summarized in Table 9–3.

ing the temporal lobe. That is, right-sided temporal lobe lesions produced prolonged responses to caloric irrigations which provoked right-beating nystagmus (40°C right/30°C left). A left-sided temporal lobe lesion produced the opposite effect. A directional preponderance was absent in the 10 cases studied with intact temporal lobes. Fitzgerald and Hallpike attributed their findings to the disruption of regions in the temporal lobe which exert some type of "tonic controlling action" on lower vestibular centers which is mediated by corticofugal fibers.

In contrast to the observations of Fitzgerald and Hallpike, several investigators reported a directional preponderance in patients with lesions localized to portions of the central nervous system (CNS) other than the temporal lobe,[146, 103] including lesions of the brain stem, cerebellar vermis and cerebellar hemisphere, and corpus callosum. Anderson[3] examined 130 patients with confirmed unilateral supratentorial lesions with and without temporal lobe involvement of varying causes (such as tumors, abscesses, thrombosis and atrophic lesions). Using duration as his measurement variable, he found that 40% of the cases demonstrated a directional preponderance for nystagmus beating toward the affected side. It is noteworthy that Anderson excluded patients with spontaneous nystagmus or unilateral weakness from his study. Kirstein and Preber[78] reported 29 cases of directional preponderance in lesions affecting the temporal lobe, frontal region, and parietooccipital region as determined by electroencephalography (EEG) abnormalities and in some cases subsequently verified by surgery. The latter authors concluded that directional preponderance in cases with cortical lesions has no unequivocal localizing value.

In addition to CNS disease, peripheral vestibular disorders have been attributed to the presence of a directional preponderance, as well. Using the frequency of nystagmus beats as the measurement variable of the caloric re-

sponse, a number of investigators employing electronystagmography (ENG) recording techniques have reported the presence of a significant directional preponderance in patients with Meniere's disease.[117 125] Using a difference of 30% or greater between left- and right-beating caloric responses, Brookler and Pulec[30] observed a significant directional preponderance in 14% of 780 patients with Meniere's disease. A significant directional preponderance was also observed in 15% of their patients with acoustic neuroma. It is notable that the direction of the directional preponderance was not of any localizing value in the latter sample for either the subjects with Meniere's disease or disease of the eighth cranial nerve. More recently, Hulshof and Baarsma[64] investigated 151 patients with unilateral Meniere's disease, in which 30.5% yielded a directional preponderance of more than 20%.

It is noteworthy that Baloh and his coworkers[10] reported that a directional preponderance was often present in patients with spontaneous nystagmus. Spontaneous nystagmus observed using ENG in the absence of fixation is known to persist for long periods of time even after spontaneous nystagmus inhibited by visual fixation can no longer be observed.[4] In this connection, a well-recognized clinical observation is that a significant directional preponderance is associated with the presence of spontaneous nystagmus. In fact, Stahle[116] regarded spontaneous nystagmus and directional preponderance as an expression of the same phenomenon. In this regard, Coats[34] stated that "directional preponderance without spontaneous or positional nystagmus is relatively uncommon. . . ." The SPV of the spontaneous nystagmus adds to that obtained from the caloric-provoked nystagmus in the same direction and subtracts from that of the caloric-provoked nystagmus in the opposite direction. For example, a right-beating spontaneous nystagmus would increase the strength of caloric responses obtained from right warm and left cool irrigations and decrease the responses obtained from left warm and right cool irrigations, thus producing a directional preponderance toward the right. In the latter case, a left peripheral vestibular deficit (and the associated right-beating spontaneous nystagmus) may have resulted in a "bias" against rightward slow-phase eye movements.

Several investigators[6, 46] have suggested that a directional preponderance may occasionally occur in patients without spontaneous nystagmus and in such instances a central disorder should be considered. This concept is a source of controversy. It is well known that patients with acute labyrinthine injury will have spontaneous nystagmus that diminishes over a few days as a function of central vestibular compensation[6, 89] Central nervous system compensation may not occur fully, however, and a "latent," easily suppressed spontaneous nystagmus may persist for several years following peripheral vestibular disease.[89] In this connection, Belal and Linthicum[19] indicated that directional preponderance probably represents a latent spontaneous nystagmus provoked by caloric irrigations. Also, Stockwell* warns the clinician that when a directional preponderance is present without spontaneous nystagmus the examiner should be suspicious of technical errors such as inadequate irrigations, insufficient patient altering, or suppression of spontaneous nystagmus. Stockwell† has suggested that a directional preponderance may result from a tonic imbalance in resting activity emanating from the peripheral vestibular system. This tonic imbalance may result in spontaneous nystagmus and/or directional preponderance.

A directional preponderance is frequently found in combination with a unilateral weakness. This is particularly apparent in patients with acute unilateral peripheral vestibular system disease and spontaneous nystagmus. Figure 9–5 displays the data obtained from a patient with uncompensated (based on rotational testing) peripheral vestibular system disease on the right. This patient yielded a unilateral weakness on the right and a directional preponderance toward the left. As CNS compensation

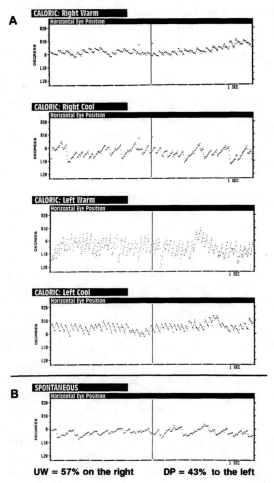

UW = 57% on the right   DP = 43% to the left

FIG 9–5.
Example of directional preponderance in the presence of a spontaneous nystagmus. This patient demonstrates a clinically significant directional preponderance to the left, with an associated left-beating spontaneous nystagmus. If the spontaneous nystagmus is abolished with visual fixation, this is "soft" evidence of a right-sided peripheral vestibular system deficit.

*Stockwell C: Directional preponderance. *ENG Report*, August 1987. ICS Medical Corp., Schaumberg, Ill.
†Stockwell C: Spontaneous nystagmus. *ENG Report*, March 1990. ICS Medical Corp., Schaumberg, Ill.

occurred over time (documented by the absence of an asymmetry and presence of a low-frequency phase deficit on rotational testing), the directional preponderance diminished yet the unilateral weakness persisted. Coats[33] evaluated 72 patients with both a unilateral weakness and directional preponderance. Based on his observation, Coats concluded that: (1) the direction of the directional preponderance had no clinical significance when patients presented with long histories of vestibular complaints and a mild directional preponderance; and (2) the directional preponderance tended to be directed toward the unimpaired ear in patients with a history of short duration vestibular deficits.

From the foregoing discussion, it is apparent that a directional preponderance has poor localizing value and is usually associated with spontaneous nystagmus. Additionally, the presence of directional preponderance indicates a tonic bias in the vestibular system which could be caused by peripheral (end organ and eighth cranial nerve) or central (brain stem and cortex) disease. In some cases a directional preponderance may be found in otologically normal subjects. The clinician may gain additional information regarding the origin of a directional preponderance by evaluating the results of neuroradiologic (such as computed tomography or magnetic resonance imaging) or electrodiagnostic (such as EEG or evoked potentials) tests.

Bilateral Weakness (Hypoactive Responses)

As noted in the beginning of this chapter, the determination of what level of dysfunction is clinically significant is a statistically based decision. Thus, the determination of what constitutes a significant bilateral weakness is no exception. Some investigators have suggested that a patient should be considered to have demonstrated a bilateral weakness if their combined caloric response SPVs are less than 30°/sec, or 40°/sec.[14, 93] Barber and Stockwell[14] have suggested that a patient will have a bilateral weakness if the total response from both sides is less than 11°/sec for warm caloric irrigations and 6°/sec for cool caloric irrigation. Similarly, it was suggested by Baloh and Honrubia[6] that because of the inherent variability in the data, absolute caloric SPVs (as opposed to relative measures such as unilateral weakness and directional preponderance) would have to decrease to extremely reduced values to be considered abnormal. For our laboratory bilateral weakness is operationally defined as total caloric response SPVs that are less than 22°/sec. An example of a bilateral weakness is shown in Figure 9–6. This patient had been placed on high doses of gentamycin for renal disease for 2 months. Note that there is a complete absence of caloric response for both cool and warm caloric irrigations. It is assumed that the known vestibulotoxic effects of this drug on the sensory epithelium of the peripheral vestibular system made it relatively insensitive to motion induced by the convection currents and, therefore, little or no nystagmus was generated following caloric stimulation. It is noteworthy that patients who have lost peripheral vestibular system function often complain of oscillopsia (the perception of movement of the surroundings) that occurs primarily during ambulation. The complaint of oscillopsia is consistent with the loss of the VOR that is needed to stabilize vision during movement.

Bilaterally reduced responses may be caused by drugs that distribute their effects bilaterally. Also, bilaterally reduced responses to caloric stimulation may be caused by systemic infections (for example, lues) that have their effects on the vestibular end organ. Alternately, CNS diseases can result in either bilateral reductions or bilateral absence of caloric responses. This may occur due to damage occurring at the level of the

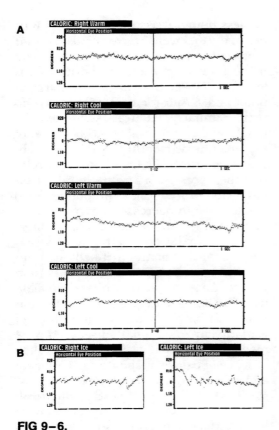

A

B

FIG 9–6.
Example of bilateral weakness. This record was obtained from a patient who was treated with medications known to have ototoxic side effects. Notice that no caloric responses could be obtained following cool or warm water irrigations. However, responses to ice water were present bilaterally, denoting residual function bilaterally.

vestibular ganglion, eighth cranial nerve, or vestibular nucleus. The effect of these lesions is to keep the flow of afferent activity from entering the brain stem. Also, motor tract disease may modulate, and if severe enough abolish, the reflex eye movements following caloric stimulation. Central nervous system diseases known to cause bilateral caloric reductions include benign intracranial hypertension (pseudotumor cerebri), and inherited and acquired brain stem and cerebellar neurodegenerative diseases (such as Friedreich's ataxia, Wernicke-Korsakoff syndrome). Additionally, bilateral vestibular hypoactivity has been reported in Lyme disease[79] and Cogan's syndrome[88] and in motor neuron dis-

ease.[119] Finally, bilateral weakness on caloric testing has been reported in subjects who demonstrate normal low-frequency rotation test results. For this subset of normal subjects it is likely that they suppress the caloric response (perhaps due to anxiety) but do not suppress rotation-induced nystagmus because the rotation stimulus is more comfortable. A listing of known causes of bilateral caloric reduction is shown in Table 9–3.

Review of Available Data on Bilateral Weakness

Simmons[110] retrospectively reviewed the ENG records of 2,500 consecutive patients. The author found that 1.7% of the patients who had bithermal caloric testing had bilateral weaknesses. Of these patients 21% had CNS neoplasms, 14% had midline posterior fossa disease, 14% had autoimmune or collagen disease, 14% had infections, 12% had drug-induced effects, and 9% had hereditary neurodegenerative diseases. It was interesting that in this sample 41% of the subjects had normal hearing sensitivity. Thus, a complete loss of caloric responsiveness was not always associated with a loss of hearing sensitivity. Additionally, oscillopsia was *not* a common complaint in this sample of subjects. What was unknown was whether this sample of subjects had preserved high-frequency vestibular system function that is required to keep the environment stationary during everyday activities such as walking.

The finding of bilateral vestibular hypoactivity has been observed in congenital and acquired syphilis (luetic vestibular disease). Wilson and Zoller[136] observed in their sample that the effects of the disease were more severe for patients with congenital luetic vestibular disease. For instance, 6 of 14 ears (43%) with congenital disease demonstrated absent caloric responses. This is to be compared with none of the ears with secondary or tertiary acquired luetic vestibular disease. The differences in the severity of the effect is attributed to the fact that patients with congenital disease acquired it before their immune systems had developed, so that the effects of the disease were more severe. Also, it is likely that the patients with congenital disease had the disease for a longer period of time.

Rosenberg et al.[106] reported two cases of patients with supratentorial brain lesions who demonstrated bilaterally absent caloric responses. Both of these patients had sustained acute cerebrovascular accidents. One patient had a large arteriovenous malformation in the right parietal lobe, and the second patient sustained a venous sinus thrombosis. Both patients were being treated with antiepileptic drugs (AEDs). The patients were examined with ice water caloric stimuli. Though the caloric responses were initially absent, the response eventually returned. It was the author's impressions that the loss of caloric responses occurred as a combined result of the acute hemispheric damage (known to extinguish fast phases of vestibular nystagmus), the effects of the AEDs, and subarachnoid blood acting on the brain stem centers responsible for the VOR.

The disorder of benign intracranial hypertension (or pseudotumor cerebri) has been associated with bilateral reductions in caloric nystagmus.[71, 111, 112] This is a disorder associated with the otologic complaints of intermittent or continuous tinnitus, hearing loss, and otic pressure and vertigo. It has been suggested that the vestibular system abnormalities are due to the distant effects of pressure distortion on the eighth cranial nerve or brain stem vestibular centers (for example, vestibular nuclei). There is no unanimity as to the origin of the increased intracranial pressure; however, the prevailing view is that there exists a disorder in the resorption of cerebrospinal fluid.[111] In the ENG studies of benign intracranial hypertension the investigators evaluated collectively 54 patients. The finding of bilateral weakness has occurred in between

5% and 17% of these patient samples. In the study by Kaaber and Zilstorff[71] bilateral weakness was defined by the duration of the caloric response (a total duration of all four calorics was less than 350 seconds). These investigators found no relationship between the degree of increased intracranial pressure and the degree of caloric weakness.

Bilateral weakness has been reported in metabolic disease affecting the brain stem. Wernicke-Korsakoff is a CNS disease often affecting alcoholics. The disease occurs as a nutritional deficiency of thiamine and is characterized by lesions in the thalamus, hypothalamus, mammilary bodies, midbrain, and at the floor of the fourth ventricle where the vestibular nuclei are located.[1] The administration of thiamine can reverse the effects of the disease if permanent damage has not occurred. Goor et al.[56] studied 39 patients with the Wernicke-Korsakoff syndrome. The investigators found bilaterally absent responses to bithermal testing in 61% of this sample. The authors also demonstrated an improvement in nystagmus velocity following thiamine treatment. Furman and Becker[52] have also reported bilateral weakness in two patients with Wernicke-Korsakoff syndrome.

Perhaps, the greatest amount of research has been conducted on the ENG manifestations of Friedreich's ataxia. This is an inherited, progressive, neurodegenerative disease, predominantly of the spinal cord. In the brain stem (at the medullocervical junction) the effects of the disease are observed in the nuclei of cranial nerves XII, X, and VIII as a decrease in the nerve cell population.[1] The caloric findings in this group of subjects have been studied by a number of investigators.[8, 45, 93, 94] Bilateral weakness has been reported to occur in a range from 20% to 29% of this group[45, 93, 94] to 80% of this group.[8] It should be noted that the variables from which bilateral weakness was calculated varied from report to report (for example, some measured duration, some measured total

SPV). As noted above, the histology of vestibular system structures has shown degeneration of Scarpa's ganglion and/or vestibular nerves.[7, 115] and, vestibular nuclei[45] with preservation of the end organs.

Bilateral weakness has been observed in 65% of 17 subjects with Cogan's syndrome.[88] Cogan's syndrome is a rare disease characterized by acute unilateral or bilateral sensorineural hearing loss, dysequilibrium, and nonsyphilitic interstitial keratitis. The disease affects the spiral ligament of the cochlea and appears to be an immune-related disorder. Finally, Steinmetz et al.[119] reported that a bilateral weakness of caloric responsiveness was observed in 12.5% of their 88 patients with motor neuron disease (amyotrophic lateral sclerosis, and progressive muscular atrophy).

It should be noted that Bell's phenomenon may complicate greatly the determination of bilateral weakness (see Chapter 8). Finally, it is possible for caloric nystagmus to be absent bilaterally due to the loss of saccadic eye movement control. In this instance, cool caloric stimulation of the left ear would result in a slow-phase eye movement toward the irrigated ear. The eye would reach its physiologic limit and stay tonically deviated until eyes open and fixation occurred. At this point the eyes normally return to midline due to the influence of the gaze system, and the caloric nystagmus may be evident. This has been misinterpreted by some as a failure of fixation suppression (because no nystagmus is evident on the chart paper during eye closure but is present during eyes-open fixation). The tonic deviation of the eyes during caloric testing has been reported to occur in patients with strokes involving the cerebral cortex.[91] Thus, if caloric testing is conducted with the patient's eyes closed, and in the presence of an absent caloric response, it is important to observe the patient's eyes when they are opened for fixation suppression testing. The finding of eyes tonically deviated in the direction of the slow phase of the induced nystagmus is an abnormal finding and suggests the presence of CNS disease, possibly occurring in the paramedian pontine reticular formation (PPRF), or cerebal cortex.

In summary, if bilateral weakness is present it is important to determine whether the patient has a saccadic system deficit, and if they have a particularly strong Bell's phenomenon. This can be accomplished by comparing caloric test results conducted with the patient's eyes closed, with test results obtained with the patient's eyes opened and wearing Frenzel's lenses in a semi-darkened room. Using Frenzel lenses makes it possible to visualize directly the eyes during caloric testing and will eliminate the contribution of Bell's phenomenon, since the test is conducted with open eyes.

Hyperactive Caloric Responses

Hyperactive caloric responses refer to caloric-induced nystagmus which exceeds the upper limits of laboratory normative data. From report to report investigators have defined hyperactivity as SPVs exceeding 40°/sec up to 80°/sec.[8, 145, 114, 120] Barber and Stockwell[14] consider hyperactive responses as SPVs which exceed 50°/sec for cool irrigations and 80°/sec for warm irrigations. For our laboratory, using statistical methods described earlier in this chapter, hyperactivity is operationally defined as total cool (for example, LC SPV + RC SPV) and total warm (for example, LW SPV + RW SPV) responses exceeding 99°/sec and 146°/sec, respectively, and a total SPV exceeding 221°/sec. An example of a hyperactive response, is shown in Figure 9–7. Hyperactive responses have been reported for a number of disorders. A listing of these disorders is shown in Table 9–3.

Review of Available Data on Hyperactive Responses

Animal studies have shown that Purkinje cells located in the flocculo-

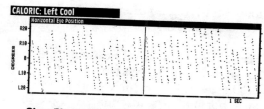

Slow Phase Velocity = 84 deg/sec

FIG 9–7.
Example of "hyperactive" caloric response. The peak SPV exceeds laboratory upper limits. The concept of abnormally brisk caloric nystagmus is controversial (see text).

nodular lobe of the cerebellum project directly to the vestibular nuclei,[42, 43, 104] having an inhibitory influence on vestibular nuclear neurons.[55] Thus, a major function of the nodulus is to inhibit the VOR.[48] Therefore, lesions of the cerebellum produce an increased excitatory state of the vestibular nuclei because of a disruption of the regulatory influence of the cerebellum.

Fredrickson and Fernandez[51] evaluated the relationship between hyperactivity of the caloric response and lesions involving the cerebellum. The investigators lesioned various portions of the cerebellum and evaluated the effects of the lesions on bithermal responses to 28° C and 48° C water caloric stimuli. Caloric stimulation produced hyperactive responses in animals with nodulus lesions in comparison to controls. Hyperactivity was manifested by an increase in amplitude and duration of the caloric response. Fredrickson and Fernandez[51] believed that destruction of the nodulus resulted in a release of the vestibular centers from cerebellar inhibition, causing an exaggerated caloric response. It is noteworthy that electro-oculographic recordings were performed with the animals, eyes open. Therefore, an interpretation of this data must be guarded, in that the latter authors may have actually observed failure of fixation suppression rather than a "true" hyperactive response.

Hyperactive caloric responses have also been associated with pathologic processes of the cerebellum in humans. Torok[128] used culmination frequency (CF) of caloric nystagmus to quantify hyperactivity. Caloric irrigations consisted of "weak" (10 mL of 20° C water over 5 seconds) and "strong" (100 mL of 20° C water over 20 seconds) stimuli. Photoelectric nystagmographic (PENG) recordings were performed in darkness. Torok identified a subgroup of 68 cases which demonstrated a higher CF than observed in the controls. Hyperactive responses were classified into three groups (Table 9–5). Based on the CF data reported in Table 9–5, Torok classified patients as "unconditionally pathologic," "more definitely pathologic," and "potentially pathologic" for groups A, B, and C, respectively. Overall, 65% of the subjects were classified as having some degree of hyperactivity according to the criteria in Table 9–5 and were found to have CNS disease. Although distinct cerebellar involvement was observed in some subjects, most patients had both acquired or congenital extracerebellar CNS disease. Thus, hemispheric lesions (such as epilepsy, or cerebral atrophy) as well as cerebellar or vestibulocerebellar pathway lesions produced hyperactive response. Hyperactivity was also found in 25% of the patients with labyrinthine disease; however, the hyperactive response often was found contralateral to the impaired ear. Interestingly, 10% of the patients with hyperactive responses showed no evidence of organic disease. Torok described this latter group of subjects as being "overanxious." It has since been

TABLE 9–5.

Classification of Hyperactive Responses Based on Culmination Frequency*

| Group | Culmination Frequency | |
	Weak Stimulation	Strong Stimulation
A	≥ 30	≥ 42
B	24–29	36–41
C	18–23	30–35

*Adapted from Torok N: Acta Otolaryngol 1970; 70:153–162.

reported that anxiety can result in either depressed or augmented caloric responses.

Baloh et al.[8] investigated whether specific deficits in ocular motility and hyperactive caloric responses could be used to classify cerebellar atrophy syndromes. Vestibular function was assessed in patients with clinically "pure," cerebellar atrophy, cerebellar and brain stem atrophy (for example, olivopontocerebellar degeneration, Ramsey Hunt syndrome), and Friedreich's ataxia. Hyperactivity was defined as caloric SPVs exceeding 45°/sec. Obvious differences between the three groups were discerned. Patients with "pure" cerebellar atrophy yielded hyperactive responses, with 1 patient showing a SPV as high as 130°/sec. In contrast, patients with Friedreich's ataxia had diminished or absent responses. Patients with both cerebellar and brain stem atrophy demonstrated mixed responses (2 out of 6 showing hyperactivity). These findings suggested that a method might exist to differentiate between clinically "pure" cerebellar atrophy and patients with Friedreich's ataxia. The authors attributed these differences to the degree of cerebellar involvement. That is, hyperactivity was associated with a release of inhibitory influence over vestibular neurons following "pure" cerebellar disease, whereas, Friedreich's ataxia primarily involves insult to the spinal cord (posterior columns and posterior spinocerebellar tracts) and low brain stem, with no cerebellar involvement.

Clinicians are advised that hyperactive responses are extremely uncommon caloric findings and may result from a number of nonorganic sources, including (1) the enhancement of caloric transfer qualities due to mastoidectomy, perforation of the tympanic membrane, atrophy, or retraction; and (2) excessive nervousness or overalertness on the part of the patient.[14, 120] Accordingly, the clinician must be aware of, and control for, these possible sources of error before classifying a patient as having cerebellar system disease.

Fixation Index and Failure of Fixation Suppression

The degree to which caloric nystagmus normally is attenuated by visual fixation has varied. Coats[35] stated that the induced nystagmus following fixation simply should be less than that observed with ENG behind closed lids. Baloh and Honrubia[6] and Katsarkas and Kirkham[77] have reported that nystagmus should be attenuated by at least 50% for fixation suppression (FS) ability to be considered normal. Alpert[2] suggested that nystagmus should be attenuated by at least 60% to 70% following visual fixation. In this vein, Sato et al.[108] have reported a normal attenuation factor of 60%, and Ödkvist[97] has reported a normal attenuation factor of at least 70% with fixation. Our laboratory upper limits suggest that physiologically normal individuals should be able to suppress caloric nystagmus 60% or more with visual fixation.[66] Examples of FS and failure of fixation suppression (FFS) are shown in Figure 9–8. The reader should be aware of the many variables that can affect FS ability that were described in the Chapter 8.

The mechanisms underlying FS are becoming better understood. The cerebellar flocculus appears to be involved intimately with the process of regulating the vestibulocular reflex. Also, the flocculus is under the efferent control of higher level centers. Takemori and Cohen[122] found that following subtotal and total destruction of the flocculus, visual suppression of caloric nystagmus was impaired in the monkey. Additionally, it has been demonstrated in animals that FS ability was affected only by large or total destruction of the flocculus. Lesser lesions resulted only in *transient* reductions in FS ability.[122]

It is known that the flocculus receives signals from at least two different routes: (1) a climbing fiber pathway

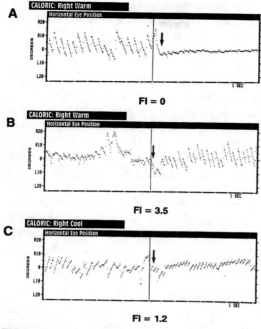

FIG 9–8.

Top, example of good fixation suppression. **Middle and bottom,** examples of failure of fixation suppression where nystagmus velocity is greater with fixation (for example, fixation indexes of 1.2 to 3.5). The middle and bottom records were obtained from patients with midline cerebellar disease.

from the inferior olive, and (2) a mossy fiber pathway from the superior colliculus. This latter pathway is responsible for adjusting the VOR during visual stimulation.[75] The flocculus also receives information about the eye position and eye velocity during pursuit activities.

It has been demonstrated that FS requires participation of the pursuit system. There is a known close relationship between the upper limits of smooth-pursuit velocity in a given individual and the upper limit of FS during rotatory stimulation.[32, 59, 108] Additionally, it has been noted by other investigators that patients who have CNS diseases affecting the cerebellar flocculus, pons, and mesencephalic visual centers have impaired smooth pursuit and FS abilities.[2, 73, 74, 121] Deficits in smooth pursuit and FS have been demonstrated in flocculectomized rabbits and monkeys.[65, 122]

Accordingly, patients who have pursuit-system deficits often demonstrate abnormalities of FS. The visual centers in the parietal lobe (areas 7 and 17) receive information from a number of areas including the superior colliculus. In turn, the parietal lobe projects to the frontal eye fields and to ipsilateral pontine nuclei.[84] It is in this manner that the pursuit system is capable of overriding the VOR during special situations. These observations have formed the support for the argument that FS is wholly or substantially mediated by the pursuit system.

Finally, it is important to note the compelling evidence that pursuit and FS are mediated by functionally distinctive pathways. For example, it is possible for animals who have poorly developed pursuit systems (for example, the cat) to suppress the VOR at head velocities of up to 60°/sec.[127] Additionally, human subjects who cannot normally generate pursuit movements in darkness (such as in the absence of a target) can suppress the VOR during rotation by "imagining" a visual stabilization point directly in front of them.[17] It is currently felt that if the pursuit system does not completely mediate FS then at least the pursuit and FS systems share common circuitry.[127]

Review of Available Data on Failure of Fixation Suppression

There appears to be unanimity with respect to the localizing and lateralizing information provided by the finding of FFS. In unilateral flocculus disease FS is impaired or absent when fast phases are directed toward the side of lesion.[41, 76, 122, 124] Fixation suppression is bilaterally absent following bilateral flocculus damage.[41] Thus, in left-sided lesions of the cerebellar flocculus, FFS would be expected to occur following irrigations yielding left-beating responses (such as left warm, right cool). An opposite trend had been observed for cortical disease. Thus, Takemori et al.[123] reported abnormal FS when fast phases were directed away from the side of lesion for patients with cerebral arteriovenous malformations and tumors. Specifically, the authors found that lesions affecting the parietal lobe (such as temporoparietal tumors, occipitoparietal tumors, and vascular lesions) decreased FS ability.

In keeping with these findings, Kato et al.[75] described three patterns of FFS abnormalities. Bilateral FFS was associated with diffuse disease involving the CNS (such as degenerative brain disease, inflammatory brain disease, and drug intoxication). Unilateral FFS (only observed following stimulation of one of the ears) was observed in the presence of extra-axial disease and specifically tumors in the cerebellopontine angle (for example, epidermoid tumors, large tumors of the eighth cranial nerve, meningiomas). The FFS was only observed following stimulation of the nonaffected side (ear), because caloric responses were absent on the affected side. The authors also observed a directional preponderance of FFS. In this case, FFS was observed when the fast phase was directed to the impaired side (discussed earlier). This pattern of abnormality was observed for cerebrovascular disorders, head trauma, and unilateral disease involving a cerebellar hemisphere.

It should be recognized that patients with saccadic system deficits may demonstrate what appears to be a total loss of caloric response during eye closure but may show a brisk nystagmus upon eye opening. This should not be interpreted as a FFS because no nystagmus was present prior to fixation. Instead, this phenomenon is caused by a gaze paralysis due to damage affecting the PPRF. This damage causes an ipsilateral tonic deviation of the eyes following closure and a concomitant absence of saccades. Visual fixation moves the eyes to midline, and nystagmus may be present.[121] This phenomenon has been observed in Wernicke's encephalopathy and in barbiturate intoxication.[13]

A large number of disorders have been identified that affect the neurophysiology of the brain stem and cerebellum and may result in FS abnormalities. These disorders are summarized in Table 9–3.

In summary, it is important to be aware that (1) most often, FS abnormalities are caused by disease affecting the cerebellar flocculus and/or the fiber connections between the vestibular nuclei and the flocculus; (2) when FS is bilateral (occurs for caloric stimulation of both ears), the implication is that brain stem or cerebellar disease is diffuse; and (3) there should be other oculomotor signs of brain stem and/or cerebellar disease (such as disordered pursuit test results).

Caloric Inversion

Caloric inversion is defined as an entire caloric response that beats in the direction opposite to that expected. A caloric inversion is a rare finding. In fact, Barber et al.[12] stated that they have identified caloric inversions "in only a handful of cases in nearly 10,000 ENG records." Caloric inversions have been associated with brain stem disease.[12, 14, 118]

Because a caloric inversion is a rare event, the clinician must consider a number of sources of error that might produce what appears at first inspection to be an abnormal central finding. The most common source of technical error occurs when the electrode leads have been plugged in incorrectly. If the horizontal electrode leads are inadvertently plugged in "backward," the caloric response will appear to be beating in the "wrong" direction (inverted). Second, the examiner must determine whether a preexisting strong positional, spontaneous, or congenital nystagmus exists that is beating opposite to the expected direction of the caloric response. Barber and Stockwell[14] presented an interesting scenerio of a patient with a right-sided vestibular neuronitis. Their patient had a strong preexisting left-beating nystagmus. When the patient's abnormal right ear was irrigated with warm water, the caloric response was not strong enough to overcome the preexisting left-beating nystagmus. Accordingly, the record showed a left-beating response (in contrast to the anticipated right-beating response) and could have been misinterpreted as a caloric inversion.

Finally, caloric inversions must be viewed with caution when air stimulation is used in the presence of a large tympanic membrane perforation. Barber et al.[12] have reported that warm air stimulation causes evaporation of moisture in the mucosal lining of the middle ear cavity, creating a cooling, rather than a warming effect. Accordingly, in this example, a warm air irrigation to the right ear with a large tympanic membrane perforation might yield left-beating nystagmus. Similar observations were also found in ears with intact tympanic membranes and moisture in the external auditory meatus. Therefore, when a caloric inversion is observed following warm air stimulation, it is incumbent on the clinician to be certain that the tympanic membrane is intact and canal wall dry prior to indicating that a caloric inversion is present.

Caloric Perversion

This term refers to the generation of an oblique or vertical nystagmus following stimulation of the horizontal semicircular canal during caloric testing.[5, 13] This phenomenon has been linked to disease affecting brain stem structures at the floor of the fourth ventricle. These structures are most likely the medial and superior vestibular nuclei. Disorders associated with the presence of perverted nystagmus are shown in Table 9–3. Perverted nystagmus may occur following caloric irrigation of the ipsilateral (medial vestibular nucleus damage) or contralateral (superior vestibular nucleus damage) ear. As noted in Chapter 8, stimulation of the horizontal canal results in activation of the lateral and medial rectus muscles that move the eyes horizontally. A vertical nystag-

mus can be generated only if the anterior or posterior semicircular canal cristae are stimulated. A number of studies have been conducted to help understand why this phenomenon exists.

Cranmer[38] was able to create a perverted nystagmus in the monkey by advancing a destructive electrical device through the lateral vestibular nucleus to the superior vestibular nucleus. The author was able to generate an opposite-beating horizontal nystagmus (destructive nystagmus) as this device was advanced into the lateral vestibular nucleus. This nystagmus changed to an oblique and then to a pure vertical nystagmus as the damaging instrument was advanced further into the superior vestibular nucleus. It was the author's feeling that a perverted nystagmus was created after partial destruction of the vestibular nuclei or brain stem. Uemura and Cohen[131] lesioned differing areas of the vestibular nuclei of rhesus monkeys and observed their responses to bithermal caloric testing. The investigators found a perverted nystagmus occurred following lesions in the rostral medial vestibular nucleus and in the superior vestibular nucleus. The perverted nystagmus was present following caloric stimulation of the ear contralateral to the lesion, although some vertical nystagmus was present following ipsilateral vestibular nucleus lesions. The authors observed that the plane of the perverted nystagmus was parallel to the plane of the anterior canal on the side of the caloric stimulation. They suggested that the vertical component originated from a disinhibition of activity originating from the anterior canal. The normal inhibition is generated by commisural fibers from the vestibular nuclei. Also, it was found that the perverted nystagmus was generated following ipsilateral warm caloric stimulation in medial vestibular nucleus lesions. Alternately the perverted nystagmus was generated following stimulation of the contralateral ear in superior vestibular nucleus lesions. Fredrickson and Fernandez[51] observed a perverted induced vestibular response in cats following lesioning of the vestibular nucleus area at the floor of the fourth ventricle. Additionally, perverted nystagmus has been reported following cerebral hemidecortication.[99]

Review of Available Data on Caloric Perversion

Few studies have evaluated prospectively the clinical significance of perverted nystagmus in humans. Riesco-MacClure[103] reviewed their experience conducting ENG examinations. The researcher noted that the presence of a rotary nystagmus following horizontal semicircular canal stimulation was not abnormal. The author noted that in his experience perverted nystagmus was observed in 16% of intracranial lesions, and that all of these patients had disease at the floor of the fourth ventricle. Baloh and Spooner,[11] in a study of downbeating gaze nystagmus, reported their caloric findings in patients with Arnold-Chiari malformation, MS, olivopontinecerebellar atrophy, and brain stem infarction. Each of these individuals generated a perverted caloric response such that a down-left-beating nystagmus was present when a left-beating nystagmus was expected and an up-right-beating nystagmus was present when a right-beating nystagmus was expected. The authors ascribed the significance of these findings to the disruption of fibers carrying excitatory (and inhibitory) impulses from the posterior and anterior canals to the inferior and superior rectus muscles. These fibers lie in the caudal pons.

A most interesting study was conducted by Barber and Stoyanoff,[15] who attempted to determine the prevalence of caloric perverted nystagmus in a clinical population. The author evaluated 112 normal subjects and 339 patients using conventional alternate binaural bithermal (ABB) caloric testing techniques. The authors found a vertical component in the caloric response for 29% of the normal subjects and 12% of the patients. These figures were reason-

ably close to those in a previous published report of Elidan et al.[44] who found a vertical nystagmus in the caloric results of 29% of 124 patients. The warm stimulus yielded the "perverted" response 66% of the time and the vertical component was usually downbeating. Further, Barber and Stoyanoff[15] found that the vertical nystagmus component was time-locked to the horizontal component although the latency of onset of the vertical component differed from the horizontal (it began approximately 13.5 seconds later), as did the maximum SPV (generally less than half of horizontal).

It has been hypothesized by Elidan et al.[44] and Norre[96] that vertical nystag-

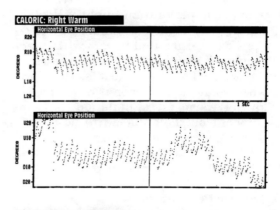

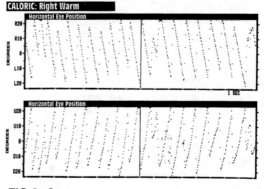

FIG 9–9.
Examples of "caloric perversion." This concept is controversial. Notice that there is significant vertical nystagmus present although the horizontal semicircular canal is in the plane of maximal stimulation. Also, note that in these two instances the vertical nystagmus was recorded following warm caloric irrigations (see text for further details). These responses were obtained from neurologically normal patients.

mus during bithermal caloric testing occurs as a result of stimulation of the posterior semicircular canal. Elidan et al.[44] stated that, whereas the superior canal is in the horizontal plane, the posterior canal is in a vertical plane during conventional caloric stimulation of the horizontal semicircular canal. Thus, thermal stimulation of the posterior semicircular canal (and the associated convection current) would lead to the generation of a vertical nystagmus. Examples of vertical nystagmus recorded during the caloric test are shown in Figure 9–9. It is important to be aware that inaccurately placed vertical electrodes also may result in the appearance of an erroneous vertical nystagmus during caloric testing.[96]

Thus, it would appear that the presence of *oblique* nystagmus in humans is not necessarily a sign of central vestibular system disease. The presence of a vertical component following conventional stimulation should be considered a sign of perverted nystagmus if (1) there is no associated horizontal component (the induced nystagmus is *purely* vertical), or (2) if the SPV of the vertical component is larger than the SPV of the horizontal component.

Dysrhythmia of Caloric Nystagmus

Dysrhythmia was originally defined by Riesco-MacClure and Stroud[104] as nystagmus that was not regular in amplitude and frequency (an example is shown in Fig 9–10). The same phenomenon was defined by Baloh and Honrubia in 1979 as a marked beat-to-beat fluctuation in the amplitude of caloric-induced nystagmus without any change in the SPV function over time. Both Riesco-MacClure and Stroud[104] and Baloh and Honrubia[5] have suggested that the cerebellum is responsible for regulating the generation of nystagmus fast components. The presence of midline cerebellar disease (effecting the flocculus) would effect the latency of onset (with respect to eye position) of saccade generation. The result would be nystagmus slow phases that would have a constant velocity; however, the time of onset of the fast phases might vary in an unsystematic way. The result would

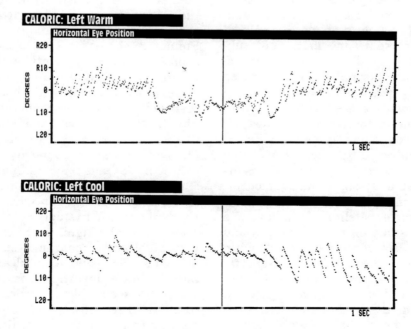

FIG 9–10.
Examples of "dysrhythmic" caloric responses (see text). These data were obtained from two neurologically normal patients.

be a dysrhythmic nystagmus pattern (some nystagmus beats would be larger than others). Nystagmus dysrhythmia requires a qualitative judgement. Thus it is one of the weaker parameters of nystagmus measurement. Just what defines nystagmus dysrhythmia? How irregular is too irregular? Since a smooth, regular eye movement is dependent on the integrity of the eye movement system, it is not surprising that dysrhythmias have been reported in patients who have motor neuron disease. Additionally, dysrhythmic caloric nystagmus may have nonpathologic origins. For example, nystagmus dysrhythmia has been reported in patients who are fatigued or anxious.

Review of Available Data on Dysrhythmic Caloric Responses

Riesco-MacClure and Stroud[104] reported the presence of dysrhythmic nystagmus in normal subjects who demonstrated slow pendular eye movements behind closed eyelids. These roving eye movements undoubtedly had an effect on the nystagmus pattern. Riesco-Mac-Clure[103] stated that dysrhythmia (defined as a nystagmus pattern consisting of fast frequencies and slow ones with periods of no nystagmus intermixed) was present sometime in normal subjects with eyes closed but never occurred when normal subjects opened their eyes (ostensibly because the roving eye movements ceased with eye opening). The finding of dysrhythmia was often observed in the presence of a hyperactive caloric response. Thus, the authors interpreted these findings as evidence that a dysrhythmia was occurring as a consequence of the loss of cerebellar control. Mehra[90] conducted a normative study on the caloric test and found that 25% of normal subjects without neurologic disease showed dysrhythmic caloric responses. Further, the author stated that eye opening had no effect on the dysrhythmic pattern. Consequently, the author did not believe that dysrhythmic nystagmus was a sign

of central vestibular system disease. Baloh et al.[8] studied patients with various types of cerebellar atrophy and found " . . . oscillations in slow component velocity" apparent in the SPV profiles of these patients. Additionally, the authors reported that this abnormality was associated with a hyperactive caloric response. Finally, Ell et al.[45] reported the appearance of a "deranged" caloric nystagmus pattern in patients with Friedreich's ataxia. It was the author's feeling that the dysrhythmic pattern was due to disease affecting neurons in the pontine reticular formation, which have been implicated in the generation of saccades following vestibular stimulation.

Dysrhythmic caloric nystagmus has been observed in the presence of motor system disease. Pialoux et al.[100] observed dysrhythmic caloric nystagmus in patients with Parkinson's disease. They recorded nystagmus before and after electrocoagulation of the subthalamic zone. The authors observed an increase in the dysrhythmia following coagulation, and that the effect was greater when the ear contralateral to the side of surgery was irrigated. At the opposite end of the motor pathway Steinmetz et al.[119] recorded caloric responses from 88 patients with motor neuron disease. These samples included patients with amyotrophic lateral sclerosis (75%), progressive muscular atrophy (15.9%), progressive bulbar palsy (3.4%), and primary lateral sclerosis (2.3%). The authors found dysrhythmic caloric nystagmus in 65% of patients.

A comprehensive listing of disorders associated with the presence of dysrhythmic caloric nystagmus is shown in Table 9–3. The significance of changes in the pattern of caloric nystagmus in animal studies is far more clear than in human clinical investigations. In animal studies it is possible to record baseline (pre-lesion) responses, and to have precise control over the recording conditions and the state of the animal. For these reasons, there seems to be disagreement over the significance of this finding in human subjects.

A dysrhythmia of caloric nystagmus can occur due to inadequate alerting of the patient. The use of inadequate alerting exercises may result in the periodic loss of the caloric response. The response will disappear when the patient is inattentive or unalert and reappear when the patient begins the alerting exercises. Also, dysrhythmic caloric responses can occur as a consequence of Bell's phenomenon (see the section on bilateral weakness in this chapter). We have found that both the vertical and the horizontal components of Bell's phenomenon contribute to nystagmus dysrhythmia. There is no doubt that the use of inadequate alerting exercises and the averting and adducting of the eyes during Bell's phenomenon are the most common causes for the transient suppression and dysrhythmias of caloric nystagmus. These findings underscore the importance of (1) adequate alerting exercises (mental tasking) during caloric testing to ensure that vertical eye deviation behind closed lids is minimal, and (2) conducting caloric testing with eyes open in complete darkness, or with eyes closed in a semi-darkened room, to minimize Bell's phenomenon as a contributor to nystagmus dysrhythmia.

Premature Reversal of Caloric Nystagmus

The caloric response usually reaches its peak approximately 45 to 90 seconds following the start of irrigation. After this peak, for most individuals, SPV diminishes and then disappears after approximately 200 seconds.[13] Some individuals may demonstrate a secondary phase nystagmus following the caloric irrigation. This secondary nystagmus beats in the opposite direction of the primary nystagmus. Milojevic and Allen[92] reported this secondary phase nystagmus in 30 of 53 normal subjects. The authors utilized the Fitzgerald-Hallpike bithermal caloric

test and reported that for 14 of the 30 subjects the secondary phase nystagmus was present for only one of the four caloric irrigations. This was usually the first irrigation of the series. It has been stated that if this secondary nystagmus begins prior to 140 seconds and if the magnitude of the SPV is greater than 6°/sec, then a premature reversal of caloric nystagmus (PCR) is said to exist.[13] This is a very rare finding in ENG examinations. In our laboratory we have observed this once in over 2,100 examinations giving the phenomenon a prevalence of less than 0.5%. An example of premature caloric reversal is shown in Figure 9–11. If a premature reversal is identified it is extremely important to determine whether

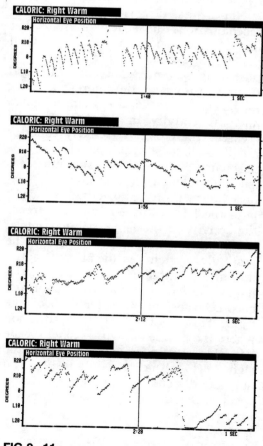

FIG 9–11.
Example of "premature caloric reversal" (see text). Note that the nystagmus changes direction approximately 2 minutes and 8 seconds (128 seconds) into the caloric test.

a preexisting opposite-beating (with reference to the caloric response) spontaneous nystagmus is present. For instance, a patient may have a right-beating spontaneous (or positional) nystagmus. A left warm caloric stimulus will yield a left-beating response. Once the caloric response begins to subside the right-beating spontaneous nystagmus may reappear. This should not be interpreted as a PCR. Indeed Milojevic and Allen[92] reported that 11 subjects in their sample with secondary phase nystagmus also had a spontaneous nystagmus that beat in the same direction as the secondary phase nystagmus. These subjects usually demonstrated a directional preponderance (in the direction of the spontaneous nystagmus) on caloric testing.

Not a great deal is known about the mechanism of the PCR. We know that for physiological stimuli the peripheral vestibular system is organized as a push-pull system. Thus, as the head turns to the right, the afferent activity in the right peripheral system increases and the activity in the left side decreases. Therefore, it is likely that for nonphysiologic stimulation (caloric testing) when activity on one side increases (such as during right warm caloric testing) interneurons connecting the right with the left vestibular nuclei decrease the activity in the left vestibular nuclei to maintain the dynamic balance in the vestibular system. As the afferent activity on the right side subsides, the activity on the left side may overadapt and become transiently greater than on the right. This would result in a situation where the degree of neural "tone" on the left side would be greater than the right.[50] This situation would result in an opposite-directed nystagmus (with respect to the direction of the primary caloric response).

Review of Available Data on Premature Caloric Reversal

Thus far, there have been four reports describing PCR in patients with neurologic disease. Disorders associated with

PCR are shown in Table 9–3. Monday et al.[93] and Monday et al.[94] reported the presence of PCR in patients with Friedreich's ataxia. Using the criteria reported by Barber and Stockwell[13] the authors reported PCR for 1 of 16 of their patients (reversal of direction in 128 seconds). Similarly, Ell et al.[145] also observed PCR in patients with Friedreich's ataxia. The authors reported that PCR in two of ten patients and described histologic findings for two patients who died. These studies showed extensive degeneration of the vestibular nuclei, with preservation of the vestibular end organs. Finally, Barber and Stockwell[13] reported a case of a patient with brain stem infarction and an internuclear ophthalmoplegia who demonstrated PCR.

Interpretation of Simultaneous Bithermal Test

Brookler and his colleagues[27, 28, 29, 63] have advocated the use of the simultaneous bithermal test (SBT) as a valuable adjunct to the alternate binaural bithermal caloric examination. In contrast to the water delivery system used for the conventional caloric test, during the SBT, water is delivered to the patient through a "Y" tube through which both ears are stimulated simultaneously. The underlying physiologic mechanism relates to the notion that if both end organ systems are responding symmetrically to the caloric irrigations there should not be any induced nystagmus because the level of excitatory and inhibitory activity resulting from bilateral stimulation within the brain stem vestibular pathway should be equal and opposite. Interpretation of the responses obtained from the SBT is based on two decisions. The first relates to whether nystagmus was produced in response to the irrigations. If nystagmus was provoked by the irrigation, the second decision concerns the determination of the direction of the nystagmus. Once these decisions have been made, the clinician can classify the responses into four major categories.

The first category is type I. According to Brookler,[28, 29] this response could be observed in cases of bilaterally normal function, bilaterally absent function, or bilaterally hyperactive function. Accordingly, type I is characterized by the absence of nystagmus in response to warm or cool water irrigation, consistent with equal vestibular function. In this case, it is imperative for the clinician to perform the ABB caloric test in order to determine whether individual nystagmus responses were within the normal range, or equally hypoactive or hyperactive. Brookler[28] studied 188 patients with a type I response. Of this group, 157 demonstrated a normal bithermal response (that is, individual responses to the alternate bithermal stimulus with SPVs ranging from 5°/sec to 25°/sec and a unilateral weakness and directional preponderance of less than 30%).

The type II response is characterized by nystagmus beating in opposing directions. That is, for example, right-beating nystagmus elicited by simultaneous warm irrigations, and a left-beating nystagmus is elicited by simultaneous cool irrigations. Conversely, type II responses also include those in which left-beating nystagmus is induced with simultaneous warm irrigations and right-beating nystagmus is elicited with simultaneous cool irrigations. This second pattern can be further described by an example. If the left end organ was impaired, the unopposed stronger right-sided simultaneous caloric responses would result in a nystagmus to the left following cool caloric irrigations and a nystagmus to the right following warm irrigations. Thus, the observation of nystagmus beating in opposite directions for each of the simultaneous irrigations was associated with a reduced peripheral vestibular system response on the side opposite the direction of the nystagmus following simultaneous warm irrigations. A type II response is usually associated with hypoactive labyrinth; however, often the conventional caloric examination is within normal limits.[28, 29]

The type III response is typified by nystagmus induced by simultaneous irrigations that beats in one direction regardless of the water temperature. For example, a left-beating nystagmus is provoked in response to simultaneous cool or warm water irrigations. Although this pattern is considered abnormal, it has no localizing value. Brookler[28, 29] indicated that a type III response is consistent with the concept of directional preponderance and is often associated with a directional preponderance obtained during the ABB test.

The type IV category is characterized by the observation of induced nystagmus for only one of the two simultaneous irrigations. For example, a cool simultaneous irrigation fails to induce a response, while a warm irrigation to both ears produces a left-beating nystagmus. Brookler[28, 29] refers to this pattern as the "wastebasket" response, suggesting its lack of localizing value. Serial testing of patients with vestibular neuronitis demonstrating a type IV response while symptomatic has revealed shifts to a type I after the patient became asymptomatic.

Hoffman and his associates[63] evaluated 53 patients with surgically confirmed acoustic tumors preoperatively, using both the conventional caloric examination and the SBT. Using the ABB test, 24 (56%) subjects had a significant unilateral weakness on the side of the tumor. The SBT producing a type II response correctly identified 35 (81%) patients. When used together, the diagnostic accuracy was increased to 86%. Moreover, Hoffman et al.[63] indicated that the SBT was particularly valuable in the diagnosis of an inferior vestibular nerve tumor, where the conventional alternate test is least accurate.

More recently, the SBT has been criticized by Furman and his colleagues.[54] These investigators, using signal detection analysis techniques, have determined that the SBT is inferior to the ABB test in detecting the presence of normal (correct rejections) or abnormal subjects (hits). Additionally, the authors described two major shortcomings of the SBT. First, the test findings were ambiguous when the induced nystagmus was of low magnitude. In these cases a low-velocity response could be interpreted either as being normal or abnormal according to the direction of the induced nystagmus. Second, if the thermal conducting properties of the middle ear and skull were different on the two sides, then it was possible for a nystagmus of one direction to be elicited at the beginning of the recording period which could change direction later in the same recording. Finally, during normal physiologic stimulation (rotation) the resulting activity from one end organ (the leading ear) is increased, in contrast to the opposite end organ (lagging ear) in which neural activity is decreased. Bilateral stimulation in the SBT results in the nonphysiologic increasing or decreasing of spontaneous activity. Because this does not represent a normal state of the vestibular system, the usefulness of the SBT is questionable.

Monothermal Caloric Testing

Monothermal Warm

Bernstein[24] and Hart[62] were among the first to suggest that the ABB caloric test could be shortened by conducting a warm caloric screening test. Barber et al.[16] were the first to investigate the efficacy of a warm monothermal screening test using ENG techniques. The authors reported a 7% false negative rate using their technique (1) when failure criteria consisted of greater than 25% interaural SPV difference, and (2) when the maximum SPV for each caloric irrigation did not exceed 11°/sec. In recent years, Dayal et al.[39] and Becker[18] reevaluated the efficiency of the monothermal warm caloric screening test. Dayal et al.[39] approached their investigation in terms of whether the monothermal cool or warm test could be used to replace the conven-

tional ABB test as opposed to using the monothermal examination as a screening test. The latter investigators made velocity measurements within the most active 10-second period, and thus did not attempt to control for the number of nystagmus beats that were used to calculate SPV. These measurements were conducted for a small number of subjects ($n = 25$) of unreported age distribution. The investigators reported an 8% false positive rate and a false negative rate that ranged from 7% to 52%, which depended on the type of balance system disease.

Becker[18] conducted a prospective study of 362 consecutive air and water caloric examinations. The authors compared results obtained with both the ABB and monothermal screening test. Using the criteria suggested by Barber et al.[16] the authors reported a 14% false negative rate and a 22% false positive rate. There was a 77% overall concurrence between the monothermal warm and ABB tests.

Longridge and Leatherdale[86] evaluated 400 consecutive patients and compared the results obtained from the ABB test with those obtained using the monothermal warm test and the failure criteria advocated by Barber et al.[16] The investigators demonstrated 0.5% false negative results using a 15% upper limit for monothermal interaural difference when the ABB test was used as the criterion measure and 25% was used as the upper limit for interaural differences for the ABB test.

Most recently Jacobson and Means[67] conducted both retrospective and prospective investigations in an attempt to determine the validity of the warm monothermal screening test as described by Barber et al.[16] The investigators evaluated the records of 69 consecutive normal ENG examinations in an attempt to determine the 95% normal upper limit (2 SD) for interaural SPV differences. The upper limit was 29.54%. In a second retrospective investigation the investigators reevaluated 62 additional ENG examinations to estimate the false negative rates associated with the monothermal warm screening test. The investigators observed a 5% false negative rate using their interaural upper limits and criteria from Barber et al.[16] regarding minimum SPV values for each of the two caloric irrigations (e.g. minimum SPV of 11°/sec.). The false negative rate improved to 3% if the failure criteria included abnormal ocular motor testing, the presence of spontaneous nystagmus, or positional or positioning nystagmus. The authors prospectively evaluated 30 consecutive patients and observed no false negative errors and 6% false positive errors using their adaptation of the monothermal warm screening test.

Each of these investigations have been associated with various levels of false positive test results (prediction is abnormal and the actual is normal). From a clinical standpoint the presence of false positive errors are not bothersome, since the prediction of abnormal findings on the monothermal warm screening test would result in the completion of the ABB test where the patient would have been found to be normal.

It is clear that there is a place for caloric screening tests in the balance function laboratory. There are a number of patients who present with vague complaints of continuous unsteadiness the origin of which is most likely extravestibular. It is for these individuals that the monothermal warm screening test was developed. The use of a screening test decreases patient discomfort and permits a more efficient use of clinical facilities. Additionally, the technique for administering the caloric stimuli for the monothermal test is identical to that for the ABB test.

Monothermal Differential Caloric Test

Despite the widespread use of the bithermal caloric irrigation test for lateralizing vestibular system deficits, it has limited value in helping to differentiate between labyrinthine (end organ) and retrolabyrinthine (eighth cranial nerve or CNS) disease. In an attempt to address this need, the monothermal differential caloric test (first described by Torok[128]) was developed to identify vestibular recruitment and vestibular decruitment. Diseases associated with vestibular recruitment and decruitment are shown in Table 9–3. Recall from Chapter 8 that vestibular recruitment is defined as an unusually rapid growth in the responsiveness of the vestibular system to increases in the intensity of the caloric stimulus. In contrast, vestibular decruitment refers to the observation of no increase or the decrease in the responsiveness of the vestibular system to increases in stimulus intensity. As indicated in Chapter 8, the intensity of the stimulus is increased by employing two separate irrigations to each ear. The first irrigation is a weak stimulus, consisting of 10 mL of water at 20°C over 5 seconds, whereas the stronger stimulus is 100 mL of water at 20°C over a 20-second time interval. Responses are quantified as the maximum nystagmus beat frequency over a 10-second interval, which Torok[129] designated the CF (see the section Hyperactive Caloric Responses earlier in this chapter).

It has been the contention of the originators of this technique[80, 130] that vestibular recruitment (like loudness recruitment of the auditory system) is observed in the presence of labyrinthine disease, whereas the decruitment phenomenon is observed in the presence of retrolabyrinthine lesions.[81] Kumar[80] stated that the normal range of CF for the weak stimulus was from 3 to 29 beats and from 10 to 39 beats for the stronger stimulus. The data are placed in a ratio as follows:

CF (strong stimulus)/CF (weak stimulus)

The normal range of the ratios are 1.2 to 3.5. When the response to the strong stimulus is a great deal larger than that to the weak stimulus (ratio exceeds 3.5) vestibular recruitment is said to exist. Alternatively, when the response following the weaker stimulus is equal to or exceeds that obtained following the stronger stimulus, vestibular decruitment is said to exist. Vestibular decruitment has been subcategorized based on the following ratios: type 1 decruitment = a ratio of 1.1 to 1.0; type 2 decruitment = a ratio of 0.9 to 0.1; and type 3 decruitment = a ratio of 0. A ratio of "0" implies that no response was obtained following either of the caloric irrigations. In this case the ear is irrigated with 100 mL of ice water over a 20-second period. If no nystagmus is elicited, then paresis of the vestibular end organ is said to exist. Additionally, a symmetry measurement is calculated as a percent difference between the ratios obtained from the left and right ear recordings. An upper limit of 25% for symmetry has been reported by Kumar.[80]

Vestibular recruitment has been observed in a number of studies employing well-defined patient samples with end organ disease. Kumar[80] studied 47 patients with Meniere's disease. All but 8 patients yielded vestibular recruitment by the monothermal differential caloric method. An example of a 43-year-old woman with Meniere's disease was presented in whom left ear calorics resulted in a CF of 3 for the 10-mL irrigation and a CF for 18 for the 100-mL irrigation, resulting in a ratio of 6.0. This ratio exceeded the criterion value of 3.5, indicating a pattern of vestibular recruitment. More recently, Bhansali et al.[26] reported 3 patients with active, well-documented Meniere's disease and 2 patients with Meniere's disease who had undergone endolymphatic sac operations for relief of vertigo. Two of the patients with active Meniere's disease demonstrated recruitment, while the third patient showed an asymmetric response between the ratios of the two ears in excess of 25%, consistent with a labyrinthine lesion in the ear with the higher ratio. The 2 patients who had undergone surgical therapy to re-

lieve dizziness showed normal responses. The authors, acknowledging their small sample size, suggested that recruitment is observable in ears with labyrinthine disease, especially when the disease process is in an active state.

In contrast to vestibular recruitment, vestibular decruitment has been associated with a variety of CNS lesions. Torok[130] reviewed 2,200 cases in which the monothermal caloric test had been performed as part of a comprehensive neurotologic evaluation. Of those patients, 139 (6%) individuals exhibited vestibular decruitment of which 75% had definite CNS or intracranial disease, including space-occupying lesions and vascular abnormalities. Among the 20 intracranial space-occupying lesions observed, 7 were acoustic neuromas. Torok reported 53 of 81 patients with type 1 decruitment (ratio of 1.0 to 1.1), and 45 of 51 patients with type 2 decruitment (0.1 to 0.9) and all 7 cases with type 3 decruitment had retrolabyrinthine disease.

In Kumar's[81] series of 54 patients demonstrating decruitment, 51 had confirmed posterior fossa disease encompassing a number of pathologic entities (vascular insufficiency, tumor, lues, infarction, malformation, epilepsy, MS), giving an identification rate of 94%. Decruitment was unilateral in 48 patients and bilateral in 6 patients (60 ears). Kumar[81] indicated, however, that the absence of decruitment did not exclude the possibility of retrolabyrinthine disease and that the presence of such a lesion may be manifested by caloric hyperactivity or other central vestibular signs.

Recently, Bhansali and his co-workers[26] evaluated 8 patients with well-documented lesions of the vestibular branch of the eighth cranial nerve or central vestibular pathways. Six of the 8 patients showed decruitment in at least one ear. Five of the 6 patients having severe intrinsic CNS disease showed hyper-responsiveness to caloric stimulation in addition to decruitment. Bhansali et al.[26] suggested that this may have possibly reflected failure of fixation suppression since the monothermal caloric test is performed with the eyes open.

It is noteworthy that the recording technique as originally outlined by Torok[128] employs photoelectric nystagmography (PENG), in which light senses movements of the eye. This technique has a sensitivity of 0.1° of eye movement.* This is in contrast to ENG recording (electro-oculography), which measures the corneoretinal potential and has a sensitivity of 1.0° of eye movement.[85] The limited sensitivity of the signal coupled with bioelectric contamination from other sources such as ECG, electroencephalographic, and electromyographic precludes small amplitude measurements in comparison to PENG. Accordingly, future study using these recording techniques should entail examination of the relationship between beat frequency and SPV in patients with vestibular system disease. In this way, it would be possible to determine whether vestibular recruitment/decruitment can be defined by SPV as readily as by nystagmus beat frequency.[135]

Ice Water Caloric Test

Within the context of the conventional ENG examination, ice water testing has been reserved primarily for instances when ABB testing yields no recordable nystagmus. Also, ice water testing is used commonly for bedside testing or in the physician's office as a screening method when ENG instrumentation is unavailable. In contrast to ABB response patterns (such as unilateral weakness, directional preponderance, bilateral weakness, hyperactivity), a qualitative approach is often taken when evaluating the ice water response. That is, when conducted by a physician in the office or at beside, ENG tech-

niques are not used. With the patient's eyes open, the duration of the response from each side is measured and an estimate of symmetry is made. Baloh and Honrubia[6] indicated that in an alert subject a burst of nystagmus following ice water infusion should develop within 30 seconds to 1 minute and last from 1 to 2 minutes.

When evaluating nystagmus obtained from the ABB test, the clinician must not assume that the absence of a response reflects no vestibular function in the horizontal semicircular canals (see the section on bilateral weakness earlier in this chapter). On the contrary, patients may demonstrate responses to ice water in the absence of responses to warm and cool irrigations, thus demonstrating that residual function remains. This point is illustrated in Figure 9–6. As can be seen, no nystagmus was observed for either the cool or warm water irrigations; however, a brisk response was seen following ice water stimulation. Although responses to standard caloric testing showed no response, ice water stimulation provoked nystagmus, indicating that residual function did indeed remain. The identification of residual vestibular function (even minimal) in an impaired system is important for a number of reasons. For instance, in a patient who is to undergo unilateral ablative surgery for intractable vertigo, the presence of some residual function allows the physician to predict that the patient will be ill following surgery. This makes it possible for the physician to anticipate the patient's need in the immediate postoperative period. Additionally, it is important to know if there is residual vestibular function when patients are being treated with medications known to be toxic to the peripheral vestibular system.

Another application of ice water caloric testing is in the documentation of the functional status of comatose patients. Several investigators[68, 95, 105] have evaluated eye movement response pat-

*Glenn Krol, BME, University of Illinois at Chicago, Department of Otolaryngology–Head and Neck Surgery, Chicago, Illinois, Personal Communication.

terns in comatose patients with CNS lesions using ice water stimulation. Although a number of patterns have emerged from the latter investigations, two important observations relating to eye movements were found. First, a bilaterally symmetrical slow deviation (originating from the vestibular system) of the eyes toward the stimulated ear was seen when there was no involvement of the VOR pathways. This finding signified that brain stem centers mediating the VOR were intact, eliminating the possibility of a serious brain stem lesion. Jadhav et al.[68] noted that bilateral conjugate deviation with a fast component away from the stimulated ear was observed in lighter stages of altered consciousness (drowsiness or stupor), whereas bilateral conjugate deviation without a fast component was found in deeper stages of unconsciousness. Vaernet[132] suggested that the tonic monophasic character of conjugate deviation without a fast component would be indicative of impaired neuronal elements of the reticular formation (the origin of the fast phase of nystagmus). Second, the finding of no response to ice water stimulation was consistent with a severe brain stem lesion that affected the VOR. Rodriguez-Barrios et al.[105] indicated that an absent response was often observed in primary or secondary pontine lesions (pontine hemorrhages secondary to cerebral hemorrhages). Jadhav et al.[68] added that this latter pattern was associated with the deepest stages of unconsciousness and prognosticated a grave outcome.

SERIAL TESTING

Serial testing using caloric methodologies may be useful for evaluating the natural course of vestibular disorders as well as monitoring the effects of ototoxicity. An important consideration prior to conducting the caloric examination in a serial fashion is to evaluate the test-retest reliability of caloric responses.

Based on test-retest data, it is possible to calculate the standard error of measurement and the standard error of measurement between successive caloric irrigations. In this way, it is possible to determine statistically the confidence interval (95%) for a true change in a caloric response between two different administrations. Unfortunately, there is a lack of studies addressing what constitutes a significant critical difference for a given individual on serial caloric testing.

Proctor and his associates[101] evaluated the degree of test-retest variability that occurred during serial caloric testing in 30 normal subjects. A short-acting caloric test was evaluated in which the temperature of the irrigation water was switched between warm and cold at specified times. Testing occurred over 3 successive days. Measurements of SPV were calculated for individual caloric tests (HR, hot right; CR, cool right; HL, hot left; CL, cool left), average responses ($\overline{X}$) on either side (HR + CR/2 = $\overline{X}$R; HL + HR/2 = $\overline{X}$L), and finally the average of all caloric responses ($\overline{X}$RESP). The investigators established a set of recommended reference values for serial caloric testing. The values were expressed as a ratio of the test in question to a previous result (R:T ratio). The following are the normal ranges of the R:T ratios for: (1) HR, CR, HL, CL (range, 0.55 to 1.7); (2) $\overline{X}$R, $\overline{X}$L (range 0.60 to 1.6) and (3) $\overline{X}$RESP (range 0.65 to 1.5). Moreover, the investigators indicated that the upper normal limits for test-retest variation for the right-left difference scores and directional preponderance of caloric responses were 24% and 22%, respectively.[101] It is important to remember that these values reflect day-to-day variation for the temperature-switching caloric test.

Bergenius et al.[23] evaluated the intra-individual difference in reactivity between ears using the standard Jongkees and Philipzoon formula described in Chapter 8. Fifteen subjects underwent a minimum of two complete caloric examinations within a 1-week interval. A caloric side difference was expressed as a ratio (CR, caloric ratio) rather than as a percentage. Accordingly, a unilateral absence of a caloric response yielded a value of 1.00, whereas complete symmetry between the two sides gave a CR of 0.00. The CR values ranged from −0.21 to 0.18. A negative sign denoted a decreased caloric response on the left side. A CR value exceeding 0.24 indicated a significant difference in caloric responses between two test sessions. The latter authors concluded that a carefully standardized caloric test seems to have low test-retest variability.

Caloric irrigations have been used to monitor disease progression. Bergenius and Magnusson[22] evaluated the relationship between tumor size and the results of caloric and oculomotor tests in 70 patients with acoustic neuromas and 9 patients with other cerebellopontine angle tumors. The authors suggested that serial caloric examinations coupled with simultaneous ocular motility studies of pursuit and gaze may provide a supplemental test for monitoring possible growth of the tumor. Matsuo and Sekitani[87] evaluated 22 patients with vestibular neuronitis using caloric stimulation over an average of 1 year and 3 months. Nine cases showed reduced responses with 30°C cool water irrigations. A number of these subjects demonstrated a recovery of caloric responses at retest.

Although serial caloric testing may provide useful information concerning the progression of, or recovery from, a disease state, it is also important to realize that in many instances it is impossible to use caloric tests for monitoring purposes because an absent response observed during the initial examination usually persists on reexamination. Accordingly, serial caloric testings coupled with rotational testing may help to monitor the natural progression of vestibular disease, especially as it relates to the process of vestibular compensation. For example, a patient with an acute unilateral peripheral vestibular system

deficit may present initially with a unilateral weakness on caloric testing and a rotary chair pattern of increased phase leads at low frequencies of sinusoidal stimulation and an asymmetry. This pattern is consistent with an uncompensated unilateral peripheral vestibular system deficit. On retest, the patient may continue to demonstrate the unilateral weakness. Although the rotational examination may still reveal a phase abnormality at low frequencies, the symmetry may have returned to normal, indicating a compensated peripheral vestibular system deficit.

Serial caloric testing also may be used to monitor the effects of ototoxic medications;[6, 40] however, serial testing using caloric stimulation may have limited value in comparison with rotational testing. That is, a bilateral reduction of caloric responses to bithermal stimulation may be observed following exposure to ototoxic drugs, yet recordable responses to rotational stimulation may be seen at higher frequencies. Furman and Kamerer[53] examined rotational responses in 1,274 patients with bilateral caloric reductions. Their findings revealed a poor correlation between the magnitude of the response to caloric irrigation (total eye speed) and the magnitude of response to rotational testing (gain at 0.05 Hz). Moreover, about half of the patients with reduced caloric responses had rotational response magnitudes that were within normal limits at 0.05 Hz and above. These investigators concluded that bilateral caloric reduction does not provide sufficient evidence for diagnosing bilateral vestibular loss, emphasizing the clinical value of serial rotational testing during periods of drug administration. Therefore, serial testing of caloric responses may show absent vestibular function, whereas serial testing using sinusoidal harmonic acceleration techniques may demonstrate a progressive reduction of vestibular function at successively higher frequencies of rotation over a period of time during which a patient is treated with a potential ototoxic agent. Further study in this area is certainly needed and would provide important information to the clinician documenting ototoxic effects.

Finally, it has been suggested that serial cold water caloric testing provides insight into a patient's changing state of consciousness.[68, 132] For example, the observation of conjugate deviation of the eyes without a fast component on the initial examination followed on retest by a conjugate deviation with a fast component is suggestive of improvement. In contrast, the reverse scenerio is indicative of deterioration. In this connection, Vaernet[132] suggested that ice water calorics may be useful in recognizing functional disturbance in neural conduction at the pontomescephalic level before functional changes progress to permanent structural damage.

It is necessary to control for a number of stimulus-related and subject-related variables (see Chapter 8) during the caloric examination in order to ensure that the obtained responses are reliable. Unless the intrasubject variability of the caloric response is low, it will be impossible to make accurate judgments about the significance of change in scores between test and retest observations.

CORRELATION BETWEEN RESULTS OF CALORIC TESTING AND OTHER BALANCE FUNCTION TEST RESULTS

Interrelationships between various measures that comprise the modern balance function test battery are seldom addressed. Table 9–6 shows the correlations between rotational (phase, gain, and asymmetry) and posturographic (sensory organization subtest) measures and caloric test variables. The data have been summarized from the results of 407 consecutive patients seen for balance function testing. Only correlations that were significant, at or better than, the .05 probability level have been displayed.

We have observed a weak but statistically significant correlation between the magnitude of unilateral weakness and the magnitude of directional preponderance. It is interesting that Coats[33] conducted an investigation in which he attempted to determine the relationship between unilateral weakness and directional preponderance in a group of 72 patients with a significant unilateral weakness on caloric testing (equal or greater than 20% difference between sides). In accordance with our findings Coats[33] reported a weak but significant correlation ($r = .335$; $p = .01$) between the two measures. The direction of the directional preponderance tended to be opposite the direction of the unilateral weakness. We have observed the same trend.

Also, it may be observed that VOR gain at 0.04- , 0.32- , and 0.64-Hz rotational frequencies demonstrated a weak positive correlation with the percent unilateral weakness. Thus, unilateral weakness (in percent) increased as gain increased at these frequencies. Additionally, rotational phase leads generally were inversely related to total cool and total caloric SPV, and were positively correlated with the magnitude of unilateral weakness and directional preponderance. These relationships were strongest for the lower rotational frequencies. Therefore, lower responsiveness of the vestibular end organ was associated with increased phase leads on rotational testing. Additionally, increases in phase lead were associated with increases in asymmetry measures on caloric testing. Finally, the magnitude of VOR asymmetry tended to be negatively correlated with the responsiveness of the peripheral system during caloric testing. Alternately, VOR asymmetry was positively correlated with asymmetry measures. Thus, increases in unilateral weakness and directional preponderance (measures of symmetry) were associated with increases in VOR asymmetry on rotational

TABLE 9–6.

Correlations Between Adjunctive Balance Function Tests and Alternate Binaural Bithermal Caloric Test*

Variable	Total Warm	Total Cool	Total	UW (%)	DP (%)
Total warm	—	—	—	—	—
Total cool	.19	—	—	—	—
Total	.28	.87	—	—	—
UW, %	—	−.26	−.31	—	—
DP, %	—	−.23	−.22	—	—
Gain .01	—	—	—	.31	—
Gain .04	—	—	—	—	—
Gain .16	—	—	—	.13	—
Gain .32	—	—	—	—	—
Gain .64	—	—	—	.13	—
Phase .01	—	—	−.11	.15	—
Phase .04	.18	−.31	−.36	.25	—
Phase .16	—	−.43	−.45	.21	.19
Phase .32	—	−.27	−.28	—	—
Phase .64	—	—	−.17	.17	.18
Asym .01	−.11	−.13	−.15	.12	.16
Asym .04	−.11	−.15	−.16	.14	.24
Asym .16	—	—	—	.17	.24
Asym .32	—	—	—	—	.14
Asym .64	—	—	—	.16	.23
Cond 1	—	—	—	—	—
Cond 2	—	—	—	—	—
Cond 3	—	—	—	—	—
Cond 4	—	—	—	—	—
Cond 5	—	—	—	—	—
Cond 6	—	—	—	—	—
Age of subject	—	−.22	−.12	.11	—

*UW, unilateral weakness; DP, directional preponderance; Asym, asymmetry; Cond, condition.

testing. Noteworthy was the finding that none of the posturographic measures correlated with caloric measures. It is interesting that the majority of significant correlations between caloric variables and phase and asymmetry measures on rotational testing occurred for low rotational frequencies. It has been stated that the velocity profile obtained from caloric testing resembles a sine wave with a frequency of approximately 0.003 Hz.[60] Therefore, it is not surprising that significant measures of association between the two test techniques should occur for low frequencies. Finally, as noted by Bruner and Norris[31] and Karlsen et al.,[72] a weak but significant negative correlation between total cool SPV and age was observed. It should be emphasized that with few exceptions all correlations were generally weak ($r \leq 0.5$) but statistically significant. In summary, results of a large correlational examination of different measures of balance function have suggested that abnormalities of rotational phase and asymmetry increase as measures of caloric responsiveness decrease and as measures of caloric asymmetry increase.

CONCLUSION

The caloric examination allows the clinician to evaluate independently each horizontal semicircular canal and the integrity of the vestibulocular reflex arc. The patterns of responses obtained following caloric irrigations often provides lateralizing information regarding a disease state and may provide localizing information as well (Table 9–7). The importance of conducting a technically precise and valid caloric examination by controlling for possible sources of error (see "Comments" in Table 9–7) can-

TABLE 9–7.

Summary of Caloric Abnormalities and Associated Clinical Significance

Caloric Abnormality[*]	Definition[*]	Location of Lesion[*]	Mechanism[*]	Comment[†]
Vestibular paresis	>22% asymmetry between right- and left-sided maximum slow-component velocity	Unilateral labyrinth, eighth nerve including root entry zone	Unilateral decrease in afferent signals to the vestibular nuclei	Rule out inadequate irrigation(s), lack of alertness
Directional preponderance	>28% asymmetry between left-beating and right-beating maximum slow-component velocity	Peripheral or central vestibular system	Interaction of spontaneous nystagmus with caloric-induced nystagmus	—
Bilateral decreased responses	Maximum slow-component velocity below normal range	Bilateral labyrinth, eighth nerve including root entry zones	Bilateral decrease in afferent signals to the vestibular nuclei	Rule out inadequate irrigation(s), CNS depressant drugs, lack of alertness, failure of fixation suppression, saccadic defect
Hyperactive responses	Maximum slow-component velocity above normal range	Cerebellum	Loss of normal inhibitory influence of cerebellum on the vestibular nucleus	—
Dysrhythmia	Marked variability in nystagmus amplitude without change in slow-component velocity profile	Cerebellum	Loss of cerebellar control on pontine saccade center	—
Impaired fixation suppression	Fixation does not produce at least 50% decrease in maximum slow-component velocity	Inferior olives, midline cerebellum	Interruption of visual signals carried to the vestibular nuclei by way of the midline cerebellum	Rule out drugs
Perverted nystagmus	Vertical or oblique nystagmus resulting from horizontal canal stimulation	Pontomedullary region	Disturbance of commissural fibers between the vestibular nuclei	Rule out superimposed preexisting or congenital nystagmus, air caloric with tympanic membrane perforation, wet ear canal
Disconjugate nystagmus	Different amplitude and waveform of nystagmus in each eye	Intrinsic brain stem usually medial longitudinal forciculus	Interruption of pathways connecting sixth and third nuclei	—

*Data from Baloh RW, Honrubia V: Clinical Neurophysiology of the Vestibular System. Philadelphia, FA Davis, 1979, p 138.
†Data from Barber HO, Stockwell CW: Manual of Electronystagmography. St Louis, CV Mosby, 1980, p 186.

not be overemphasized. Only in this way can the clinical significance derived from the caloric test be viewed with confidence.

REFERENCES

1. Adams RD, Victor M: *Principles of Neurology.* New York, McGraw-Hill, 1981.

2. Alpert J: Failure of fixation suppression: A pathologic effect of vision on caloric nystagmus. *Neurology* 1974; 24:891–896.

3. Anderson HC: Directional preponderance in some intracranial disorders. *Acta Otolaryngol* 1954; 44:563–573.

4. Aschan G, Bergstedt M, Stahl J: Nystagmography. *Acta Otolaryngol* 1956; 46:1–103.

5. Baloh RW, Honrubia V: *Clinical Neurophysiology of the Vestibular System.* Philadelphia, FA Davis, 1979.

6. Baloh RW, Honrubia V: *Clinical Neurophysiology of the Vestibular System,* ed 2. Philadelphia, FA Davis, 1990.

7. Baloh RW, Jenkins HA, Honrubia V, et al: Visual-vestibular interaction and cerebellar atrophy. *Neurology* 1979; 29:116–119.

8. Baloh RW, Konrad HR, Honrubia V: Vestibulo-ocular function in patients with cerebellar atrophy. *Neurology* 1975; 25:160–168.

9. Baloh RW, Konrad HR, Dirks D, et al: Cerebellar-pontine angle tumors: Results of quantitative vestibulo-ocular testing. *Arch Neurol* 1976; 33:507–512.

10. Baloh RW, Sills AW, Honrubia V: (1977). Caloric testing: Patients with peripheral and central vestibular lesions. *Ann Otol Rhinol Laryngol [Suppl]* 1977; 43:24–30.

11. Baloh RW, Spooner JW: Downbeat nystagmus: A type of central vestibular nystagmus. *Neurology* 1981; 31:304–310.

12. Barber H, Harmand W, Money K: Air caloric stimulation with tympanic membrane perforation. *Laryngoscope* 1978; 88:1117–1126.

13. Barber HO, Stockwell CW: *Manual of Electronystagmography.* St Louis, CV Mosby, 1976.

14. Barber HO, Stockwell CW: *Manual of Electronystagmography.* St Louis, CV Mosby, 1980.

15. Barber HO, Stoyanoff S: Vertical nystagmus in routine caloric testing. *Otolaryngol Head Neck Surg* 1986; 95:574–580.

16. Barber HO, Wright G, Demanuele F: The hot caloric test as a clinical screening device. *Arch Otolaryngol* 1971; 94:335–337.

17. Barr CC, Schultheis LW, Robinson DA: Voluntary, non-visual control of the human vestibulo-ocular reflex. *Acta Otolaryngol* 1976; 81:365–375.

18. Becker GD: The screening value of monothermal caloric tests. *Laryngoscope* 1979; 89:311–314.

19. Belal A Jr, Linthicum FH Jr: Pathologic correlates of electronystagmographic tracings. *Am J Otolaryngol* 1980; 1:213–223.

20. Benitez JT, Bouchard KR: Electronystagmography: Significant alterations in tumors of the cerebellopontine recess. *Ann Otol Rhinol Laryngol* 1974; 83:399–402.

21. Bergenius J, Borg E: Audio-vestibular findings in patients with vestibular neuritis. *Acta Otolaryngol* 1983; 96:389–395.

22. Bergenius J, Magnusson M: The relationship between caloric response, oculomotor dysfunction and size of cerebellopontine angle tumors. *Acta Otolaryngol* 1988; 106:361–377.

23. Bergenius J, Perols O, Lofqvist L: Some considerations on caloric test results. *Acta Otolaryngol [Suppl]* 1988; 455:21–23.

24. Bernstein L: Simplification of the clinical caloric test. *Arch Otolaryngol* 1965; 81:347–349.

25. Beyer WH: *Basic Statistical Tables.* Cleveland, Chemical Rubber Co., 1971.

26. Bhansali SA, Stockwell CW, Bojrab DI, et al: Evaluation of the monothermal caloric test. *Laryngoscope* 1989; 99:500–504.

27. Brookler KH: Simultaneous bilateral bithermal caloric stimulation in electronystagmography. *Laryngoscope* 1971; 81:1014–1019.

28. Brookler KH: The simultaneous binaural bithermal: A caloric test utilizing electronystagmography. *Laryngoscope* 1976; 86:1241–1250.

29. Brookler KH: Electronystagmography. *Neurol Clin* 1990; 8:235–259.

30. Brookler KH, Pulec JL: Computer analysis of electronystagmography records. *Trans Am Acad Ophthalmol Otolaryngol* 1970; 74:563–575.

31. Bruner A, Norris TW: Age related changes in caloric nystagmus. *Acta Otolaryngol [Suppl]* 1979; 282:1–17.

32. Chambers BR, Gresty MA: The relationship between disordered pursuit and vestibulo-ocular reflex suppression. *J Neurol Neurosurg Psychiatr* 1983; 46:61–66.

33. Coats AC: Directional preponderance and unilateral weakness as observed in the electronystagmographic examination. *Ann Otol Rhinol Otolaryngol* 1965; 74:655–668.

34. Coats AC: Directional preponderance and

spontaneous nystagmus as observed in the electronystagmographic examination. *Ann Otol Rhinol Laryngol* 1966; 75:1135–1159.

35. Coats AC: Central electronystagmographic abnormalities. *Arch Otolaryngol* 1970; 92:43–53.

36. Cohen B, Uemura T: Ocular changes in monkeys after lesions of the superior and medial vestibular nuclei and the vestibular nerve roots; in Naunton RF (ed): *The Vestibular System*. New York; Academic Press, 1975, pp 187–202.

37. Corvera J, Davalos RL: Neurotologic evidence of central and peripheral involvement in patients with vestibular neuronitis. *Otolaryngol Head Neck Surg* 1985; 93:524–528.

38. Cranmer R: Nystagmus related to lesions of the central vestibular apparatus and the cerebellum. *Ann Otol Rhinol Laryngol* 1951; 60:186–196.

39. Dayal VS, Farkashidy J, Kuzin B: Clinical evaluation of the hot caloric test as a screening procedure. *Laryngoscope.* 1973; 83:1433–1439.

40. Dayal VS, Farkashidy J, Tarantino L, et al: End-organ and drug-induced vestibular nystagmus. *Ann Otol Rhinol Laryngol* 1977; 86:89–93.

41. Dionne J, Wright G, Barber HO, et al: Oculomotor and vestibular finding in autosomal recessive spastic ataxia. *Can J Neurol Sci* 1979; 6:177–184.

42. Dow RS: The filter connections of the posterior parts of the cerebellum in the rat and cat. *J Comp Neurol* 1936; 63:527.

43. Dow RS: Efferent connections of the flocculo-nodular lobe in Macaca mulatta. *J Comp Neurol* 1938; 68:297.

44. Elidan J, Gay I, Lev S: On the vertical caloric nystagmus. *J Otolaryngol* 1985; 14:287–292.

45. Ell J, Prasher D, Rudge P: Neuro-otological abnormalities in Friedreich's ataxia. *J Neurol Neurosurg Psychiatr* 1984; 47:26–32.

46. Eviatar A, Wassertheil S: The clinical significance of directional preponderance concluded by electronystagmography. *J Laryngol Otol* 1971; 85:355–367.

47. Eviatar L: Vestibular testing in basilar artery migraine. *Ann Neurol* 1980; 9:126–130.

48. Fernandez C: Interrelations between flocculondular lobe and vestibular system, in Rasmussen GL, Wendle WF (eds): *Neural Mechanisms of Auditory and Vestibular System*. Springfield, Ill, Charles C Thomas, 1960, pp 285–296.

49. Fitzgerald G, Hallpike CS: Studies in human vestibular function. I: Observations on the directional preponderance ("nystagmusbereitschaft") of caloric nystagmus resulting from cerebral lesions. *Brain* 1942; 62(part 2):115–137.

50. Fluur E, Mendel L: Habituation, efference and vestibular interplay. *Acta Otolaryngol* 1962; 55:65–80.

51. Fredrickson JM, Fernandez C: Vestibular disorders in fourth ventricle lesions. *Arch Otolaryngol* 1964; 80:521–540.

52. Furman JM, Becker JT: Vestibular responses in Wernicke's encephalopathy. *Ann Neurol* 1989; 26:669–674.

53. Furman JM, Kamerer DB: Rotational responses in patients with bilateral caloric reductions. *Acta Otolaryngol* 1989; 108:355–361.

54. Furman JM, Wall C, Kamerer DB: Alternate and simultaneous binaural bithermal caloric testing: A comparison. *Ann Otol Rhinol Laryngol* 1988; 97:359–364.

55. Gilman S, Bloedel JR, Lechteberg R: *Disorders of the Cerebellum*. Philadelphia, FA Davis, 1981.

56. Goor C, Endtz LJ, Muller-Kobold MJ: Electro-nystagmography for the diagnosis of vestibular dysfunction in the Wernicke-Korsakow syndrome. *Clin Neurol Neurosurg* 1975; 78:112–116.

57. Grad A, Baloh RW: Vertigo of vascular origin. Clinical and electronystagmographic features in 84 cases. *Arch Neurol* 1989; 46:281–284.

58. Grenman R, Aantaa E, Katevuo VK, et al: Otoneurological and ultra low field MRI findings in multiple sclerosis patients. *Acta Otolaryngol [Suppl]* 1988; 449:77–83.

59. Halmagyi GM, Gretsy MA: Clinical signs of visual-vestibular interaction. *J Neurol Neurosurg Psychiatry* 1979; 42:934–939.

60. Hamid MA, Hughes GB, Kinney SE: Criteria for diagnosing bilateral vestibular dysfunction, in Graham MD, Kemink JL (eds): *The Vestibular System: Neurophysiologic and Clinical Research*. New York, Raven Press, 1987, pp 115–118.

61. Harder H: Audiovestibular tests in the diagnosis of cerebellopontine angle tumors. *Acta Otolaryngol [Suppl]* 1988; 452:12–15.

62. Hart CW: The ocular fixation index. *Ann Otol Rhinol Laryngol* 1973; 82:848–851.

63. Hoffman RA, Brookler KH, Baker AH: The accuracy of the simultaneous binaural bithermal test in the diagnosis of acoustic neuroma. *Laryngoscope* 1979; 89:1046–1052.

64. Hulshof JH, Baarsma EA: Vestibular investigations in Meniere's disease. *Acta Otolaryngol* 1981; 92:75–81.

65. Ito M, Shiida T, Yagi N, et al: Visual influence on rabbit horizontal vestibulo-ocular reflexes presumably effected via the cerebellar flocculus. *Brain Res* 1974; 65:170–174.

66. Jacobson GP, Henry KG: Effect of temperature on fixation suppression ability in normal subjects: The need for temperature and age-dependent values. *Ann Otol Rhinol Laryngol* 1989; 98:369–372.

67. Jacobson GP, Means ED: Efficacy of a monothermal warm water caloric screening test. *Ann Otol Rhinol Laryngol* 1985; 94:377–381.

68. Jadhav WR, Sinha A, Tandon PN, et al: Cold caloric test in altered states of consciousness. *Laryngoscope* 1971; 81:391–402.

69. Johnsen NJ, Dam M, Thomsen J, et al: Multiple sclerosis: The value of clinical vestibular examination. *Clin Otolaryngol* 1976; 1:225–232.

70. Jongkees LBW: Value of the caloric test of the labyrinth. *Arch Otolaryngol* 1948; 48:402–417.

71. Kaaber EG, Zilstorff K: Vestibular function in benign intracranial hypertension. *Clin Otolaryngol* 1978; 3:183–188.

72. Karlsen EA, Hassanein RM, Goetzinger CP: The effects of age, sex, hearing loss and water temperature on caloric nystagmus. *Laryngoscope* 1981; 91:620–627.

73. Kato I, Kimura Y, Aoyagi M, et al: Visual suppression of caloric nystagmus in normal individuals. *Acta Otolaryngol* 1977; 83:245–251.

74. Kato I, Nakamura T, Kimura Y, et al: Visual-vestibular interaction in central nervous system disorders. *Ann NY Acad Sci* 1981; 374:764–773.

75. Kato I, Sato Y, Aoyagi M, et al: Caloric pattern test with special reference to failure of fixation-suppression. *Acta Otolaryngol* 1979; 88:97–104.

76. Kato I, Watanabe J, Nakamura T, et al: Diagnostic confirmation of lesions in cerebellar peduncles by combined use of otokinetic nystagmus and fixation-suppression of caloric nystagmus. *Adv Otorhinolaryngol* 1988; 42:63–70.

77. Katsarkas A, Kirkham TH: Failure of suppression of post-caloric nystagmus by fixation. *J Otolaryngol* 1982; 11:57–59.

78. Kirstein L, Preber L: Directional preponderance of caloric nystagmus with organic brain diseases. An electroencephalographic study. *Acta Otolaryngol* 1954; 44:256–273.

79. Krejcova H, Bojar M, Jerabek J, et al: Oto-neurological symptomatology in lyme disease. *Adv Otorhinolaryngol* 1988; 42:210–212.

80. Kumar A: Diagnostic advantages of the Torok monothermal differential caloric test. *Laryngoscope* 1981; 91:1679–1694.

81. Kumar A: Reliability of central vestibular signs in identification of posterior fossa pathology. *Adv Neurol* 1981; 30:291–299.

82. Kuritzky A, Toglia JU, Thomas D: Vestibular function in migraine. *Headache* 1981; 21:110–112.

83. Laird FJ, Harner SG, Laws ER Jr, et al: Meningiomas of the cerebellopontine angle. *Otolaryngol Head Neck Surg* 1985; 93:163–167.

84. Leigh RJ, Zee DS: *The Neurology of Eye Movements*. Philadelphia, FA Davis, 1983.

85. Leigh RJ, Zee DS: *The Neurology of Eye Movements*, ed 2. Philadelphia, FA Davis, 1991.

86. Longridge NS, Leatherdale A: Caloric screening tests. *J Otolaryngol* 1980; 9:478–481.

87. Matsuo T, Sekitani T: Vestibular neuronitis: Neurotological findings and progress. *Ann Otol Rhinol Laryngol* 1985; 47:199–206.

88. McDonald TJ, Vollertsen RS, Young BR: Cogan's syndrome: Audiovestibular involvement and prognosis in 18 patients. *Laryngoscope* 1985; 95:650–654.

89. McGee M: Electronystagmography in peripheral lesions. *Ear Hear* 1986; 7:167–175.

90. Mehra YN: Electronystagmography: A study of caloric tests in normal subjects. *J Laryngol Otol* 1964; 78:520–529.

91. Merwarth H, Feiring E: Modifications of induced nystagmus by acute cerebral lesions. *Brooklyn Hosp J* 1939; 1:99–106.

92. Milojevic B, Allen T: Secondary phase nystagmus: The caloric test. *Laryngoscope* 1966: 77:187–201.

93. Monday LA, Lemieux B, St-Vincent H, et al: Clinical and electronystagmographic findings in Friedreich's ataxia. *Can J Neurol Sci* 1978; 5:71–73.

94. Monday L, Lesperance J, Lemieux B, et al: Follow-up study of electronystagmographic findings in Friedreich's ataxia patients and evaluation of their relatives. *Can J Neurol Sci* 1984; 11(suppl 4):570–573.

95. Nathanson M, Bergman PS, Anderson PJ: Significance of oculo-cephalic and caloric responses in the unconscious patient. *Neurology* 1957; 7:829–832.

96. Norre M: Caloric vertical nystagmus: The vertical semicircular canal in caloric testing. *J Otolaryngol* 1987; 16:36–39.

97. Ödkvist LM: Value of vestibular function tests in the differential diagnosis of vertigo. *Acta Otolaryngol* 1988; 460:122–127.

98. Parker SW, Weiss AD: Some electronystagmographic manifestations of central nervous system disease. *Ann Otol Rhinol Laryngol* 1976; 85:127–130.

99. Pasik P, Pasik T, Bender M: Oculomotor function following cerebral hemidecortication in the monkey: A study with special reference to optokinetic and vestibular nystagmus. *Arch Neurol* 1960; 3:298–305.

100. Pialoux P, Fontelle P, Burgeat M: Electronystagmographic study of vestibular apparatus in Parkinson's disease before and after coagulation of thalamus. *Acta Otolaryngol* 1969; 68:215–223.

101. Proctor L, Glackin R, Shimizu H, et al: Reference values for serial vestibular testing. *Ann Otol Rhinol Laryngol* 1986; 95:83–89.

102. Reed AH, Henry RJ, Mason WB: Influence of statistical method used in the resulting estimate of a normal range. *Clin Chem* 1971; 17:275–284.

103. Riesco-MacClure JS, Stroud M: Dysrhythmia in the post-caloric nystagmus. Its clinical signifiance. *Laryngoscope* 1960; 70:697–721.

104. Reisco-MacClure JS: Caloric tests: Methods and interpretation. *Ann Otol Rhinol Laryngol* 1964; 73:829–837.

105. Rodriguez-Barrios R, Botinelli MD, Medoc J: The study of ocular motility in the comatose patient. *J Neurol Sci* 1966; 3:183–206.

106. Rosenberg M, Sharpe J, Hoyt WF: Absent vestibulo-ocular reflexes and acute supratentorial lesions. *J Neurol Neurosurg Psychiatry* 1975; 38:6–10.

107. Royston, P, Matthews JNS: Estimation of reference ranges from normal samples. *Stat Med* 1991; 10:691–695.

108. Sato Y, Kato I, Kawasaki T, et al: Failure of fixation suppression of caloric nystagmus and ocular motor abnormalities. *Arch Neurol* 1980; 37:35–38.

109. Shapiro SS, Wilk MB, Chen HJ: A comparative study of various tests for normality. *J Am Stat Assoc* 1968; 63:1343–1372.

110. Simmons FB: Patients with bilateral loss of caloric response. *Ann Otol Rhinol Laryngol* 1973; 82:175–178.

111. Sismanis A: Otologic manifestations of benign intracranial hypertension syndrome: Diagnosis and management. *Laryngoscope* 1987; 97:1–17.

112. Sismanis A, Hughes GB, Abedi E, et al: Otologic symptoms and findings of the pseudotumor cerebi syndrome: A preliminary report. *Otolaryngol Head Neck Surg* 1985; 93:398–402.

113. Snedecor GW, Cochran WG: *Statistical Methods*, ed 8. Ames, Iowa; Iowa State University Press, 1989.

114. Spector M: Electronystagmographic findings in central nervous system disease. *Ann Otol Rhinol Laryngol* 1975; 84:374–378.

115. Spoendlin H: Optic and cochleovestibular degenerations in the hereditary ataxias. II: Temporal bone pathology in two cases of Friedreich's ataxia with vestibulo-cochlear disorders. *Brain* 1974; 97:41–48.

116. Stahle J: Electro-nystagmography in the caloric and rotary tests. *Acta Otolaryngol [Suppl]* 1958; 137:5–83.

117. Stahle J, Bergman B: The caloric reaction in Meniere's disease: An electronystagmographical study in 300 patients. *Laryngoscope* 1967; 77:1629–1643.

118. Steenerson R, Van De Water S, Systma W, et al: Central vestibular findings on electronystagmography. *Ear Hear* 7:176–181.

119. Steinmetz EF, Lebo CP, Norris FH Jr: Electronstagmographic findings in motor neuron disease. *Laryngoscope* 1974; 84:281–289.

120. Stockwell CW: Vestibular function tests, in Cummings CW (ed): *Otolaryngology—Head and Neck Surgery* vol 4. St Louis, CV Mosby, 1986, pp 2743–2763.

121. Takemori S, Aiba R, Shizawa R: Visual suppression of caloric nystagmus in brain-stem lesions. *Ann NY Acad Sci* 1981; 374:846–854.

122. Takemori S, Cohen B: Loss of visual suppression of vestibular nystagmus after flocculus lesions. *Brain Res* 1974; 72:213–224.

123. Takemori S, Ono M, Maeda T: Cerebral contribution to the visual suppression of vestibular nystagmus. *Arch Otolaryngol* 1979; 105:579–581.

124. Takemori S, Suzuki M: Cerebellar contribution to oculomotor function. *Otorhinolaryngol* 1977; 39:209–217.

125. Thomas K, Harrison MS: Long-term follow-up of 610 cases of Meniere's disease. *Proc R Soc Lond [Med]* 1971; 64:853–856.

126. Toglia JU, Thomas D, Kuritzky A: Common migraine and vestibular function: Electronystagmographic study and patholgenesis. *Ann Otol Rhinol Laryngol* 1981; 90:267–271.

127. Tomlinson RD, Robinson DA: Is the vestibulo-ocular reflex cancelled by smooth pursuit? in, Fuchs AF, Becker W (eds): *Progress in Oculomotor Research*. New York, Elsevier/North Holland, 1981, pp 533–539.

128. Torok N: The hyperactive vestibular response. *Acta Otolaryngol* 1970; 70:153–162.

129. Torok N: Standard evaluation of the reactive nystagmus. *Arch Otolaryngol* 1972; 96:448–452.

130. Torok N: Vestibular decruitment in central nervous system disease. *Ann Otol Rhinol Laryngol* 1976; 85:131–135.

131. Uemura T, Cohen B: Vestibular nuclei lesions. *Acta Otolaryngol [Suppl]* 1973; 315: 5–71.

132. Vaernet K: Caloric vestibular reactions in transtentorial herniation of the brainstem. *Neurology* 1957; 7:833–836.

133. Wennmo C, Hindfelt B: Eye movements in brainstem lesions. *Acta Otolaryngol* 1980; 90:230–236.

134. Wennmo C, Pyykkö I: Vestibular neuronitis: A clinical and electro-oculographic analysis. *Acta Otolaryngol* 1982; 94:507–515.

135. Wexler DB: The caloric test in electronystagmography. *ENTechnology*, 1989, September, pp 6–17.

136. Wilson W, Zoller M: Electronystagmography in congenital and acquired syphilitic otits. *Ann Otol Rhinol Laryngol* 1981; 90:21–24.

PART III

Rotational Testing

CHAPTER 10

Background and Technique of Rotational Testing

Charles W. Stockwell, Ph.D
Dennis I. Bojrab, M.D.

Rotational tests have been widely used to evaluate vestibular function since the beginning of this century. Various testing methods have been used, but nearly always the patient is positioned so that the rotational axis is vertical and passes through the center of the head, thus stimulating only the patient's horizontal semicircular canals and none of the other labyrinthine receptors. Horizontal eye movements are monitored. These rotational tests evaluate a specific component of vestibular function, *the horizontal canal-ocular reflex.*

Rotational tests can be classified into two types. There are *passive* rotational tests, in which the patient's whole body is rotated without any relative movement between the head and body, and *active* rotational tests, in which the patient rotates his or her own head back and forth while the body remains stationary.

PASSIVE ROTATIONAL TESTS

Passive rotational tests differ from one another primarily in the particular stimulus employed. Two types of stimulus, *velocity steps* and *sinusoidal oscillations*, are widely used.

Tests Employing Velocity Steps

Early Velocity-Step Tests

Barany[4] first described the velocity-step test in 1907. The patient was seated in a rotating chair with his or her head tilted forward by 30° to bring the horizontal semicircular canals into the plane of rotation. The patient was then manually rotated at approximately 180°/sec for long enough to let the response to the initial acceleration subside. Then the patient was suddenly stopped facing the examiner, who timed the nystagmus response generated by the sudden deceleration by using a stopwatch. This procedure was performed both in the clockwise and in the counterclockwise directions. The examiner noted two features of each response: its *strength* and its *symmetry*. Weak or absent responses generally denoted bilateral loss of vestibular function. Asymmetric responses, that is, responses that were stronger in one direction than in the other, often denoted unilateral vestibular loss on the side of the weak response.

In 1948, Van Egmond et al.[34] described an elaboration of this test, which they called *cupulometry*. The patient was slowly accelerated to a series of different rotational velocities before being suddenly stopped. The durations of the nystagmus responses were measured, and a "cupulogram" was then generated by plotting nystagmus response duration versus the log of stimulus magnitude.

These tests are rarely performed today. They have proved to be highly unreliable and insensitive to detection of lesions, primarily because of the difficulty in producing repeatable stimuli and making accurate response measurements.

Modern Velocity-Step Tests

The modern era of rotational testing began in the 1960s when methods became available for generating precise, repeatable rotational stimuli and for making quantitative measurement of eye movements. Today all aspects of rotational testing—including stimulus generation, response measurement, and data analysis—are controlled by computer.

Test procedures vary somewhat among laboratories, but generally the patient is subjected to a series of velocity steps, both to the right and to the left, while seated in a chair mounted on a servo-controlled torque motor. The whole apparatus is enclosed within a small lightproof booth whose walls are concentric with the axis of chair rotation. An example of a modern rotary chair system is shown in Figure 10–1. The patient is tested with eyes open in total darkness. For safety, the patient wears a seatbelt and is in two-way voice communication with the examiner. In addition, the patient is usually monitored with an infrared video camera. The patient continuously performs mental arithmetic or some other task to maintain alertness.

The signal from the chair's tachometer measures chair motion, and since the patient's head is firmly restrained by a headband, head motion is inferred from the chair tachometer signal. The patient's horizontal eye position is detected by the method of electro-oculography from electrodes placed near the

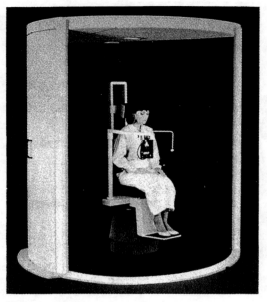

FIG 10–1.
A system for administering passive rotational tests. The patient is seated in a rotary chair enclosed within a lightproof booth. *(Courtesy of ICS Medical Corporation, Schaumburg, Ill.)*

outer canthi of his or her eyes. The eye movement signal is amplified on-board the chair and then sent by way of slip rings to the signal processor.

The clinician examines the relationship between the patient's head and eye motion. Head and eye motion data for a normal individual during a single trial are shown in Figure 10–2. In this example, the person underwent a leftward velocity step, with an angular acceleration of $100°/sec^2$ lasting for 1 second (see Fig 10–2,A). At the end of the acceleration, the patient was rotating at a constant velocity of 100°/sec to the left (see Fig 10–2,B). This velocity was maintained for the remainder of the trial.

In response to this stimulus, the person displayed a burst of horizontal nystagmus (see Fig 10–2,C). This nystagmus began with a fast phase to the left, followed by a slow phase that brought the eyes back toward center. Subsequent fast phases kept the eyes deviated to the left, that is, in the direction of rotation. Presumably, in real life, this deviation enables the eyes to pick up newly arriving visual targets quickly in

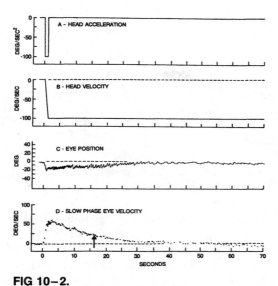

FIG 10-2.
Head and eye motion of a healthy individual during a leftward velocity step (discussed in text). Upward deflection indicates rightward motion. *Vertical arrow* in *D* indicates the point at which the response dropped to 37% of its peak value. *(Adapted from Baloh RW, Honrubia V: Clinical Neurophysiology of the Vestibular System. Philadelphia, FA Davis, 1990.)*

order to hold fixation on them for as long as possible during the subsequent slow phase.[24] The eyes gradually returned to center gaze as the response died away and was followed by a few beats of nystagmus in the opposite direction.

After the test, the computer differentiates the eye position signal and removes the nystagmus fast phases, yielding a plot of slow-phase eye velocity (see Fig 10-2,D). This plot shows a rapid rise to a peak, an exponential decline back to zero, and finally a weak reversal.

To understand the relationship between head velocity (Fig 10-2,B) and slow-phase eye velocity (Fig 10-2,D), it is important first of all to realize that the canal-ocular reflex is designed to provide ocular stabilization during head movements: that is, to generate slow-phase eye movements that are equal and opposite to head movements. It performs this function with remarkable accuracy for natural head movements that occur in everyday life. However the sys-

tem does not perform well in this test situation. If it were generating eye movements that were exactly equal and opposite to head movements, the slow-phase eye velocity plot in Figure 10-2,D would be the mirror image of the head velocity plot in Figure 10-2,B, but it is not. Slow-phase eye velocity does not match the step in head velocity; it initially rises to a peak that is lower than head velocity and then declines exponentially back to zero, even as the head continues to rotate. This test situation is wholly unnatural, and the canal-ocular reflex was not designed to operate under these circumstances. Nevertheless the clinician finds it useful to test the reflex in this situation because it allows clinically relevant characteristics of the reflex to be defined.

The response is described by two parameters. The first is response *gain*, which is the ratio of peak eye velocity to head velocity. In this example head velocity is 100°/sec, whereas peak eye velocity is only about 60°/sec, for a gain of 0.60. The second parameter is response *time constant*, which is the time, in seconds, for the response to decline to 37% of its peak value. In this example, the time constant is about 16 seconds. The clinician compares gain and phase values for rightward and leftward accelerations. As we shall see in the Chapter 11, these comparisons are useful in distinguishing between normal individuals and patients with vestibular lesions.

Over the years, a large number of studies in both animals and humans have led to a fairly clear understanding of the response to velocity-step stimuli. The response is made up of three distinct processes (Fig 10-3). The first process is the *mechanical response* of the cupulae of the horizontal semicircular canals (*a* in Fig 10-3). The canals respond specifically to the impulse of head angular acceleration shown in Figure 10-2,A. This impulse almost immediately displaces the endolymph within the canals, which in turn deflects the cupula and bends the sensory hairs imbed-

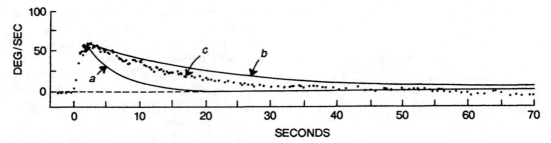

FIG 10–3.
Components of the response to a velocity step: *a*, response of peripheral labyrinthine afferents; *b*, perseveration of response by velocity storage mechanism; *c*, observed response, modified by adaptation.

ded within it, inducing a change in the firing rates of afferent vestibular neurons. The leftward acceleration shown here increases the firing rates of afferent neurons of the left horizontal canal and decreases the firing rates of those of the right horizontal canal. The acceleration lasts for only 1 second, and once it ceases, the cupulae swing back to their neutral positions following an exponential time course, and accordingly the firing rates of afferent neurons return to their resting rates. The time constant of vestibular afferent response decline has not been measured in humans, but is presumed to be similar to that measured in vestibular afferent neurons in the squirrel monkey, which has been reported to be about 6 seconds.[7, 9] (A concise and highly readable mathematical description of cupular mechanics is provided by Baloh and Honrubia.[2])

The second process is *velocity storage*,[28] which is a positive feedback loop located within the central vestibular system. This mechanism performs the equivalent of a mathematical integration of the labyrinthine inputs and yields a response with a time constant longer than that generated by the vestibular afferents (*b* in Fig 10–3).

The third process is *adaptation*, which can be conceptualized as a "zero-velocity reference level" located within the central vestibular system that gradually shifts during sustained stimulation in the direction of the ongoing response.[23, 30, 35] Adaptation progressively reduces the strength of a unidirectional

response and, after the response finally subsides, induces a response reversal.

The net result of these three processes is the observed nystagmus response (*c* in Fig 10–3).

Tests Employing Sinusoidal Oscillations

Torsion Swing Test

The torsion swing test was employed for clinical vestibular testing for many years and was popular because instrumentation costs were relatively modest. The patient was seated in a chair fitted with a calibrated spring. When the chair was displaced and then released, the spring caused it to oscillate back and forth, with progressively decreasing amplitude, and finally to come to rest. In one version of the test,[22] the spring was calibrated so that the patient underwent about 15 sinusoidal oscillations at 0.05 Hz. The patient's head was positioned so that the horizontal semicircular canals were in the plane of rotation, and horizontal eye movements were monitored by the method of electro-oculography in total darkness. The nystagmus response changed in direction with each half cycle. The intensities of right-beating and left-beating nystagmus were separately calculated and plotted as a function of peak angular acceleration of the stimulus.

The torsion swing test could be used to detect severe bilateral loss of vestibular function and showed asymmetries as a result of unilateral peripheral lesions in some patients. However it is rarely performed today because, like early velocity-step tests, it has proved to be relatively unreliable and insensitive to lesion detection.

Modern Sinusoidal Oscillation Tests

Today, the most widely used rotation test is the slow harmonic acceleration test.[36, 37] The testing equipment is the same as that employed in modern velocity-step tests—the patient is seated in a chair mounted on a servo-controlled torque motor enclosed within a light-proof booth. The horizontal semicircular canals are in the plane of rotation, and horizontal eye movements are monitored by the method of electro-oculography. The patient is tested with eyes open in total darkness while performing mental arithmetic. He or she undergoes sinusoidal oscillation about a vertical axis at several different frequencies. The test protocol varies somewhat among laboratories, but a commonly used procedure employs oscillation frequencies of 0.01, 0.02, 0.04, 0.08, 0.16, 0.32, and 0.64 Hz, with peak angular velocities of 50°/sec at each frequency.[29] The patient undergoes multiple cycles of oscillation at each frequency.

The relationship between head and eye movement during several cycles of sinusoidal oscillation for a normal individual is shown in Figure 10–4. The oscillation frequency in this example was 0.16 Hz, which is near the middle of the test frequency range. Figures 10–4,A and 10–4,B show head angular acceleration and velocity, respectively. Figure 10–4,C shows horizontal eye position. The patient had nystagmus with leftward slow phases when his head was moving rightward and nystagmus with rightward slow phases when his head was moving leftward. The computer differentiated the eye position signal, removed the fast phases of nystagmus, and displayed slow-phase eye velocity, shown in Figure 10–4,D. Recall that the function of the canal-ocular reflex is to

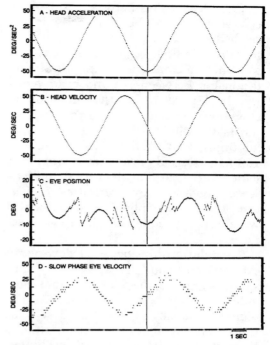

FIG 10–4.
Head and eye motion of a normal individual during oscillation at 0.16 Hz. Upward deflection denotes rightward motion.

produce eye movements that compensate for head movements. If the reflex had been performing perfectly, the slow-phase eye velocity plot in Figure 10–4,D would have been the mirror image of the head velocity plot in Figure 10–4,B. However compensation was less than perfect. The gain of slow-phase eye velocity with respect to head velocity was only about 0.6. In other words, the eyes did not move quite fast enough during the nystagmus slow phases to compensate entirely for head movements.

The gain of the canal-ocular reflex during oscillation at low frequencies has been shown to be dependent on the subject's ideation.[5] If persons imagine an earth-fixed visual scene moving past them as they are rotated, gain is high, about 0.9. If they imagine a visual scene moving along with him, gain is low, about 0.1. If they are distracted by performing mental arithmetic, gain is intermediate between the two, as seen in Figure 10–4.

The relationship between slow-phase eye velocity and head velocity is described by two parameters in addition to gain. The first parameter is *phase angle*, which is a measure of the timing relationship between eye and head velocity. In Figure 10–4, the direction of slow-phase eye velocity was exactly opposite the direction of head velocity at all times; that is, the phase angle was 180°. The second parameter is *symmetry*, which is the ratio of rightward and leftward slow-phase eye velocities. In Figure 10–4, slow-phase eye velocities were roughly equal in the two directions.

The relationships between slow-phase eye velocity and head velocity are shown in Figure 10–5 for a normal individual at four test frequencies. At the higher frequency of 0.64 Hz, these relationships were about the same as at 0.16 Hz, but when the person was oscillated at progressively lower frequencies of 0.04, and finally 0.01 Hz, these relationships showed progressive change. Slow-phase eye velocities exhibited progressively lower gains, and they were no longer exactly opposite in phase, but rather displayed progressively larger phase leads; that is, changes in slow-phase eye velocity occurred more and more in advance of head velocity. To understand the low-frequency gain reduction and phase lead, it is important to realize that the canal-ocular system functions as an integrating angular accelerometer. It detects angular acceleration of the head and produces an output related to head angular velocity. Part of this integration is performed mechanically within the semicircular canal itself, and further integration is performed by the velocity storage mechanism within the central vestibular system, extending the low-frequency sensitivity of the canal-ocular system. However, even with this integration, the system performs well only for relatively fast head motions. The oscillation frequencies used in the slow harmonic acceleration test are at the lower end of its operating range, and therefore, as oscil-

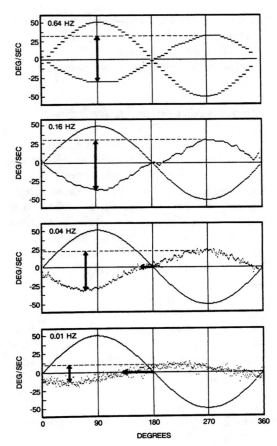

FIG 10–5.
Head and slow-phase eye velocities of a normal individual during oscillation at four different frequencies. Upward deflection denotes rightward velocities. Response gains *(vertical arrows)* are 0.61 at 0.64 Hz, 0.67 at 0.16 Hz, 0.52 at 0.04 Hz, and 0.25 at 0.01 Hz. Phase leads *(horizontal arrows)* are 0° at 0.64 and 0.16 Hz, 15° at 0.04 Hz, and 45° at 0.01 Hz.

lation frequency decreases, the system becomes less sensitive to the head motions and fails to integrate the head acceleration signal completely, yielding lower gains and greater phase leads.

In Figure 10–6, graphic plots of phase, gain, and symmetry data for a normal individual are displayed over the entire range of test frequencies. Phase and gain values show the progressive phase lead and gain reduction as oscillation frequency decreases. Symmetry values are approximately zero at all frequencies.

Note that there is a correspondence between the gain and phase values measured by the slow harmonic acceleration

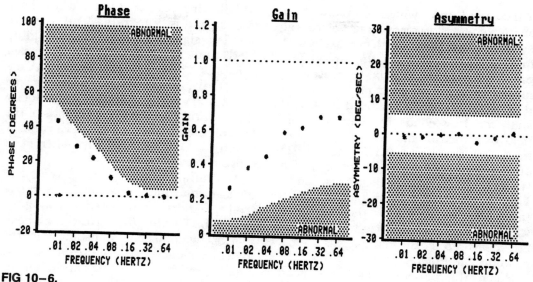

FIG 10–6.

Phase, gain, and asymmetry values in relation to oscillation frequency for a normal individual. Note that, for convenience, the eye velocity signal is inverted during the analysis, so that a phase angle of 180° is expressed as a phase angle of 0°.

test and the gain and time constant values measured by the velocity-step test described earlier. In both cases, gain is the ratio of peak eye velocity to peak head velocity. The phase lead (θ) at low oscillation frequencies is inversely related to the time constant (T_c) of response decay following a velocity-step stimulus by

$$T_c = 1/2\pi f \tan\theta$$

where T_c is the response time constant, f is oscillation frequency, and θ is phase lead at that frequency. In practice, time constants measured by the velocity-step test are somewhat shorter than those calculated from phase values measured by the slow harmonic acceleration test, because adaptation affects velocity-step responses more than it does the responses to oscillation even at low frequencies.[13]

ACTIVE ROTATIONAL TESTS

Many clinicians have been dissatisfied with passive rotation tests for two reasons: (1) expensive equipment is required to rotate an adult human with satisfactory precision, and (2) passive tests do not evaluate vestibular responses to strong head motions such as those encountered in everyday life. Therefore clinicians have sought to test vestibular function by monitoring eye movements while the patient simply shakes the head back and forth. Patients can shake their heads quite briskly, generating angular accelerations far in excess of those achieved by available passive rotational devices.

Two types of active rotational test are in current clinical use: (1) the so-called *vestibular autorotation test*, in which eye movements are monitored *during* active head rotation, and (2) the so-called *head-shaking test*, in which eye movements are monitored *after* active head rotation.

Vestibular Autorotation Test

Over the years, various methods have been used to evaluate the canal-ocular response during active head rotation.[1, 10, 14, 32, 33] Today the most widely used method is one devised by O'Leary and his colleagues,[8, 21, 26, 27] who coined the term "vestibular autorotation test." The patient is seated in a chair wearing a headband upon which is mounted an accelerometer for measuring horizontal head motion. Horizontal eye motion is monitored by electro-oculography. The patient is instructed to fixate on a target placed directly in front of him. He is then asked to shake his head back and forth for 18 seconds in time with the ticks of a metronome. The frequency of ticks increases from 0.5 Hz to 0.8 Hz during the first 6 seconds, and from 0.8 Hz to 6 Hz during the last 13 seconds. This procedure is performed three times. The entire test is then repeated while vertical eye and head movements are measured as the patient shakes his head up and down.

When the patient shakes his head while fixating a visual target, both the canal-ocular and pursuit reflexes participate in generating eye movements. However, the pursuit system is effective only for head movements at velocities below about 60°/sec and frequencies below about 1 Hz,[25] so it may be assumed that the canal-ocular reflex is primarily responsible for the eye movements generated by this test, especially at the higher frequencies.

Following testing, the head acceleration signal is integrated and the eye position signal differentiated, yielding head and eye velocity signals. Fast phases are removed, and the eye velocity signal is calibrated by matching its amplitude with that of the head velocity signal during the first few seconds of the trial on the assumption that eye velocity exactly follows head velocity when head movements are slow.

An example of head and eye velocities for a normal individual during a single trial of horizontal head shaking is shown in Figure 10–7. Note that head motion was nearly sinusoidal at the lower frequencies, but tended to become smaller and more irregular at the higher frequencies. Nevertheless eye motion was equal and opposite head motion throughout the frequency range. From the eye and head velocity data, values for phase, gain, and symmetry are estimated at various frequencies in the same manner as these parameters are estimated in the slow harmonic acceleration test. For normal individuals, phase values are approximately zero at the lower frequencies and lag somewhat

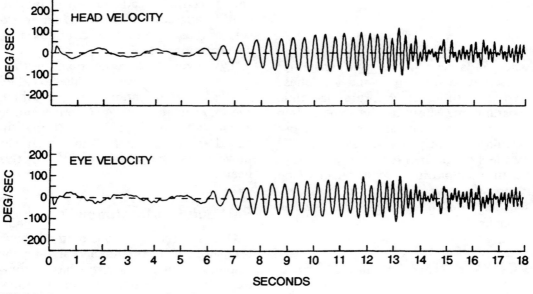

FIG 10–7.
Head and eye velocities for a normal individual during autorotation. *(Redrawn from Kitsigianis G-A, O'Leary DP, Davis LL:* Otolaryngol Head Neck Surg 1988; 98:82–87.)

at the higher frequencies. Gain values are approximately 0.9 at lower frequencies and decline somewhat at the higher frequencies. Symmetry values are approximately zero at all frequencies.[8]

Several considerations dictate that caution be used when interpreting the results of the vestibular autorotation test. First, measurement of head and eye motion at high frequencies is technically difficult. The head motion sensor is mounted on a headband, which tends to slip when the head is shaken vigorously. Vigorous head motion also introduces artifact into the electro-ocular signal due to electrode and lead wire movement, and this problem is exacerbated by the fact that low-pass filtering must be applied with the care to avoid introducing errors in estimating phase and gain. Furthermore, the eye motion signal generally contains saccades as well as the canal-ocular response, and the two have similar velocities at high frequencies of head oscillation, making them nearly impossible to distinguish. Finally, there is evidence that, in addition to the canal-ocular reflex, the cervico-ocular reflex and motor programming associated with volitional head movements also contribute to compensatory eye movements during active head oscillation.[11, 20]

Head-Shaking Test

The head-shaking test is a provocative test designed to evoke a nystagmus response in patients with vestibular lesions. Clinicians have looked for nystagmus following vigorous head shaking for many years as part of the physical examination of the dizzy patient. Kamei and his colleagues[15-19] described a version of this test using electro-oculography to monitor eye movements. The test is administered in a darkened room with the patient wearing Frenzel's lenses (Fig 10–8), which are +20 to +30 D lenses mounted with two small lights in a goggle-like frame that fits snugly against the patient's head. Frenzel's

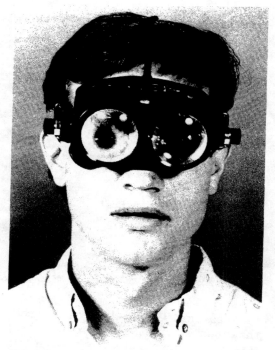

FIG 10–8.
A subject wearing Frenzel's lenses *(From Jacobson GP, Newman CW: Semin Hear 1991; 12:218. Used by permission.)*

lenses magnify and illuminate the patient's eyes and, when used in a darkened room, reduce the patient's ability to fixate. Thus outfitted, the patient is asked to shake the head back and forth vigorously in the horizontal plane for about 20 seconds, then abruptly stop shaking the head. Eye movements are monitored for the presence of nystagmus for at least 30 seconds. In many patients with severe unilateral peripheral vestibular lesions, vigorous head shaking induces horizontal nystagmus. The intensity of the response varies widely among patients, lasting from just a few seconds to up to 30 seconds. The nystagmus generally begins immediately after head shaking ceases, with slow phases that are toward the side of the lesion and gradually die away. If the initial response is strong, it may be followed by a secondary response with slow phases away from the side of the lesion. An example is shown in Figure 10–9.

Hain et al.[12] have offered an hypothe-

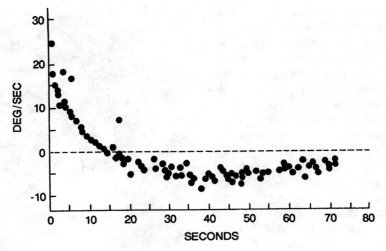

FIG 10–9.
Slow-phase velocity of head-shaking nystagmus in a patient with a severe right peripheral vestibular lesion. *(Adapted and redrawn from Hain TC, Fetter M, Zee DS: Am J Otolaryngol 1987; 8:36–47.)*

sis regarding the mechanism of head-shaking nystagmus. They proposed that this nystagmus is due to asymmetric charging of the velocity storage mechanism. When a patient with only one functioning labyrinth shakes his or her head vigorously, rotation toward the side of the intact labyrinth increases the firing rates of its horizontal canal afferents, and rotation away from that side decreases their firing rates. During strong stimulation like that generated by vigorous head shaking, the response of a single horizontal canal becomes asymmetric. The tonic firing rates of canal afferents are in the lower portion of their operating ranges, so that strong excitatory stimuli can increase their firing rates to high levels, whereas inhibitory stimuli can only decrease their firing rates to zero.[3] Thus during head shaking, there is a net preponderance of input during rotation toward the side of the intact labyrinth. Hain and his colleagues argue that this directionally asymmetric input causes asymmetric charging of the velocity storage mechanism.[12] When head shaking stops, the velocity storage mechanism discharges, inducing head-shaking nystagmus.

Demer[6] presented an alternative hy-pothesis. He described a patient with strong head-shaking nystagmus who had no evidence of a unilateral peripheral vestibular lesion, but who did have asymmetric time constants on the passive step-velocity test. Takahashi et al.[31] have reported similar cases. Demer argued that head-shaking nystagmus in such cases cannot be due to asymmetric vestibular input, so it must be due to asymmetric velocity storage itself.

REFERENCES

1. Atkin A, Bender M: Ocular stabilization during oscillatory head movements. *Arch Neurol* 1968; 19:599–605.

2. Baloh RW, Honrubia V: *Clinical Neurophysiology of the Vestibular System.* Philadelphia, FA Davis, 1990.

3. Baloh RW, Honrubia V, Konrad HR: Ewald's second law re-evaluated. *Acta Otolaryngol* 1977; 83:474–479.

4. Barany R: Physiologie und Pathologie des Bogengangsapparates beim Menschen. Vienna, Deuticke, 1907.

5. Barr CC, Schultheis LW, Robinson DA: Voluntary, non-visual control of the human vestibulo-ocular reflex. *Acta Otolaryngol* 1976; 81:365–375.

6. Demer JL: Hypothetical mechanism of head-shaking nystagmus (HSN) in man: Asymmet-

rical velocity storage. *Soc Neurosci Abstr* 1985; 11:1038.

7. Fernandez C, Goldberg JM: Physiology of peripheral neurons innervating semicircular canals of the squirrel monkey. II: Response to sinusoidal stimulation and dynamics of peripheral vestibular system. *J Neurophysiol* 1971; 34:661–675.

8. Fineberg R, O'Leary DP, Davis LL: Use of active head movements for computerized vestibular testing. *Arch Otolaryngol Head Neck Surg* 1987; 113:1063–1065.

9. Goldberg JM, Fernandez C: Physiology of peripheral neurons innervating semicircular canals of the squirrel monkey. I: Resting discharge and response to constant angular accelerations. *J Neurophysiol* 1971; 34:635–660.

10. Gresty MA, Hess K, Leech J: Disorders of the vestibulo-ocular reflex producing oscillopsia and mechanisms compensating for loss of labyrinthine function. *Brain* 1977; 100:693–716.

11. Grossman GE, Leigh RJ: Instability of gaze during locomotion in patients with deficient vestibular function. *Ann Neurol* 1990; 27:528–532.

12. Hain TC, Fetter M, Zee DS: Head-shaking nystagmus in patients with unilateral peripheral vestibular lesions. *Am J Otolaryngol* 1987; 8:36–47.

13. Honrubia V, Jenkins HA, Baloh RW, et al: Evaluation of rotatory vestibular tests in peripheral labyrinthine lesions, in Honrubia V, Brazier MAB (eds): *Nystagmus and Vertigo. Clinical Approaches to the Patient with Dizziness.* New York, Academic Press, 1982, pp 57–78.

14. Jell RM, Guedry FE, Hixson WC: The vestibulo-ocular reflex in man during voluntary head oscillations under three visual conditions. *Aviat Space Environ Med* 1982; 53:541–548.

15. Kamei T: The two-phase occurrence of head-shaking nystagmus. *Arch Otorhinolaryngol* 1975; 209:59–67.

16. Kamei T: Two types of head-shaking test in vestibular examination. *Acta Otolaryngol [Suppl]* 1988; 458:108–112.

17. Kamei T, Kimura K, Kaneko H, et al: Revaluation of the head-shaking test as a method of nystagmus provocation. Part I: Its nystagmus eliciting effect. *Jpn J Otolaryngol* 1964; 67:1530–1534.

18. Kamei T, Kornhuber HH: Spontaneous and head-shaking nystagmus in normals and in patients with central lesions. *Can J Otolaryngol* 1979; 3:372–280.

19. Kamei T, Takahashi S, Kamada H, et al: Re-valuation of the head-shaking test as a method of nystagmus provokation. P2: Its diagnostic significance for site of lesion. *Equil Res* 1984; 43:236–242.

20. Kasai T, Zee DS: Eye-head coordination in labyrinthine-defective human beings. *Brain Res* 1978; 144:123–141.

21. Kitsigianis G-A, O'Leary DP, Davis LL: Active head-movement analysis of cisplatin-induced vestibulotoxicity. *Otolaryngol Head Neck Surg* 1988; 98:82–87.

22. Leliever WC, Calhoun, KH, Correia MJ: Diagnostic accuracy of rotation testing vs. standard vestibular test battery: A long-term study. *Laryngoscope* 1984; 94:896–904.

23. Malcolm R, Melvill Jones G: A quantitative study of vestibular adaptation in humans. *Acta Otolaryngol* 1970; 43:304–308.

24. Melvill Jones G: Predominance of anticompensatory oculomotor response during rapid head rotation. *Aerospace Med* 1964; 35:965–968.

25. Meyer CH, Lasker AG, Robinson DA: The upper limit of human smooth pursuit velocity. *Vision Res* 1985; 25:561–563.

26. O'Leary DP, Davis LL: Vestibular autorotation testing of Meniere's disease. *Otolaryngol Head Neck Surg* 1989; 103:66–71.

27. O'Leary DP, Davis LL: High-frequency autorotational testing of the vestibulo-ocular reflex. 1990; *Neurol Clin* 8:297–312.

28. Raphan T, Matsuo V, Cohen B: Velocity storage in the vestibulo-ocular reflex arc (VOR). *Exp Brain Res* 1979; 35:229–248.

29. Stockwell CW: Computerized vestibular function tests. *Hear J* 1988; 41:20–29.

30. Stockwell CW, Gilson RD, Guedry FE: Adaptation of horizontal semicircular canal responses. *Acta Otolaryngol* 1973; 75:471–476.

31. Takahashi S, Fetter M, Koenig E, et al: The clinical significance of head-shaking nystagmus in the dizzy patient. *Acta Otolaryngol* 1990; 109:8–14.

32. Takahashi M, Uemura T, Fujishiro T: Studies of the vestibulo-ocular reflex and visual-vestibular interactions during active head movements. *Acta Otolaryngol* 1980; 90:115–124.

33. Tomlinson RD, Saunders GE, Schwartz DWF: Analysis of human vestibulo-ocular reflex during active head movements. *Acta Otolaryngol* 1980; 90:184–190.

34. Van Egmond AAJ, Groen JJ, Jongkees LBW: The turning test with small regulable stimuli. I: Method of examination: Cupulometria. *J Laryngol Otol* 1948; 2:63–69.

35. Young LR, Oman CM: Model for adaptation to horizontal rotation. *Aerospace Med* 1969; 40:1076–1080.

36. Wolfe JW, Engelken EJ, Kos CM: Low-frequency harmonic acceleration as a test of labyrinthine function: Basic methods and illustrative cases. *Trans Am Acad Ophthalmol Otolaryngol* 1978; 86:130–142.

37. Wolfe JW, Engelken EJ, Olson JE, et al: Vestibular responses to bithermal caloric and harmonic acceleration. *Ann Otol Rhinol Laryngol* 1978; 87:861–865.

CHAPTER 11

Interpretation and Usefulness of Rotational Testing

Charles W. Stockwell, Ph.D.
Dennis I. Bojrab, M.D.

In Chapter 10, four rotational tests were described: two passive rotational tests (the *velocity-step test* and the *slow harmonic acceleration test*), and two active rotational tests (the *vestibular autorotation test* and the *head-shaking test*.) Interpretation of the four rotational tests is the subject of this chapter.

The primary purpose of rotational tests is to detect and locate lesions of the vestibular system. However, because these tests evaluate vestibular *function*, it is natural to interpret test results in terms of function. Because a great deal is known about the anatomic sites of functional components of the vestibular system, it is often possible to infer the site of lesion on the basis of functional abnormalities. It is more difficult to relate test results to specific pathologic causes, except insofar as these are implied by site of lesion. Reference to specific pathologic causes will be made when appropriate.

PASSIVE ROTATIONAL TESTS

Velocity-Step Test

Patients with unilateral peripheral vestibular lesions show directional asymmetries in response to velocity-step stimuli.[4, 6, 7] An example is shown in Figure 11–1 for a patient who was tested shortly after suffering a sudden right peripheral vestibular lesion. The velocity step to the left (away from the side of the lesion) induced a nystagmus response with rightward slow phases. Its gain was about 0.95, and its time constant was about 11 seconds. The velocity step to the right (toward the side of the lesion) induced an attenuated response with leftward slow phases. Its gain was only about 0.50, and its time constant was about 6 seconds.

This asymmetry can be explained on the basis of three processes. The first is spontaneous nystagmus, which results from the vestibular imbalance induced by cessation of tonic input from the damaged labyrinth. At the time of testing, this patient had spontaneous nystagmus in darkness with rightward slow phases at velocities of about 10°/sec. This nystagmus added to rotation-induced nystagmus with rightward slow phases and subtracted from rotation-induced nystagmus with leftward slow phases. However spontaneous nystagmus only partially accounts for the gain asymmetry. A second process—saturation of inhibitory responses of the intact labyrinth during rotation toward the side of the lesion—increases the gain asymmetry by attenuating nystagmus with leftward slow phases. Finally, a third process—an asymmetric loss of velocity storage—shortens the response time constant, especially for the re-

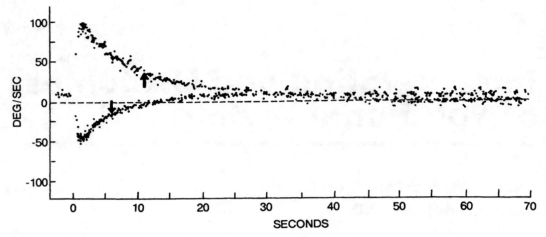

FIG 11–1.
Responses of a patient with an acute right peripheral vestibular lesion to leftward and rightward velocity steps of
100°/sec. Angular acceleration in both cases was 140°/sec.[2] *(Data adapted from Baloh RW, Honrubia V:* Clinical
Neurophysiology of the Vestibular System. *Philadelphia, FA Davis, 1990.)*

sponse to rotation toward the side of the lesion. Recall that the time constant of horizontal canal input is about 6 seconds and that the time constant of the canal-ocular response is lengthened in normal individuals to about 16 seconds by velocity storage. In this patient, velocity storage has been partially lost for the response to rotation to the left (away from the side of the lesion), yielding a response time constant of about 11 seconds, and it has been completely lost for the response to rotation to the right (toward the side of the lesion), yielding a response time constant of only about 6 seconds, the same as the time constant for peripheral input.

Compensation occurs even if the lesion is permanent. Spontaneous nystagmus subsides, and gain asymmetry decreases. However, gain asymmetry never entirely disappears, because saturation of inhibitory responses of the intact labyrinth persists. Phase asymmetry also decreases as a result of partial recovery of velocity storage, but it also never entirely disappears.

Baloh et al.[7] subjected 48 patients with unilateral peripheral lesions (that is, patients with significantly reduced caloric responses in one ear) to a series of rightward and leftward velocity steps

ranging in amplitude from 16°/sec to 256°/sec. They found that asymmetries were detected most consistently in patients with the most severe lesions using the largest velocity-step stimuli. Such stimuli revealed significant asymmetries, with attenuated responses for rotation toward the side of the lesion, in 20 of 23 patients with unilateral absence of caloric response, but in only 10 of 25 patients with unilateral reduction, but not absence, of caloric response. They concluded that the caloric test is more sensitive than the velocity-step test in detecting unilateral peripheral vestibular lesions.

Baloh et al.[7] also subjected 15 patients with bilateral absence of caloric response to velocity-step stimuli. Five of these patients showed no response even to large-amplitude velocity steps. Surprisingly, 6 patients did show responses, although they were abnormally weak, and 4 patients even had normal responses. This result indicates that an absence of caloric response does not necessarily mean an absence of vestibular function, a fact that would be important to clinicians evaluating the effects of vestibular ablative surgery or ototoxic drugs.

Asymmetry of velocity-step responses

can occur in patients without unilateral peripheral vestibular lesions. Takahashi et al.[25] reported such asymmetry in 10 of 47 dizzy patients with normal caloric responses.

Slow Harmonic Acceleration Test

The slow harmonic acceleration test shows abnormalities primarily at the lowest and at the highest oscillation frequencies. Low frequencies reveal abnormal phase leads and gain reductions. High frequencies reveal asymmetries.

Patients with acute unilateral peripheral lesions show the most severe abnormalities. Figure 11–2 shows test results in a patient who underwent the slow harmonic acceleration test shortly after the sudden onset of severe vertigo. The eventual diagnosis was vestibular neuritis. Electronystagmography (ENG), performed at the same time, showed spontaneous nystagmus with rightward slow phases as well as absent caloric responses bilaterally.

At the lower oscillation frequencies, this patient displayed progressively greater-than-normal phase leads, reflecting a loss of velocity storage that is normally provided by the central

vestibular system to enhance the low-frequency response of the canal-ocular system. Loss of velocity storage seems to represent habituation to the strong tonic asymmetry produced by the unilateral peripheral vestibular lesion.[8, 11, 14, 20] This loss is not an exclusive feature of unilateral peripheral vestibular lesions. It is seen in a variety of vestibular disorders, both peripheral and central, and has also been observed in normal individuals who have undergone prolonged rotation.[2]

Loss of response to low-frequency stimulation probably explains why caloric responses were absent in this patient, even in the uninvolved ear. The caloric stimulus is a very low frequency stimulus, approximately an octave below the lowest frequency tested by the slow harmonic acceleration test. If low-frequency responses of the vestibular system are attenuated by a unilateral peripheral vestibular lesion, then it is not surprising that caloric responses are weak or even absent.

This patient also had a rightward asymmetry; that is, nystagmus with rightward slow phases was stronger than nystagmus with leftward slow phases. At low-oscillation frequencies,

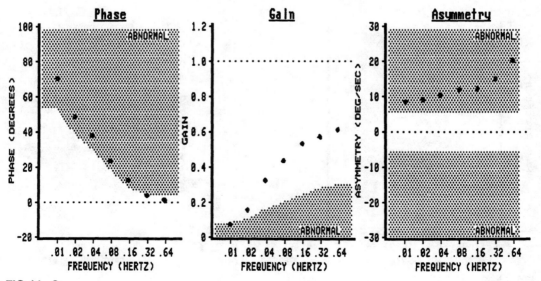

FIG 11–2.
Phase, gain, and asymmetry values in relation to oscillation frequency in a patient with an acute right peripheral vestibular lesion.

the asymmetry was about equal to the slow-phase velocities of the patient's spontaneous nystagmus with eyes closed, but at higher frequencies, the asymmetry was greater than could be accounted for by this bias. This additional asymmetry is presumed to be due to saturation of inhibitory responses of the intact labyrinth during rotation toward the side of the lesion.

This response pattern—abnormal low-frequency phase leads and high-frequency asymmetry—is observed routinely in patients with acute unilateral peripheral vestibular loss, and the asymmetry is always toward the side of the loss.[22, 23]

A second type of abnormality consists solely of greater-than-normal phase leads at the lower oscillation frequencies. An example is seen in Figure 11–3 from a patient with a left acoustic neuroma. Electronystagmography showed a severe left caloric weakness in this patient.

The abnormality seen here is presumed to reflect the same loss of velocity storage that is seen in patients with acute vestibular disorders. The velocity storage loss is persistent, remaining for years following vestibular malfunc-

tion,[11, 14, 20] although there is nearly always partial recovery. The reason for the persistence of velocity storage loss is not understood. Honrubia et al.[11] have argued that velocity storage loss is inconsequential because visual input alone can provide eye stabilization at low frequencies of head motion, although, if one accepts this argument, one must ask why the velocity storage mechanism exists in the first place.

The absence of tonic asymmetry in this patient illustrates the effect of vestibular compensation. If a peripheral vestibular lesion develops slowly, as it generally does in a patient with acoustic neuroma, the compensation process is able to rebalance the tonic asymmetry continuously and therefore to prevent the vertigo and spontaneous nystagmus that would otherwise occur. Even when the lesion develops suddenly, as it did in the previous patient with vestibular neuritis, compensation would quickly rebalance the tonic asymmetry over a period of days.[8, 14, 20] Thus the response pattern in a patient with an acute lesion like that shown in Figure 11–2 would evolve into a pattern like that shown in Figure 11–3 if the patient were tested after a few weeks. The high-frequency

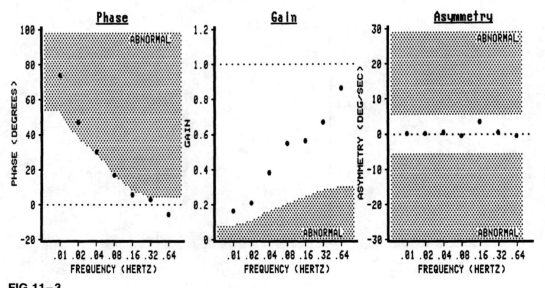

FIG 11–3.
Phase, gain, and asymmetry values in relation to oscillation frequency in a patient with a chronic left peripheral vestibular lesion.

asymmetry, presumably due to saturation, was also absent in this patient, suggesting that compensation also causes an increase in the saturation level.

This response pattern—abnormal low frequency phase leads—is by far the most common abnormality seen in the slow sinusoidal rotation test. Stockwell[22] reported abnormal low-frequency phase leads as the sole abnormality on the slow harmonic acceleration test in 109 of 305 dizzy patients. Twenty-seven of these patients showed no abnormalities on ENG; eight had a diagnosis of unilateral Meniere's disease, and the rest were scattered across diagnostic categories. Fifty-five of these patients showed evidence of a chronic unilateral peripheral vestibular lesion (that is, a significant unilateral caloric weakness without significant spontaneous nystagmus), and most were diagnosed as having either Meniere's disease or acoustic neuroma. The caloric weaknesses in these patients was nearly always greater than 50%. Patients with unilateral caloric weaknesses of less than 50% generally did not show abnormal phase leads. The remaining 27 patients showed various abnormalities on ENG, mostly either evidence of central nervous system dysfunction or a combination of abnormalities.

The slow harmonic acceleration test also shows abnormalities in patients with bilateral loss of vestibular function. An example is shown in Figure 11–4 from a patient with total bilateral absence of caloric response of unknown cause. Rotation confirmed the bilateral caloric loss. The patient failed to show a clear nystagmus response at any oscillation frequency.

The result shown in Figure 11–4 is actually quite uncommon. Most patients with bilateral absence of caloric response show absent responses or reduced response gains at the lower oscillation frequencies, but normal gains at the highest frequencies. An example is shown in Figure 11–5 from a patient who developed unsteadiness following a course of gentamycin therapy and

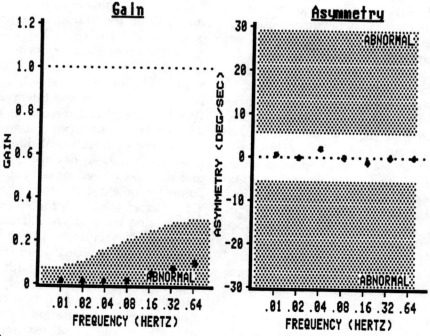

FIG 11–4.
Gain and asymmetry values in relation to oscillation frequency in a patient with bilateral absence of caloric response, showing absent responses at all oscillation frequencies. Phase values are not plotted due to low response gains.

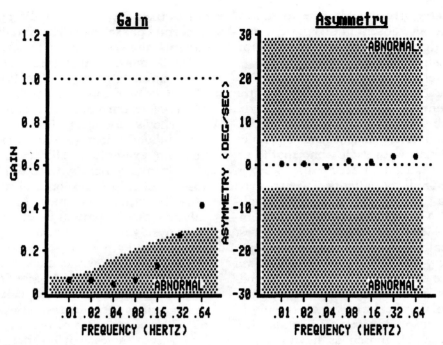

FIG 11–5.
Phase, gain, and asymmetry values in relation to oscillation frequency in a patient with bilateral absence of caloric response, showing a normal response gain at highest frequency. Phase values are not plotted due to low response gains.

showed a bilateral absence of caloric response. Baloh et al.[5] reported that rotation testing often demonstrates normal vestibular function at high frequencies even when ice water irrigations have failed to provoke a response from either ear. In these cases, the results of caloric and rotation tests are not contradictory, because the caloric response is a response to low-frequency stimulus and therefore should be similar to responses to low-frequency rotational stimuli. However, in other cases, rotation testing shows normal response gains at all frequencies despite absent caloric responses, indicating a false positive caloric test result. Clearly the slow harmonic acceleration test is the procedure of choice in evaluating patients suspected of having bilateral loss of vestibular function. The caloric test, even with ice water, does not define the extent of the loss and sometimes yields false positive results.

One shortcoming of the slow harmonic acceleration test is its failure to

lateralize peripheral vestibular lesions. The test does show asymmetries toward the side of the lesion in acute cases (such as that shown in Fig 11–2), but generally provides no evidence regarding side of lesion in chronic cases (such as that shown in Fig 11–3). It is well known that stronger rotatory stimulation does reveal asymmetries in patients with unilateral peripheral lesions. Such testing presents technical difficulties. A powerful rotation device is required, and analysis of eye movement data becomes problematic, since nystagmus slow phases approach the speed of fast phases, and the two are difficult to distinguish.[5] Nevertheless, several investigators have succeeded in detecting asymmetries in patients with chronic unilateral lesions using very strong stimuli. Istl et al.[12] used sinusoidal and other types of stimulation between 0.5 and 3.0 Hz and found asymmetries at the higher frequencies in patients with total chronic unilateral peripheral vestibular lesions. Paige[21] showed consistent asymmetries in patients with such lesions using sinusoidal rotation at 0.25 Hz with peak velocities of 300°/sec. Interestingly, Paige failed to find evidence of saturation of inhibitory responses during rotation toward the side of the lesion at high head velocities. He concluded that the observed response asymmetries were better explained by an asymmetry of velocity storage.

ACTIVE ROTATIONAL TESTS

Vestibular Autorotation Test

There have as yet been few clinical studies of eye movements during active head rotation. Atkin and Bender[1] found that two patients with bilateral peripheral vestibular lesions showed normal responses below 60°/sec and steadily lower gains at velocities exceeding this range. One patient with a unilateral lesion showed low gains at high frequencies, but only when the head moved toward the side of the lesion.

Gresty et al.[9] tested three patients with total bilateral absence of caloric response, one who experienced oscillopsia during fast head movements and two who did not. All three patients showed poor ocular stabilization only during fast head oscillations. The patient who suffered from oscillopsia showed severely impaired stabilization. The two patients without oscillopsia showed better, but not normal, stabilization. Gresty and associates[9] tested patients with lesions of the central nervous system, who showed poor ocular stabilization at all head frequencies.

Nogami et al.[18] tested six patients with unilateral peripheral vestibular lesions and three patients with bilateral lesions at frequencies below 1.0 Hz. Patients with unilateral lesions showed low response gains during rotation toward the lesioned side. Patients with bilateral lesions showed low response gains during both directions of head rotation, especially at the higher oscillation frequencies.

Using the vestibular autorotation test procedure described in the previous chapter, Kitsigianis et al.[16] tested nine patients before and after treatment with cisplatin, which is known to have ototoxic effects. They found consistent reductions in response gain and increases in phase lag following treatment, especially at the higher head oscillation frequencies. Post-treatment head and eye movements for one of the subjects is shown in Figure 11–6. Eye velocities followed head velocities quite well at the lower oscillation frequencies, but decreased markedly at frequencies above 3 Hz.

O'Leary and Davis[19] tested 10 patients with unilateral Meniere's disease. They found that gain and phase values were normal in these patients during horizontal head oscillation, but that gain values were significantly higher than normal and phase lags less than normal during vertical oscillation at high frequencies.

Head-Shaking Test

Vigorous head shaking seems to produce nystagmus with slow phases toward the side of the lesion fairly consistently in patients with pure and severe unilateral peripheral vestibular lesions as demonstrated by a significant unilateral caloric weakness without additional abnormalities. Such head-shaking nystagmus was reported in 13 of 16 patients with unilateral lesions by Takahashi,[24] in 6 of 6 patients with total unilateral lesions due to acoustic neuroma removal or labyrinthectomy by Hain et al.[10] and in 30 of 36 patients with unilateral lesions by Takahashi et al.[25] Jacobson et al.[13] reported a much lower incidence. They elicited head-shaking nystagmus in only 14 of 51 patients with unilateral peripheral dysfunction, although not all of these patients had unilateral caloric weakness.

The slow phases of head-shaking nystagmus are not always toward the lesioned ear. Takahashi[24] reported head-

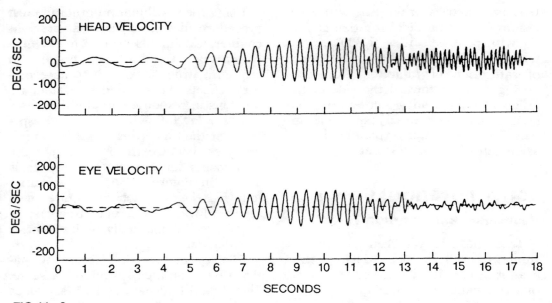

FIG 11–6.
Head and eye velocities during autorotation in a patient after treatment with cisplatin. *(Redrawn from Kitsigianis G-A, O'Leary DP, Davis LL: Otolaryngol Head Neck Surg 1988; 98:82–87.)*

shaking nystagmus with slow phases away from the side of the lesion in 3 of 16 patients, and Takahashi et al.[25] reported such nystagmus in 2 of 36 patients. Most of these patients had Meniere's disease, suggesting that head-shaking nystagmus in these patients may be due to a central vestibular imbalance and not to unilateral peripheral hypofunction. However, head-shaking nystagmus in the unexpected direction is not pathognomonic of Meniere's disease. Some patients with Meniere's disease displayed head-shaking nystagmus with slow phases toward the side of the lesion.

Head-shaking nystagmus is also present in some patients with central vestibular disorders. Kamei and Kornhuber[15] observed head-shaking nystagmus in 15 of 60 patients with a variety of central nervous disorders. Takahashi et al.[25] reported head-shaking nystagmus in 5 of 7 patients with signs of central vestibular dysfunction, either alone or in combination with a unilateral peripheral lesion. In patients with both central and peripheral lesions, head-shaking nystagmus had slow phases away from the

side of the peripheral lesion. Head-shaking nystagmus has also been observed in some individuals with no evidence of vestibular disorder, either peripheral or central.[25]

It seems that the clinician cannot rely solely on the head-shaking test to detect and lateralize peripheral vestibular lesions. Although the test seems to be sensitive to such lesions when they are severe and uncomplicated, it does not enable detection of them all. If one accepts the hypothesis of Hain et al.[10] that head-shaking nystagmus is caused by an imbalance of the velocity storage mechanism due to asymmetric peripheral input, there are at least two instances in which one would not expect unilateral peripheral lesions to induce head-shaking nystagmus: (1) when the lesion is mild, because then the input asymmetry would be relatively minor; and (2) when the lesion is acute, because acute severe lesions greatly reduce or abolish velocity storage.[17] Furthermore, head-shaking nystagmus lateralizes poorly in patients with Meniere's disease or concomitant central vestibular dysfunction. It may also occur in patients with central vestibular disease without unilateral peripheral lesions and even in some individuals with no evidence of vestibular dysfunction. In general, the presence of head-shaking nystagmus seems to be closely (but not perfectly) related to the presence of asymmetric time constants as measured by the velocity-step test,[25] an example of which is shown in Figure 11–1.

CONCLUSION

Rotational tests in one form or another are used by a growing number of clinicians, who seem to find them useful. There exists considerable overlap between rotational tests and conventional ENG. Many patients exhibit abnormalities on both tests. However, the overlap is not complete. A significant percentage of dizzy patients, perhaps 10%, show abnormalities on rotational testing without showing any abnormalities on ENG. These rotational test abnormalities show that something is wrong with the vestibular system but, unfortunately, are nonspecific. They do not localize the dysfunction or identify a cause.

Rotational tests and their interpretation are a still-evolving discipline, with active research being done to further define their functional implications and clinical usefulness. Recent studies indicate that sensitivity to vestibular lesions is highest in tests that employ strong stimuli—high-amplitude steps in the velocity-step test, high frequencies and high peak velocities in the slow harmonic acceleration test, and the strong stimuli induced by active head shaking—although interpreting eye movement recordings made during strong stimulation remains a challenge.

At their present stage of development, none of these tests replaces any component of the standard workup of the dizzy patient: a careful history and a thorough physical examination, as well as conventional laboratory studies, including ENG. Today it appears that the primary role of rotational tests is to help the experienced and thoughtful clinician to gain further insight into the vestibular dysfunction of patients who suffer from dizziness.

REFERENCES

1. Atkin A, Bender M: Ocular stabilization during oscillatory head movements. *Arch Neurol* 1968; 19:599–605.

2. Baloh RW, Henn V, Jager J: Habituation of the human vestibulo-ocular reflex by low frequency harmonic acceleration. *Am J Otolaryngol* 1982; 3:235–241.

3. Baloh RW, Honrubia V: *Clinical Neurophysiology of the Vestibular System.* Philadelphia, FA Davis, 1990.

4. Baloh RW, Honrubia V, Konrad HR: Ewald's second law re-evaluated. *Acta Otolaryngol* 1977; 83:475–479.

5. Baloh RW, Honrubia V, Yee RD, et al: Changes in the human vestibulo-ocular reflex after loss of peripheral sensitivity. *Ann Neurol* 1984; 16:222–228.

6. Baloh RW, Konrad HR, Dirks D, et al: Cerebellar-pontine angle tumors: Results of quantitative vestibulo-ocular testing. *Arch Neurol* 1976; 33:507–512.

7. Baloh RW, Sills AW, Honrubia V: Impulsive and sinusoidal rotatory testing: A comparison with results of caloric testing. *Laryngoscope* 1979; 89:646–654.

8. Fetter M, Zee DS: Recovery from unilateral labyrinthectomy in rhesus monkey. *J Neurophysiol* 1988; 59:370–393.

9. Gresty MA, Hess K, Leech J: Disorders of the vestibulo-ocular reflex producing oscillopsia and mechanisms compensating for loss of labyrinthine function. *Brain* 1977; 100:693–716.

10. Hain TC, Fetter M, Zee DS: Head-shaking nystagmus in patients with unilateral peripheral vestibular lesions. *Am J Otolaryngol* 1987; 8:36–47.

11. Honrubia V, Jenkins HA, Baloh RW, et al: Vestibulo-ocular reflexes in peripheral labyrinthine lesions. I: Unilateral dysfunction. *Am J Otolaryngol* 1984; 5:15–26.

12. Istl YE, Hyden D, Schwarz DWF: Quantification and localization of vestibular loss in unilaterally labyrinthectomized patients using a precise rotatory test. *Acta Otolaryngol* 1983; 96:437–445.

13. Jacobson GP, Newman CW, Safadi I: Sensitivity and specificity of the head-shaking test

for detecting vestibular system abnormalities. *Ann Otol Rhinol Laryngol* 1990;99:539–542.

14. Jenkins HA: Long-term adaptive changes of the vestibulo-ocular reflex in patients following acoustic neuroma surgery. *Laryngoscope* 1985; 95:1224–1234.

15. Kamei T, Kornhuber HH: Spontaneous and head-shaking nystagmus in normals and in patients with central lesions. *Can J Otolaryngol* 1979; 3:372–280.

16. Kitsigianis G-A, O'Leary DP, David LL: Active head-movement analysis of cisplatin-induced vestibulotoxicity. *Otolaryngol Head Neck Surg* 1988; 98:82–87.

17. Leigh RJ, Zee DS: *The Neurology of Eye Movements.* Philadelphia; FA Davis, 1991, p 47.

18. Nogami K, Uemura T, Iwamoto M: VOR gain and phase in active head rotation tests of normal subjects and patients with peripheral labyrinthine lesions. *Acta Otolaryngol* 1989; 107:333–337.

19. O'Leary DP, Davis LL: Vestibular autorotation testing of Meniere's disease. *Otolaryngol Head Neck Surg* 1989; 103:66–71.

20. Olson JE, Wolfe JW, Engelken EJ: Responses to low-frequency harmonic acceleration in patients with acoustic neuromas. *Laryngoscope* 1981; 91:1270–1277.

21. Paige GD: Nonlinearity and asymmetry in the human vestibulo-ocular reflex. *Acta Otolaryngol* 1989; 108:1–8.

22. Stockwell CW: Vestibular function testing: 4-year update, in Cummings CW et al. (eds): *Otolaryngology–Head and Neck Surgery: Update II.* St Louis, Mosby-Year Book, 1989; pp 39–53.

23. Stockwell CW: Vestibular function tests, in Paparella MM, et al. (eds): *Otolaryngology,* ed 3. Philadelphia, WB Saunders, 1991, pp 921–948.

24. Takahashi S: Clinical significance of biphasic head-shaking nystagmus. *Auris Nasus Larynx* 1986; 13:199–204.

25. Takahashi S, Fetter M, Koenig E, et al: The clinical significance of head-shaking nystagmus in the dizzy patient. *Acta Otolaryngol* 1990, 109:8–14.

PART IV

Posturographic Testing

CHAPTER 12

Practical Biomechanics and Physiology of Balance

Lewis M. Nashner, Sc.D.

Balance is a complex process involving the coordinated activities of multiple sensory, motor, and biomechanical components. The position of the body in relation to gravity and the surrounds is sensed by combining visual, vestibular, and somatosensory inputs. Balance movements involve motions of the ankle, knee, and hip joints, which are controlled by the coordinated actions of ankle, thigh, and lower trunk muscles.

The aim of this chapter is to describe the principal biomechanical, sensory, and motor components of balance, and their interactions within a systematic model of balance control. Chapter 13 describes a method for assessing the sensory and motor components of balance based on this model. Chapter 14 demonstrates the clinical applicability of the method in patients with a variety of otologic and neurologic disorders affecting balance.

BIOMECHANICS OF BALANCE

Definition of Balance

To balance with the feet in-place, the position of the body's center of gravity (COG) must be maintained vertically over the base of support.[29, 33, 45] When this condition is met, a person can both resist the destabilizing influence of gravity and actively move the COG. If the COG is positioned outside the perimeter of the base of support, the person has exceeded the in-place limits of stability. At this point a rapid step or stumble to reestablish the base of support beneath the COG, or additional external support, is required to prevent a fall.

The state of a person's balance is best described in terms of angular displacement of the COG from the gravitational vertical. Center of gravity sway is then defined as the angle formed by the intersection of a first line from the center of the base of support through the COG and a second line extending vertically from the center of support as shown in Figure 12–1. This definition of balance pertains, whether the person moves about the ankles, the hips, or about both joints, and also takes height into account.[53] Thus, a given sway angle indicates a comparable state of balance for all body movement patterns and heights. This definition of balance is further discussed in the section on limits of stability.

Base of Support

The base of support for standing on a flat, firm surface is defined as the area contained within the perimeter of contact between the surface and the two feet. The base of support area is nearly square when the feet are placed comfortably apart while the person is quietly standing. Similarly, a diagonal

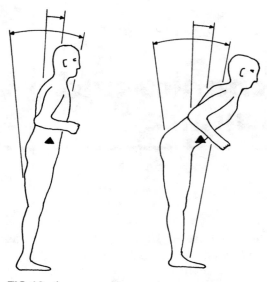

FIG 12–1.
Center of gravity (COG) sway angle in relation to the "limits of stability" cone. The figure on the *left* is moving about the ankles; the figure on the *right* is moving about the hips. The COG sway angles of the two figures are approximately the same, although the joint motions are much larger using the hip strategy. Filled diamonds show the body COG positions.

stance produces a parallelogram-shaped base of support extending forward on one side and backward on the other, while a tandom stance position creates a long but very narrow base of support.

When the support surface area is smaller than the feet, or when surface irregularities limit the contact between the feet and the surface, the base of support is reduced. Standing sideways on a narrow beam, for example, provides a base with a normal width but very short length. Thus, the person's limits of stability are effectively reduced in the anterior-posterior (AP) but not the lateral dimensions.

Limits of Stability

The limits of stability (LOS) is a two-dimensional quantity defining the maximum possible COG sway angle as a function of sway direction from the center position.[33, 39] The LOS depends on the placement of the feet and the base of support. In normal adults standing on a flat, firm surface with feet spaced com-

fortably apart, the LOS perimeter can best be described as an ellipse as shown in Figures 12–1 and 12–3. The AP dimension of this ellipse is approximately 12.5° from the backwardmost to the forwardmost points on the perimeter.[53] While height of the COG above the surface and foot length affect the AP limits of stability, these two features co-vary, resulting in approximately the same AP limits for people of various heights.[23]

The lateral LOS depends on the person's height relative to the spacing between the feet. When the feet of a person 70 inches tall are placed 4 inches apart, for example, the lateral dimension of the LOS ellipse is approximately 16° from the left to the rightmost points on the perimeter. For taller individuals, a wider spacing between the feet is required to produce a 16° elipse, while shorter people can place their feet closer together.

The biomechanical properties that determine the LOS are similar while standing in-place, walking, and sitting without trunk support, as shown in Figure 12–2. During in-place standing the COG moves randomly within an LOS perimeter determined by the base of support and the placement of the feet. During walking, the COG progresses forward through the LOS in a smooth, rhythmic movement.[48, 52] At heel strike, an LOS is established with the COG positioned at the posterior perimeter. As the step progresses, the COG moves forward within the LOS. As the COG approaches the anterior perimeter of the LOS, the next step establishes a new LOS and the rhythmic process is repeated. When sitting without trunk support, the height of the COG above the support surface is less and the base area is larger. Therefore, the LOS perimeter is larger when one is seated than in quiet standing.

Limits of Sway

It is impossible to maintain the COG motionless, because in-place standing is

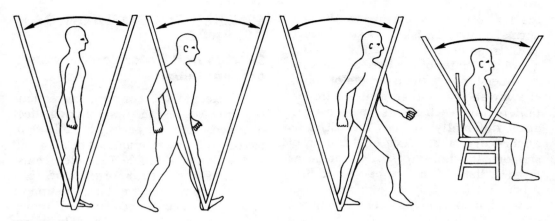

FIG 12–2.
Limits of stability boundaries during standing, walking, and sitting.

an inherently unstable task requiring periodic corrections to overcome the destabilizing influence of gravity.[4, 14, 17, 63] Thus, a person attempting to maintain balance spontaneously sways back and forth and from side to side. The limits of sway is a two-dimensional quantity defining the maximum spontaneous COG sway angle as a function of the sway direction, as shown in Figure 12–3. A person's limits of spontaneous sway vary with the sensory conditions and the configuration of the base of support. But,

unless the person loses balance, the limits of sway is always well within the LOS.

Center of Gravity Alignment

A point at the center of the area contained within the limits of sway perimeter defines the COG alignment, as shown in Figure 12–3. This definition of COG alignment is based on the assumption that a person is attempting to maintain a COG position which is at the center of

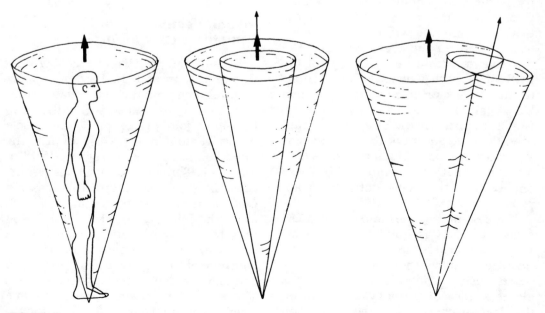

FIG 12–3.
Relations between the LOS, the sway envelope, and the COG alignment. The *middle* figure shows the COG alignment centered within the LOS. The *right* figure shows the COG aligned forward relative to the center.

the limits of sway perimeter. When a normal person is asked to stand erect, COG alignment is placed accurately above the center of the base of support.

Understanding the concepts of limits of sway and COG alignment are important, because each effects a person's balance differently. When the COG is aligned over the center of the base of support, the limits of sway can be as large as the LOS before balance is lost. A person whose COG alignment is offset forward, backward, or to one side of the center of support is not as stable as a person whose COG alignment is centered, even when the limits of sway are similar in the two. The person with the offset COG alignment is less stable, because smaller sway angles in the direction of the offset will move the COG beyond the LOS perimeter.

Limits of Stability and Sway Frequency

In addition to placement of the feet and size of the base of support, the actual LOS depends on the COG sway frequency.[56] When COG sway is slow, gravity is the only significant destabilizing force that must be overcome, and the COG can be moved within the full range of the LOS. For the average adult, COG movements within the full range of the LOS are possible when sway oscillations (front to back or side to side and then back again) last 2 to 3 seconds or longer. In contrast, when the COG moves rapidly, the momentum of the body acts as an additional destabilizing force. When a sway oscillation is completed in 1 second or less, the LOS contracts to approximately 3°.

Understanding the impact of COG sway frequency is important in assessing a person's balance. As higher frequencies reduce the effective LOS, a person using fast sway movements is closer to exceeding the LOS than an individual swaying slowly though a comparable arc.

SENSING THE POSITION OF BALANCE

Sensory and Motor Components of Balance

To execute the constant corrections required to resist the destabilizing effect of gravity and the perturbing effects of purposeful motor actions while standing and walking, the balance system must determine the position of the COG relative to gravity and the base of support and then execute coordinated movements to correct any COG deviations. Although the neural processes for determining COG position and moving the COG are highly integrated, the two are separated here for purposes of developing a systematic model of balance control. From a clinical perspective, separating the sensory and motor processes of balance means that a patient may have impaired balance for one or a combination of two reasons: (1) the position of the COG relative to the base of support is not accurately sensed, and (2) the automatic movements required to bring the COG to a balanced position are not timely or effectively coordinated.

Visual, Vestibular, and Somatosensory Inputs

Sensing the position of the COG relative to gravity and the base of support requires a combination of visual, vestibular, and somatosensory (tactile, deep pressure, joint receptor, and muscle proprioceptor) inputs. Utilization of the three balance senses is reviewed in Table 12–1. Three senses are required because no single sense directly measures COG position. Vision measures the orientation of the eyes and head in relation to surrounding objects. Somatosensory inputs provide information on the orientation of the body parts relative to one another and to the support surface. The vestibular system does not provide orientation information in relation to external objects. Rather, it measures

TABLE 12–1.

Utilization of the Senses for Balance

Sense	Reference	Conditions Favoring Use	Conditions Disrupting Use
Somatosensory	Support surface	Fixed support surface	Irregular or moving support
Visual	Surrounding objects	Fixed visible surrounds and irregular or moving support	Moving surrounds, darkness
Vestibular	Gravity and inertial space	Irregular or moving support and moving surrounds or darkness	Unusual motion environments

gravitational, linear, and angular accelerations of the head in relation to inertial space.

Neither is there a single combination of the three senses providing accurate COG information under all conditions. This is because one or more of the senses may provide information that is misleading or inaccurate for purposes of balance control. For example, when a person stands next to a large bus that suddenly begins to move forward, momentary disorientation or unsteadiness may result. A fraction of a second is required for the brain to determine whether the resulting visual stimulus indicates backward sway of the person or forward movement of the bus. If a downwardly tilted support surface is encountered, the brain must determine whether the surface is tilted downward or the surface is level and the body is tilted back. During sensory conflict situations, the brain must quickly select the sensory inputs providing accurate orientation information and ignore the misleading ones. The process of selecting and combining appropriate sensory information is called sensory organization.

Somatosensory Input

Somatosensory input derived from the contact forces and motions between the feet and the support surface is the dominant sensory input to balance under normal (fixed) support surface conditions.[1, 16, 18, 22, 27] When a person

stands on a firm, level surface, the extent of COG sway is very small relative to the LOS. Closing the eyes to eliminate vision causes little if any functionally significant increase in COG sway. Even a well-compensated patient with a bilateral vestibular loss sways well within the LOS with the eyes closed.[7, 8, 50, 64] In contrast, ischemic disruption of somatosensory input from the ankle muscles increases COG sway significantly when the eyes are closed.[18, 32]

Visual Input

Vision plays a significant role in balance, especially when the support surface is unstable.[4, 19, 35, 60, 61] For example, when toes up and toes down tilting of the surface in direct relation to the AP sway disrupts somatosensory input useful for balance, COG sway is significantly less with eyes open than with eyes closed.[7, 8, 50] The stabilizing effect of vision is also illustrated by comparing eyes open and eyes closed sway while a person stands on a compliant foam rubber pad. Vision also influences COG alignment. When a person is exposed to a constant linear or rotational movement of the visual field, for example, the alignment of the COG over the base of support shifts in the direction of the visual field motion.[12, 36]

The reader may have experienced the effect of vision on balance, for example, at the seashore when a wave causes a large area of the surrounding water to move in or out at constant velocity. If a person is attending to the moving water, there is a tendency to sway and sometimes even stumble in the direction of the moving water. Alterations in body alignment also occur when subjects are exposed to a room with tilted walls. Similar visual illusions are sometimes used in carnival fun-houses to throw participants off balance.

Vestibular Input

When functionally useful somatosensory and visual inputs are available, vestibular inputs play a minor role in controlling COG position.[10, 50, 64] This is because the somatosensory and visual inputs are more sensitive to body sway than the vestibular system.[56] The primary role of vestibular input under these conditions is most probably to allow independent and precise control of head and eye positions. Precise head and eye control is critical in the execution of many complex motor activities such as running and either kicking or catching a moving ball.

Vestibular input is, however, critical for balance when both the somatosensory and visual inputs are misleading or unavailable.[2, 9, 26] The patient with a profound bilateral vestibular loss, for example, is unsteady standing in darkness on a compliant or irregular surface. Because vestibular input is seldom if ever misleading (except in cases of disease or other disorder and unusual motion environments), vestibular information is critical for balance when conflicting visual and/or somatosensory information requires a person to identify and quickly ignore a misleading input.[7, 8] This is why patients with peripheral vestibular deficits frequently complain of dizziness and/or unsteadiness during exposure to conflicting visual and support surface stimuli.

Exposure to zero gravity or to a simulation of zero gravity is believed to cause changes in the way the brain interprets orientation input from the vestibular system. The utricular otoliths normally sense both the linear acceleration of the head and the tilt angle of the head with respect to gravity. Under zero gravity conditions, the brain must adapt to an absence of the tilt angle component of the otolith input. The adaptive changes in interpretation of the vestibular input following zero gravity exposure may be viewed as a temporary, environmentally induced pathologic condition.[58, 65] These maladaptive changes are most potent immediately after return to normal terrestrial conditions, and are most pronounced when the returning astronauts are exposed to conflicting visual conditions.[58]

MOTOR CONTROL OF BALANCE

Anatomy and Physiology of Movement

During erect standing with the arms at the side or folded at the waist, the COG is located in the area of the lower abdomen, with the exact position at a given moment dependent on the relative positions of the ankle, knee, and hip joints.[39] Because there are three principle joint systems—ankles, knees, and hips—between the base of support and the COG during standing, a wide variety of different postures can be assumed with the COG over the center of the base of support,[46] as illustrated in Figure 12–4. For similar reasons, a wide variety of active ankle, knee, and hip movement patterns can be used to produce similar shifts in COG position. Examples of this diversity of postures and balance movement patterns can be observed in individuals performing highly trained dance or martial arts routines.

A detailed description of the large number of muscles controlling ankle, knee, and hip joint motions is beyond the scope of this chapter. Instead, this section focuses on the key muscle groups involved in balance and on the

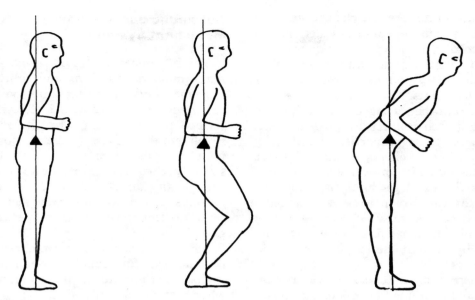

FIG 12–4.
Examples of the variety of different postures during which the body COG is centered over the base of support.

general physiologic principles governing coordination of these muscles during postural movements.

Motions about a given joint are controlled by the combined actions of at least one pair of muscles working in opposition. All leg and lower trunk joints have multiple pairs of opposing muscles. Furthermore, many leg muscles act about two neighboring joints. At the ankle joint, the gastrocnemius and tibialis anterior are the major extensor (plantar flexor) and flexor (dorsiflexor) muscles, respectively. The quadriceps is the major knee extensor, while the hamstrings and gastrocnemius are both knee flexors. The hamstrings and lower back muscles are hip extensors, while hip flexion is controlled by quadriceps and abdominals.

An isolated muscle acts like a spring, tending to resist attempts to stretch the muscle beyond a resting length.[30] The degree of the muscle's resistance to stretch is called muscle stiffness. Both the rest length of the muscle and the muscle stiffness vary depending on how strongly the muscle is being activated. An inactive muscle has an extended rest length and offers little resistance to stretching. The rest length of a highly active muscle is shorter, and the muscle vigorously resists stretching.

When the forces exerted by pairs of opposing muscle about a joint are combined, the effect is to resist rotation of the joint relative to a resting position. The degree to which the joint resists rotation is called joint stiffness. The resting position and the stiffness of the joint are each altered independently by changing the activation levels of one or both muscles. Joint resting position and joint stiffness, however, are by themselves an inadequate basis for controlling postural movements. This is because the stiffness properties of muscle are highly nonlinear. While resistance to a small displacement from the resting position is strong, the resistance breaks down over larger displacements unless the activation level is increased.[34]

The myotatic stretch reflex is the earliest mechanism for increasing the activation level of the muscles of a joint following an externally imposed rotation of the joint. This response component is initiated by inputs from muscle spindles, tiny stretch sensitive receptors imbedded within the muscle. Output fibers from the muscle spindles enter the spinal cord and, by way of single synapses within the cord, activate muscle fibers within the same muscle originating the spindle inputs.[34]

Current theory suggests that the myotatic stretch reflexes improve the nonlinear stiffness properties of muscle in controlling the effects of external disturbances during movement control.[34] Thus, during larger joint displacements, reflexes rapidly increase activation of the stretching muscles, decrease activation of the shortening antagonists, and thereby prevent the breakdown of joint stiffness.

There are, however, several reasons why the combined effects of the muscle stiffness properties and the stretch reflexes are still insufficient to maintain standing balance. First, the level of ankle joint stiffness resulting from these two mechanisms does not fully counteract the destabilizing force of gravity during sway.[24, 43] Second, because rotations of the support surface can elicit stretch reflexes inappropriate for balance control, other response mechanisms not dependent on local stretch inputs are required.[43]

Automatic and Volitional Movement Systems

The influences of stretch reflex, automatic movement system, and volitional movement system on standing balance are reviewed in Table 12–2. As described previously, the stretch reflexes regulate the stiffness properties of the joints involved in maintaining postural stability. Stretch reflexes, however, play little if any direct role in mediating a person's active postural movements in response to external balance perturbations.[24, 28]

Automatic postural movements are the earliest functionally effective responses helping to maintain stability when a standing individual's balance is perturbed.[43, 44, 57] Automatic postural movements resemble reflex responses in some respects, and voluntary movements in others. Like reflexes, automatic movements are triggered by external stimuli, occur at fixed latencies, and are relatively stereotyped. Like voluntary postural movements, automatic responses involve the coordinated actions of many leg and trunk muscles, and the amplitudes and patterns of automatic responses adapt to the task conditions.

TABLE 12–2.

Properties of the Three Movement Systems

Property	Movement Systems		
	Reflex	Automatic	Voluntary
Mediating pathways	Spinal cord	Brain stem and subcortical	Brain stem and cortical
Mode of activation	External stimulus	External stimulus	Self-generated or external stimulus
Response properties	Localized to point of stimulus and highly stereotyped	Coordinated among leg and trunk muscles, and stereotyped but adaptable	Limitless variety
Role in posture control	Regulate muscle forces	Coordinate movements across joints	Generate purposeful behaviors
Response times	Fixed at 40 msec	Fixed at 100 msec	Varies with difficulty, 150+ msec

Although the pathways mediating automatic postural movements have not been fully elucidated, the 90- to 100-msec latencies of electromyographic (EMG) responses are sufficient to include significant brain stem and subcortical involvement.[25, 37, 40]

Voluntary postural movements can occur either in the presence or absence of external stimuli, and the variety of voluntary patterns is almost limitless, in theory at least. When elicited by external stimuli, voluntary movement latencies are 150 msec or much longer, depending on the person's level of attention and extent of practice, and on the complexity of the required movement response.[51] When a freely standing person exerts a voluntary force against an external object, automatic and voluntary activities are closely coordinated to provide a stable base of support for the voluntary movement.[5, 13] In these instances, automatic postural reactions occur first, and the onset of the voluntary component is delayed accordingly.[51]

Automatic Postural Movements

When an automatic postural movement is initiated by an external stimulus, the onset of muscular EMG activity occurs within 90 to 100 msec, and the resulting patterns of activation among leg and lower trunk muscles are directionally specific and relatively stereotyped. The onset of active movement force is delayed an additional 20 to 40 msec, because there is a delay between electrical activation and force generation in a muscle.[3]

Local somatosensory input from the feet and ankle joints is by itself sufficient to trigger an automatic postural movement.[32] The direction of the automatic movement is also determined by the triggering somatosensory stimulus.[31, 44, 57] A backward movement is triggered by forward displacement of the body's COG, as for example, when

the support surface moves backward or when the subject pulls backward on a rigid object. A forward movement follows a backward COG displacement, caused by forward movement of the surface or pushing against a rigid object.

Although the amplitude of the automatic movement is related to the intensity of the triggering somatosensory stimulus,[20] visual input, vestibular input, and the past experiences of the individual also influence the amplitude of the response.[43, 49, 64] The pattern of movement response among leg and lower trunk muscles, in contrast, is determined not by the triggering stimulus but by the configuration of the support surface and the previous experience of the individual.

COORDINATION OF AUTOMATIC POSTURAL MOVEMENTS

Biomechanics of Coordinated Movement

The major joint and muscle systems controlling the COG during standing are illustrated in Figure 12–5. Postural movements involve the coordinated actions of the ankle, knee, hip joints, and frequently also the neck. The motions about each of these joints, however, are not determined simply by the muscles acting directly about the joint. This is because leg and trunk muscles also exert indirect forces on neighboring joints through the inertial interaction forces among body segments.[47, 53] For example, when the ankle muscles contract to extend the lower leg segments backward, the hips will flex unless thigh and lower trunk muscles are activated to stabilize these joints. The hips will flex in the absence of additional stabilizing forces, because the inertia of the trunk tends to make its movements lag behind those of the legs.

Because of the indirect inertial effects of muscular forces, the function of leg

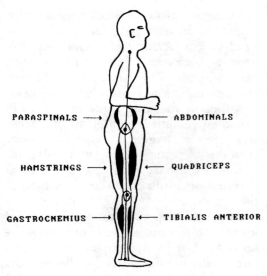

FIG 12–5.
Functional anatomy of the major joint and muscle systems controlling movements of the body's COG during standing balance.

and trunk muscles during posture control can differ quite dramatically from their traditional anatomic classification, as summarized in Table 12–3. When a person is standing on a rigid surface, contraction of the tibialis anterior (anatomically classified as an ankle dorsiflexor) also causes knee flexion, even though there is no anatomic insertion of this muscle at the knee. As dorsiflexion of the ankle moves the lower leg forward, inertia causes the thigh to lag behind and the knee flexes as a result. Although the gastrocnemius is anatomically classified as an ankle extensor and knee flexor, its functional effect on the knee during standing is extension rather than flexion. The knee extends because of inertial interactions similar to the others mentioned.

Contractions of thigh and lower trunk muscles exert similar indirect effects on the knee and ankle joints. The quadriceps muscle is not only a hip flexor and knee extensor by direct action, but also an ankle extensor by indirect action. The hamstrings muscle is an indirect ankle flexor in addition to its direct knee flexor and hip extensor functions.

One common example of an abnormal movement pattern is the destabilization of a proximal knee or hip joint during postural movement. This problem is often called proximal joint instability. While it is tempting to attribute an unstable knee or hip joint to weakness or inactivity in the muscles acting directly about these joints, the instability can also be caused by the indirect effects of delayed ankle muscle activation.[54]

Coordination of Postural Movements Into Strategies

When a person's balance is disrupted by an external perturbation, one or a combination of three different strategies can be used to coordinate movement of the COG back to a balanced position.

TABLE 12–3.
Functional Anatomy of Muscles Involved in Balance Movements

	Extension		Flexion	
Joint	Anatomic	Functional	Anatomic	Functional
Hip	Paraspinals Hamstrings	Paraspinals Hamstrings Tibialis	Abdominal Quadriceps	Abdominals Quadriceps Gastrocnemius
Knee	Quadriceps	Paraspinals Quadriceps Gastrocnemius	Hamstrings Gastrocnemius	Abdominals Hamstrings Tibialis
Ankle	Gastrocnemius	Abdominals Quadriceps Gastrocnemius	Tibialis	Paraspinals Hamstrings Tibialis

Properties of the three strategies are reviewed in Figure 12–6. A step or stumbling reaction is the only movement strategy effective in preventing a fall when the perturbation displaces the COG beyond the LOS perimeter. When the COG remains within the LOS, two different strategies or combinations of strategies can be used to move the COG while maintaining the initial placement of the feet on the support surface. The following sections describe the biomechanical and physiologic properties of these two in-place movement strategies.

Ankle Strategy

The ankle strategy shifts the COG while maintaining the placement of the feet by rotating the body as an approximately rigid mass about the ankle joints, as shown in Figure 12–6. This is accomplished by contracting the ankle joint muscles to generate torque about the ankle joints. At the same time, contractions of thigh and lower trunk muscles are required to resist the destabilization of these proximal joints due to the indirect effects of the ankle muscles on the proximal joints (see Table 12–3).

Ankle movements are generated by EMG responses which begin at 90 to 100 msec in the directionally appropriate ankle joint muscles.[31, 44, 57] The gastroc-nemius muscles are activated for backward postural movements, while contractions of the tibialis anterior produce forward movements. Electromyographic activity then radiates in sequence to the thigh and then the lower trunk muscles on the same dorsal or ventral aspect of the body. Activation of the thigh and lower trunk muscles stabilizes the knees and hips, allowing the body to move as a unit about the ankles. Thigh and trunk muscle EMG onsets average 10 to 30 msec later than those of the ankle. Activation of the ankle muscles first provides proximal muscles with a stable movement base.

Hip Strategy

Movements organized into the hip strategy are centered about the hip joints with smaller opposing ankle joint rotations, as shown in Figure 12–6. The COG shifts in the direction opposite to the hip because of the inertia of the trunk (moving in one direction), generating an opposite horizontal (shear) reaction force against the support surface.[53] The tendency for destabilization of the knee joints is resisted by coordination of the muscular actions about the ankle, knee, and hip joints.

Hip strategy movements are generated by activation of the directionally

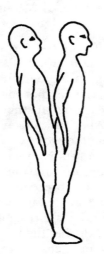 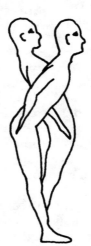 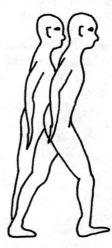

FIG 12–6.
Three strategies for moving the COG relative to the base of support during postural sway, and their functional properties.

appropriate thigh and lower trunk muscles at 85- to 95-msec latencies.[31] Quadriceps and abdominal muscles are activated to flex the hips and move the COG backward. The knee remains relatively stable, because these two muscles have opposite functional effects about this joint (see Table 12–3). Paraspinal and hamstring activation extends the hips and moves the COG backward. Opposing functional effects of these two muscles also stabilize the knees. During movements in both directions, the ankle muscles are relatively inactive.

Appropriate Use of Postural Movement Strategies

The relative effectiveness of ankle, hip, and stepping strategies in repositioning the COG over the base of support depends on the configuration of the base of support, the COG alignment in relation to the LOS, and the speed of the postural movement.[31, 38, 53] For example, the ankle strategy is most effective in executing relatively slow COG movements when the base of support is firm and the COG is well within the LOS perimeter. The ankle strategy is also effective in maintaining a static posture with the COG offset from the center.

The amplitude and speed of ankle movements are biomechanically limited by the torque that can be exerted about the ankles before the feet lift off the support surface.[56] The reader can experience this biomechanical constraint by increasing the amplitude and frequency of sway about the ankles to the point where the feet begin to lift off the floor. The strengths of the ankle joint muscles are not the limiting factors. Gastrocnemius strength is determined by the force requirements for running and jumping, and therefore far exceeds the requirements for executing ankle movements. The maximum force capabilities of the tibialis anterior muscles, in contrast, are more closely matched to the requirements for balance. Thus, reductions in ankle muscle strength are more likely to impair a person's use of ankle movements to recover from backward displacements of the COG.

Hip movements rely on horizontal shear forces rather than ankle torques to shift the COG and are therefore not limited by constraints on ability to exert torque about the ankles. Thus, hip movements are effective when the COG is positioned near the LOS perimeter, and when the LOS boundaries are contracted by a narrowed base of support. The reader can experience the conditions requiring the use of hip movements by attempting to shift posture while standing on tiptoes or with the feet placed laterally heel to toe.

Hip movements also have biomechanical limitations in that they cannot produce large shifts in COG position. In addition, because hip movements rely on inertial reaction forces, they cannot be used to maintain balance effectively with the COG offset from the center.

When the COG is displaced beyond the LOS, a step or stumble is the only effective strategy for preventing a fall. While stepping and stumbling are subject to fewer biomechanical limitations, they are inefficient, disruptive, and usually inappropriate when simpler ankle or hip movements are effective.

Selecting the Postural Movement Strategy

The strategy selected for responding to an external perturbation is set in advance depending on the person's immediate past experience, not on a conscious decision made at the time of response.[31, 38] When a person is well practiced at standing on a particular support surface, a relatively pure example of the appropriate movement strategy described in the preceding sections is observed. In contrast, a more complex movement combining the two pure strategies is observed during the initial practice trials following a change in support surface conditions. After 10 to 15 practice trials on the new surface, however, the less appropriate component is progressively reduced, and reliance on the well-practiced pure strategy increases. Movement strategies are not voluntarily changed by instruction alone, even if a person is familiar with and motivated to change the pattern quickly.

COORDINATION OF HEAD AND BODY MOVEMENTS

Head Movement Strategies

Movements of the head relative to the trunk have a relatively minor effect on the COG position during standing. This is because the mass of the head is substantially smaller than that of the trunk. Motions of the head during postural sway are important, nevertheless, because they have a strong influence on two of the three principal senses of balance: vision and the vestibular system. The head and body movement strategies reviewed in Figure 12–7 can affect the ability to determine the position of the COG accurately during postural sway.[46, 64]

Trunk-Fixed Strategy

Strategies for coordinating movements of the head relative to the trunk can be classified in three categories: trunk-fixed, gravity-fixed, and combinations of the two. In the trunk-fixed strategy, the head and trunk move as a unit. The neck muscles stiffen to resist the inertial and gravitational forces tending to rotate the head opposite to the trunk. Thus, this strategy fixes movements of the head to those of the trunk.

Gravity-Fixed Strategy

The gravity-fixed strategy rotates the head in opposition to the trunk so that the head remains level relative to the gravitational vertical. This strategy requires coordinated neck and trunk muscular actions to eliminate head rotations correlated with COG sway, while preserving the linear translational components of head motion.

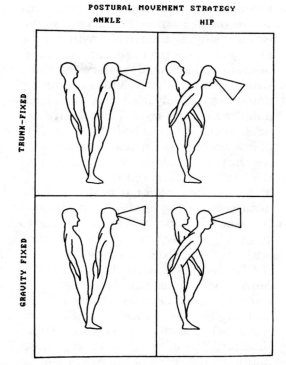

FIG 12–7.
Strategies for moving the head relative to the trunk during postural sway, and their functional properties. *Visual "rays"* show the direction of the gaze. Note that when the head position is trunk-fixed, the gaze direction is disturbed substantially more by the hip than the ankle strategy. When head position is gravity-fixed, gaze direction is not disturbed by either strategy.

INTERACTIONS BETWEEN SENSORY AND MOTOR COMPONENTS OF BALANCE

Sensory Effects of Body and Head Movement Strategies

The pattern of ankle, knee, hip, and head movements strongly influences the visual and vestibular inputs to balance.[46] If a person is swaying about the ankles while holding the head fixed to the trunk, for example, the head and body move as a unit and the linear and rotational motions of the head and the body COG are similar. In theory at least, this strategy simplifies the brain's task of interpreting input from the visual and vestibular systems.

Moving the head and body as a unit, however, is disadvantageous whenever independent head and eye movements are required, such as in tracking an object or scanning the terrain. Without the ability to move the head and eyes independently, backward or forward sway will move the head and eyes up or down, respectively, and thus away from a desired visual target. The negative impact on vision of the body-fixed strategy of head control is particularly great during hip movements, when motions of the trunk are large and rapid.

Fixing the rotational position of the head relative to gravity has two potential benefits. First, the eyes are freer to track objects in the visual surround with the head fixed in relation to gravity. Second, the gravity-fixed strategy of head coordination has the potential for reducing the confusion between linear and angular accelerations, a shortcoming of all inertial-gravitational systems including the vestibular system. An example of this type of confusion can be experienced when a wide-bodied jet brakes immediately after touching down on the runway. A passenger looking straight ahead will sometimes sense that the cabin is tilting downward, even to the point of dipping below the level of the runway. This illusion occurs even though the plane remains level, because the brain incorrectly interprets the linear deceleration inputs from the vestibular system as being caused by forward tilting.

There is the potential for misinterpretation of tilt and linear acceleration inputs to the vestibular system during sway, because the head both tilts and moves linearly.[59] Fixing the rotational position of the head relative to gravity reduces the confusion between tilting and linear motions, because this strategy eliminates the tilt component of the vestibular input. When a gravity-fixed strategy is used, linear acceleration input from the vestibular system can be safely interpreted as actual linear head acceleration.

This theoretical analysis of the senses suggests that selection of head and body movement strategies is based not only on surface conditions and COG position within the LOS, as described previously, but also on the need to simplify the interpretation of vestibular input to balance. There is no conclusive experimental proof that sensory processes influence a person's choice of head and body movement strategies. The following section describes results with healthy individuals and patients with sensory balance problems which are consistent with this conclusion.

Integration of Head and Body Movement Strategies

In normal individuals, movements of the head and body are coordinated when a hip strategy is used during in-place standing, and when running, jumping, and hopping.[55, 62] During these tasks, the head is approximately stabilized relative to the gravitational vertical, as shown in Figure 12–7. Analysis of leg, lower trunk, and neck muscle EMG activity during automatic postural movements indicates that the motions of the head and body are coordinated at the automatic level of control. During forward automatic hip movements, for example, rectus abdominus (hip flexor) and sternocleidomastoid (neck flexor) are simultaneously activated at 90 to 100 msec. The sternocleidomastoid activation prevents the large nose-up rotation of the head that would occur in the absence of active head control.

When normal individuals use the ankle strategy, head and body movements are not tightly coordinated. Instead, the head moves passively in the direction opposite to the body, rotating nose up and then nose down in relation to gravity over a range of approximately 10°. These opposing head rotations occur as predicted by biomechanics in the absence of active head control. Analysis of leg, lower trunk, and neck muscle EMG activities during automatic ankle movement confirms that neck muscle actions are not correlated with those of the legs and lower trunk.[64]

In contrast to normal individuals, patients with bilateral loss of vestibular inputs avoid hip movements under all conditions, even though they have no motor deficits that impair their hip motor control.[64] These patients also tend to fix the position of the head relative to the trunk. Subjects deprived of somatosensory inputs from the feet by transient ischemia prefer hip movements under all support surface conditions, even though the sensory loss does not impair their ability to execute ankle movements.

Head-body coordination during in-place hip movements and during running, hopping, and jumping is consistent with the need for head stabilization during complex movements. As suggested in the section on sensory effects of head and body movement strategies, the COG position is more difficult to determine from vestibular and visual inputs during complex movements. This process is simplified by stabilizing the position of the head relative to gravity.

Voluntary Movements Influence Balance

A standing person's voluntary motor activities, as well as gravity and external perturbing forces, can destabilize balance. Excluding movements having a direct effect on the base of support (shifting weight; raising or changing the placement of a foot), the voluntary actions summarized in Table 12–4 are classified in two categories based on their effects on balance.

The first category of voluntary actions includes movements involving manipulation of external objects. These actions have the greatest destabilizing effects on balance. For example, when pulling open a heavy door, the backward force required to move the door generates an equal and opposite forward force on COG of the body. If this destabilizing force is not compensated by an appropriate postural reaction, the person falls forward into the opening door.

The second category includes voluntary actions not involving external objects. These actions change body posture but have only indirect and relatively minor effects on COG position. Raising an arm from the side to a forward pointing position, for example, does not substantially alter the COG position, because the force required to accelerate the arm forward produces an equal and opposite force accelerating the trunk slightly backward. The net result is little if any change in balance.

Students of physics will recognize that voluntary actions are distinguished based on the presence or absence of ex-

TABLE 12–4.

Functional Properties of Two Types of Voluntary Actions

	Voluntary Actions	
Property	Object Manipulations	Free Body Movements
Effect on center of gravity	Direct equal and opposite force	Little if any direct force
Coordination during free standing	Anticipatory postural response and delayed voluntary onset	Less postural activity and rapid voluntary onset
Coordination with the body supported	Little postural activity and rapid voluntary onset	Little postural activity and rapid voluntary onset
Examples	Pull or push on object, grasp and lift object	Lift arm, reach or point

ternal and internal forces. External forces have a direct effect on the COG position of a body, while internal forces acting between body parts tend to reorient the parts relative to one another with little net effect on COG position. "Real world" situations, however, are never quite so simple. Because the body is supported by contact with a surface, rapid elevations of an arm can have minor effects on balance.

Coordination of Voluntary and Automatic Postural Movements

When a freely standing person performs a voluntary action involving external forces (for example, pulling on a heavy external object), an automatic postural movement is initiated in advance of the voluntary arm movement to compensate for the disturbance in balance.[5, 13, 51] The anticipatory automatic postural movement minimizes any disturbance to balance and provides a stable base for the voluntary action.

The properties of an anticipatory postural movement depend on the requirements for balance at the time of the voluntary action. Removing the need to maintain balance by providing trunk support during a voluntary action, for example, abolishes the anticipatory postural movement. In this instance, the voluntary action itself can actually be initiated sooner. This later observation indicates that, to meet the requirements of balance in a free standing task, voluntary actions with the potential for disrupting balance are actively delayed so that a stable base of support is established first.

CONCLUSIONS

Balance is a multicomponent and highly adaptable control process. When the balance of a healthy individual is challenged, the sensory inputs determining the COG position and the pattern of movement correcting the pertur-

bation depend on the task conditions and the person's immediate past experience. An individual with one or more impaired sensory input or motor output component will attempt to compensate by adapting both the impaired and normally functioning components to suit the demands of the balance task.

When a patient complains of unsteadiness, the problem is seldom caused by the absence of balance-related activities. More frequently, some components are functioning normally and others abnormally, the interactions of which lead to functionally inappropriate or ineffective balance responses. Because of these multiple interactions, focusing the diagnostic assessment or treatment on isolated component(s) of the balance system is frequently ineffective. In these cases, understanding the patient's abnormality requires an assessment approach that systematically examines all components and their interactions under a variety of task conditions. A test battery designed to generate a systematic description of the patient's balance problem, called computerized dynamic posturography, is described in Chapter 13.

REFERENCES

1. Aggashyan RV, Gurfinkel VS, Mamasakhlisov GV, et al: Changes in spectral and correlation characteristics of human stabilograms at muscle afferentation disturbance. *Agressologie* 1973; 14:5–9.
2. Allum JHJ, Honegger F, Pfaltz CR: The role of stretch and vestibulo-spinal reflexes in the generation of human equilibrating reactions; in Allum JHJ, Hulliger M (eds): *Progress in Brain Research*, vol 80. New York, Elsevier, 1989, pp 399–409.
3. Bawa P, Stein RB: Frequency response of human soleus muscle. *J Neurophysiol.* 1976; 39:788–793.
4. Begbie JV: Some problems of postural sway, in deReuck AVS, Knight J (eds): *CIBA Foundation Symposium on Myotatic, Kinesthetic and Vestibular Mechanisms.* London, Churchill, 1967, pp 80–92.
5. Belen'kii VY, Gurfinkel VS, Pal'tsev YI: On

the elements of voluntary movement control. *Biophysics* 1967; 12:135–141.

6. Berthoz A, Pozzo T: Intermittent head stabilization during postural and locomotory tasks in humans; in Amblard B, Berthoz A, Clarac F (eds): *Posture and Gait: Development, Adaptation and Modulation.* New York, Elsevier 1988, pp 189–198.

7. Black FO, Nashner LM: Vestibulospinal control differs in patients with reduced versus distorted vestibular function. *Acta Otolaryngol* 1984; 406:110–114.

8. Black FO, Nashner LM: Postural control in four classes of vestibular abnormalities, in Igarashi M, Black FO (eds): *Vestibular and Visual Control of Posture and Locomotor Equilibrium.* Basel, S Karger, 1985, pp 271–281.

9. Bles W, de Jong JMBV: Uni- and bilateral loss of vestibular function, in Bles W, Brandt T (eds): *Disorders of Posture and Gait.* New York, Elsevier, 1986, pp 127–139.

10. Bles W, de Jong JMBV, de Wit G: Somatosensory compensation for loss of labyrinthine function. *Acta Otolaryngol* 1984; 97:213–221.

11. Bouisset S, Zattara M: A sequence of postural movements precedes voluntary movement. *Neurosci Lett* 1981; 22:263–270.

12. Brandt T, Paulus W, Straube A: Vision and posture, in Bles W, Brandt T (eds): *Disorders of Posture and Gait.* New York, Elsevier, 1986, pp 157–175.

13. Cordo PJ, Nashner LM: Properties of postural adjustments associated with rapid arm movements. *J Neurophysiol* 1982; 47:287–302.

14. Dichgans J, Diener HC: Different forms of postural ataxia in patients with cerebellar diseases, in Bles W, Brandt T (eds): *Disorders of Posture and Gait.* New York, Elsevier, 1986, pp 207–215.

15. Dichgans J, Held R, Young LR, et al: The moving visual scenes influence the apparent direction of gravity. *Science* 1972; 178:1217–1219.

16. Diener HC, Dichgans J: On the role of vestibular, visual, and somatosensory information for dynamic postural control in humans, in Pompeiano O, Allum JHJ (eds): *Progress in Brain Research,* vol 76. New York; Elsevier, 1988, pp 253–262.

17. Diener HC, Dichgans J, Bacher B, et al: Quantification of postural sway in normals and patients with cerebellar diseases. *Electroencephlogr Clin Neurophysiol* 1984; 57:134–142.

18. Diener HC, Dichgans J, Guschlbauer B, et al: Role of visual and static vestibular influences on dynamic posture control. *Hum Neurobiol* 1986; 5:105–113.

19. Diener HC, Dichgans J, Guschlbauer B, et al:

The significance of proprioception on postural stabilization as assessed by ischemia. *Exp Brain Res* 1984; 296:103–109.

20. Diener HC, Horak FB, Nashner LM: Influence of stimulus parameters on human postural responses. *J Neurophysiol* 1988; 59:1888–1895.

21. Dietz V: Afferent and efferent control of posture and gait, in Bles W, Brandt T (eds): *Disorders of Posture and Gait.* New York, Elsevier, 1986, pp 69–81.

22. Dietz V, Horstmann GA, Berger W: Significance of proprioceptive mechanisms in the regulation of stance, in Allum JHJ, Hulliger M (eds): *Progress in Brain Research,* vol 80. New York; Elsevier, 1989, pp 419–423.

23. Duncan PW, Weiner DK, Chandler J, et al: Functional reach: A new clinical measure of balance. *J Gerentol* 1990; 45:192–197.

24. El'ner AM, Popov KE, Gurfinkel VS: Changes in stretch reflex system concerned with the control of postural activity of human muscle. *Agressologie* 1972; 13:19–23.

25. Evarts EV, Tanjii J: Gating of motor cortex reflexes by prior instruction. *Brain Res* 1974; 71:479–494.

26. Fregly AR: Vestibular ataxia and its measurement in man, in Kornhuber HH (ed): *Handbook of Sensory Physiology,* vol 6, no. 2. Berlin, Springer-Verlag, 1974, pp 321–360.

27. Gurfinkel VS, Lipshits MI, et al: The state of the stretch reflex during quiet standing in man, in Homma H (ed): *Progress in Brain Research,* vol 44. New York; Elsevier 1976, pp 473–490.

28. Gurfinkel VS, Lipshits MI, Popov KY: Is the stretch reflex the main mechanism in the system of regulation of the vertical posture of man? *Biophysics* 1974; 19:744–748.

29. Gurfinkel VS, Osevets M: Dynamics of the vertical posture in man. *Biophysics* 1972; 17:496–506.

30. Hill AV: (1953). The mechanics of active muscle. *Proc R Soc Lond* 1953; 141B:104–117.

31. Horak FB, Nashner LM: Central programming of postural movements: Adaptation to altered support surface configurations. *J Neurophysiol* 1986; 55:1369–1381.

32. Horak FB, Nashner LM, Diener HC: Postural strategies associated with somatosensory and vestibular loss. *Exp Brain Res* 1990; 82:167–177.

33. Koozekanni SH, Stockwell CW, McGhee RB, et al: On the role of dynamic models in quantitative posturography. *IEEE Trans Biomed Eng* 1980; 27:605–609.

34. Houk JC: Regulation of stiffness by skeleto-

motor reflexes. *Annu Rev Physiol* 1979; 41:99–114.

35. Lee DN, Lishman JR: Visual proprioceptive control of stance. *J Hum Movement Stud* 1975; 1:87–95.

36. Lestienne F, Soechting J, Berthoz A: Postural readjustments induced by linear motion of visual scenes. *Exp Brain Res* 1977; 28:363–384.

37. Marsden CD, Merton PA, Morton HB: Latency measurements compatible with a cortical pathway for the stretch reflex in man. *J Physiol* 1973; 230:58–59.

38. McCollum G, Horak FB, Nashner LM: Parsimony in neural calculations for postural movements, in Bloedel J, Dichgans J, Precht W (eds): *Cerebellar Functions.* Berlin, Springer-Verlag, 1984, pp 52–66.

39. McCollum G, Leen TK: Form and exploration of mechanical stability limits in erect stance. *J Motor Behav* 1989; 21:225–244.

40. Melvill Jones G, Watt DGD: Observations on the control of stepping and hopping movements in man. *J Physiol* 1971; 219:709–727.

41. Nashner LM: *Sensory Feedback in Human Posture Control.* Massachusetts Institute of Technology Report MVT-70-3. Cambridge, Mass, MIT, 1970.

42. Nashner LM: A model describing vestibular detection of body sway motion. *Acta Otolaryngol* 1971; 72:429–436.

43. Nashner LM: Adapting reflexes controlling the human posture. *Exp Brain Res* 1976; 26:59–72.

44. Nashner LM: Fixed patterns of rapid postural responses among leg muscles during stance. *Exp Brain Res* 1977; 150:403–407.

45. Nashner LM: Analysis of stance posture in humans, in Towe AL, Luschei ES (eds): *Handbook of Behavioral Neurobiology,* vol 5. New York, Plenum Press, 1981, pp 527–565.

46. Nashner LM: Strategies for organization of human posture, in Igarashi M, Black FO (eds): *Vestibular and Visual Control of Posture and Locomotor Equilibrium.* Basel, S Karger, 1985, pp 1–8.

47. Nashner LM: A functional approach to understanding spasticity, in Struppler A, Weindl A (eds): *Electromyography and Evoked Potentials.* Berlin, Springer-Verlag, 1985, pp 22–29.

48. Nashner LM: The organization of human postural movements during standing and walking, in Grillner S, Stein PSG, Stewart DG, et al: (eds): *Neurobiology of Posture and Locomotion.* London, MacMillan, 1986, pp 637–648.

49. Nashner LM, Berthoz A: Visual contribution to rapid motor responses during posture control. *Brain Res* 1978; 150:403–407.

50. Nashner LM, Black FO, Wall C: Adaptation to altered support and visual conditions during stance: Patients with vestibular deficits. *J Neurosci* 1982; 2:536–544.

51. Nashner LM, Cordo PJ: Relation of automatic postural responses and reaction-time voluntary movements of human leg muscles. *Exp Brain Res* 1981; 43:395–405.

52. Nashner LM, Forssberg H: Phase-dependent organization of postural adjustments associated with arm movements while walking. *J Neurophysiol* 1986; 55:538–548.

53. Nashner LM, McCollum G: The organization of human postural movements: A formal basis and experimental synthesis. *Behav Brain Sci* 1985; 8:135–172.

54. Nashner LM, Shumway-Cook A, Marin O: Stance posture control in select groups of children with cerebral palsy: Deficits in sensory organization and muscular coordination. *Exp Brain Res* 1983; 49:393–409.

55. Nashner LM, Shupert CL, Horak FB: Head-trunk coordination in the standing posture, in Pompeiano O, Allum JHJ (eds): *Progress in Brain Research,* vol 76. New York, Elsevier 1988, pp 243–251.

56. Nashner LM, Schupert CL, Horak FB: et al: Organization of posture controls: An analysis of sensory and mechanical constraints, in Allum JHJ, Hulliger M (eds): *Progress in Brain Research,* vol 80. New York, Elsevier, 1989, pp 411–418.

57. Nashner LM, Woollacott M, Tuma G: Organization of rapid responses to postural and locomotor-like perturbations of standing man. *Exp Brain Res* 1979; 36:463–476.

58. Paloski WH, Reschke MF, Doxey DD, et al: Neurosensory adaptation associated with postural ataxia following space flight, in Woollacott M, Horak F (eds): *Posture and Gait: Control Mechanisms, Vol. I.* Eugene, University of Oregon Books, 1992, pp 311–314.

59. Parker DE, Reschke MF, Arrott AP, et al: Otolith tilt-translation reinterpretation following prolonged weightlessness: Implications for preflight training. *Aviat Space Environ Med* 1985; 56:601–606.

60. Paulus WM, Straube A, Brandt T: Visual stabilization of posture: Physiological stimulus characteristics and clinical aspects. *Brain* 1984; 107:1143–1163.

61. Paulus WM, Straube A, Brandt T. Visual postural performance after loss of somatosensory and vestibular function. *J Neurol Neurosurg Psychiatry* 1987; 50:1542–1545.

62. Pozzo T, Berthoz A, Lefort L: Head kinematics during various motor tasks in humans, in Allum JHJ, Hulliger M (eds): *Progress in Brail Research*, vol 80. New York, Elsevier 1989, pp 377–383.

63. Scott DE, Dzendolet E: Quantification of sway in standing humans. *Agressologie* 1972; 13:35–40.

64. Shupert CL, Black FO, Horak FB, et al: Coordination of head and body in response to support surface translations in normals and patients with bilaterally reduced vestibular function, in Amblard B, Berthoz A, Clarac F (eds): *Posture and Gait: Development, Adaptation and Modulation*. New York, Elsevier 1988, pp 281–289.

65. Young LR, Oman CM, Watt DGD, et al: Spatial orientation in weightlessness and readaptation to earth's gravity. *Science* 1984; 225:202–208.

CHAPTER 13

Computerized Dynamic Posturography

Lewis M. Nashner, Sc.D.

BACKGROUND

Historical Development of Posturography

Computerized dynamic posturography (CDP) is a quantitative method for assessing upright balance function under a variety of tasks that effectively simulate the conditions encountered in daily life. The test protocols are designed to isolate the principle sensory, motor, and biomechanical components contributing to balance, and to analyze the patient's ability to effectively use these components singularly and in concert to maintain balance. The protocols and data analysis techniques employed in CDP are based on a systems model of human posture derived from the experimental research on normal and abnormal human balance and movement control reviewed in Chapter 12.

Performance Measures of Posture Control

Historically, assessment of human posture control has developed using two complementary methodologies summarized in Table 13–1. The first method had its beginning with the nineteenth century work of Romberg,[38] who compared spontaneous sway under eyes open and eyes closed body conditions to identify peripheral somatosensory system deficits. Implicit in Romberg's interpretation of the eyes open and eyes closed performance of the patient is the assumption that the somatosensory input should dominate the control of balance whenever one is standing on a fixed support surface, and that visual input is the primary backup whenever the somatosensory input is disrupted. Based on this assumption, a substantial increase in sway under eyes closed relative to eyes open conditions is indicative of impairment of the dominant somatosensory input.

With forceplate technology, the use of so called "static" posturography has expanded Romberg's original concept by enabling examiners to acquire more quantitative measurement and analysis of the patient's postural sway.[4, 5, 7, 24, 33, 39] The typical forceplate consists of a flat, rigid surface supported on three or more points by independent force-measuring devices. As the patient stands on the forceplate surface, the vertical forces recorded by the measuring devices are used to calculate the position of the center of the vertical forces exerted on the forceplate surface over time.

The center of vertical force movements themselves provide an indirect measure of postural sway activity. This measure, however, is limited by the fact that motions of the center of vertical force produced by an equivalent angle of sway are larger in taller and/or

TABLE 13–1.

Methodologies for Assessing Human Posture Control

Method	Data Obtained	Advantages	Disadvantages
Performance tests	Postural stability	Correlates with daily life functional capabilities	Influenced by conscious effort
	Movement strategies	Quantifies adaptive capabilities	Dependent on patient cooperation
Posture-evoked response tests	Latency	Provides diagnostic information	Uncorrelated with daily life functional capabilities
	Pattern		
	Strength	Uneffected by patient motivation	No adaptive capability information

heavier individuals than in shorter and lighter persons. Furthermore, the excursion of the center of vertical force produced by a given angle of sway increases dramatically as the frequency of sway increases.[31]

When the height and weight of the patient on the forceplate is known, a computer model of body dynamics can be used to derive the center of gravity (COG) sway angle over time from the center of vertical force movements. To produce a measure of COG sway in real time, however, this approach requires considerable computational speed.

The forceplate can also be used to measure the horizontal shear forces exerted by the patient's feet against the support surface. Horizontal shear forces measure the accelerations of the body COG in the antero-posterior (AP) and lateral directions. These acceleration forces are extremely small when the body moves slowly, but increase dramatically as the frequency of COG motion increases. For this reason, horizontal shear forces are useful in identifying the pattern of body motion being used to produce COG sway.

Measurement of Discrete Postural Responses

A second approach used by investigators to study posture control has involved the use of brief and unexpected disturbances in balance to quantify the characteristics of the resulting discrete postural responses. With this method, balance is disturbed by briefly translat-ing the support surface in the anterior or posterior direction[26, 27, 32] or by rotating the surface toes up or toes down.[1, 9, 11, 15, 26] The major emphasis of these studies has been analyzing the latency, strength, and pattern of response to variations in disturbance size and direction.

Relative Value of Discrete and Performance Measures

Computerized dynamic posturography combines the discrete response and continuous performance methods for assessing balance function. The motor control test (MCT) includes protocols which use various types of brief displacements in the support surface to evoke discrete postural responses. In the standard MCT protocol, the patient's postural responses are recorded with forceplate technology and comprise the classic "motor control test" of CDP. When combined with surface electromyography (EMG) recordings, the data set is expanded to include the posture-evoked responses (PER) which directly reflect activation of the segmental, spinal, and long-loop response pathways as well as the coordination of ankle, thigh, and lower trunk muscles.

In general, the MCT protocols offer two distinct advantages. First, the approach is similar to that used in traditional clinical "reflex" tests and is therefore conceptually familiar to most clinicians. Second, because evoked postural responses are not under conscious control, the test results are relatively unaffected by patient motivation and effort. The MCT protocols, however, have limitations. First, they do not characterize a patient's functional status relative to daily life tasks. Second, because the evoked postural responses are discrete events, they do not reveal the patient's adaptive ability to combine the various individual components under more complex task conditions.

The sensory organization test (SOT) assesses the patient's balance performance during a sequence of progressively more difficult task conditions. Continuous performance measures of balance have several advantages. First, performance measures correlate with a patient's functional status. Second, knowledge of the task conditions leading to poor performance help isolate the cause of instability to an individual balance component (or components) and document a patient's strategy for utilizing the components of balance under varying task conditions. Third, improvements in balance performance with repeated practice can help identify those patients for whom a course of balance therapy may be appropriate.

The disadvantage of measuring balance performance is the potential influence of nonphysiologic factors such as patient motivation and cooperation. Computerized dynamic posturography overcomes this limitation by combining the evoked response and performance methodologies. "Nonphysiologic" influences such as poor motivation, anxiety, and deliberate exaggeration of symptoms lead to inconsistencies in the results generated by the two types of protocols and can therefore be readily identified.

SELECTION, INSTRUCTION, AND PREPARATION OF PATIENTS FOR CDP TESTING

Minimum Physical Requirements for CDP Testing

Patients must be able to stand erect with eyes open and unassisted for peri-ods of at least 1 minute. Little useful information will be obtained from those who spontaneously lose their balance in less than a minute while standing eyes open on a fixed support surface. Special care should be taken with patients who have severe arthritic or orthopedic conditions affecting the ankles, knees, hips, or back. These conditions might be aggravated by the abrupt movements associated with "falls" into the supporting harness. The test administrator should take note of any musculoskeletal abnormalities affecting the relative lengths of the two legs; the ranges of ankle, knee, and hip joint motion; the strengths of leg and lower trunk musculature; and the postural orientation of limb and or trunk. While these types of musculoskeletal disorders do not preclude CDP testing, the interpretation of, especially, the motor coordination results relative to central nervous system and peripheral sensory functions must be qualified in these cases.

Patient Instructions

Prior to the day of testing, patients should be instructed to abstain from drugs that may affect their balance function. Ideally, drugs should be withheld for a period of 24 to 48 hours. Patients should also refrain from alcohol and caffeine during this period. Of course, the treating physician should be consulted to assure that the patient continues life-sustaining drugs such as insulin, blood pressure, heart, and seizure-control medications. Women should be asked to wear loose-fitting slacks to permit easier mounting of the safety harness.

On the day of testing, the aim of pretest instructions is to minimize anxiety and assure the best possible patient performance. The purpose and general features of the test should be explained to the patient. The patient should be reassured that testing begins with easy tasks and only slowly progresses to more difficult tasks and that the safety harness is available in case one's balance is lost.

Also it should be explained that CDP is a sensitive test which best documents the extent of any abnormality when the patient gives his or her best performance.

Preparation for Testing

To eliminate the risk of falls when balance is lost, the patient is fitted with a parachute-type safety harness connected to an overhead bar, as shown in Figure 13–1. The shoulder, waist, and leg straps of the harness are adjusted to assure that any patient weight on the harness is transferred through the lower trunk rather than the upper trunk and shoulders. It is essential that the straps connecting the harness to the overhead bar are adjusted to allow complete freedom of motion within the normal limits of stability. An overly tight harness may provide the patient with external postural support and result in inappropriately high scores under the more difficult SOT conditions. An overly tight harness also will interfere with the for-

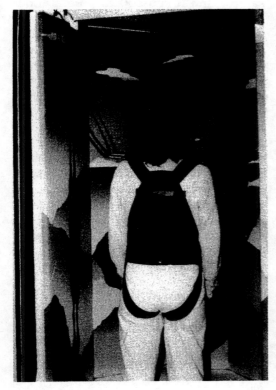

FIG 13–1.
Fitting the overhead harness.

ceplate measurements of the patient's movement strategy.

Proper placement of the feet on the forceplates is essential for accurate scoring of COG alignment during the SOT and MCT. To assure proper scoring of AP alignment, the medial maleolis of the ankle joint (the protruding ankle bone on the inside of the foot) is centered directly over a marking stripe that laterally transects the two forceplates. Accurate scoring of lateral alignment requires that the feet are laterally centered relative to the line dividing the left and right forceplates. Although the SOT equilibrium and strategy scores, and all MCT scores, are unaffected by foot placement, proper alignment of the ankle joints with the platform rotation axis gives the most accurate results.

Operator Administration of Testing

During administration of the test, the operator should observe the patient for signs of anxiety and fatigue. If either of these problems arise, the test can be interrupted for brief rest periods. In some cases of anxiety, the patient should be calmed by the operator who should describe each test protocol more thoroughly. Because the automatic posture control system is relatively unaffected by the patient's conscious efforts, results are not compromised by providing the patient a detailed description of the test protocol. When the patient is suspected of exaggerating symptoms for secondary gain, the best approach is to repeat the test and look for inconsistent results. When inconsistent CDP results are obtained, the finding can be further supported by repeating the test components in a random order.

The operator is provided a continuous display of the position of the patient's COG relative to the center of the support surface during all CDP protocols. During the SOT, the patient must be properly aligned on the forceplate and should be encouraged to stand as vertically as possible. The patient, however, should not be given feedback by the operator when the COG position is displaced from the center. Under no circumstances should the patient's foot placement on the forceplate be adjusted to center the COG curser. This is because abnormalities in COG alignment relative to center are one of the clinically useful measures provided by the SOT.

The purpose of the MCT and the PER tests is to detect abnormalities in the long-loop automatic pathways controlling balance movements. In contrast to the SOT, COG alignment errors in these tests can introduce artifacts in the results. Specifically, automatic responses may be suppressed in a leg bearing substantially less than the normal one-half share of body weight. Furthermore, forward or backward motor responses can be suppressed when the patient's COG is aligned substantially forward or backward of the center, respectively. For these reasons, the operator should determine that the patient is centered during administration of the MCT and PER tests. If the patient is forward, backward, or to one side, the operator can inform the patient and encourage him or her to correct the error. Again, however, the COG curser should not be centered by adjusting the placements of the patient's feet on the forceplate.

CDP RESULTS IN A CLINICALLY NORMAL POPULATION

CDP results have been gathered in samples of asymptomatic normal individuals. A sample of 145 individuals, 58 distributed between 20 and 59 years of age, 54 between 60 and 69 years, and 28 between 70 and 79 years, received the complete SOT and MCT battery. An additional 54 individuals between 20 and 59 years of age were included only in the SOT portion of the assessment. A sample of 49 adult individuals between the ages of 20 and 69 received the complete PER test battery.*

The clinically normal samples consisted of unpaid volunteers recruited by ordinary means. Each subject was examined by a trained audiologist or neurotologist prior to testing. All subjects had normal vision (corrected with lenses, if necessary) and normal oculomotor function. No clinical vestibular or neurologic signs were present. Subjects with a history of vestibular, neurologic, or orthopedic disorders were excluded. Any subject taking medication affecting the central nervous system or known to affect balance and coordination were also excluded. Individuals above 65 years of age were also screened to exclude those with diabetes; symptoms of depression; and those with history of falls, blackouts, head or back injury, or joint surgery.

For all age ranges and CDP measures, the limits of clinically normal performance are defined to include the scores achieved by 95% of the asymptomatic sample. In the subsequent presentations of results, the reader will note that some CDP scores are considered clinically abnormal only when they deviate in one direction from the population average (one-sided distributions), while deviations of other scores in either direction from the average are considered clinically abnormal (two-sided distributions). For scores considered clinically abnormal in one direction from the mean, the normal limit is established at ± 1.67 SD from the sample average. For scores considered clinically abnormal in either direction from the mean, or upper and lower normal limits, are established at ± 2 SD from the sample average.

The CDP results of the above asymp-

---

* The MCT and SOT data from samples of asymptomatic normal subjects were provided to NeuroCom International Inc. by: Jules Friedman, M.D., Braintree Hospital, Braintree Mass.; Susan Herdman, Ph.D., Johns Hopkins University Hospital, Baltimore; David Cyr, Ph.D., Boys Town National Institute, Omaha; and Neil Shepard, Ph.D., University of Michigan Hospitals, Ann Arbor Mich.

tomatic normal samples are statistically summarized in the Appendix. A number of other laboratories have collected SOT, MCT, and PER results on independent samples of asymptomatic normal individuals.[2, 8, 21, 22, 25, 35, 36, 40] These studies used similar criteria for defining the clinically normal range, and in all cases their results compare favorably with those presented in this chapter.

POSTURE-EVOKED RESPONSE TEST

Support Surface Rotation as Stimulus

When the support surface rotates significantly faster than the body can move, the COG initially remains stationary and the ankle joints rotate. For example, toes-up rotation of the support surface dorsiflexes the ankles and stretches the gastrocnemius muscles. Toes-down rotation plantarflexes the ankles and stretches the tibialis anterior muscles. Brief and rapid rotations of the support surface are commonly used to elicit the PER.

In the standardized PER protocol, responses are elicited by a series of 10 to 20 toes-up or toes-down surface rotations. To assure that the segmental reflex and automatic systems are saturated by the ankle "stretch" stimuli, high-velocity support surface rotations (50°/sec for 80 msec) are used.[11, 25] The addition of a random time interval between rotations serves to minimize anticipation by the patient and further enhance response amplitude. Because forward and backward leaning postures can influence the results, care must be taken to ensure that the patient is tested in an approximately centered stance position.[9]

Presentation of PER Results

During support surface rotations, the relation between the directions of in-

duced COG sway and ankle rotation is opposite that which occurs in physiologic sway while a subject is standing on a fixed support surface, as illustrated in Figure 13-2. The earliest two components of response to support surface rotation, termed short latency (SL) and medium latency (ML) responses, occur in the stretching ankle joint muscles. Rather than having a stabilizing effect on posture, in the stretching ankle joint these two responses serve to exaggerate the COG sway disturbance.[25] However, healthy subjects do not lose balance. This is because a later stabilizing component, termed the long latency (LL) response, occurs in the ankle muscles initially shortened by the rotations.[1, 12]

To measure the three response components, surface EMG signals are recorded simultaneously from the gastrocnemius and tibialis anterior muscles of the two legs. Each of the four raw EMG signals is full-wave rectified, low-pass filtered, and then averaged over the 10 to 20 trials relative to the onset times of the individual rotational stimuli. Figure

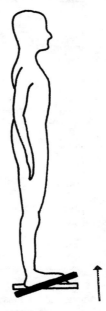

FIG 13-2.
Stimulus paradigm for the PER. The support surface is rapidly rotated toes-up (or toes-down) while the body remains initially stationary. Note that the amplitude of the support surface rotation is exaggerated for purposes of illustration.

13–3 shows the graphical and raw data components obtained from a typical PER test in which a sequence of 10 toes-up rotations of the support surface was imposed. The top trace shows the rotational stimulus waveform. The subsequent four traces show the EMG waveforms of the four ankle muscles, each averaged relative to the stimulus onset times.

PER Results in Clinically Normal Subjects

In asymptomatic normal subjects, toes-up rotations of the support surface elicit the SL and ML responses in the gastrocnemius muscles of both legs (see Figure 13–3). The average latencies of the SL responses are approximately 32 msec. Latency variations among indi-

viduals are less than a few milliseconds. These SL responses are attributed to the monosynaptic stretch reflex system.[6, 25]

Medium latency responses are identifiable in some but not all clinically asymptomatic subjects. In those subjects with identifiable ML components, average latencies in the gastrocnumius muscles are approximately 80 msec. ML responses are attributed to polysynaptic segmental reflex mechanisms.[14, 15] Because the SL and ML responses both resist the rotation of the ankle joints, they exaggerate rather than help compensate for the associated COG sway disturbances.

Following toes-up rotation, well-defined LL responses are recorded in the tibialis anterior muscles of both legs of all subjects. Average LL response latencies are approximately 110 msec. The

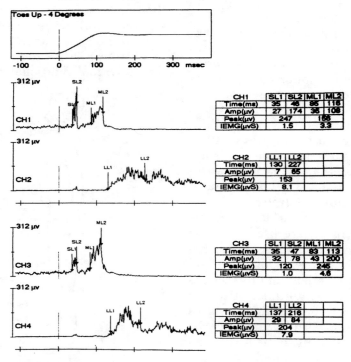

FIG 13–3.
Averaged data summaries of the toes up PER test of a clinically normal 28 year old man. The EMG traces are full-wave rectified EMG signals averaged over 20 trials. Channel 1 is right gastrocnemius; channel 2, right tibialis; channel 3, left gastrocnemius; and channel 4, left tibialis. *Arrows* show the marked beginning *(1)* and ending *(2)* times of the *SL, ML,* and *LL* component. Numerical data use similar labels to show beginning and ending times of the three components. Additional numerical data show the signal amplitude at each marker, the signal peak between pairs of markers, and the integrated area *(IEMG)* between pairs of markers. *(Courtesy of Neuro Com International.)*

LL responses are mediated by requirements for postural stability rather than local stretch inputs.[10, 25, 26] Long latency responses observed during PER testing are thought to be equivalent to the automatic postural responses that are the main line of defense against many types of unexpected postural disturbances.[19, 28, 32]

Toes-down rotations of the support surface stretch the tibialis anterior muscles and displace the COG forward. Because myotatic stretch reflexes are relatively inactive in the flexor leg muscles of humans, SL responses are typically not observed in the stretching tibialis anterior muscles. However, the ML and LL components in the tibialis anterior and gastrocnemius muscles, respectively, are observed with latencies simular to those reported for toes-up rotations.

The short, medium, and long response latencies reported for asymptomatic normal samples are summarized in the Appendix. Similar PER results in clinically normal samples of subjects have been reported by other laboratories.[2, 8, 21, 25] Because only delayed response latencies are considered abnormal, one-sided distributions are used to identify the upper limits of clinically normal latencies for the SL, ML, and LL components.

Except for one factor, the results presented in the Appendix are consistent. In three of the older studies the latencies reported for all three components were approximately 10 to 15 msec greater in comparison to those in more recent investigations. The probable cause for the 10 to 15 msec differences in latencies was the use of the command signal onset, rather than the actual onset time of the surface rotation, as the benchmark time.

Potential Problems With PER Testing

The principle technical problem with PER testing is obtaining accurate and reliable EMG recordings from the ankle joint musculature. Sources of EMG inaccuracy include electrical resistance between skin and electrodes too high to be compatible with the recording amplifiers, external electrical noise contamination, and inprecise placement of the electrodes. The first two sources can be minimized by thorough skin preparation for EMG recording, proper placement and spacing of electrodes, differential amplifiers with high common mode rejection, and adequate patient grounding. Errors in electrode placement can be minimized by palpating the skin to ensure electrode placement over the belly of the muscle rather than neighboring bony areas.

A potential physiologic problem with PER testing is suppression of the LL response component. Suppression will occur only when the patient is not actively controlling balance during the test. To minimize this source of error, the safety harness must not be overly tight. In addition, the operator must motivate the patient to avoid falls into the harness if at all possible.

In many patients, identification of the ML component is difficult. This component is absent in some patients and is combined with the SL component in others. While there are no technical remedies for this problem, the test results are valid without the ML component. This is because most of the diagnostic value of the PEP is obtained by determining the latency characteristics of the SL and LL components.

STANDARD MOTOR CONTROL TEST

Horizontal Support Surface Displacement

In the MCT, automatic postural responses are elicited by translating the support surface in the horizontal direction. When the support surface translates horizontally more rapidly than the body COG, the COG remains approximately stationary and becomes offset relative to the base of support as illustrated in Figure 13–4.[27, 32] Backward translation stretches the gastrocnemius muscles and displaces the COG forward in relation to the base of support. The COG is re-centered over the base of support by a backward-directed automatic postural response. Similarly, forward surface translation stretches the tibialis anterior muscles and displaces the COG backward. This disturbance to posture is corrected by a forward directed automatic postural response.

In contrast to the responses elicited by surface rotations during the PER, activation of the stretching ankle joint muscles in response to horizontal translation is helpful in compensating for the COG sway disturbance. Compared to the rapid rotation used in PER testing, support surface translation rotates the body about the ankle joints at a significantly much slower speed ranging between 3°/sec and 8°/sec. At these slower

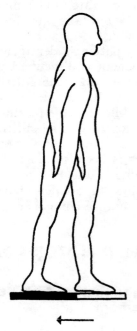

FIG 13–4.
Stimulus paradigm for the MCT. The support surface is translated backward (or forward) while the position of the upper body remains initially stationary. Note that the amplitude of the translation is exaggerated for purposes of illustration.

rotational speeds SL responses in the stretching ankle muscles are seldom observed.[26, 27, 32] Rather, the earliest responses occur in the stretching ankle joint muscles and correspond in time to the LL responses observed in the PER. These compensatory postural movements are termed automatic postural responses. This is because their latencies are too long to be mediated by the segmental stretch reflex pathways but too short to be initiated under voluntary control of the subject.[29]

The MCT protocol is summarized in Table 13–2. In the protocol, the automatic postural response system is analyzed over a range of velocities and directions using forward and backward translations varying in magnitude (threshold, intermediate, and saturating) and timing (random intervals between stimuli). Translations of the same direction and size are always imposed in groups of three. Results from the three trials are then averaged to obtain a stable characterization of the active force responses.

Responses to forward and backward translations are analyzed separately, because the flexor and extensor pathways mediating automatic postural responses are anatomically separate and may be effected differently by a disease process. Responses of the left and right legs are analyzed separately, because the pathways mediating responses on the two sides can also be selectively effected by disease. The random intertrial intervals minimize the likelihood that the patient can anticipate the onset of displacements.

In the standard MCT protocol, the support surface translates at a constant velocity over a fixed interval of time to achieve a predetermined velocity and amplitude of COG displacement.[13] Using a 180 cm tall patient as an example, a small translation of 1.25 cm over a 250-msec interval rotates the COG about the ankle joints at 2.8°/sec for a total distance of 0.7°. This is approximately the threshold displacement re-

TABLE 13–2.

Protocol for the Motor Control Test

Stimulus	Number of Trials	Measurements
Backward translation 1.25 cm in 250 msec (height scaled)	3	
Backward translation 3.15 cm in 300 msec (height scaled)	3	Active force responses: latency, strength symmetry
Backward translation 5.7 cm in 400 msec (height scaled)	3	
Toes-up rotation 4.0° in 500 msec	5	Sway energy
Forward translation 1.25 cm in 250 msec (height scaled)	3	
Forward translation 3.15 cm in 300 msec (height scaled)	3	Active force responses: latency, strength symmetry
Forward translation 5.7 cm in 400 msec (height scaled)	3	
Toes-up rotation 4.0° in 500 msec	5	Sway energy

quired to elicit an automatic postural response. A medium translation of 3.15 cm over a 300-msec interval rotates the COG about the ankle joints at 6°/sec for a total distance of 1.8°. Finally, a large translation of 5.70 cm over a 400-msec interval rotates the COG about the ankle joints at 8°/sec for a total distance of 3.2°. This stimulus produces an approximately maximum amplitude automatic response in the healthy subject.[18]

For individuals shorter or taller than 180 cm, the translation amplitude is adjusted to produce the same velocity and amplitude of COG sway. For individuals shorter or taller than 180 cm, the distance the surface translates is proportionately smaller or larger, respectively, while the durations of the translations are the same.

Recording Active Force Responses

Automatic postural responses to support surface translations are recorded using separate forceplates for each foot, each of which measures the active compensatory force exerted by the foot against the support surface. When each foot is properly positioned on the forceplate, the forceplate measures the portion of total body weight carried by the foot and the AP position of the center of vertical force exerted by the foot relative to the ankle joint position. The weight and position quantities are used to calculate the active torque exerted by the musculature of leg about the ankle joint.[27, 32]

Presentation of MCT Results

Real Time MCT Display

The cathode ray tube (CRT) display presents a real time summary of the raw COG sway data and the resulting active force latency scores during administration of the MCT. The latency plot on the left side of the display indicates the current movement direction, amplitude, and trial number, and also plots the latency scores of all completed trials. Green bars show latencies falling within the normal range. Red bars show latencies falling above the normal limits established for the age-matched clinically normal sample. Numbers on each bar indicate the confidence level of the automatic scoring algorithm. If the operator chooses to repeat a previously executed and scored trial, the replacement bar is striped.

The right section of the CRT plots the AP and lateral positions of the COG in real time. This display accurately indicates COG position relative to the center of the base of support when the patient's feet are properly placed on the support surface. Because accurate scoring of MCT latencies and strengths depends on weight bearing within the normal range, alignment of the COG (lateral, forward, or backward) should be corrected if possible with the following pro-

cedure. The positions of the patient's feet should be checked first to assure that inaccurate foot placement is not the cause. Each foot should not be positioned away from the proper position on the forceplate as the means to correct the COG misalignment. Instead, the patient should be encouraged by the operator to shift the upper body to center the COG.

Weight Symmetry

The graphic and raw data components of a typical MCT result are shown for one movement direction in Figure 13–5. In the complete MCT printout, an identical series of plots are included for

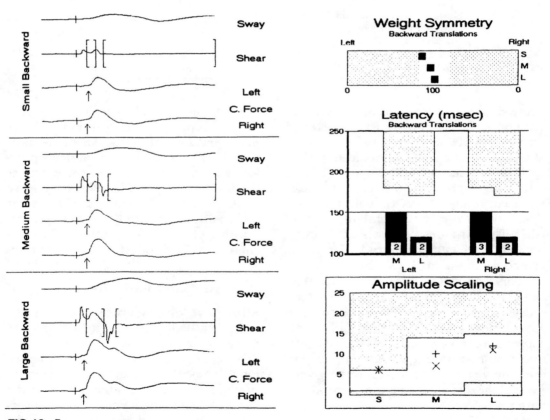

FIG 13–5.
Graphical and raw data summaries of MCT results of a typical clinically normal adult for backward support surface translations. Traces on the *left* show COG sway, horizontal shear force, and left and right center of vertical force (COF) (torque) responses averaged over three trials each for the three sizes of perturbations. *Vertical lines* show onset of surface translations. *Arrows* on the COF traces show onset times of the active force responses. Plots on the *right* show the relative bearing of weight between the two legs (100 equals perfect symmetry), the active force response latencies for left and right legs and the two larger sized translations, and the active force response strengths for the left (x) and right (+) legs. *Shaded areas* show scores falling outside the clinically normal limits, based on the normal population study.

backward and forward movement responses on the left and right sides of the page, respectively. For each movement direction, separate plots show weight symmetry, active force response latency, and active force response strength scores. In all of the plots, open areas encompass the range of scores considered to be within the clinically normal limits based on results from the asymptomatic sample.

A weight symmetry plot for each movement direction indicates the percentage of total body weight borne by each leg during the automatic postural response. Weight symmetry is displayed as a nondimensional quantity, with a score of 100 indicating that weight is borne equally by the two legs. The weight symmetry score decreases to zero or increases to 200 when all the weight is borne by the left or right leg, respectively. Weight symmetry scores are important, because the onset latencies and the strengths of automatic postural responses in each leg are influenced by the fraction of total body weight supported by the leg.

Active Force Latency

The automatic postural response elicited by a support surface translation compensates for COG sway by exerting active torque about the ankle joints. As the patient's COG moves forward (or backward) in response to horizontal surface translation, the initial resistance due to the inherent stiffness of the ankle joints is small and insufficient to stabilize the COG sway.[17, 26] The myotatic reflexes are either too weak or inhibited during standing to have a significant overall impact on the active force response.[16, 17] Active force increases abruptly within 30 to 40 msec following onset of the automatic component of the postural response at 90 to 100 msec latencies as recorded by EMG.[26, 27, 32] This is indicated by an abrupt and rapid increase in force resistance as measured by the forceplates. This sequence of events is illustrated

in the raw data components of Figure 13–5.

The active force response latencies are calculated automatically for each leg and for each direction and magnitude of displacement, along with a quality factor indicating the reliability of the latency score. To produce each latency score, four separate slope detection algorithms are used to identify the active force "takeoff point." The four results are then compared. If results of none of the algorithms agree within a 10-msec tolerance, the longest of the four latency scores is used, and a quality factor of 1 is indicated. If two or more scores are within 10 msec, the longest of these scores is used, and a quality factor of 2 to 4 indicates the number scores within the tolerance. Thus, a quality factor of 4 indicates the highest level of consistency, while a 1 indicates the least consistency. Latency scores for each leg and translation size are presented as separate bars in the latency plot.

The second page of the MCT printout shows the active force response traces of each leg and the COG sway averaged over the three trials. The latency takeoff points identified by the computer for the left and right leg active force responses are marked with arrows as shown in Figure 13–5. If the operator disagrees with the placement of one or more arrows, a magnified view of the force traces in question can be displayed on the monitor and the takeoff points manually marked by the operator. In these cases the quality factor is displayed as an "*M*" on the graphic printout page.

Because the active force response elicited by a small translation is near the automatic response threshold, the associated latency is quite variable and in some instances impossible to identify. Medium and large translations, in contrast, elicit vigorous active force responses with a high degree of latency symmetry between left and right legs, and between forward and backward translations of the same magnitude. Thus, latency results from medium and large translations can be of significant value in identifying motor system abnormalities in patients with imbalance or postural instability.

Active Force Strength

Adjusting the size of support surface translations for variations in patient height assures that the velocity and amplitude of COG sway is the same for all patients. In physical terms, this means that a given size translation imparts the same sway momentum to all patients, regardless of individual variations in body height and weight. To counteract the sway momentum produced by the translation, the patient must exert a restoring force that imparts approximately twice the momentum in the opposite direction. Half of the restoring momentum is required to stop the COG sway; the other half, to return the body to the original equilibrium position. For this reason, the magnitude (strength) of the active force response is best characterized by the momentum generated by the active force.

Following onset of the active force response, the support surface continues to translate, displace the COG, and stretch the ankle joint muscles. This requires the continued exertion of active force by the two legs to regain balance. The magnitude (strength) of this active force is quantified relative to the rate of increase of ankle torque exerted by each leg over a 150-msec interval following the latency onset.[13] Dividing the raw scores by patient height and weight compensates for differences in patient stature and produces strength scores with the appropriate units of (sway) angular momentum.

For each movement direction, active force strength is plotted as a function of translation size for each leg and translation size. In the clinically normal individual, strength scores for equivalent sized translations in the two directions are similar. In addition, lateral strength symmetry is demonstrated when the active force responses for a given size translation are similar in the two legs. When differences in strength between the two legs exceed the normal range, the data points in question are enclosed by a box.

MCT Results in a Clinically Normal Sample

Selected results from the asymptomatic normal sample of individuals are described in Appendix A. For all age ranges, the average weight symmetry scores are near 100, indicating that weight is borne equally by the two legs. Because scores both significantly above and below 100 (weight bearing to the right and left of center, respectively) are considered abnormal, the clinically normal limits for symmetry are set at ± 2 SD from the average.

In all age groups and in both movement directions, onset latencies are slightly longer for the medium than for the large translations. Furthermore, the response latencies show the expected slight increases with age. Other research studies have also shown subtle variations in EMG latencies that are dependent on the velocity and magnitude of the evoking translation.[10, 25] These latencies have been shown to increase in latency with age.[36, 40]

Only those latency scores significantly longer than the averages of the asymptomatic normal sample are considered clinically abnormal. Thus, the upper limits for clinically normal latencies are set at 1.67 SD above the sample averages.

In all age groups, the height and weight compensated response strengths are symmetrical for the two legs and movement directions. For all translation magnitudes, the average strength scores are sufficient to return the COG to the centered position without excessive undershoot or overshoot. Specifically, the angular momenta imparted to the body by the small, medium, and large translations are 2.8°/sec, 6.0°/sec, and 8.0°/sec, respectively. To return the COG to center, the total angular momentum generated by the two legs must be twice that produced by the translation. One half of the response momentum is needed to arrest the sway, the other half to return the body COG to the center position. This is accomplished when each leg generates angular momentum equal to that of the translation. Figure 13–6 shows that, on average, asymptomatic normal individuals produce the amount of active force necessary to accurately return the body COG to the original centered position.

Response strengths significantly weaker or stronger than the averages of the asymptomatic normal sample are considered clinically abnormal. Thus, the normal limits of the strengths for each age group are set at ± 2 SD from the sample averages.

Potential Problems With MCT Results

The greatest potential sources of error in the MCT are latency and strength changes in one leg caused by a substan-

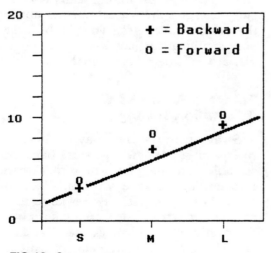

FIG 13–6.
Active force strengths in a clinically normal sample of persons 20 to 59 years of age as functions of translation size and direction. The *heavy line* shows the response strengths needed to exactly re-center the COG. Vertical units of measurement refer to angular momentum per unit of body mass (degrees/sec/kg). Horizontal notations refer to amplitude of displacement (S = small; M = medium; L = large).

tial unweighting of that leg during testing. Errors in one leg are readily recognized by the combination of delayed latencies, low response strengths, and weight bearing toward the opposite leg. The problem can only be remedied during testing. The operator should monitor the real time COG cursor during MCT testing and instruct the patient to center the COG cursor within the normal limits whenever a substantial lateral displacement of the cursor is noted.

Weak response strengths create the potential for latency scoring errors. This problem is minimized by reviewing the raw data and determining that the marker arrows are appropriately placed at the active force response take-off points. Questionable scores can be manually rescored by the operator. In the case of a very weak response, an accurate determination of latency may not be possible.

The response take-off point and strength may be difficult to identify in highly unstable patient, because responses are obscured by the high level of background sway activity. Manual review of the raw data is sometimes helpful in these cases.

AUTOMATIC RESPONSE ADAPTATION

Slow Support Surface Rotations

The adaptation protocol exposes the patient to a series of five identical toes-up or toes-down rotations of the support surface. In contrast to the PER test, the rotations are imposed at a relatively slow 8°/sec. These relatively slower stimulus velocities rotate the ankle joints at velocities similar to those generated by the large support surface translations during the MCT. Because these slower stimulus velocities do not saturate the automatic posture control system, it is possible to measure adaptive changes in the patient's responses over the course of the five rotations.

A series of five identical rotations is

typically interposed between sets of support surface translations. When the first unexpected surface rotation is imposed after a set of surface translations, the automatic posture control system is initially prepared to actively resist ankle joint rotation as a means to stabilize COG sway. Because resisting the ankle joint rotation is destabilizing when the surface rotates, the COG sway is frequently increased during the recovery period following the first surface rotation. Asymptomatic subjects, however, do not typically lose their balance. By the fourth and fifth rotations of the series, the automatic system attenuates the ankle joint resistance. This adaptive change enhances the subject's stability during the recovery period.[26]

The adaptive mechanisms responsible for attenuating ankle joint resistance and reducing COG sway during the recovery period following support surface rotation are complex and probably involve both reduction in the amplitude of the stretch-evoked (destabilizing) responses and enhancement of the later stabilizing responses. Nevertheless, when the patient makes these adaptive changes, COG sway is reduced during the recovery periods following the last few rotational trials of the series.

Presentation of Adaptation Results

Sway energy is used as a nonspecific but quantitative measure of the magnitude of COG sway during the recovery period following a support surface rotation. Sway energy is a weighted sum of the root mean square COG sway velocity and sway acceleration measured over the 2.5-second interval immediately following rotation. While this measure does not reflect changes within the individual response components described previously, it is an accurate measure of the overall functional effect of these adaptive changes.

Adaptation results are presented by plotting a separate sway energy score

for each of the five rotations. The display of results of toes-up rotation, which elicits a backward COG displacement, is displayed under the backward movement response results of the MCT. Similarly, the results of toes-down rotations are displayed under the forward movement results of the MCT.

Adaptation Results in the Clinically Normal Sample

Asymptomatic normal individuals show progressive reductions in sway energy over the course of five repeated exposures to toes-up or toes-down rotations, as shown in Figure 13–7. While the sway energy scores of younger and older subjects are similar during the first toes-up and toes-down trials, improvements in stability are significantly greater in the younger subjects by the fourth and fifth trials. Poorer adaptation in the elderly may be caused by a slowing of central adaptation, musculoskeletal factors which increase mechanical stiffness at the ankles, or a combination of these factors.[20, 40]

The upper limits for clinically normal sway energies are set at 1.67 SD above the sample averages. This is because only significantly increased sway energies are considered abnormal.

Potential Problems With Adaptation Testing

Sway energy scores may be inaccurate when a patient falls, steps back, or stumbles on the platform rather than maintaining balance with the feet in place. When the patient's response to a rotation is a free-fall, step, or stumble, the operator should mark the trial as a fall. The maximum sway energy score is assigned to these trials. If a free-fall is not marked as a fall by the operator, a deceptively low sway energy score will usually result. In contrast, unmarked steps and stumbles usually result in more appropriately high sway energy scores.

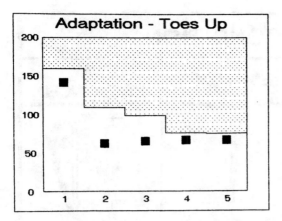

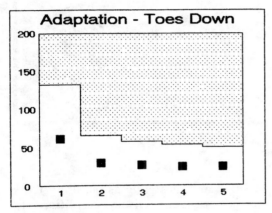

FIG 13–7.
Graphical summary of the adaptation results of a typical clinically normal subject. The *vertical axes* show the sway energy expended during corrective responses. The *horizontal axes* show trial numbers. *Shaded areas* show scores falling outside the clinically normal limits, based on the normal population study.

SENSORY ORGANIZATION TESTING

Sensory Conditions

The six conditions of the SOT protocol are designed to assess the patient's ability to effectively use visual, vestibular, and somatosensory inputs to maintain balance, and to select the input(s) providing the functionally most appropriate orientation information under a variety of conditions. Sensory organization is evaluated by selectively disrupting somatosensory and/or visual information regarding body COG orientation in relation to vertical and then measuring the patient's ability to maintain balance.

Somatosensory and/or visual information is disrupted by a method commonly referred to as "sway-referencing." This method involves the tilting of the support surface and/or the visual surround about an axis co-linear with the ankle joints to directly follow the patient's COG sway in the AP direction.[28] Under sway-referenced conditions, the orientation of the support surface and/or the visual surround remains constant in relation to the COG sway angle. Although the somatosensory and visual systems continue to provide information during sway-referenced conditions, these inputs contain no functionally useful information relating the orientation of the body COG relative to the gravity vertical.

Information derived from a sense subjected to sway-referencing (vision/proprioception), indicates that the orientation of the body COG relative to gravity is not changing when in fact it is. Healthy subjects ignore a sway-referenced sensory input that is functionally inaccurate and maintain balance using other sensory inputs. In addition to sway-referencing, eyes closed conditions are used to further isolate the somatosensory and vestibular systems. Unfortunately, there is no noninvasive way to selectively disrupt vestibular orientation information.

Protocol for the Sensory Organization Test

The SOT exposes the patient to the six sensory conditions illustrated in Figure 13–8. The six conditions consist of all combinations of normal (fixed), eyes closed, and sway-referenced visual and support surface sensory conditions.[4, 28] The six conditions are presented beginning with the simplest, eyes open on a fixed support surface, and ending with the most challenging in which the sup-

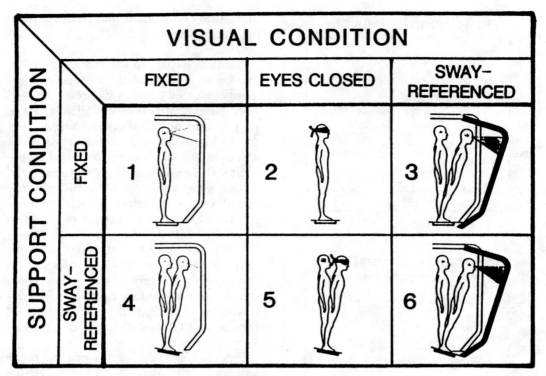

FIG 13–8.
The SOT protocol showing the six sensory test conditions.

port surface and the visual surround are both sway-referenced.

During sensory conditions 1 and 2, the support surface and visual surround are fixed, and the patient stands with eyes open and eyes closed, respectively. These trials provide baseline measures of the patient's postural stability. Under sensory condition 3, the surface remains fixed while the patient stands with eyes open in a sway-referenced visual surround. In the last three test conditions, the support surface is sway-referenced while the patient stands with eyes open and with the visual surround fixed (condition 4), eyes closed (condition 5), and eyes open and the visual surround sway-referenced (condition 6).

The complete protocol consists of eighteen, 20-second trials, three consecutive trials for each of the six sensory conditions. During each trial, the patient is instructed to ignore any surface or visual surround motion and remain upright and as steady as possible. Three trials for each sensory condition improves the reliability of the resulting measures. The repeated measures also provide an opportunity to determine whether the patient's performance improves under a given condition with practice.

Equilibrium Scores

During each trial, the COG sway angle is calculated in real time based on the biomechanical relations between the position of the center of vertical force (COF) exerted by the feet against the support surface, the position of the COG, and the limits of stability.[23, 37] When the frequency of COG sway is below 0.5 Hz, the COG is located vertically above the COF. As COG sway frequency increases, movements of the COG lag behind the COF and decrease in relative size.[31, 37] A real time, multiple pole digital filter is used to approximate these amplitude and frequency relations between the COF and COG motions.

A separate measure of stability, called the equilibrium score, is calculated for each trial. As shown in Figure 13–9, the equilibrium score is a nondimensional percentage which compares the patient's peak amplitude of AP sway to the theoretical AP limits of stability (LOS). The patient's theoretical LOS is the maximum forward and backward COG sway angles that can be achieved by a normal individual of similar height and weight. Equilibrium scores near 100% indicate little sway, while scores approaching zero indicate that sway is nearing the LOS. Trials in which the patient exceeds the LOS and loses balance

are arbitrarily assigned equilibrium scores of zero.

Center of Gravity Alignment

For each SOT trial, separate AP and lateral alignment scores are calculated by averaging the AP and lateral positions of the COG sway angle over the 20-second test interval. These calculations are based on the assumption that the patient's spontaneous COG swaying over the course of the trial occurs symmetrically about the point of COG alignment.

Ankle vs. Hip Movements

When ankle movements are used to control sway, the associated low-fre-

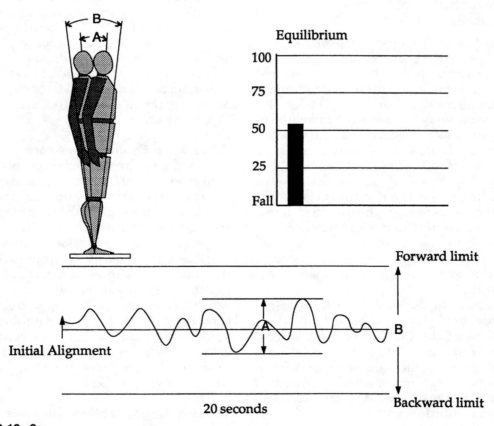

FIG 13–9.
Graphic illustration of the method for calculating the equilibrium score from the raw COG sway data of a 20-second trial. The equilibrium score compares the maximum patient anteroposterior sway angle (A) to the patient's theoretical limits of stability (B). As *A* increases from 0 toward *B*, the equilibrium score decreases from 100 (perfect stability) toward 0 (loss of balance).

quency motions of the COG generate relatively little horizontal shear force against the support surface. Higher frequency hip and upper body movements, in contrast, generate small but rapid shifts in COG position and much larger horizontal shear forces.[19, 30] Based on this biomechanical principle, the relative amounts of ankle and hip movement are determined by comparing the peak-to-peak amplitude of the horizontal shear force to a theoretical limit for normal of similar weight. Although this method provides an accurate measure of the extent of hip and upper body movement activity, this score does not measure the time-dependent trajectory of the actual body motion.

Presentation of Sensory Organization Test Results

Real Time Display of Results

The CRT display presents a real time summary of the raw COG sway data and the resulting equilibrium scores during administration of the SOT. The left side of the display indicates the currently selected sensory condition and trial number, and also plots the equilibrium scores of all completed trials. Green bars show scores of completed trials falling within the normal range, while red bars show scores below the fifth percentile relative to the age-matched clinically normal sample. If the operator chooses to repeat a previously executed and scored trial, the replacement bar is striped.

The right section of the CRT provides a real time plot of the AP and lateral positions of the COG. This display accurately indicates COG position relative to the center of the base of support when the patient's feet are properly placed on the support surface. If lateral, forward, or backward alignment of the COG is noted during testing, the positions of the patient's feet should be rechecked for accurate placement. Under no circumstances, however, should the patient be coached to reposition the feet away from

their proper positions or to shift the COG, as these procedures will invalidate the COG alignment scores.

Raw Sway Data and Equilibrium Scores

The raw data and graphic components of a typical SOT result are shown in Figures 13–10 and 13–11, respectively. The first graphic plot summarizes the equilibrium scores obtained from a maximum of three trials under each of the six sensory conditions. Each equilibrium score is presented as a bar. All areas of the plot in which equilibrium scores fall below the fifth percentile relative to the age-matched clinically normal sample are indicated by stippling.

The raw data traces for each 20-second trial are presented using the two formats (Fig 13–10). One format plots the AP sway angle (heavy trace) and the horizontal shear force (light trace) signals as concurrent functions of time. The second format (not illustrated) plots the AP versus the lateral component of the COG sway angle.

Composite Equilibrium Score

A patient's overall level of performance on the SOT is best characterized by the composite equilibrium score, which is the average of the following 14 equilibrium scores: the condition 1 average score, the condition 2 average score, and the three scores from each of the conditions 3 through 6 trials. Note that the resulting composite score is a weighted average which emphasizes the conditions 3 through 6 equilibrium scores. This weighting is used because sensory balance deficits are more readily reflected under the more difficult sensory conditions.

Sensory Organization Analysis

The specific nature of a patient's sensory balance problem is best characterized by quantifying relative differences in the equilibrium scores among the six sensory conditions. Differences in equi-

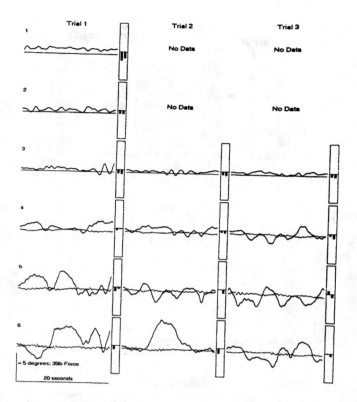

FIG 13–10.
Raw data summary of the SOT results shown in Figure 13–9. The *numbered rows* show COG sway responses during each of the six sensory test conditions. The *numbered columns* show trials one through three responses for each sensory test condition. Note that conditions *1* and *2* were tested at only one trial each. *Heavy traces* show the COG sway (up indicates forward and down indicates backward). *Fine traces* show the horizontal shear force. *Bars* to the right of each trace show COG alignment. *Shaded areas* show scores falling outside the clinically normal limits, based on the normal population study.

librium scores are shown in the sensory organization analysis plot of Figure 13–11. Relative differences in scores are quantified using ratios in which the three-trial average equilibrium score of one sensory condition is divided by the three-trial average score of another condition. The four equilibrium score ratios and their physiologic meaning are summarized in Figure 13–12.

The Somatosensory ratio, which compares the condition 2 to the condition 1 equilibrium score, quantifies the extent of stability loss when the patient closes the eyes. Since eye closure eliminates the visual input, an atypically low ratio is interpreted as dysfunction of the remaining somatosensory input, which normally dominates the control of balance during stance on a fixed support surface. Although the vestibular input is

potentially a second alternative to vision during eye closure, this alternative is substantially less sensitive than the somatosensory input in controlling sway. Therefore, use of the vestibular input rather than the somatosensory input during eye closure on a fixed surface significantly increases the COG sway. This is the same interpretation originally proposed by Romberg.[7, 38]

The visual ratio compares the condition 4 score with the condition 1 score. This ratio quantifies the extent of stability loss when the normally dominant somatosensory input is disrupted by sway-referencing of the support surface. Although COG sway usually increases slightly when the somatosensory input is disrupted, the increase in sway is small when the alternative visual input is functioning normally. For reasons

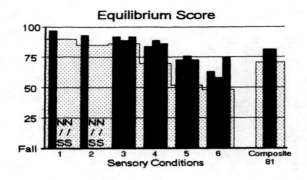

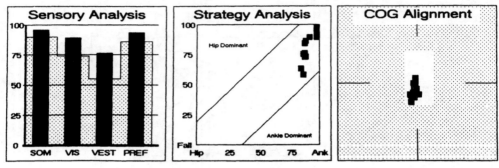

FIG 13-11.
Graphical summary of the SOT results of a typical clinically normal subject. The *upper plot* shows the equilibrium scores for the six sensory conditions (up to three trials per condition) and the composite equilibrium score. The *lower plots* show the four sensory analysis ratios, the analysis of movement pattern versus equilibrium score, and the COG alignment. *Shaded areas* show scores falling outside the clinically normal limits, based on the normal population study.

similar to those presented previously, sway increases will be abnormally large if the vestibular input rather than the visual input is used. Therefore, a lower than normal ratio in this case is interpreted as dysfunction of the visual sense of balance.

The vestibular ratio comparing the condition 5 score with the condition 1 score reflects a relative reduction in stability when visual and somatosensory inputs are simultaneously disrupted. Although COG sway increases significantly under condition 5 for the reasons described previously, clinically normal individuals maintain their balance well within the LOS using the remaining vestibular inputs. A lower than normal ratio is therefore interpreted as a dysfunctional vestibular sense of balance.

The vision preference ratio comparing the sum of conditions 3 and 6 scores

to the sum of conditions 2 and 5 scores reflects a relative reduction of stability under sway-referenced visual conditions compared with the equivalent eyes closed conditions. The stability of clinically normal individual is similar when eyes are closed and when presented with a functionally inappropriate visual input. In both cases, no visual information useful for controlling balance is available. Thus, a lower than normal ratio in this case is interpreted as an abnormal preference for using vision. In other words, the patient attempts to orient himself or herself to the sway-referenced (conflicting) visual input and sways more in comparison to the equivalent eyes closed conditions.

COG Alignment

Center of gravity alignment is analyzed by plotting for each of the 18 SOT

SENSORY ANALYSIS			
RATIO NAME	**TEST CONDITIONS**	**RATIO PAIR**	**SIGNIFICANCE**
SOM Somatosensory	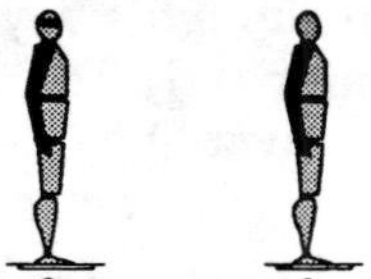 2 1	Condition 2 / Condition 1	**Question:** Does sway increase when visual cues are removed? **Low scores:** Patient makes poor use of somatosensory references.
VIS Visual	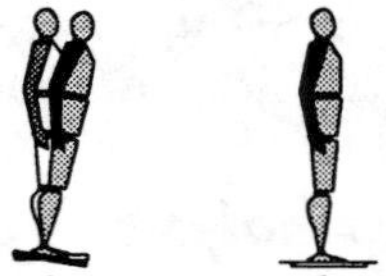 4 1	Condition 4 / Condition 1	**Question:** Does sway increase when somatosensory cues are inaccurate? **Low scores:** Patient makes poor use of visual references.
VEST Vestibular	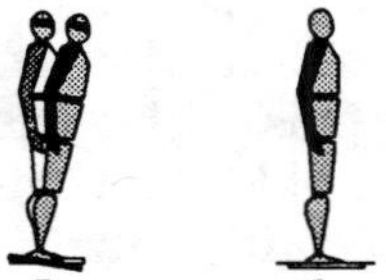 5 1	Condition 5 / Condition 1	**Question:** Does sway increase when visual cues are removed and somatosensory cues are inaccurate? **Low scores:** Patient makes poor use of vestibular cues, or vestibular cues unavailable.
PREF Visual Preference	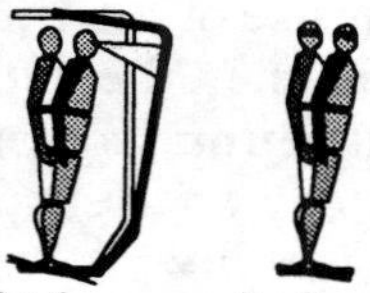 3 + 6 2 + 5	Condition 3 + 6 / Condition 2 + 5	**Question:** Do inaccurate visual cues result in increased sway compared to no visual cues? **Low scores:** Patient relies on visual cues even when they are inaccurate.

FIG 13–12.
Sensory analysis ratios and their functional meaning.

trials the average AP and lateral positions of the COG (see Fig 13–9). When the patient's COG is aligned over the center of the base of support, the points corresponding to each trial are clustered near the center of the plot. Points above the center indicate an alignment forward of center, while points below the center of the plot indicate a backward COG alignment. Points to the left or right of the center indicate a laterally misaligned COG in the corresponding direction. Areas of the alignment plot falling outside the fifth percentile relative to the clinically normal sample are indicated by stippling.

Strategy Analysis

The patient's movement strategy during each SOT trial is analyzed by plotting the resulting movement strategy score against the corresponding equilibrium score as shown in Figure 13–9. Points falling in the upper left quadrant of the strategy plot indicate trials in which the COG sway excursions are small but the amplitude of hip and upper body movements is large. This region of the plot is therefore labeled "hip dominant." Points in the lower right quadrant indicate trials in which COG sway excursions are large, but the movements are primarily about the ankle joints. This region is therefore labeled "ankle dominant." Points falling along an upper right to lower left diagonal indicate trials in which the amplitude of hip and upper body movements increase in proportion to the amplitude of the COG sway.

SOT Results in the Clinically Normal Sample

Equilibrium Scores and Sensory Analysis Ratios

In the Appendix to this chapter, Tables 13–A1 through 13–A6 show the ranges of equilibrium scores, composite scores, and sensory organization ratios for the sample of asymptomatic subjects. Equilibrium scores for each sensory condition are based on the average of scores for the three trials. Equilibrium scores of zero are used for trials in which subjects lost balance. Sizable normal population studies in children to elderly by other groups have yielded similar SOT results.[22, 35, 40, 44]

Because the distributions of equilibrium scores are skewed toward the higher values, the limits for clinically normal scores are determined by calculating the lowest fifth percentile of equilibrium scores for each age range and condition. Because the sensory analysis ratio scores are normally distributed, scores below 1.67 SD of the population means define the lower limits of the clinically normal range.

The equilibrium scores of clinically normal subjects of all ages are the highest for the first three sensory conditions. This is because somatosensory inputs dominate balance when the support surface is fixed, regardless of the status of visual and vestibular inputs. Although equilibrium scores decrease when the functionally useful somatosensory input is disrupted (sway-referenced support surface) during conditions 4 through 6, clinically normal subjects continue to maintain balance well within the LOS. The sensory condition 4 scores are the highest of these three conditions, because normal visual inputs are available. The lowest equilibrium scores occur under conditions 5 and 6, when both somatosensory and visual inputs are disrupted and subjects must rely on vestibular inputs alone to maintain balance.

Center of Gravity Alignment

Clinically normal subjects align the COG very near to the center of the base of support under all six sensory conditions. Even though sway amplitudes increase significantly under conditions 5 and 6, the average COG positions remain very nearly centered. Because offset positions in all directions are considered abnormal, alignment values beyond ± 2 SD in lateral and AP directions are considered abnormal.

Strategy Analysis

In the strategy analysis plots of our normal subject population, points corresponding to individual trials fall along a diagonal. This is because normal subjects use ankle movements when the COG is well within the limits of stability (high equilibrium scores) and will increase their use of hip movements as the COG approaches the limits of stability (low equilibrium scores). When points in the strategy analysis plot fall along a nearly vertical line, the patient is abnormally dependent on ankle movements. Points along a horizontal line indicate that the patient is abnormally dependent on hip movements.

Repeatability of Sensory Organization Test Results

Recently several investigators have performed multiple SOT evaluations on samples of clinically normal individuals.[41, 43] For example, Coogler et al.[42] evaluated 45 subjects who received SOT evaluations on three separate days.[42] A comparison of the mean equilibrium scores from each session showed small but statistically significant improvements in equilibrium scores between the first to the third session on the more difficult sensory conditions. The mean equilibrium score improved approximately 5% for sensory condition 4, while improvements in sensory condition 5 and 6 scores were less than 10%. Most improvements were noted between the first and second sessions. This result suggests that the multiple administrations of the SOT can be used to follow the progress of the patient over time.

As part of an ongoing study of space motion sickness, astronauts participating in the NASA space shuttle program received preflight SOT evaluations at regular intervals, and then received serial postflight evaluations beginning within hours of their return from zero gravity.[34] The average equilibrium scores on SOT condition 6 for the first 10 returning astronauts dropped from the preflight range of 70% to 80% ("supernormal" values relative to the sample of asymptomatic normal individuals) to the 35% to 45% range immediately after flight (considered borderline "abnormal" compared to the clinically normal sample). Although not specifically documented in the report, results of the first five sensory conditions were reported to show much smaller postflight reductions. In all cases, equilibrium scores improved to their preflight values within several days.

The returning astronauts demonstrated a significant and specific reduction in sensory balance control, despite the fact that they were familiar with the SOT prior to space flight, and despite the fact that they were also highly motivated individuals. This suggests that the SOT can be used to track progress during treatment, because prior knowledge of the test will not mask a sensory organization abnormality.

Potential Problems With the SOT

Equilibrium scores may be higher than the actual functional capabilities when a tight safety harness "catches" a patient who would otherwise have fallen. Falls into the safety harness, however, can be identified on the raw shear force trace. While the shear forces generated by free swaying are very brief and symmetrical about zero axis, harness bumps cause large and prolonged deflections of the shear force trace in one direction.

As already discussed for the PER and MCT, results are most accurate when the patient gives his or her best performance without outside help. Poorly motivated patients, or patients who exaggerate symptoms, may produce equilibrium scores below their best functional capabilities. In these cases, the equilibrium scores are frequently inconsistent. Physiologically inconsistent patterns of scores are discussed in detail in Chapter 14, on CDP interpretation. Surprised and overly anxious patients also perform below their maximum functional capabilities. In these cases, the test protocols can be carefully explained to reassure the patient. As already discussed in relation to repeatability and reliability, detailed knowledge of the test is generally not a problem, because the functions being assessed are automatic rather than consciously controlled.

As is also true with the MCT, inaccurate placement of the feet on the forceplates effects the COG alignment and weight symmetry scores. However, as long as both feet are completely on the forceplates, the equilibrium and strategy scores will not be affected.

Finally, small movements and changes in position by the patient can artificially lower the equilibrium score on a trial. This problem is especially true during the first three sensory conditions, when scores are normally very high. The operator should watch the patient for evidence of head turns, postural shifts, coughs, and sneezes. Data obtained on these trials should be deleted and the trials repeated.

SUMMARY

Computerized dynamic posturography is an objective means for assessing the major sensory and motor components of balance, and uses a multiplicity of independent test protocols. All protocols are based on documented physiologic principles of human balance. Some protocols provide information relative to the patient's functional capacity within a variety of daily life tasks. Others provide information which can help localize the cause of a balance system disorder. The ability to identify inconsistencies among independent test results is an additional advantage in identifying nonphysiologic causes of unsteadiness such as anxiety and deliberate exaggeration of symptoms. Experimental studies with various populations of clinically normal individuals indicate that CDP can provide reliable and repeatable test results.

REFERENCES

1. Allum JHJ, Keshner EA: Vestibular and proprioceptive control of sway stabilization, in Bles W, Brandt T (eds): *Disorders of Posture and Gait*. New York, Elsevier, 1986, pp 19–40.

2. Beckley DJ, Bloem BR, van Dijk JG, et al: Electrophysiological correlates of postural instability in Parkinson's disease. *Electroencephalogr Clin Neurol* 1991; 81:263–268.

3. Black FO, Wall C III, Nashner LM: Effect of visual and support surface references upon postural control in vestibular deficit subjects. *Acta Otolaryngol* 1983; 95:199–210.

4. Black FO, Wall C III, O'Leary DP: Computerized screening of the human vestibulospinal system. *Ann Otol Rhinol Laryngol* 1978; 87:853–861.

5. Black FO, Wall C III: Normal subject postural sway during the Romberg test. *Am J Otolaryngol* 1982; 3:309–318.

6. Dichgans J, Diener HC: Clinical evidence for functional compartmentalization of the cerebellum; in Bloedel JR, Dichgans J, Precht W (eds): *Cerebellar Functions*. New York, Springer-Verlag, 1985, pp 126–147.

7. Dichgans J, Mauritz KH, Allum JHJ, et al: Postural sway in normals and ataxic patients: Analysis of the stabilizing and destabilizing effects of vision. *Agressologie* 1976; 17:15–24.

8. Diener HC, Ackermann H, Dichgans J, et al: Medium- and long-latency responses to displacements of the ankle joint in patients with spinal and central lesions. *Electroencephalography Clin Neurophysiol* 1985; 60:407–416.

9. Diener HC, Bootz F, Dichgans J, et al: Vari-

ability of postural "reflexes" in humans. *Exp Brain Res* 1983; 52:423–428.

10. Diener HC, Dichgans J, Bacher M, et al: Characteristic alterations of long-loop "reflexes" in patients with Friedreich's disease and late atrophy of the cerebellar anterior lobe. *J Neurol Neurosurg Psychiatry* 1984; 47:679–685.

11. Diener HC, Dichgans J, Bootz F, et al: Early stabilization of human posture after sudden disturbance: Influence of rate and amplitude of displacement. *Exp Brain Res* 1984; 56:126–134.

12. Diener HC, Dichgans J, Scholz E, et al: Long loop reflexes in a standing subject and their use for clinical diagnosis; in Igarashi M, Black FO (eds): *Vestibular and Visual Control on Posture and Locomotor Equilibrium*. Basel, S Karger, 1985, pp 290–294.

13. Diener HC, Horak FB, Nashner LM: Influence of stimulus parameters on human postural responses. *J Neurophysiol* 1988; 59:1888–1905.

14. Dietz V, Quintern J, Berger W: Corrective reactions to stumbling in man: Functional significance of spinal and transcortical reflexes. *Neurosci Lett* 1984; 44:131–135.

15. Dietz V, Quintern J, Berger W, et al: Cerebral potentials and leg muscle EMG responses associated with stance perturbation. *Exp Brain Res* 1985; 57:348–354.

16. El'ner AM, Popov KE, Gurfinkel VS: Changes in stretch reflex system concerned with the control of postural activity of human muscle. *Agressologie* 1972; 13:19–23.

17. Gurfinkel VS, Lipshits MI, Popov KY: Is the stretch reflex the main mechanism in the system of regulation of the vertical posture of man? *Biophysics* 1974; 19:744–748.

18. Horak FB, Diener HC, Nashner LM: Influence of central set on human postural responses. *J Neurophysiol* 1989; 62:841–853.

19. Horak FB, Nashner LM: Central programming of postural movements: Adaptation to altered support surface configurations. *J Neurophysiol* 1986; 55:1369–1981.

20. Horak FB, Shupert CL, Mirka A: Components of postural dyscontrol in the elderly: A review. *Neurobiol Aging* 1989; 10:727–738.

21. Huttunen J, Homberg V: EMG responses in leg muscles to postural perturbations in Huntington's disease. *J Neurol Neurosurg Psychiatry* 1990; 53:55–62.

22. Jackson RT, Epstein CM: Effect of head extension on equilibrium in normal subjects. *Ann Otol Rhinol Laryngol* 1991; 100:63–67.

23. Koles ZJ, Casttelein RD: The relationship between body sway and foot pressure in normal man. *J Med Eng Technol* 1980; 4:279–285.

24. Kapteyn TS, de Wit G: Posturography as an auxiliary in vestibular investigation. *Acta Otolaryngol* 1972; 73:104–111.

25. Nardone A, Giordano O, Corra T, et al: Responses of leg muscles in humans displaced while standing. *Brain* 1990; 113:65–84.

26. Nashner LM: Adapting reflexes controlling the human posture. *Exp Brain Res* 1976; 26:59–72.

27. Nashner LM: Fixed patterns of rapid postural responses among leg muscles during stance. *Exp Brain Res* 1977; 150:403–407.

28. Nashner LM, Black FO, Wall C: Adaptation to altered support and visual conditions during stance: Patients with vestibular deficits. *J Neurosci* 1982; 2:536–544.

29. Nashner LM, Cordo PG: Relation of automatic postural responses and reaction-time voluntary movements of human leg muscles. *Exp Brain Res* 1981; 43:395–405.

30. Nashner LM, McCollum G: The organization of human postural movements: A formal basis and experimental synthesis. *Behav Brain Sci* 1985; 8:135–172.

31. Nashner LM, Shupert CL, Horak FB, et al: Organization of posture controls: An analysis of sensory and mechanical constraints, in Allum JHJ, Hulliger M (eds): *Progress in Brain Research*, vol 80. New York, Elsevier, 1989, pp 411–418.

32. Nashner LM, Woollacott M, Tuma G: Organization of rapid responses to postural and locomotor-like perturbations of standing man. *Exp Brain Res* 1979; 36:463–476.

33. Njiokiktjien C, De Rijke W: (1972). The recording of Romberg's test and its application in neurology. *Agressologie* 1972; 13(C):1–7.

34. Paloski WH, Reschke MF, Doxey DD, et al: Neurosensory adaptation associated with postural ataxia following spaceflight, in Woollacott M, Horak F (eds): *Posture and Gait: Control Mechanisms*, vol I. Eugene, University of Oregon Books, 1992, pp 311–314.

35. Peterka RJ, Black FO: Age-related changes in human posture control: Sensory organization tests. *J Vestibular Res* 1990; 1:73–85.

36. Peterka RJ, Black FO: Age-related changes in human posture control: Motor coordination tests. *J Vestibular Res* 1990; 1:87–96.

37. Riley P, Mann RW, Hodge A: Modelling of the biomechanics of posture and balance. *J Biomech* 1990; 23:503–506.

38. Romberg MH: *Manual of Nervous System Disease of Man*. London, Sydenham Society, 1853 pp 395–401.

39. Terekhov Y: Stabilometry as a diagnostic tool in clinical medicine. *Can Med Assoc J* 1976; 115:631–633.

40. Wolfson L, Whipple R, Derby C, et al: A dynamic posturography study of balance in healthy elderly. *Neurology*. (in press).

41. Barin K, Seitz CM, Welling DB: Effect of head orientation on the diagnostic sensitivity of posturography in patients with compensated unilateral lesions. *Otolaryngol Head Neck Surg*, 1992; 106: 355–362.

42. Coogler CE, Wolf S: Consistency of postural responses in elderly individuals, in Woollacott M, Horak F (eds): *Posture and Gait: Control Mechanisms*, vol II. Eugene, University of Oregon Books, 1992, pp 239–242.

43. Epstein CM, Jackson RT: Head extension and sway in normal volunteers, in Woollacott M, Horak F (eds): *Posture and Gait: Control Mechanisms*, vol I. Eugene, University of Oregon Books, 1992, pp 171–174.

44. Ledin T: Dynamic posturography in childhood and senescence, in Woollacott M, Horak F (eds): *Posture and Gait: Control Mechanisms*, vol II. Eugene, University of Oregon Books, 1992, pp 279–282.

APPENDIX

TABLE 13–A1.

Normal Subject Posture-Evoked Response Latencies*

Reference	No. of Subjects	Short Latency	Medium Latency	Long Latency
2	10	42.9 ± 3.3	86.6 ± 6.4	128.6 ± 10.1
8	50	43.5 ± 4.2	89.5 ± 10.0	125.3 ± 17.8
21†	26	34 ± 3	86 ± 6	114 ± 16
† and ‡	74	30.0 ± 4.6	73.3 ± 11.2	104.2 ± 17.0

*All studies used 50-degrees/sec 4-degree toes-up rotations.

†In these studies, time was determined by the actual platform movement onset rather than the movement command, reducing latencies by 10 to 15 msec.

‡Data provided to NeuroCom International, Inc. by Chris Diener, Universitat Essen, Germany.

TABLE 13–A2.

Mean (+ 1.67 SD) Latency Scores as Functions of Translation Size, Direction, and Subject Age

Movement	Population Latency Scores (msec)		
	20–59 yrs (n = 58)	60–69 yrs (n = 54)	70–79 yrs (n = 28)
Medium back	156 (182)	160 (187)	168 (200)
Large back	137 (168)	148 (171)	155 (178)
Medium forward	164 (194)	164 (184)	170 (196)
Large forward	153 (167)	155 (173)	159 (177)

TABLE 13–A3.

Mean (± 2 SD) Active Force Strengths as Functions of Translation Direction, Size, and Subject Age*

Movement	Population Strength Scores		
	20–59 yrs (n = 29)	60–69 yrs (n = 54)	70–79 yrs (n = 28)
Small back	03.4 ± (1.4)	04.1 ± (4.6)	04.2 ± (4.5)
Medium back	07.1 ± (5.8)	07.8 ± (5.5)	07.9 ± (7.0)
Large back	08.7 ± (5.2)	09.9 ± (5.5)	10.4 ± (7.4)
Small forward	03.6 ± (3.9)	05.1 ± (4.5)	05.2 ± (4.2)
Medium forward	08.4 ± (4.9)	09.0 ± (5.0)	08.6 ± (4.2)
Large forward	10.0 ± (5.7)	10.1 ± (5.3)	09.7 ± (6.0)

*All values are in units of angular momentum normalized for differences in body mass.

TABLE 13–A4.

Mean (+ 1.67 SD) Sway Energy Scores as Functions of Toes-Up and Toes-Down Trial Numbers and Subject Age*

Motion	Population Adaptation Scores		
	20–59 yrs (n = 64)	60–69 yrs (n = 54)	70–79 yrs (n = 28)
Toes up			
1	85 (160)	76 (125)	75 (132)
2	67 (109)	68 (97)	74 (118)
3	62 (99)	62 (91)	74 (103)
4	54 (76)	59 (81)	72 (111)
5	53 (75)	60 (83)	66 (91)
Toes down			
1	76 (134)	75 (120)	72 (113)
2	45 (66)	59 (88)	66 (112)
3	40 (58)	52 (81)	61 (95)
4	37 (54)	49 (77)	60 (99)
5	36 (50)	49 (76)	60 (99)

*All values are in units of sway energy normalized for differences in body mass.

TABLE 13–A5.

Mean (fifth percentile) Equilibrium Scores as Functions of Age and Sensory
Test Condition

	Population Equilibrium Scores		
Condition	20–59 yrs (*n* = 112)	60–69 yrs (*n* = 54)	70–79 yrs (*n* = 28)
1	94(90)	94(90)	89(70)
2	92(85)	91(86)	86(63)
3 Average	91(86)	89(80)	88(82)
4 Average	82(70)	85(77)	78(69)
5 Average	69(52)	65(51)	61(45)
6 Average	67(48)	65(49)	53(27)
Composite	798(704)	776(676)	729(638)

TABLE 13–A6.

Mean (± 2 SD) COG Alignment Scores as Functions of Sensory Test
Conditions and Age*

	Population Alignment Scores		
Condition	20–59 yrs (*n* = 77)	60–69 yrs (*n* = 54)	70–79 yrs (*n* = 28)
Initial	0.3 ± (1.8)	−0.1 ± (2.0)	0.0 ± (1.8)
Dynamic			
1	0.2 ± (2.0)	−0.3 ± (1.9)	−0.2 ± (1.9)
2	0.3 ± (1.6)	−0.1 ± (2.0)	0.0 ± (1.7)
3	0.3 ± (1.6)	0.0 ± (2.1)	−0.2 ± (1.7)
4	0.3 ± (1.6)	−0.1 ± (2.1)	−0.1 ± (1.7)
5	0.7 ± (1.8)	0.1 ± (2.2)	0.2 ± (2.2)
6	0.8 ± (1.9)	0.4 ± (2.3)	0.3 ± (1.7)

*All values are in units of degrees from the center position.

CHAPTER 14

Computerized Dynamic Posturography: Clinical Applications

Lewis M. Nashner, Sc.D.

BACKGROUND

Challenge of Treating Balance Disorders

The medical management of patients whose chief complaints are "dizziness" and "unsteadiness" must focus on two fundamental goals. The first is to differentiate the central and/or peripheral processes underlying the disorder, since peripheral pathologic conditions are frequently self-limiting and seldom life-threatening.[33] Central nervous system (CNS) problems, in contrast, are potentially progressive and terminal. Thus, the diagnostic effort must continue until potentially life-threatening CNS diseases are ruled out. In addition, while disease processes associated with balance disorders are usually self-limiting, they frequently cannot be resolved. The second goal, then, is to manage the patients's symptoms, minimizing discomfort and maximizing the functional capabilities that enhance the quality of life.

Several attributes of the balance system make these goals a unique challenge. First, balance involves multiple sensory, musculoskeletal, and CNS components. Problems in one component frequently cause secondary adaptive changes in others. Hence, the primary pathologic process may be difficult to distinguish from the secondary adaptive changes, particularly in the patient with chronic balance problems. Second, balance is largely an automatic subconscious process. Hence, the patient's subjective impressions are sensitive overall indicators of abnormality but are frequently inadequate to describe the specific details of the problem.

Patient Selection

The clinical applicability of computerized dynamic posturography (CDP) assessment varies with the chief complaints of the individual patient and the physician's clinical goals. The current literature has shown CDP to have the maximum clinical value in patients with symptoms of unsteadiness, disorientation, and/or vertigo, in whom the history and physical examination do not suggest an obvious localized cause. In such cases, the underlying disease process is unknown, and the initial clinical goal is to identify the process and differentiate it as to central or peripheral origins. Examples of such patient histories include:

1. Disequilibrium of unknown origin;
2. History of falls;
3. Vertigo or dizziness that does not respond to the usual medications;

4. Persistent disequilibrium with normal electronystagmography (ENG) and/or rotary chair test results;

5. Gait or postural disorders with the neurologic examination either within normal limits or revealing only "soft" signs that do not account for the symptoms;

6. Persistent symptoms following aminoglycoside therapy, chemotherapy, or inner ear surgery; and

7. Progressive rigidity or spasticity.

In other complex cases in which the underlying pathologic process is known, the goal is to manage the symptoms and enhance the patient's daily life functional capabilities. However, knowledge of the cause is frequently, by itself, an insufficient foundation on which to base a treatment program and to monitor the results. Patient disorders in this latter category include:

1. Balance dysfunction secondary to head trauma;

2. Stroke-related balance and mobility problems;

3. Developmental disorders such as cerebral palsy and certain learning disorders involving balance and motor coordination; and

4. Age-related balance problems in an otherwise clinically normal individual.

In patients whose history and symptoms suggest a well-localized disease process, specific localizing tests will frequently provide more information than CDP for making the diagnosis. For example, classical vestibular function tests such as ENG and the rotary chair examination may be more useful in confirming the presence and localizing a peripheral vestibular lesion in the patient whose history and symptoms suggest a unilateral process such as vestibular neuronitis or Meniere's disease.

Role of Computerized Dynamic Posturography

Computerized dynamic posturography addresses the aforementioned goals and challenges by providing quantitative information specific to the individual sensory, motor, and central coordinating elements that comprise the balance system. As suggested by Table 14–1, some components of CDP results correlate with specific types of disease processes and therefore are applicable during the diagnostic process. Other components of the CDP results identify

TABLE 14–1.

Applications of Information From Computerized Dynamic Posturography

Test Modality	Applications	
	Diagnostic	Functional
Response latencies	Peripheral nerve, spinal cord, and brain stem lesions	None documented
Response strengths	Cerebellar deficits (muscle weakness, nerve injuries)	Automatic motor adaptation
Sensory organization test patterns	Vestibular system dysfunction, positive evidence for symptoms exaggeration	Overall balance and sensory adaptive capabilities
Strategy analysis	None documented (ankle muscle weakness, distal sensory losses)	Movement control adaptive capabilities
Center of gravity alignment	None documented (reduced range)	Perception of vertical

the patient's adaptive strategies for coping with the balance disorder. These results are most useful in designing a course of treatment and monitoring the outcome. Still other CDP components correlate with the patient's functional capabilities in daily life. These latter results are applicable to the objective assessment of the patient's disability. Applications enclosed by parentheses in Table 14–1 have been reported anecdotally but are not substantiated by clinical studies. In all instances, however, the clinical value of the posture-evoked response (PER), motor control test (MCT), and sensory organization test (SOT) results are greatest in combination with the patient's history and the results of other clinical tests.

This chapter begins by describing the clinical applications of the individual CDP test components. Later sections describe the ways in which CDP results can be combined with the patient's history and other clinical results in the complex process of diagnosis, treatment design, and monitoring of outcomes.

DIAGNOSTIC APPLICATION OF THE SENSORY ORGANIZATION TEST

Normal vs. Abnormal Sensory Organization Test: The Composite Equilibrium Score

An overall description of a patient's ability to organize and utilize sensory information while balancing is best obtained by examining the composite equilibrium score. When the composite score is within the normal range, the patient has also scored within the normal range on most if not all of the individual sensory conditions. Occasionally, the equilibrium score on one sensory condition may be slightly below normal when the composite is in the low-normal range. This occurs when the patient performs well on the remaining sensory conditions, and suggests borderline normal sensory organization. When the compos-

ite score is below the normal range, the patient's balance will be significantly below normal on at least one of the sensory conditions.

Abnormal Results: Physiologically Inconsistent

Internally Inconsistent Results

Table 14–2 reviews the criteria for judging an SOT result as being inconsistent (see also Hamid et al.[21]). In one form of inconsistent pattern, a patient with an abnormal composite score obtains equilibrium scores on the more difficult sensory conditions, 4, 5, and 6, which are equal to or better than those obtained in the easier conditions, 1, 2, and 3. In a variation of this inconsistent pattern, the equilibrium scores on sensory conditions 5 and 6 are both within the normal range, while scores on the easier conditions 1, 2, and 3 and the composite score are abnormal. In any of these instances, the SOT is internally inconsistent, and the patient's sensory organization should be considered normal. Physiologically inconsistent results of these types occur, for example, when the patient exhibits a regular but well-controlled sway oscillation that does not increase as the task becomes more difficult, or when the patient simply exaggerates sway during the easier conditions.

An example of an internally physiologically inconsistent SOT result is shown in

TABLE 14–2.

Criteria for Judging Physiologically Inconsistent
Sensory Organization Test Results

Types of CDP* Inconsistencies	Distinguishing Characteristics
Internally inconsistent	Stability does not decline as difficulty increases
Inconsistent between test modalities	Performance results poor relative to evoked response results
Inconsistent relative to clinical status	CDP results much poorer relative to functional status

CDP, computerized dynamic posturography.

Figure 14–1. The patient in question is a 33-year-old woman with a history of minor, work-related head injury. She reports constant dizziness since the accident, and is seeking compensation. The patient either falls or scores between 50% and 75% under all sensory conditions 3 through 6. Emphasizing the extent of inconsistency, scores on all three of the condition 6 trials are equal to or better than the three condition 3 scores. The raw sway data show regular, high-frequency oscillations leading to occasional and sudden falls during some of the trials. The MCT results of this patient (not shown) are within the normal limits. The inconsistent SOT results and normal MCT results are interpreted as positive evidence that the patient is exaggerating her symptoms.

When either one or both of the conditions 5 and 6 scores are abnormal but high relative to the conditions 1, 2, and 3 scores, the SOT result is considered partially inconsistent. A partially inconsistent pattern suggests that the patient's sensory organization is either normal or mildly impaired. It further suggests, however, that the patient is exaggerating the extent of any impairment.

SOT Results Inconsistent With Other Clinical Findings

Another form of inconsistency occurs when a very poor SOT result is seen in a patient whose daily life balance and locomotor capabilities are not obviously impaired. Specifically, substantially abnormal conditions 1 and 2 scores are physiologically inconsistent when observed in a patient who is not ataxic and who ambulates without the use of balance aids. These types of results are judged inconsistent because research has shown a strong correlation between SOT findings and other clinical measures of balance system disability.[30]

Confirming an Inconsistent Result

Patients with physiologically inconsistent results can be retested after careful instructions are given to assure full cooperation. If deliberate exaggeration of symptoms is suspected, a retest can be given in which the order of sensory conditions is randomized. Based on research studies with clinically normal subjects, the retest results should be substantially similar, with no greater than 5% to 10% improvement in scores on the more difficult sensory conditions. Substantially greater variations in results between the tests can provide additional evidence for physiological inconsistency.

Abnormal SOT Results: Sensory Organization Analysis

When a patient's composite equilibrium score is in the abnormal range and there is no evidence of inconsistency, the ratio scores determined by sensory

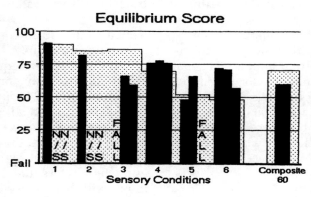

FIG 14–1.
Example of a physiologically inconsistent SOT result. The composite score is abnormal. The condition 3 scores, however, are substantially lower than the more difficult condition 6 scores, which are well within the normal range.

organization analysis are examined to identify the dysfunctional sense(s). A sense is said to be dysfunctional when the patient either cannot or does not effectively use information from the sense to maintain balance. A dysfunctional sense may be caused by loss of the associated peripheral input, disruption of CNS pathways processing the input, adaptive suppression of the input, or a combination of these factors. Figure 13–12 in Chapter 13 describes the four sensory analysis ratios and their physiological meaning. The clinical significance of the four sensory analysis ratios are summarized as follows.

Somatosensory Dysfunction

The use of the somatosensory input is reflected by the ratio between the eyes open and eyes closed equilibrium scores obtained from conditions 1 and 2. This ratio is equivalent to the classic "Romberg quotient" and is interpreted in the same manner.[42] In clinically normal subjects standing on a fixed, regular support surface, the somatosensory input dominates the control of balance under both eyes open and eyes closed conditions. Hence, a normal individual shows little if any increase in sway when the eyes are closed.[7, 10]

The patient who relies on the visual rather than somatosensory input to maintain balance under fixed surface conditions shows significantly increased sway with eye closure. Sway increases with eye closure, even if the vestibular input is functioning normally. This is because the vestibular input is not as sensitive in controlling sway as the somatosensory or visual inputs. The patient who has somatosensory dysfunction and therefore depends on vision is expected to show ataxia and instability during normal ambulation, because use of vision can be difficult when the subject is moving.

Vision Dysfunction

The ability to make effective use of the visual input to maintain balance is reflected by the ratio between the sensory conditions 4 and 1 equilibrium scores. This ratio extends the concept of the Romberg quotient to the visual system, which is isolated using a sway-referenced support surface (condition 4) to remove the useful somatosensory input. If the patient cannot or does not make effective use of vision in the absence of useful somatosensory inputs, sway increases abnormally during condition 4 testing.

Patients with visual dysfunction ambulate normally on a fixed and level support surface. The patient with vision dysfunction, however, is destabilized by compliant, irregular, and moving support surfaces.

Vestibular Dysfunction

A patient's ability to make effective use of the vestibular input is reflected by the ratio between the sensory conditions 5 and 1 equilibrium scores. Condition 5 provides the most definitive assessment of the vestibular input (see Chapter 13), because useful somatosensory inputs are disrupted by sway-referencing, and vision is removed by eye closure. The patient with vestibular dysfunction experiences instability when both the support surface and visual inputs are reduced by conditions such as darkness in conjunction with an irregular or compliant support surface.

Vision Preference

A patient's ability to suppress input from the visual system when it is available but functionally inaccurate is reflected by the ratio comparing the sum of conditions 3 and 6 with the sum of conditions 2 and 5 equilibrium scores. When functionally inaccurate (sway-referenced) visual inputs are presented, the normal individual ignores the visual input and performs as if the eyes were closed. In contrast, the patient who balances normally in the absence of vision but who prefers the conflicting visual input will be less stable under sway-referenced visual conditions 3 and 6, compared to the comparable eyes closed conditions 2 and 5 (see Chapter 13). Patients with an abnormal vision preference experience unsteadiness and disorientation in environments containing many moving visual stimuli.

Additional Information Provided by SOT Raw Data

When a patient loses balance during an SOT trial, examination of the raw sway traces can determine the type of fall. When loss of balance is the result of a free-fall, the sway trace deviates from center in one direction and at an accelerating rate as shown in Figure 14–2. The loss of balance after a corrective action is identified by one or more changes in the direction of sway prior to loss of balance.

Free-falls are associated with the most severe forms of sensory dysfunction, indicating that the patient is making little if any use of the involved sense(s). In addition, the presence of free-falls is usually a contraindication for exaggeration of symptoms, because it is

difficult for a patient to completely suppress a physiologically functional balance reaction.

The raw data also reflect certain types of technical operating errors. When a trial is prematurely stopped and marked as a fall by the operator, the sway trace remains relatively close to the centered position at the time of termination. When a tight harness or other external constraint catches a patient and prevents what would otherwise have been a loss of balance, a large and sustained offset in the horizontal shear trace documents when the patient is supported by the harness.

A recent clinical study used the raw SOT data to compute an additional quantity related to the level of effort (energy) expended by clinically normal subjects and patients with balance disorders.[29] Their results suggest that the sensitivity of the SOT is increased by identifying patients who maintain the COG within normal limits but who exert an abnormally high level of effort in doing so. When the raw sway data are

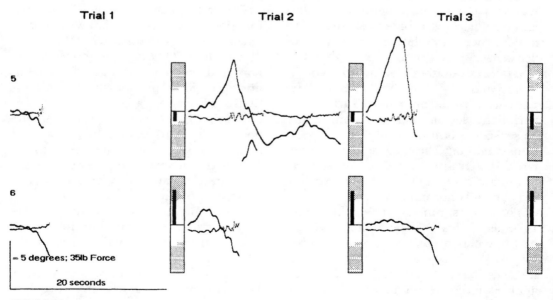

Trial 1   Trial 2   Trial 3

5

6

= 5 degrees; 35lb Force

20 seconds

FIG 14–2.

Center of gravity sway traces recorded during the SOT test. *Rows* show results recorded under one sensory test condition. *Columns* show trials one through three results for each sensory condition. *Heavy traces* show COG sway during each 20-second trial. *Fine traces* show horizontal shear forces. Under sensory condition 5, the patient free-falls on the first trial. On the second and third trials, the patient falls after attempting to regain equilibrium. Under sensory condition 6, the patient free-falls during all three trials.

inspected, patients expending the higher levels of energy at a given amplitude of sway show higher sway frequencies.

Diagnostic Significance of SOT Patterns

The most useful diagnostic information provided by the SOT is the pattern of normal and abnormal sensory organization ratios and the associated normal and abnormal equilibrium scores.[21, 37] A sensory organization analysis using the SOT ratios should not be attempted, however, whenever the results are determined to be inconsistent according to the criteria described previously. Physiologically inconsistent results in the absence of other abnormal indications invalidate the SOT analysis, because they suggest that the patient is either normal or is exaggerating symptoms of imbalance.

Vestibular Dysfunction and Vision Preference Patterns

Vestibular dysfunction patterns are seen in virtually all patients with bilateral peripheral vestibular deficits. These patients perform relatively normally under sensory conditions 1 through 4 but free-fall repeatedly under sensory conditions 5 and 6.[9, 24, 34, 35, 49, 61, 66] Similarly, patients with uncompensated unilateral peripheral lesions perform abnormally on sensory condition 5 only, or on conditions 5 and 6.* These patients may free-fall, fall after attempts to regain balance, or remain standing but score well below the clinically normal limits.

The SOT summary shown in Figure 14–3 is typical of the patient with a poorly compensated peripheral vestibular loss. Sensory analysis shows primarily vestibular dysfunction. Strategy analysis indicates an abnormal reliance on ankle movements during large amplitude sway, while the COG alignment

plot shows a bias to the left. Results of this patient's MCT (not shown) are normal in all respects. This 35-year-old woman complained of mild and intermittent spatial disorientation and unsteadiness. Results of the physical examination were normal. Vestibular function tests revealed a vestibular-ocular reflex (VOR) asymmetry consistent with unilateral loss.

Because the SOT tests the patient's ability to effectively use sensory inputs rather than the peripheral senses themselves, the vestibular dysfunction pattern does not distinguish between peripheral and central vestibular system lesions.[21] Similar vestibular dysfunction patterns are seen in patients with peripheral vestibular lesions and CNS lesions affecting central pathways of the vestibular system; for example, patients with cerebellar ataxia.[38] For similar reasons, the SOT does not detect well-compensated unilateral vestibular lesions. Patients who compensate following unilateral injuries typically return to normal SOT performance within 2 to 4 weeks of the initial insult.[8, 19, 20]

Figure 14–4 shows the vestibular dysfunction pattern of a patient with disease affecting the CNS pathways of the vestibular system. This patient shows an abnormal dependence on ankle movements during large amplitude sway, while the COG is biased forward of the center. The patient's COG alignment shows a pronounced forward leaning bias. The MCT results for this patient (not shown) are within the normal range. This 51-year-old man complained of spontaneous, episodic spells of ataxia and vertigo of mild intensity. Balance, gait, motor, and sensory functions are normal in the clinical examination. Rotary chair testing shows a VOR asymmetry and phase abnormalities, and failure of VOR suppression. Magnetic resonance imaging reveals a cerebellar disorder resulting from an Arnold Chiari malformation.

An abnormal preference for vision, either alone or in combination with vestibular dysfunction, is most frequently

*References 2, 8, 11, 14, 16, 19, 20, 26, and 54.

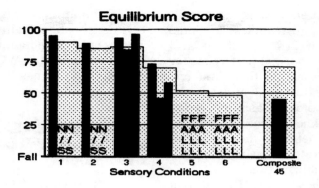

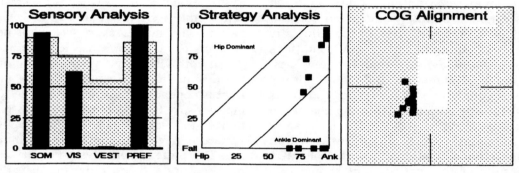

FIG 14–3.
Results of SOT of a patient with peripheral vestibular loss.

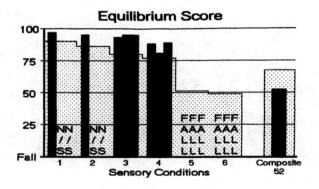

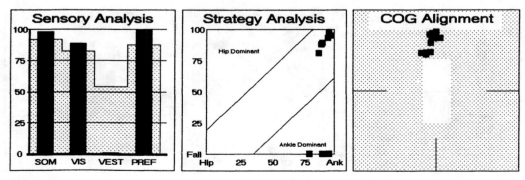

FIG 14–4.
Results of SOT in a patient with central vestibular system pathology.

observed in patients with post-traumatic vertigo and unsteadiness.[5, 6] Some elderly patients with unsteadiness also demonstrate an abnormal preference for vision, especially during their first few exposures to conditions 3 and 6.[57] Although the pathologic basis for vision preference is unknown, the above data suggest that the deficit is more likely to occur in the central processing of vestibular and visual information.

Figure 14–5 shows an SOT result of a patient with symptoms of disorientation secondary to mild head trauma. The patient scores well below the clinically normal limits under sensory conditions 3, 5, and 6. Sensory analysis shows vestibular dysfunction and an abnormal preference for vision. Strategy analysis shows the patient relying too heavily in hip motions as the amplitude of sway increases. His COG alignment is within the clinically normal limits. The MCT results of this patient (not shown) are again normal in all respects. The physi-

cal examination of this 21-year-old man reveals no abnormalities. The ENG is also normal, although rotary chair testing reveals a mild VOR phase abnormality. The diagnosis is mild post-traumatic vestibulopathy.

Vestibular and Vision or Vestibular and Somatosensory Dysfunction

A patient with two of the three senses dysfunctional exhibits what is generally called multisensory pattern.[21, 37] The patient with multisensory pattern is dependent on a single sense for balance. When both visual and vestibular inputs are dysfunctional, for example, the patient is dependent at all times on the somatosensory input for balance. This patient is unsteady whenever the support surface is irregular, compliant, or moving. The patient with dysfunctional somatosensory and vestibular inputs is dependent on vision at all times for

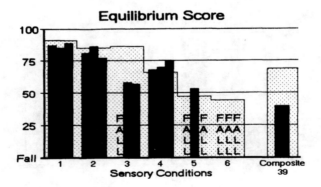

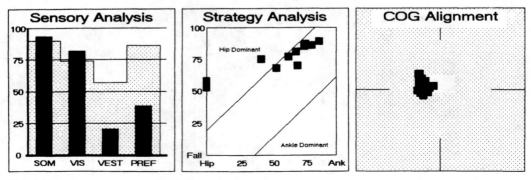

FIG 14–5.
Results of SOT in a patient with complaints of disequilibrium following head trauma.

balance, and, is unsteady whenever the visual surround is obscured or in motion.

Clinical research has shown that multisensory patterns occur principally in patients with CNS lesions extending beyond the peripheral and/or central vestibular system.[51, 55] In support of this conclusion, many patients with multisensory SOT patterns also demonstrate

prolonged MCT latencies, another CDP finding consistent with CNS pathology.[51, 55]

Figure 14–6 shows the test results of a 35-year-old male patient with somatosensory and vestibular dysfunction, and with prolonged MCT latencies. Equilibrium scores are below the clinically normal limits under sensory conditions 2, 3, 5, and 6. Sensory analysis

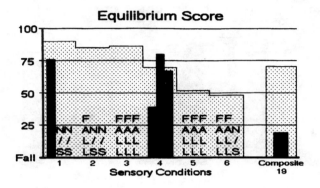

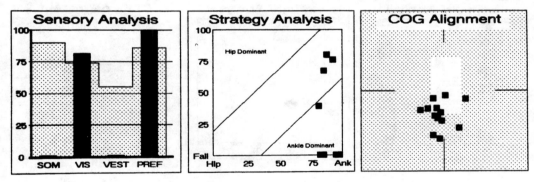

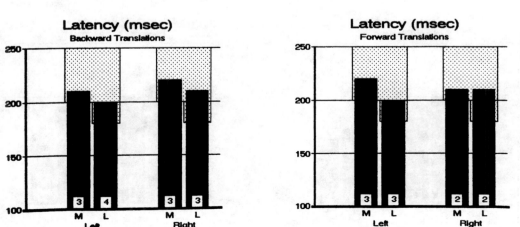

FIG 14–6.
Results of SOT and MCT testing in a patient with sensory and motor deficits following head trauma.

shows only the vision function to be normal. The patient relies almost exclusively on ankle movements. The COG alignment is within the clinically normal limits. The patient complains of both dizziness and unsteadiness following an accident-related head injury. The ENG shows unilateral vestibular weakness. The combination of a multisensory SOT pattern and abnormally prolonged MCT latencies, however, indicates that the injury extends beyond the vestibular system to include portions of the motor control pathways. This lesion could be in the spinal cord, brain stem, and/or subcortical sensorimotor areas.

Figure 14–7 shows the CDP results of a 76-year-old woman with a 2-week history of unsteadiness. The SOT results indicate a visual and vestibular

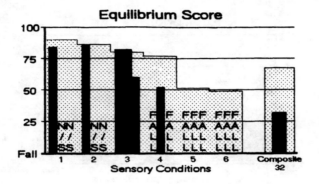

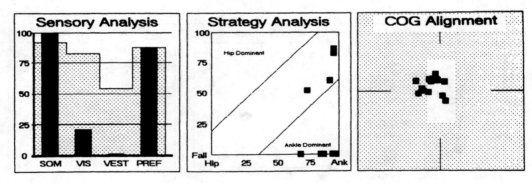

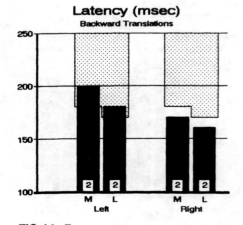

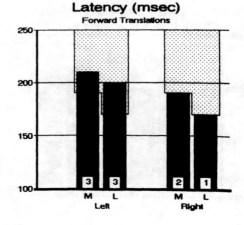

FIG 14–7.
Results of SOT in an elderly patient with unsteadiness.

dysfunction pattern, while the MCT results show prolonged latencies on the left side and borderline normal latencies on the right. This patient's ENG results are normal. This patient does have cataracts which reduce her vision, although this slowly progressive problem does not account for the recent and relatively sudden onset of unsteadiness. Additional tests are needed to rule out peripheral neuropathy as the cause of the latency prolongation although this problem is more likely to be bilateral. Peripheral neuropathy, however, is also a slowly progressive problem, and therefore will probably not account for the sudden onset of symptoms. The most likely conclusion, based on the history and unilateral latency abnormality, is a recent localized central brain stem/subcortical injury which might have been caused by a stroke.

Additional SOT Diagnostic Information Provided by Head Positioning

As described previously, the conventional SOT (performed with head facing forward) is relatively insensitive to detecting chronic, compensated unilateral peripheral vestibular disorders.[8,19] The results of three recent studies suggest that the sensitivity and specificity of the SOT in detecting unilateral compensated peripheral deficits can be significantly enhanced when the SOT is repeated with the patient's head in different positions.

In the first study, 24 patients with known unilateral vestibular lesions and 24 age-matched normal controls were retested under sensory condition 5 (sway-referenced surface and eyes closed) while the patient tilted the head 45 degrees to the left and then to the right.[58] These lateral head tilts did not affect the SOT results of the normal controls relative to the normal head position, nor did tilting the head to the side of the vestibular lesion affect the results of the patients. In the patients, however,

head tilts away from the side with the lesion reduced the SOT condition 5 scores to a 95% level of confidence. A second study of 30 normal subjects and 19 patients with unilateral vestibular deficits used a modified SOT in which subjects turned the head 45 degrees to the left or right.[60] This study reported no changes in SOT results related to the head-turned positions in the normals. In contrast, for patient's with unilateral lesions, asymmetries in SOT results related to left/right head positions were noted when the same manuevers were applied.

A third study has shown that SOT testing with backward head extension was found to significantly increase the percentage of abnormal SOT results in a group of 28 patients with chronic Meniere's disease relative to a population of normal controls tested with the head-extended position.[59, 63] While only 25% of the patients had abnormal SOT results on the conventional SOT, 86% were abnormal relative to the normal controls in the head-extended testing position.

Additional Diagnostic Information Provided by Strategy Analysis and COG Alignment

Inappropriate use of ankle and hip movements can be caused by many different types of disorders. Weakness of the ankle joint muscles, for example, limits the torsional forces that can be exerted about the ankles and forces the patient to rely on hip movements. Ankle muscle weakness is more likely to affect the tibialis anterior (dorsiflexor) and the associated forward body movements. Because the strengths of the gastrocnemius and soleus muscles (ankle plantarflexors) are determined by requirements for running and jumping, their strengths are normally many times greater than those required for balance.[24]

Loss of ankle joint mobility forces a patient to rely more heavily on hip joint movements, while loss of hip joint mobility leads to an increased reliance on ankle movements. The patient experiencing pain with movement about the ankles or hips may also alter their movement strategy to minimize movements about the affected joints. Finally, research suggests that patients who have lost sensations in the feet and ankle joints modify their patterns to rely more heavily on hip movements.[24]

Many disorders can result in lateral shifts in COG alignment. Examples include pain with weight bearing, limb weakness due to orthopedic injury, unilateral neurologic deficits affecting limb sensations and motor responses, and disease of the central vestibular system that disrupts the sense of vertical.[46] The MCT information alone may not differentiate among the other possible causes of an asymmetry in weight bearing. When localized brain stem conditions such as stroke causes a lateral shift in COG alignment, prolonged MCT latencies, reduced response strengths, or both latency and strength abnormalities are likely to occur in one of the two legs. In cases of localized brain stem disease, however, the resulting latency and strength abnormalities may occur in either leg relative to the lateral shift in COG alignment.

DIAGNOSTIC APPLICATIONS OF THE MOTOR COORDINATION TEST

Normal Vs. Abnormal MCT Latencies

A determination as to normal versus abnormal MCT latency is made separately for each leg and movement direction. When making this determination, the latencies of one leg associated with the medium and large size translations in one direction will occasionally disagree. Latency for medium translations that is in the abnormal range and the latency for large translations that is in the normal range may indicate a subtle increase in response threshold, although

this determination has not been verified by clinical trials. When only the latency associated with the large translations is in the abnormal range, the result can be considered borderline normal.

Normal versus abnormal latency scores can only be interpreted relative to the age-matched clinically normal sample when the weight bearing between the two legs is within its normal range during testing. This is because automatic response strengths can decrease in a leg bearing substantially less than half the body weight, even in healthy subjects.

Patterns of Abnormal MCT Latencies

Because the efferent spinal and brain stem pathways mediating long-loop responses are anatomically distinct for the two legs and movement directions, abnormally prolonged MCT latencies can occur in a variety of patterns. The distribution of prolonged MCT latencies can provide the following additional information relative to the location of the lesion:

1. Bilateral and bidirectional prolongations of MCT latencies are most likely the result of global CNS deficits such as polyneuropathy, neurotoxic exposure, or multiple sclerosis.

2. Unilateral prolongations of MCT latencies are indicative of localized CNS lesions, which may be peripheral (for example, orthopedic nerve abnormality) or central (for example, brain stem stroke). Weight bearing should be examined prior to interpreting these patterns, because substantial unloading of a leg can result in prolongation of what would otherwise be normal latencies.

3. Unidirectional prolongations of MCT latencies are most likely caused by CNS deficits localized to efferent branches of the long-loop system, although this has not been verified by clinical trials. This is because the muscle proprioceptor inputs responsible for trig-

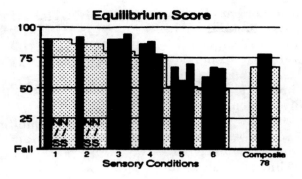

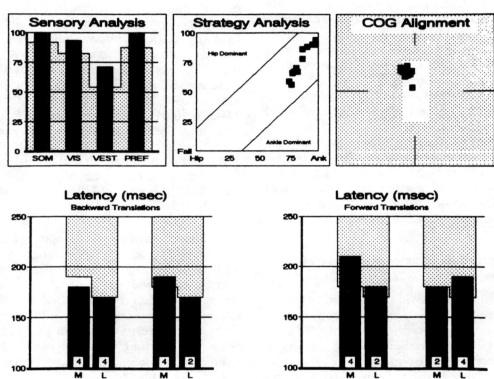

FIG 14–8.
Results of SOT and MCT in a patient suspected of being in the early stages of developing multiple sclerosis.

gering automatic responses are bidirectionally sensitive, and delay or disruption of sensory input limited to one direction of movement is unlikely.

Diagnostic Significance of Prolonged MCT Latencies

Prolonged MCT latencies are evidence for abnormality in any one or a combination of components comprising the long-loop automatic system and therefore are strong indications for nonvestibular, spinal cord, brain stem, and/or subcortical involvement.[4, 32, 41, 51, 67] Long-loop pathway components include the sensory and motor peripheral nerves, the ascending and descending sensory and motor pathways of the spinal cord, and the brain stem and subcortical sensory and motor pathways.

Peripheral neuropathy,[32] multiple sclerosis,[41] and age-related disorders[57] are commonly associated with bidirectional and bilateral prolonged MCT latencies. More localized brain stem lesions such as those associated with stroke[36] and cerebral palsy[38] commonly cause unilateral latency abnormalities, while more global brain stem disorders result in bilaterally prolonged latencies.[51] Prolonged latencies associated with orthopedic nerve injuries also have been reported, but this has not been formally verified by clinical trials. Prolonged latencies, in contrast, are not commonly associated with cerebellar deficits and Parkinson's disease,[3, 15, 23, 25] although the cerebellum and basal ganglia influence other characteristics of the automatic responses.

Figure 14–8 shows SOT and MCT results of a 35-year-old woman suspected of having very early stage multiple sclerosis. The MCT results show that the long-loop motor pathways have been selectively impaired, while the SOT results indicate normal organization and utilization of sensory inputs, movement strategies, and COG alignment.

Additional Diagnostic Information Provided by MCT Strength

Abnormalities in the strengths of automatic responses occur in patterns similar to those described for the MCT latencies. Bilateral and bidirectional strength abnormalities are more likely caused by adaptive deficits in the modulation of automatic response strengths. Large, bilateral strength elevations, for example, are observed in patients with cerebellar deficits.[23] Less dramatic bilateral elevations are seen in patients with profound bilateral vestibular losses who (presumably) increase their reliance on the alternative somatosensory input.[23]

Unilateral reductions in strength are likely in the presence of more localized CNS and orthopedic lesions. For example, patients with hemiplegia secondary to brain stem stroke show not only increased latencies but also reduced strengths on the affected side.[36]

DIAGNOSTIC APPLICATIONS OF POSTURE-EVOKED RESPONSE AND ELECTROMYOGRAPHY

Prolonged Electromyography Responses

In patients exhibiting prolonged MCT latencies, analysis of the electromyography (EMG) responses assessed by the PER protocol provides additional information that can assist one in localizing pathologic processes within the long-loop automatic pathways. Further localization is possible, because each of the three EMG components assessed by the PER is mediated by a different component of the long-loop system.[15] Table 14–3 reviews the patterns of PER results and their probable clinical interpretations.

Abnormal PER results occur in the following patterns, each of which suggests a different probable site for the CNS lesion.

1. Short latency (SL) component delays (see Chapter 13) are strongly suggestive of peripheral nerve pathology. The SL component is equivalent to the myotatic tendon reflex, based on the clinical observations that myotatic and short latency responses occur at similar latencies, and that both components are delayed in patients with known peripheral neuropathies.[15]

2. Long latency (LL) component delays are suggestive of lesions at the level of brain stem and/or subcortical pathways.[17, 18, 28] Normal SL responses and delayed medium latency and/or LL responses have been reported in patients with multiple sclerosis,[18] posterior column lesions,[17] and Huntington's disease.[51] Additional research suggests that PER and electroencephalographic scalp recordings can be combined to further isolate delays in the third component to the afferent (sensory) or the efferent (motor) branches of the long-loop system.[1]

TABLE 14–3.

Clinical Interpretation of Posture-Evoked Response Patterns

Pathology Type and Distribution	Latency Pattern		
	Short Latency	Medium Latency	Long Latency
Peripheral nerve, nerve roots L5, S1: unilateral	Prolonged unilateral	Prolonged unilateral	Normal
Polyneuropathy demylination: bilateral	Prolonged bilateral	Prolonged bilateral	Normal (occasionally prolonged)
Spinal cord, brain stem, pyramidal tract, thalamus, cortex: unilateral	Normal	Normal	Prolonged unilateral
Spinal cord, brain stem, pyramidal tracts, thalamus, cortex: bilateral	Normal	Normal	Prolonged bilateral
Multilevel: bilateral	Prolonged bilateral	Prolonged bilateral	Prolonged bilateral
Cerebellar	Normal	Normal	Normal

3. The SL and LL component delays might be caused by peripheral nerve disease alone, if the peripheral nerve disease delays the input signals to both systems. A combination of peripheral nerve and central disease, however, cannot be ruled out on the basis of this pattern.[15]

4. Results showing LL normal with SL delays can occur in patients with peripheral nerve injuries. This pattern is seen because the LL system draws on sensory inputs from a much broader range of receptor types and locations. Thus, the LL component continues to receive timely input from proximal muscles and joints less impacted by the neuropathy, while the distal muscle receptor inputs driving the SL system are delayed.

DIAGNOSTIC APPLICATIONS COMBINING CDP AND OTHER CLINICAL RESULTS

Decision Matrix for Combining Clinical Test Results

In patients exhibiting complex symptoms of disorientation and/or unsteadiness, combined use of traditional vestibular function tests and CDP aids in the differential diagnosis of peripheral and central disease.[37] Diagnostic inferences based on the combined use of such a test battery can best be described by a three-dimensional decision matrix shown in Table 14–4, where the dimensions are determined by the outcome of

1. Vestibular function tests,
2. The SOT pattern of the CDP test, and
3. The MCT latency of the CDP test

The diagnostic inferences suggested by the matrix are based on the known physiology of the balance system and the published results of the many heretofore referenced clinical studies comparing the findings from vestibular and/or neurologic function tests with those from CDP.

When the outcome on two of the three test dimensions is within normal limits and a single dimension is abnormal, it can be assumed that the deficit is within the abnormal dimension (for example, the vestibulo-ocular, sensory balance, or automatic motor system). When abnormal data are encountered on multiple dimensions, the diagnostic inferences drawn from the matrix are based on the following key assumptions which account for the possible interactions among the systems.

1. The interpretation of an inconsistent SOT pattern as indicative of normal function is modified if other abnor-

TABLE 14–4.

Diagnostic Decision Matrix for Combining Information From Computerized Dynamic Posturography (CDP) and Other Clinical Test Results

Vestibular Function Tests	CDP TEST RESULTS				
	Normal	Vestibular Dysfunction	Multisensory Dysfunction	Prolonged Latencies	Physiologically Inconsistent
Normal	Normal	Central vestibular	Central vestibular	Spinal/brain stem	Normal
Peripheral vestibular	Peripheral vestibular (compensated)	Peripheral vestibular (uncompensated)	Peripheral and central vestibular	Peripheral vestibular and spinal/brain stem	Exaggerating symptoms
Central vestibular	Central vestibular	Central vestibular	Central vestibular	Central vestibular and spinal/brain stem	Exaggerating symptoms

mal vestibular test results are found, or if inspection of the raw data indicates that the patient consistently free-falls on some of the sensory conditions. In these cases, an inconsistent SOT pattern suggests that the patient has an abnormality but is nevertheless exaggerating the symptoms.

2. In the presence of a substantial MCT latency abnormality, an inconsistent determination should not be made. This is because underlying disease within the long-loop system can distort the SOT results.

3. Evidence of a multisensory SOT pattern and/or prolonged MCT latencies modifies the interpretation of a unilateral vestibular weakness documented by ENG testing, because neither of these CDP results are commonly seen with peripheral vestibular disorders, whereas these patterns are common in patients with CNS deficits.

4. A central vestibular system problem is the most likely cause when the SOT pattern consistent with vestibular dysfunction is seen in conjunction with negative vestibular function test results. The possibility of a peripheral otolithic or vertical canal lesion, however, cannot be ruled out.

5. The presence of a well-compensated unilateral, peripheral vestibular lesion is probable when vestibular test results are abnormal and consistent with a peripheral lesion, and CDP results are within normal limits. This is because patients with well-compensated lesions typically perform normally on CDP.

Clinical Demonstration of the Decision Matrix

The validity of the decision matrix in identifying the cause of a balance disorder has been tested by conducting independent clinical and CDP evaluations on a diverse group of 96 patients (mean age 51 ± 21 years), all of whose symptoms included balance disorders.[36] The patient sample included those with stroke, mild to moderate head injury, and vestibular system disorder. Results of CDP, the physical examination, and other neurologic and vestibular tests were interpreted independently and then correlated.

All patients could stand independently for periods of 1 minute or more and had no biomechanical or orthopedic injuries that might confound the CDP results. The clinical evaluation included ocular motility, visual acuity, Romberg, rotary chair, sensory/motor neurologic tests, and gait assessment.

Patients were grouped into three categories of abnormality based on the clini-

TABLE 14–5.

Correlations (%) Between Computerized Dynamic Posturography and Clinical Examination Results in 96 Patients With a Combination of Vestibular System and Central Nervous System Deficits*

Abnormal Systems Identified by Clinical Examination	Patient Category According to Posturography		
	% Abnormal Sensory Organization (normal movement results) (n = 57)	% Movement Latency Delay/Lateral Asymmetry (± sensory organization) (n = 17)	% Normal Sensory and Movement Results (n = 24)
Peripheral/central vestibular only	91	18	38
Brain stem/spinal cord/peripheral nerves (± vestibular)	3	82	10
Normal and uncertain	6	0	52

*Each patient was placed into one of three clinical categories based on clinical examination results, and independently placed into one of three CDP categories based on the posturography results. Numbers of patients in each CDP category are shown in the column headings. Percentages under each CDP category show the numbers of patients who fell into each of the three indicated clinical categories.

cal results: peripheral/central vestibular, brain stem/spinal cord CNS, and normal. The CDP categories included abnormal SOT only, prolonged latencies (unilateral or bilateral), and normal. The results tabulated in Table 14–5 showed a good correlation between the clinical and CDP categories. A substantial majority of patients with abnormal SOT results only (91%) had vestibular system disease. In contrast, a substantial majority of patients with prolonged latencies (82%) had brain stem/spinal cord disorders. Among the patients with normal CDP results, the majority (52%) also were clinically normal. Of those who were not clinically normal (38%), the majority had compensated peripheral vestibular abnormalities which were usually not detected by CDP.

CDP APPLICATIONS IN PREDICTING TREATMENT OUTCOME

Importance of Higher Level Adaptive Functions

Understanding a patient's higher level adaptive function is critical to predicting the outcome of a particular treatment approach, whether the treatment includes surgery, drugs, physical therapy, or a combination of approaches. This is be-

cause adaptation and motor learning are a primary means by which a patient optimizes performance in the presence of both temporary and irreversible changes in the nervous system. Of course, other factors extending beyond the scope of this chapter also must be considered before undertaking treatment. These include the following: (1) the probable course of the disease process; (2) the presence of other exacerbating conditions; and (3) the patient's lifestyle and treatment expectations.

The purpose of some CDP tests is to provide information relative to the patient's higher level adaptive function. These tests are designed to quantify the impact of a balance disorder on the patient's ability to perform daily life tasks, and to determine the patient's ability to develop compensatory strategies for improving performance. Tests of adaptive functions are generally less useful in the diagnostic process, because correlations between specific forms of disease and higher level adaptive functions are either unknown or poorly understood at the present time.[16, 49]

The process of predicting the outcome of a treatment approach usually is very complex, because balance capabilities are influenced by the interactions of multiple components and adaptive strategies, and because the correlations between any known disorder and the nature and extent of the individual's functional balance disability are frequently weak. In some cases, consideration of all the factors can lead to an adequate understanding of the patient's problem in advance of treatment. In other cases, the patient's underlying disease is never well understood. In either case, a treatment aimed at reducing symptoms and improving performance must be undertaken if possible.[12, 22, 44, 45, 47]

Higher Level Adaptive Information Provided by CDP

Vision Preference Pattern

In the patient with an abnormal preference for vision, none of the three senses are dysfunctional. The first three sensory ratios shown in Figure 13-12 of Chapter 13 are within the normal range, indicating normal performance under sensory conditions 2, 4, and 5. Rather, the patient has an adaptive problem determining when to ignore the visual balance information as indicated by the fourth sensory ratio. Scores are below the normal range under the sway referenced visual conditions 3 and 6 relative to the equivalent eyes closed conditions 2 and 5. Thus, when visual information is functionally useful (for example, a fixed and visible surround), the patient makes effective use of vision and balances normally even when somatosensory inputs are disrupted. Alternatively, however, the patient, uses the visual input when it provides erroneous balance information.

Movement Strategy

Factors that can render a patient incapable of producing a movement pattern already have been described. Most patients with balance problems are physically capable of performing the necessary body movement patterns. However, under some conditions, patients in this latter group select body movement patterns that are inefficient or ineffective for maintaining balance.

The strategy analysis plot described in Figure 13-11 can assist in the identification of patients who select inefficient or ineffective strategies, and can help the examiner determine the conditions under which inappropriate selections occur.

A normal individual moves primarily about the ankles when sway amplitudes are well within the limits of stability (see Chapter 12), and increases the use of hip movement as sway approaches the limits of stability. Balance movements are ineffective in the patient who uses ankle strategy movements to control large amplitude sway displacements. The patient dependent on ankle movements falls prematurely when sway amplitudes are large. The patient using hip movements to control small amplitude sway is inefficient and expends a needlessly high level of energy to maintain a centered COG position.

Center of Gravity Alignment

A normal individual maintains the COG very nearly centered over the base of support. Although sway increases significantly during the more difficult sensory conditions, these individuals continue to maintain the COG alignment near the center. The patient whose COG is maintained forward, backward, or to one side of the center of the base of support cannot tolerate larger COG displacements in the direction of the misalignment without losing balance. For example, smaller dynamic movements in the backward direction will move the patient to the limits of stability when the COG is aligned substantially backward from the center.

Motor Response Strength

Abnormally weak automatic responses can be caused by reduced ankle muscle mass or by neuromuscular deficits affecting these muscles. When the weakness is unilateral, the cause is more likely to be musculoskeletal or neuromuscular. In the patient with a balance disorder, however, automatic responses are more frequently bilaterally reduced by central adaptive changes in the modulation of strength. A central adaptive change in modulation is always the cause when the automatic responses are abnormally strong or when patients such as those with Parkinson's disease fail to appropriately scale response strength in relation to the stimulus.[64] The MCT response strength plots shown in Figure 13–5 of Chapter 13 quantify whether the patient's automatic responses are appropriately scaled to return the COG to the centered position without excessive undershoot (weakness) or overshoot (overly strong) following perturbations of the support surface.

Response Adaptation

The response adaptation test is designed to determine whether the patient can suppress automatic responses to support surface inputs under conditions in which they have a disruptive rather than stabilizing influence. Patients who are unable to suppress automatic responses are more likely to experience difficulties with balance when walking over irregular surfaces and when walking or standing on an unstable surface.

Patients can exhibit a number of types of abnormal adaptation patterns. Some patients are destabilized on the early trials but adapt into the normal range by the fifth trial. Other patients show high sway energy scores and no adaptation across the five trials. Still other patients show a normal adaptation curve but with all scores biased above the normal range.

Clinical Example: Predicting the Outcome of Vestibular Nerve Section

An acute unilateral loss of vestibular function frequently causes periods of nausea, dizziness, and unsteadiness. After several weeks, however, the typical patient with a stable lesion compensates and the symptoms diminish. Compensation may not occur when the status of the lesion fluctuates, or when additional complications prevent adaptation. When compensation fails to occur, therapeutic surgery may be considered to either repair the affected ear or interrupt the signals from the ear.

Most types of vestibular system disorders are not reversible with surgery. Sectioning the vestibular nerve is therapeutic when the input from an organ providing conflicting and inappropriate motion signals is eliminated. Conflicting motion signals prevent the patient from using other sensory inputs and prevents adaptation. If all other components of the balance system are functioning normally, removal of the conflicting signals allows an otherwise normal system to compensate.

The challenge to the clinician considering an irreversible vestibular nerve section, however, is to predict whether or not the patient will compensate once the disruptive signals are removed. Two recent studies of patients undergoing vestibular nerve section suggest that preoperative CDP results may help predict the extent to which improvements in symptoms can be expected following vestibular nerve section.

In the first study of 24 patients undergoing vestibular nerve sections, 20 (83%) of 24 showed CDP results in the normal range during the preoperative assessment.[13] Following an early period of compensation in which approximately half of the patients tested within 7 days of surgery displayed the vestibular dysfunction pattern in the SOT, 18 (90%) of 20 of preoperatively normal group showed a return to normal SOT results during long-term follow-up testing. In contrast, of the patients with abnormal preoperative SOT results, 3 (75%) of the 4 displayed abnormal SOT results during follow-up testing 3 to 20 months after surgery.

The second study examined the long-term recovery of 14 patients following unilateral vestibular nerve sections using both VOR and CDP tests.[8] The recovery of eye movement and postural functions followed separate time courses, suggesting that both systems must be examined to understand the mechanisms of compensation. In agreement with the first study, most patients showed vestibular dysfunction patterns in the SOT during the immediate post-operative period, while 11 (78%) of 14 displayed SOT results in the normal range after 3 to 30 months. Of the 3 patients with abnormal SOT results after 3 to 30 months, 2 (66%) of 3 had shown abnormal preoperative SOT results.

In the latter two studies, patients with normal adaptive capabilities would be expected to have normal preoperative CDP results. In the first study, a majority of the patients had Meniere's disease, a condition resulting in a fluctuating deficit. Typically, Meniere's patients adapt and show normal balance function or only mild CDP deficits during periods of remission. In the second study, 10 patients had Meniere's or hydrops and the remaining 4 had acoustic neuromas, which cause very slow progressive changes in vestibular function. Typically, because of the slow tumor development, patients with early-stage neuromas adapt and do not show CDP deficits.

Based on these findings, one can conclude that patients with Meniere's disease or acoustic neuroma who show abnormal preoperative CDP results are more likely to have problems with central adaptation, whereas normal preoperative CDP results during periods of remission are a strong indication of normal adaptive capability. Furthermore, patients with defects in central adaptation are more likely to experience problems adapting following surgery.

A cautionary note is necessary, however, before extending this conclusion to other patient populations. In some populations, an abnormal CDP result is expected in the well-adapted patient. For example, in the patient with a bilateral vestibular deficit, a vestibular dysfunction pattern is expected. In well-adapted patient populations with abnormal CDP patterns, it is necessary to show addi-tional CDP abnormalities suggestive of abnormal adaptation. Additional findings suggestive of an adaptive deficit might include multisensory SOT patterns, inappropriate movement strategies, and/or response adaptation abnormalities.

CDP APPLICATIONS IN PHYSICAL THERAPY

Patients Likely to Benefit From Physical Therapy

Physical therapy focused on improving dysfunctional components of balance can have a positive impact on the overall performance capabilities of patients with dizziness and/or unsteadiness. Patients likely to benefit from physical therapy are identified by the history, diagnosis, psychologic profile, and other lifestyle factors. A thorough description of the positive indications for balance physical therapy have not been articulated fully, because this is a relatively new approach (see Chapter 18). However, the evidence to date, suggests that the elderly with balance problems,[44] vestibular deficit patients with symptoms of dizziness and unsteadiness,[22, 47, 48, 50, 62, 68] and those with brain injuries due to trauma and stroke[46] are among the appropriate candidates who can benefit from physical therapy specialized to treat the specific functional problems of the individual.

Setting Goals for Physical Therapy

Once the decision has been made to treat a patient with physical therapy, additional information is needed to identify which of the patient's functions can be improved by therapy and which are best managed by adjusting the patient's lifestyle and expectations. This is because preliminary clinical research indicates that balance therapy focused on the specific functional problems of the patient is more effective than generalized balance conditioning.[12, 22, 44, 45, 47] For example, a normally sighted person making ineffective use of vision or having an abnormal preference for vision under conflict conditions oftentimes can be trained to make more effective use of vision. A patient with profound bilateral loss of vestibular dysfunction, in contrast, cannot regain the vestibular balance capability and must be counseled to avoid environments with inadequate lighting and unstable surfaces.

Many of the component functions assessed by CDP are amenable to physical therapy, while others are unlikely to be affected. The following describes the CDP findings that suggest that physical therapy can be beneficial.

Vestibular Dysfunction and/or Vision Preference

Patients with these abnormal SOT patterns gain improvement from physical therapy, depending on the diagnosis of the underlying disorder.[22, 48, 50, 62, 68] In patients with profound bilateral loss of vestibular function, physical therapy cannot be used to restore normal balance in the absence of useful visual and somatosensory inputs. Physical therapy, in contrast, can be a primary mode of treatment in patients with vestibular dysfunction patterns caused by incomplete compensation for partial peripheral and/or central vestibular system lesions. Physical therapy is also a useful adjunct when drugs or surgery are also used to treat these latter conditions.

Multisensory Disorders With and Without Prolonged Latencies

Vestibular and vision dysfunction, vestibular and somatosensory dysfunction, and either of these patterns combined with prolonged MCT latencies are all indicative of additional CNS pathology which may or may not be documented by other clinical tests (see for example, reference 54). Although clinical studies to substantiate the experiences of these patients are incomplete, anecdotal evidence suggests that the prognosis for improvement with physical therapy may be more limited, especially when the MCT latencies are also prolonged.

Physiologically Inconsistent

Inconsistent results in the absence of other clinical findings suggest that the patient's balance is physiologically normal but is impaired either by intense anxiety or by deliberate exaggeration of the symptoms. In the presence of other clinical findings, an inconsistent SOT pattern suggests that the patient's balance problems are aggravated by anxiety or exaggeration. A diagnosis of exaggerated symptoms is further substantiated in patients who refuse to cooperate with physical therapy. If the patient improves with therapy, deliberate exaggeration may be ruled out, although the actual cause might never be determined.

Inappropriate Movement Strategy

Ineffective use of movement strategies may be caused by an abnormal adaptation or by an inability to produce one of the two movement patterns. Inappropriate use of hip movements during small amplitude sway, for example, might be an abnormal adaptation caused by anxiety or misperception of the limits of stability. In these cases, training aimed at teaching the appropriate conditions for using ankle movements can have a positive impact. In contrast, weakness of ankle joint muscles, loss of ankle sensation, reduced mobility about the ankles, or combinations of these factors prevent the patient from generating effective ankle movements and are contraindications for movement strategy training, unless the underlying physiologic factors are also addressed.

Inappropriate use of ankle movements during large amplitude sway might be an abnormal adaptation used to minimize head movements and associated stimulation of the vestibular system. When inappropriate use of ankle movement is an abnormal adaptation, training is likely to have a positive effect. Contraindications to teaching appropriate use of hip movements might include weakness or loss of mobility about the hip joints. There is also clinical evidence suggesting that patients with profound bilateral loss of peripheral vestibular function cannot effectively coordinate hip movements and that training is ineffective.[49]

Center of Gravity Alignment

A displaced COG increases the risk for falls, especially when displacement is in the backward direction. Like inappropriate movement strategies, abnormal COG alignment can be the result of either an abnormal adaptation or an underlying musculoskeletal deficit. When there are no deficits preventing normal COG alignment, biofeedback therapy in which the patient's COG position is displayed relative to the LOS can be successful in teaching patients to monitor their COG position.[46] Examples of disorders inhibiting normal COG alignment include muscular weakness or contractures and orthopedic disorders.

Response Adaptation

Patients with response adaptation abnormalities tend to make inappropriate use of somatosensory input for balance when the support surface is irregular or moving. Failure to suppress functionally inappropriate input from the destabilized support surface is commonly seen in individuals of advanced age[27, 57] and may indicate an abnormal adaptation, a central disorder, or loss of mobility at the ankle joints. Relatively little has been documented regarding the physiologic basis and the treatment of this component of balance control.

APPLICATIONS OF CDP IN DISABILITY AND RISK ASSESSMENT

The Elderly

While many factors contribute to loss of mobility in the elderly, impaired balance is an important component.[39, 56] In addition, fall-related injury is a major cause for morbidity in this age group. Due to the prevalence of balance and mobility disorders which have a major negative impact on their quality of life and independence,[52] the elderly are an appropriate population for fall risk assessment and intervention.

While aging can affect a wide range of factors contributing to abnormal balance, including the biomechanical, musculoskeletal, and sensorimotor systems, recent evidence suggests that the ability to adapt quickly to unexpected conditions and challenges provides a sensitive indication for the risk of impending falls.[31, 43, 57, 65] Recent clinical results suggest that certain elements of CDP can be appropriate objective tools for assessing the potential impact of impaired balance on safe mobility in the elderly. Recent results further indicate that physical therapy training can improve substantially balance function, even in the advanced elderly.[31]

Occupations Requiring Exceptional Balance Skills

Assessment of balance function can be a major challenge in occupations such as commercial and military flying, both of which require exceptional spatial orientation and coordination skills. Given the time and expense of training pilots, methods are being sought to more quickly identify those unlikely to qualify. Similarly, when a qualified pilot develops a medical problem involving the balance system, accurate information is needed to determine when, and if, the individual should return to work.

To date, no standards have been established for occupational assessment of balance. However, recent investigations indicate that the more stressful and life-like balance function tests (particularly those requiring subjects to perform in a variety of tasks and environments) do provide an accurate and objective measure of the individual's overall performance capabilities. For example, a recent retrospective study of the Royal Danish Air Force concluded that the vestibular autorotation test is more sensitive than the traditional caloric test in setting minimum vestibular function test standards for high-performance pilots.[53] Similarly, the SOT protocol of CDP consistently shows the inability of astronauts to suppress inappropriate visual cues to balance during the early phases of re-adaptation after prolonged exposure to zero-gravity and zero-gravity simulator conditions.[40] Military pilots who are required to suppress vestibular cues and rely on vision during high performance maneuvers also tended to not suppress inappropriate visual cues during the SOT.[69] In addition, the results of the SOT component correlates well with the Dizziness Handicap Inventory results in patients with documented balance disorders.[30]

Medical-Legal Cases Involving Balance Disorders

Medical-legal cases involving complaints of unsteadiness and/or dizziness can be very difficult to settle equitably, because there are no well-established correlations between the traditional hard clinical signs of disease and the actual extent of a patient's symptoms and functional impairment. While suspicion that the patient is exaggerating symptoms for secondary gain is raised by negative results on the classic clinical tests, these tests provide only indirect circumstantial evidence. That is, they are not based on the patient's functional capabilities in an interactive test situation. Thus, the information gained from CDP can be of significant assistance in two ways. First, CDP test protocols provide an objective assessment of the patient's balance function that can be related to their capabilities in daily life. Second, when CDP results are physiologically inconsistent, they can provide positive evidence for exaggeration of symptoms.

CONCLUSIONS

Balance is a complex process involving the integration of multiple biomechanical, sensory, muscular, and neural components. In a few instances, a patient's imbalance is caused by the lack of responses which, in turn, can be traced to disruption of a specific function, such as a bilateral peripheral vestibular loss. In the majority of cases, however, balance problems are complex, chronic, and are provoked only under specific conditions. Complex balance problems usually result from the patient's adopting an inappropriate or maladaptive strategy rather than an absence of one or more responses. In these later cases, diagnosis and treatment of the primary disorder does not assure that the patient's symptoms and performance problems will be improved.

The model of human posture control presented in Chapter 12, and the methodologies used to measure balance and clinically interpret the results presented in Chapter 13, provide a means to identify the principle sensorimotor abnormalities affecting balance. Additionally, this information may be used to design and monitor treatment protocols aimed at improving the patient's functional capabilities and enhancing his or her quality of life.

REFERENCES

1. Ackermann H, Diener HC, Dichgans J: Mechanically evoked cerebral potentials and long-latency muscle responses in the evaluation of afferent and efferent long-loop pathways in humans. *Neurosci Lett* 1986; 66:233–238.

2. Asai M, Watanabe Y, Ohashi N, et al: Clinical evaluation of the EquiTest system in peripheral vestibular patients, in Brandt T, Paulus W, Bles W, et al. (eds): *Disorders of Posture and Gait.* New York, Georg Thieme, 1990, pp 202–205.

3. Beckley DJ, Bloem BR, van Dijk JG, et al: Electrophysiological correlates of postural instability in Parkinson's disease. *Electroencephalogr Clin Neurophysiol* 1991; 81:263–268.

4. Beckley DJ, Bloem BR, Remler MP: The effect

of perturbation size and cognitive set on long latency response in Parkinson patients, in Agnoli A (ed): *European Conference on Parkinson's Disease and Extrapyramidal Disorders.* Rome, John Libbey, 1991, pp 507–512.

5. Black FO, Nashner LM: Vestibulospinal control differs in patients with reduced versus distorted vestibular function. *Acta Otolaryngol* 1984; 406:110–114.

6. Black FO, Nashner LM: Postural control in four classes of vestibular abnormalities, in Igarashi M, Black FO (eds): *Vestibular and Visual Control of Posture and Locomotor Equilibrium.* Basel, S Karger, 1985; pp 271–281.

7. Black FO, Shupert CL, Horak FB, et al: Abnormal postural control associated with peripheral vestibular disorders, in Pompeiano O, Allum JHJ (eds): *Progress in Brain Research*, vol 76. New York; Elsevier, 1988, pp 263–276.

8. Black FO, Shupert C, Peterka RJ, et al: Effects of unilateral loss of vestibular function on the vestibulo-ocular reflex and posture control. *Ann Otol Rhinol Laryngol* 1989; 98:884–889.

9. Black FO, Wall III C, Nashner LM: Effect of visual and support surface references upon postural control in vestibular deficit subjects. *Acta Otolaryngol* 1983; 95:199–210.

10. Black FO, Wall III C, Rockette HE, et al: Normal subject postural sway during the Romberg test. *Am J Otolaryngol* 1982; 3:309–318.

11. Bowman CA, Mangham CA: Clinical use of moving platform posturography. *Semin Hear* 1989; 10:161–170.

12. Brandt T, Daroff RB: Physical therapy for benign paroxysmal positional vertigo. *Arch Otolaryngol* 1980; 106:484–485.

13. Cass SP, Kartush JM, Graham MD: Clinical assessment of postural stability following vestibular nerve section. *Laryngoscope* 1991; 101:1056–1059.

14. Cyr DG, Moore GF, Moller CG: Clinical application of computerized dynamic posturography. *ENTechnology* 1989; 9:36–47.

15. Dichgans J, Diener HC: Clinical evidence for functional compartmentalization of the cerebellum; in Bloedel JR, Dichgans J, Precht W (eds): *Cerebellar Functions.* New York, Springer-Verlag, 1985, pp 126–147.

16. Dichgans J, Diener HC: The contribution of vestibulospinal mechanisms to the maintenance of human upright posture. *Acta Otolaryngol* (in press).

17. Diener HC, Dichgans J, Bacher M, et al: Characteristic alterations of long-loop "reflexes" in patients with Friedreich's disease and late atrophy of the cerebellar anterior lobe. *J Neurol Neurosurg Psychiatry* 1984; 47:679–685.

18. Diener HC, Dichgans J, Hulser P-J, et al: The significance of delayed long-loop responses to ankle displacement for the diagnosis of multiple sclerosis. *Electroencephalogr Clin Neurophysiol* 1984; 57:336–342.

19. Fetter M, Diener HC, Dichgans J: Recovery of postural control after an acute unilateral vestibular lesion in humans. *J Vestibular Res* 1991; 1:373–383.

20. Goebel JA, Paige GD: Dynamic posturography and caloric test results in patients with and without vertigo. *Otolaryngol Head Neck Surg* 1989; 100:553–558.

21. Hamid MA, Hughs GB, Kinny SE: Specificity and sensitivity of dynamic posturography: A retrospective analysis. *Acta Otolaryngol [Suppl]* 1991; 481:596–600.

22. Herdman SJ: Management of balance disorders in vestibular deficiency. *Rehab Management* 1991; 4:68–73.

23. Horak FB: Comparison of cerebellar and vestibular loss on scaling of postural responses, in Brandt T, Paulus W, Bles W, et al. (eds): *Disorders of Posture and Gait.* New York, Georg Thieme, 1990, pp 370–373.

24. Horak FB, Nashner LM, Diener HC: Postural strategies associated with somatosensory and vestibular loss. *Exp Brain Res* 1990; 82:167–177.

25. Horak FB, Nutt JG, Nashner LM: Postural dyscoordination in Parkinsonian subjects. *J Neurol Sci* (in press).

26. Horak FB, Shumway-Cook A, Crowe TK, et al: Vestibular function and motor proficiency of children with impaired hearing, or with learning disability and motor impairment. *Dev Med Child Neurol* 1988; 30:64–79.

27. Horak FB, Shupert CL, Mirka A: Components of postural dyscontrol in the elderly: A review. *Neurobiol Aging* 1989; 10:727–738.

28. Huttunen J, Homberg V: EMG responses in leg muscles to postural perturbations in Huntington's disease. *J Neurol Neurosurg Psychiatry* 1990; 53:55–62.

29. Jackson RT, Epstein CM, Boyette JE: Enhancement of posturography testing with head tilt and energy measurements. *Am J Otol* 1991; 12:420–425.

30. Jacobson GP, Newman CW, Hunter L, et al: Balance function test correlates of the dizziness handicap inventory. *J Am Acad Audiol* 1991; 2:253–260.

31. Ledin T, Kronhed AC, Moller C, et al: Effects of balance training in elderly evaluated by clinical tests and dynamic posturography. *J Vestibular Res* 1991; 1:129–138.

32. Ledin T, Odkvist LM, Vrethem M, et al: Dynamic posturography in assessment of polyneuropathic disease. *J Vestibular Res* 1991; 1:123–128.

33. McCabe BF, Ryu JH: *Vestibular Physiology in Understanding the Dizzy Patient.* Washington DC, American Academy of Otolaryngology Head and Neck Surgery, 1987.

34. Mirka A, Black FO: Clinical application of dynamic posturography for evaluating sensory integration and vestibular dysfunction, in Arenberg IK, Smith DB (eds): *Neurologic Clinics: Diagnostic Neurotology.* Philadelphia, WB Saunders, 1990, pp 351–359.

35. Nashner LM, Black FO, Wall C: Adaptation to altered support and visual conditions during stance: Patients with vestibular deficits. *J Neurosci* 1982; 2:536–544.

36. Nashner LM, Friedman J, Wusteney E: Dynamic posturography assessment of patients with peripheral and central vestibular system deficits: Correlations with results from other clinical tests. Uppsala, Sweden, Barany Society Abstracts, 1988.

37. Nashner LM, Peters JF: Dynamic posturography in the diagnosis and management of dizziness and balance disorders, in Arenberg IK, Smith DB (eds): *Neurologic Clinics: Diagnostic Neurotology.* Philadelphia, WB Saunders, 1990, pp 331–349.

38. Nashner LM, Shumway-Cook A, Marin O: Stance posture control in selected groups of children with cerebral palsy: Deficits in sensory organization and muscular coordination. *Exp Brain Res* 1983; 197:393–409.

39. Overstall PW, Exton-Smith AN, Imms FJ, et al: Falls in the elderly related to postural imbalance. *Br Med J* 1977; 1:261–264.

40. Paloski WH, Reschke MF, Doxey DD, et al: Neurosensory adaptation associated with postural ataxia following spaceflight, in Woollacott M, Horak F (eds): *Posture and Gait: Control Mechanisms vol I.* Eugene, University of Oregon Books, 1992, pp 311–314.

41. Panzer VP, Smith ME, Martin R, et al: Functional evaluation of clinical status in multiple sclerosis. *Neurology* 1992; 42(S3):446.

42. Paulus W, Straube A, Brandt T: Visual postural performance after loss of somatosensory and vestibular function. *J Neurol Neurosurg Psychiatry* 1987; 50:1542–1545.

43. Peterka RJ, Black FO: Age-related changes in human posture control: Sensory organization tests. *J Vestibular Res* 1990; 1:73–85.

44. Shepard NT: The clinical use of dynamic posturography in the elderly. *Ear Nose Throat J* 1989; 68:940–957.

45. Shepard NT, Telian SA: Balance disorders (the dizzy patient), in Jacobson JT, Northern (eds): *Diagnostic Audiology.* Austin, Tex, Pro Ed, 1991, pp 267–294.

46. Shumway-Cook A, Anson D, Haller S: Postural sway biofeedback: Its effect on reestablishing stance stability in hemiplegic patients. *Arch Phys Med Rehabil* 1988; 69:395–400.

47. Shumway-Cook A, Horak FB: Vestibular rehabilitation: An exercise approach to managing symptoms of vestibular dysfunction. *Semin Hear* 1989; 10:196–209.

48. Shumway-Cook A, Horak FB: Vestibular rehabilitation: an exercise approach to managing symptoms of vestibular dysfunction. *Neurol Clin North Am* 1990; 8:444–457.

49. Shupert CL, Black FO, Horak FB, et al: Coordination of head and body in response to support surface translations in normals and patients with bilaterally reduced vestibular function, in Amblard B, Berthoz A, Clarac F (eds): *Posture and Gait: Development, Adaptation and Modulation.* New York, Elsevier, 1988, pp 281–289.

50. Smith-Wheelock M, Shepard NT, Telian SA: Physical therapy program for vestibular rehabilitation. *Am J Otol* 1991; 12:218–225.

51. Tian J-R, Herdman SJ, Zee DS, Folstein SE: Postural instability in patients with Huntington's disease. *Neurology* 1992; 42:1232–1238.

52. Tinetti M, Speechley M, Ginter SF: Risk factors for falls among elderly persons living in the community. *N Engl J Med* 1988; 319:1701–1707.

53. Vesterhauge S, Mansson A: The vestibular autorotation test (VAT): Its application in Danish aviation medicine, in Haid CT (ed): *Vestibulare Diagnosis and Neuro-Otosurgical Management of the Skull Base.* Grateifing, Demeter, 1991.

54. Voorhees RL: The role of dynamic posturography in neurotologic diagnosis. *Laryngoscope* 1989; 99:995–1001.

55. Voorhees RL: Dynamic posturography findings in central nervous system disorders. *Otolaryngol Head Neck Surg* 1990; 103:96–101.

56. Wolfson L, Whipple R, Amerman P, et al: Stressing the postural response: A quantitative method for testing balance. *J Am Geriatr Soc* 1986; 34:845–850.

57. Wolfson L, Whipple R, Derby C, et al: A dynamic posturography study of balance in healthy elderly. *Neurology* (in press).

58. Barin K, Seitz CM, Welling DB. Effect of head orientation on the diagnostic sensitivity of posturography in patients with compensated unilateral lesions. *Otolaryngol Head Neck Surg* 1992; 106:355–362.

59. Epstein CM, Jackson RT: Head extension and sway in normal volunteers, in Woollacott M, Horak F (eds): *Posture and Gait: Control Mechanisms, vol I.* Eugene, University of Oregon Books, 1992, pp 171–174.

60. Fox CR, Paige GD: Effect of head orientation on human postural stability following unilateral vestibular ablation. *J Vestib Res* 1992; 1: 153–160.

61. Freyss G, Semont A, Vitte E, et al: Dynamic body stabilization: EquiTest system in patients with bilateral vestibular caloric areflexia, in Woollacott M, Horak F (eds): *Posture and Gait: Control Mechanisms vol I.* Eugene, University of Oregon Books, 1992, pp 292–295.

62. Horak FB, Jones-Rycewicz C, Black FO, Effects of vestibular rehabilitation on dizziness and imbalance. *Otolaryngol Head Neck Surg* (in press).

63. Jackson RT, Epstein CM: Posturography patterns in Meniere's disease, in Woollacott M, Horak F (eds): *Posture and Gait: Control Mechanisms, vol I.* Eugene, University of Oregon Books, 1992, pp 300–303.

64. Nutt JG, Horak FB, Frank JS: Scaling of postural responses in Parkinson's disease, in Woollacott M, Horak F (eds): *Posture and Gait: Control Mechanisms, vol II.* Eugene, University of Oregon Books, 1992, pp 4–7.

65. Panzer VP, Kaye J, Edner A, et al: Standing postural control in the elderly and very elderly, in Woollacott M, Horak F (eds): *Posture and Gait: Control Mechanisms, vol II.* Eugene, University of Oregon Books, 1992, pp 220–223.

66. Parker SW, Krebs DE, Gill KM, et al: Varying sway-referencing gain to quantify measurement of standing balance in patients with bilateral vestibular hypofunction, in Woollacott M, Horak F (eds): *Posture and Gait: Control Mechanisms, vol I.* Eugene, University of Oregon Books, 1992, pp 315–318.

67. Pratt CA, Horak FB, Herndon RM: Differential effects of somatosensory and motor system deficits on postural dyscontrol in multiple sclerosis, in Woollacott M, Horak F (eds): *Posture and Gait: Control Mechanisms, vol II.* Eugene, University of Oregon Books, 1992, pp 118–121.

68. Rycewicz C, Horak FB, Shumway-Cook A, Comparisons of exercises and medication for the treatment of peripheral vestibular dysfunction, in Woollacott M, Horak F (eds): *Posture and Gait: Control Mechanisms, vol II.* Eugene, University of Oregon Books, 1992, pp 419–422.

69. Vitte E, Diard JP, Freyss M, et al: Dynamic posturography: EquiTest in evaluation of pilots aptitudes, in Woollacott M, Horak F (eds): *Posture and Gait: Control Mechanisms, vol I.* Eugene, University of Oregon Books, 1992, pp 246–251.

PART V

Special Issues

CHAPTER 15

Medical and Surgical Treatment of Vertigo

Michael J. LaRouere, M.D.

Michael D. Seidman, M.D.

Jack M. Kartush, M.D.

Vertigo is a term used to describe a sensation of motion. The patient suffering from vertigo often uses the term "dizzy" to describe this sensation. Dizziness can also refer to such feelings as lightheadedness, unsteadiness, confusion, giddiness, or nausea. It is the purpose of this chapter to discuss the medical and surgical treatments of vertigo.

The prevalence of vertigo is difficult to ascertain. Disequilibrium has been found to be the first or second most common diagnosis in the short-stay hospital diagnosis related groups (DRGs), with an average hospital stay of 4 days.[120] In 1984, the National Health Interview Survey Supplements on Aging found that 18% of people over the age of 65 and 25% over the age of 75 have falls.[41] When asked, "does dizziness prevent you from doing things you otherwise could do?" 34% of the population between 65 and 74 answered yes, increasing to 37% over the age of 75 years. This would place 12.5 million persons over the age of 65 years as having serious dizzy complaints in 1984.[41] The National Ambulatory Medical Care Survey in 1981 found the most common presenting symptom in patients 75 years or older was dizziness.[61] This information is particularly impressive because, in 1980, 11% of the population was age 75 or older. This number is expected to increase to nearly 21% by the year 2030.[55]

Causes of vertigo can be divided into peripheral, and central and systemic etiologies. Diseases which affect the peripheral vestibular system include Meniere's disease, vestibular neuritis, benign paroxysmal positional vertigo, perilymphatic fistula, trauma, infection, and autoimmune inner ear disease. Central causes of vertigo include vascular loops, vertebrobasilar insufficiency, multiple sclerosis, migraine, and cervical vertigo. Finally, systemic disorders such as hyperglycemia, hyperlipidemia, hypothyroidism, drug effects, and allergy can cause symptoms of disequilibrium.

CASE HISTORY

The most important aspect in the evaluation of vertigo is the patient's history. There are four critical areas that must be examined: (1) vestibular-related symptoms; (2) auditory symptoms; (3) general neurologic symptoms; and (4) past medical history.

Vestibular Symptoms

The most common dizzy sensation associated with a primary vestibular disorder is vertigo; however, a pulsion sensation, unsteadiness, lightheadedness, or "wooziness" may be caused by a vestibular lesion. Central nervous system disorders are usually characterized by the latter three symptoms, with vertigo being much less common.

The duration of the episode is important. Dizzy spells that last minutes to hours are more often associated with a vestibular disorder, in contrast to episodes lasting seconds or to continuous disequilibrium. The onset of the dizziness may help in distinguishing peripheral from central disease and in determining a cause. Typically dizziness associated with vestibular disease is abrupt in onset. Its time course may be short (a few days for vestibular neuritis), recurrent (as in Meniere's disease), or occur after specific head movements (as in benign paroxysmal positional vertigo). Associated symptoms such as nausea and vomiting frequently accompany disequilibrium caused by a vestibular lesion and are uncommonly associated with other causes of dizziness.

After detailing the primary episode, subsequent dizzy spells should then be elaborated upon. Their similarity or difference compared to the first attack should be documented as well as the patients status between attacks. With Meniere's disease and benign paroxysmal positional vertigo the patient is generally well between spells of dizziness. With vestibular neuritis or central nervous system disease, the disequilibrium may be continuous.

Auditory Symptoms

Auditory symptoms, occurring in conjunction with vestibular symptoms, point to a peripheral or vestibular cause of the dizziness and are helpful in isolating the offending ear. Foremost among auditory symptoms is hearing loss. Aspects of hearing that need to be elucidated include the following: Is the hearing loss unilateral or bilateral, progressive, fluctuating, or associated with the dizziness? Meniere's disease is characterized by a fluctuating sensorineural hearing loss, most often unilateral. Autoimmune inner ear disease can also be accompanied by a fluctuating hearing loss. A sudden decrease in hearing occurs with a viral labyrinthitis, whereas a progressive hearing loss may occur with an acoustic neuroma or syphilis.

In addition to hearing loss, ear pressure or fullness and tinnitus help in localizing the problem to the peripheral vestibular system. Fullness, generally fluctuating, is a hallmark of Meniere's disease (cochlear-vestibular hydrops).

General Neurologic Symptoms

In addition to recording symptoms of inner ear dysfunction, the history should be directed toward the patient's general neurologic status. A loss of consciousness with the attacks implicates a central nervous system cause, possibly vertebrobasilar insufficiency. Headaches, if present, may suggest migraine disease. Changes in vision or motor and sensory function could be additional manifestations of a neoplastic, demyelinating, ischemic, or vasculitic process within the central nervous system.

Past Medical History

The patient's general medical condition should be documented. Acute problems such as viral or bacterial illnesses could be a cause of disequilibrium. Chronic diseases that could cause dizziness include diabetes, thyroid dysfunction, cardiac disease, or blood pressure disorders. Medication, drug use, or alcohol use could be the cause of the patient's dizziness. Medication can affect the central nervous system, the peripheral vestibular system, or other organ systems such as the cardiovascular system, with resultant disequilibrium.

CAUSES OF VERTIGO

Peripheral Causes of Vertigo

Meniere's Disease

Vertigo is most commonly caused by disease of the peripheral vestibular system. Prosper Meniere,[72] in 1861, expanded the work of Pierre Flourens and described an otogenic disorder, erroneously referred to as a triad, consisting of four symptoms: vertigo, tinnitus, fluctuating sensorineural hearing loss, and aural fullness.

Meniere's disease usually begins between the ages of 20 and 60 years and is estimated to affect 2.4 to 4.8 million Americans.[73] Typically the disease is unilateral, however up to 40% of patients develop symptoms in the opposite ear.[7] Clinically, Meniere's disease is characterized by the sudden onset of vertigo often accompanied by pallor, diaphoresis, nausea, and vomiting. The attacks are usually associated with tinnitus and/or aural fullness. The episodes may last from minutes to several hours. Rarely, some patients may experience explosive attacks, precipitating a fall. These drop attacks, termed Crisis of Tumarken or utricular crises, usually occur in the later stages of the disease.

More than a century has passed, yet there continues to be debate as to the pathophysiology of this disorder. Schuknecht[96] states that Meniere's disease is a symptom complex caused by different diseases that share the same pathophysiology of endolymphatic hydrops. Hydrops, an increase in endolymphatic fluid pressure, is thought to result from endolymphatic sac dysfunction (decreased resorptive capabilities) secondary to infection, congenital hypoplasia, trauma, inflammatory causes, or an idiopathic cause. Schuknecht classifies Meniere's disease as an idiopathic endolymphatic hydrops. He has proposed a five-step mechanism that leads to the development of Meniere's disease.[97]

1. *Decreased endolymph resorption.* This may be caused by labyrinthitis, trauma, or hypoplasia.
2. *Endolymphatic hydrops.* This occurs because of overaccumulation of endolymph, which distorts Reisner's membrane.
3. *Membrane rupture.* Endolymph

then mixes with perilymph which temporarily paralyzes the auditory and vestibular system.

4. *Healing of ruptures.* The breaks of Reisner's membrane heal, thus allowing the entire process to repeat itself.
5. *Distortion and atrophy.* With disease progression, permanent changes in the membranous labyrinth and eighth cranial nerve occur, causing persistent disequilibrium and/or hearing loss.

Vestibular Neuritis

Vestibular neuritis is characterized by the sudden onset of disabling vertigo often associated with nausea and vomiting without auditory symptoms. Typically the onset of symptoms occurs after an upper respiratory tract infection. Vestibular neuritis most often affects patients in the 3rd to 5th decades without a sex predilection. Vertiginous symptoms are often worse with head motion. Clinically, horizontal nystagmus toward the uninvolved ear may be detected during the acute phase. Caloric testing typically reveals a reduced response in the involved ear. Routine audiometry is usually normal. Recovery is generally expected within 1 to 3 months.

Histopathologic studies have suggested involvement of the superior vestibular nerve and vestibular ganglion, often with little or no involvement of the actual end organ. Infection has long been considered a causative factor in vestibular neuritis.[24] Intracytoplasmic particles have been found in human vestibular ganglia which support a viral cause. These particles are thought to be dormant forms of a virus, which may produce infection with resultant inner ear disease.[44, 59] Other causes such as occlusion of the anterior vestibular artery, cerebellar infarctions, and acute diabetic neuropathy have been implicated in the etiology of vestibular neuritis.[92] Toxic and allergic causes are also thought to play a role in the disease process.[104]

It has been claimed that vestibular

neuritis affects only the vestibular portion of the eighth cranial nerve and that the cochlear portion is left unaffected. However, Rahko and Karma[90] found that the involved ear has a 14 to 24 dB sound pressure level (SPL) threshold difference compared to the unaffected ear at 20 kHz, implicating some degree of damage to the auditory system in patients with vestibular neuritis.

Benign Paroxysmal Positional Vertigo

Benign paroxysmal positional vertigo (BPPV) was first described by Barany[9] in 1921 as a brief, violent vertiginous episode occurring within seconds after a change in head position. Usually the attacks resolve if the patient remains in that position. In 1981, the Research Committee for Peripheral Disorders in Japan proposed diagnostic criteria for BPPV.[74] These include (1) whirling vertigo induced by a specific head position or movement; (2) a characteristic burst of positioning nystagmus that is rotary in nature, fatigable, and occurs within seconds after position changes; and (3) exclusion of central nervous system disorders, cervical disorders, and cochlear disorders associated with vertigo. The nystagmus is typically induced by turning the involved ear downward. Although the nystagmus is usually rotary and in the direction of the downturned ear, Stahle and Gerins[113] noted that the nystagmus pattern can vary. Caloric tests are normal in over two thirds of the patients.

In many series, BPPV is the most frequent cause of vertigo. It is most commonly seen in people over the age of 40, and women outnumber men affected by a ratio of 1.6:1.[8] The process lasts for weeks to months, with spontaneous recovery in 90%. These episodes may recur.[113] Longridge and Barber[63] have demonstrated bilaterality in up to 15% of affected individuals.

The cause of BPPV has been a source of controversy. Baloh and co-workers studied 240 cases of BPPV and found that the most common cause was idiopathic (118 of 240 patients), followed by post-traumatic cause (43 patients), viral neurolabyrinthitis, (37 patients) and miscellaneous causes (42 patients). Benign paroxysmal positional vertigo may occur in association with other disorders such as central nervous system disease and Meniere's disease. Schuknecht and Ruby[99] observed basophilic deposits in the cupula of the posterior semicircular canal in two patients with BPPV. He proposed that otoconia are released from a degenerating utricular macula and settle on the cupula of the posterior canal, causing it to become heavier than the surrounding endolymph.

Perilymphatic Fistula

A perilymphatic fistula is the result of an abnormal communication between the inner ear and middle ear spaces. It generally occurs as a result of stapedectomy, head trauma, barotrauma, chronic ear surgery, congenital anomalies, or spontaneously.[101] This disease continues to be a focal point for debate because the presenting symptoms are similar to other otologic disorders and because of the difficulty in objectively diagnosing a perilymph fistula.

Symptoms due to a perilymphatic fistula may be similar to those of Meniere's disease or endolymphatic hydrops.[4, 27] Usually patients complain of fluctuating unilateral sensorineural hearing loss, tinnitus, aural fullness, and vertigo. One or more of these symptoms usually exists. Occasionally, *Hennebert's* (a positive fistula test especially with negative pressure) or *Tullio's sign* (vertigo and nystagmus induced by loud noise) are seen.[25, 110] In a symptomatic individual with a clear history of barotrauma, closed head injury, or prior otologic surgery, a perilymphatic fistula may be suspected.

Once the diagnosis of perilymphatic fistula is considered, there are several tests that can be supportive. Only exploratory tympanotomy with direct observation can confirm the diagnosis and this can be subject to error as local anesthetics may seep into the middle ear space, or minimal manipulation on the promontory may cause microvascular disruption with release of vessel exudate. Noninvasive tests, such as pneumo-otoscopy (positive and negative pressure applied to the tympanic membrane) can produce nystagmus and vertigo. Vertigo is most often seen during the application of negative pressure. Daspit and Linthicum[21] coupled electronystagmography testing with pneumo-otoscopy, adding more objective evidence as compared to the standard fistula test. Platform posturography testing has been recommended by Black.[12] Recently Schweitzer et al.[100] identified six "best amino acid markers" which differentiate perilymph from serum, plasma, or cerebrospinal fluid.

Trauma

Trauma is a frequent cause of vertiginous symptoms. Any insult that disrupts the labyrinth or ossicular chain may lead to vertigo. Transverse temporal bone fractures typically involve the otic capsule and cause labyrinthine dysfunction. Longitudinal temporal bone fractures less commonly cause vertigo but may do so either from head trauma itself, otic capsule injury, or ossicular disruption. A concussive effect on the central nervous system (CNS) may result in post-traumatic disequilibrium. Central nervous system concussion may affect the brain stem, cerebellum, or higher centers. Schneider et al.[93] described damage to the superior temporal gyrus caused by an injury to the occiput which disrupts a vestibular projection area and may be one reason for post-traumatic dizziness.

Infection

Acute and chronic infection may affect the middle or inner ears, which may lead to a spectrum of clinical symptoms. The occurrence of vertigo with acute suppurative otitis media, acute suppurative labyrinthitis, and chronic suppurative otitis media with or without cholesteatoma is well known. Less commonly appreciated is the occurrence of vertigo in childhood related to eustachian tube dysfunction with resultant middle ear effusion. In a study of 27 children with dizziness, Blayney and Colman[13] found that 5 had serous otitis media and, when treated appropriately, their dizziness resolved. Involvement of the labyrinth secondary to infection may be caused by toxins, by actual bacterial invasion by way of emissary veins, or by erosion of the semicircular canal.[122]

There exist a variety of viral causes of inner ear disease including mumps, measles, varicella zoster, cytomegalovirus, and influenza B. Delayed onset vertigo may occur because of these viral disorders. For example, mumps causing a severe sensorineural hearing loss in childhood may not affect the vestibular system until years later, perhaps due to delayed endolymphatic hydrops. While viruses are felt to be important etiologic agents, evidence is mostly circumstantial. At present, only cytomegalovirus and the mumps virus have been cultured from the perilymph of affected ears.[22, 121]

Autoimmune Inner Ear Disease

Autoimmune disease affecting the inner ear, with resultant vertigo, sensorineural hearing loss, aural fullness, and tinnitus, has been an area of intensive research. It was first highlighted by McCabe in 1979[65] and elaborated by Hughes and co-workers.[46] The latter group stated that autoimmune mediated inner ear disease is diagnosed by clinical findings (progressive or fluctuating sensorineural hearing loss, fullness, tinnitus), positive immunologic laboratory testing, and positive treatment response. The typical patient is middle aged, a woman, and exhibits bilateral progressive sensorineural hearing loss (may be asymmetric) with or without dizziness, aural fullness, or tinnitus. Symptoms often progress over weeks to months, although sudden hearing loss has been reported.[51] Occasionally, the patient may have a systemic immune disease such as rheumatoid arthritis.[46, 47, 65] Hughes et al.[46] examined 52 patients suspected of having autoimmune inner ear disease and found 7 to have Cogan's syndrome, 4 to have rheumatoid arthritis, and 1 to have systemic lupus erythematosus. Cogan's syndrome is a rare disease characterized by nonsyphilitic interstitial keratitis associated with tinnitus, vertigo, and hearing loss.[19] The cause is uncertain, but evidence suggests that immunologic or infectious causitive factors are likely.[118]

Central Causes of Vertigo

Vascular Loop

The idea that vascular compression of cranial nerves may lead to clinically significant symptoms dates back to Dandy's[20] first description of trigeminal neuralgia secondary to a vascular loop. It is now well accepted that the cause of tic douloureux and hemifacial spasm is a loop of the anterior inferior cerebellar artery or nearby veins pulsating on the trigeminal or facial nerves.[52]

More recently, vascular loops compressing the vestibulocochlear nerve have been considered a possible cause of hearing loss, vertigo, and tinnitus.[2] The symptoms often mimic those of cerebellopontine angle tumors. Examinations such as air contrast computed tomography and magnetic resonance imaging have, occasionally, demonstrated prominent vascular loops penetrating into the internal auditory canal.[2, 83] Unilateral delays observed in auditory brain stem evoked response testing have also been correlated with compression of the eighth cranial nerve complex by a vascular loop.[75]

Anatomic dissections indicate that approximately 65% of specimens have vascular loops approaching the seventh and eighth cranial nerves.[36] McCabe and Harker[66] described eight patients with discrete spells of true vertigo who were previously diagnosed with Meniere's disease or an unknown cause. All patients underwent vestibular nerve section, and in each case a vascular loop extending far into the internal auditory canal with compression of the superior vestibular nerve was found. Janetta and co-workers[54] have suggested that patients with vascular loops are more apt to present with constant positional vertigo or disequilibrium associated with nausea. They generally do not have the typical hearing loss of Meniere's disease, and vestibular function testing often shows normal results.

Vertebrobasilar Insufficiency

Vascular insufficiency may occur in the vertebrobasilar system secondary to obstruction, stenosis, or "steal" flow patterns. Ischemia is responsible for over 80% of central vestibular disturbances.[117] The variable history and clinical findings associated with vertebrobasilar insufficiency (VBI) occur because of the complexity and high numbers of sensory and motor pathways that are supplied by the posterior circulation. Carotid insufficiency secondary to stenosis may cause blood flow reversals in the posterior communicating artery, with a resultant "steal phenomenon" from the vertebrobasilar system.[117]

Grad and Baloh[32] examined a series of 84 patients with posterior circulation problems and found that there was a high prevalence of isolated episodes of vertigo associated with vertebrobasilar insufficiency. They also described a 42% prevalence of unilateral caloric weakness, concluding that the vestibular labyrinth is vulnerable to ischemia from disorders in the vertebrobasilar system. Visual dysfunction, drop attacks, unsteadiness, and extremity weakness were the symptoms most commonly associated with VBI.

In Valvassori's[117] study of 200 patients with VBI, 87% complained of dizziness. He suggested that if computed tomographic dynamic examinations suggested flow aberrations, angiography should be performed to confirm the flow abnormality.

Multiple Sclerosis

Multiple sclerosis is a demyelinating disorder characterized by a variety of neurologic signs and symptoms that have a tendency toward remission and exacerbation. Typically, it is a disease of young adult white women. The cause is unknown; however, based on epidemiologic and virologic studies, it is suggested that the disease may be caused by an abnormal immunologic response to previous viral exposure.[49] Recent studies show wide discrepancies in the percentage of patients with symptoms of vertigo or disequilibrium, ranging from 5% to 51%.[48] A gaze-induced horizontal nystagmus is thought to occur in up to 65% of patients with the disease.[38, 77] Vertical nystagmus occurs in approximately one third of multiple sclerosis patients.[48, 49] Demyelination occurs in the white matter in the periventricular region, optic tracts, brain stem, cerebellum, and spinal cord, including the dorsal columns. For significant disequilibrium to occur, two or more of these areas are generally involved.

Migraine

Migraine was first described by Hippocrates 25 centuries ago. It is a common disorder that affects approximately 25% of women, 20% of men, and 2% to 5% of children.[85, 119] Typically, migraine is characterized by periodic headaches that are associated with nausea, vomiting, and neurologic symptoms. In common migraine, absence of neurologic symptoms is the rule, whereas in classic migraine an aura typically precedes the headaches.[1] It is also well documented that neurologic symptoms termed "migraine equivalent" can occur in the interval between headaches.[39] Of 200 patients with migraine examined by Kayan and Hood,[57] 53 complained of vertigo. Vertigo was noted as an aura in 8 patients, during the headache in 25 patients, after the headache in 1 patient, and between headaches in 19 patients.

Bickerstaff was the first to describe basilar artery migraine.[38] This was characterized by an aura of scotomata, transient blindness, vertigo, dysarthria, parasthesias, ataxia, and tinnitus.

Cervical Vertigo

Cervical vertigo was first documented by Claude Bernard in 1858.[11] Gait disorders which resemble cerebellar ataxia occur after severing cervical muscles in several animal species. There are several theories as to the cause of cervical vertigo, including inflammatory and degenerative changes in the cervical spine or neck musculature which can lead to altered neck proprioceptive input. These reflexes or impulses are important for cervical righting reflexes. Barre[10] injected 1% procaine into deep cervical tissues and found not only vertigo, horizontal contralateral nystagmus, ipsilateral past pointing, and falling toward the injected side, but also observed tinnitus and an ipsilateral Horner's syndrome. Vascular insufficiency may be another cause of cervical vertigo. It is well known that turning the head leads to decreased flow in vertebral vessels;[79] however, general cardiovascular causes such as atherosclerosis appear more important. Irritation of the cervical sympathetic system has also been implicated as a potential cause of cervical vertigo.[76]

Miscellaneous Causes of Vertigo

Multiple metabolic derangements have been implicated as causative factors in inner ear disease. According to Rubin,[91] five major organ systems are responsible for inner ear homeostasis. These include the adrenal and pituitary glands, the hormonal and immune systems, and the hypothalamus.

The most frequent laboratory abnormality associated with vestibular dysfunction is hyperglycemia. Frequently, dietary manipulation will lead to a beneficial response.[17] Spencer[111] reported on 1,400 patients with hearing loss and vertigo who were diagnosed with hyperlipidemia. Hypothyroidism has also been implied as a potential cause of neuro-otologic dysfunction.[17]

Many drugs are known to produce vertigo, including alcohol, phenobarbital, dilantin, chlorpromazine, adrenocorticotropic antagonists, cholinomimetics, cholinesterase inhibitors, and γ-aminobutyric acid agonists.[124] Medications, especially in the elderly, may act chiefly on the peripheral vestibular system, producing vestibular toxicity, or may suppress the central nervous system, causing ataxia. In addition, medication may affect other organ systems and cause such side effects as postural hypotension. It has also been suggested that food allergies or inhalant allergies may be a contributing factor in the development of endolymphatic hydrops.[104] Shambaugh and Wiet[104] currently encourage dietary management of food allergens for relief of symptoms of Meniere's disease.

MEDICAL TREATMENT OF VERTIGO

Meniere's Disease

Treatment options for Meniere's disease are diverse. Initial medical treatment includes a salt-restricted diet, often in combination with a diuretic. Other dietary adjustments proposed by Strome et al.[114] and Kinney[58] are a reduction of carbohydrate and lipid intake.

Non-osmotic diuretics (thiazide diuretics, chlorthalidone, potassium-sparing drugs, and furosemide) are used in the treatment of Meniere's disease. This type of therapy tends to reduce the number and severity of the vertiginous attacks, but has not been shown to have a long-term effect on hearing.[26, 60] In contrast, osmotic diuretics have shown dramatic, albeit temporary, improvement in hearing in approximately 60% of patients with Meniere's disease.[112] Examples of osmotic diuretics include

glycerin, mannitol, urea, and isosorbide. The intent of these drugs is to dehydrate the labyrinth.

Vasodilator therapy has been used with some success. This class of medication may be effective in alleviating acute exacerbations, stabilizing hearing, and reducing vertigo. Vasodilatory agents currently in use are nicotinic acid,[103] intravenous histamine,[103] and betahistine[82] (an oral histamine preparation). Carbon dioxide with oxygen (carbogen), a potent vasodilator, has been reported to improve hearing.[40] Hearing improvement is more likely to be seen in early stages of Meniere's disease.[103, 112, 115]

Pressure chamber therapy has been touted to be successful in providing long-lasting improvement in both hearing and vertigo in 45% of Meniere's patients.[116] The decompression chamber causes a reduction in air pressure, which creates a relative positive pressure in the middle ear, decreasing venous congestion and reducing endolymphatic hydrops.

McCabe et al.[67] has demonstrated that vestibular suppressants, specifically diazepam, are effective in reducing the vestibular symptoms associated with Meniere's disease. Daily therapy is considered important in reducing the likelihood of recurrent vertigo. Anticholinergics are also helpful in ameliorating associated nausea and vomiting. There is some controversy regarding the prolonged use of vestibular suppressants in that by using vestibular suppressants, long-term central nervous system compensation may take longer to occur or may not occur to its full extent.[71]

Graham and co-workers[35] were able to demonstrate preservation of or improvement in hearing as well as alleviation of vertiginous episodes in patients with bilateral intractable Meniere's disease using titration streptomycin therapy. The purpose of this treatment is to eliminate vertigo without causing oscillopsia or hearing loss. This is achieved by frequent assessment of audiologic and vestibular function during treatment.

Vestibular Neuritis

Treatment for vestibular neuritis is essentially symptomatic. During the acute phase it is important to provide the patient relief from the intense vertigo, nausea, and vomiting. This includes the use of a vestibular suppressant such as diazepam or meclizine combined with an antiemetic. Short-term use of steroids has also been effective.[5]

Benign Paroxysmal Positional Vertigo

Treatment for BPPV is primarily symptomatic. During acute exacerbations vestibular suppressants such as benzodiazepines and antihistamines are used. However, in order to habituate the vestibular system rather than suppress it, head exercises or customized vestibular exercises[78] are used which reduce symptoms and lessen the severity of recurrences.

Perilymphatic Fistula

The mainstay in the medical management of perilymphatic fistula is bedrest for 7 to 10 days.[105] Vestibular suppressants may be effective in alleviating vertigo in the early stages of this disease. Failure of bedrest to resolve the vertigo, or a progression of the sensorineural hearing loss, are indications for surgical intervention.

Autoimmune Inner Ear Disease

Glucocorticoids have been the primary treatment for autoimmune inner ear disease and Cogan's syndrome.[42] Cyclophosphamide and azathioprine have also been used with some success.[68] Plasmapheresis has led to good results, as demonstrated by Luetje.[64] Plasma-

pheresis entails the removal of plasma from withdrawn blood, thereby removing antibodies, antigens, immune complexes, and blocking antibody. Leutje[64] studied eight patients diagnosed with autoimmune inner ear disease and concluded that plasmapheresis can be used as alternative or adjunctive therapy in these patients, as it stabilizes or improves auditory and vestibular symptoms in selected patients.

Migraine

Medical intervention for vertigo associated with migraine includes the typical treatments for migraine headaches. During an attack, ergotamine tartrate helps alleviate symptoms.[39] Propranolol has been effective in long-term control of migraine symptoms including vertigo,[23] as have been the calcium channel blockers amitriptyline, Periactin, and methysergide maleate.[39, 81, 123]

SURGICAL TREATMENT OF VERTIGO

Surgical therapy for vertigo is considered when conservative management (diet and medical) fails. Prior to surgery, the disorder needs to be isolated to the peripheral vestibular system and the diseased ear needs to be identified through history, and by auditory and vestibular testing. Various other factors such as hearing level, severity and frequency of symptoms, physiologic age, and employment must also be considered. Two types of surgical procedures exist which offer relief of vertigo: preservation procedures (endolymphatic sac surgery, cochleosacculotomy, microvascular decompression, and perilymphatic fistula repair) and ablative procedures (labyrinthectomy, vestibular nerve section, singular neurectomy, posterior semicircular canal occlusion, and streptomycin perfusion of the labyrinth).

Endolymphatic Sac Surgery

Several surgical procedures have been proposed to treat vertigo associated with Meniere's disease[15, 33, 62, 87] and delayed onset of vertigo (delayed endolymphatic hydrops).[3, 43] In those patients refractory to medical management, endolymphatic sac surgery can be offered as an attempt to decompress the hydropic condition (increased endolymphatic fluid) thought to exist in the diseased ear.

Various techniques of decompression include endolymphatic sac-subarachnoid shunts,[15] endolymphatic sac-mastoid shunts,[3] and wide bony decompression of the endolymphatic sac.[33, 62] Despite the technique used, the success rate for endolymphatic sac surgery has ranged from 60% to 85%,* with respect to a reduction in or a cure of vertigo. Hearing improvement occurs in 10% to 56% of cases.[3, 16, 102] Aural pressure is often reduced, and occasionally tinnitus is lessened.

These results are comparable to those of Bretlau et al.[16] who evaluated 23 patients with active Meniere's disease. In their double blind study, approximately 70% of patients receiving either a simple mastoidectomy or endolymphatic-mastoid shunt experienced an elimination of or a significant reduction in their vertigo. These results were reported after a 9-year follow-up period. The authors argued for a strong placebo effect of sac surgery and suggested that the effect of surgery was not specifically related to manipulation of the sac.

Several authors offer endolymphatic sac decompression-shunting as an early alternative in Meniere's patients hoping to reduce or eliminate vertigo and stabilize hearing. Brown[18] reviewed 245 patients who underwent endolymphatic sac surgery and found that in the early stages of Meniere's disease 75% of patients had relief of vertigo, while 50% had continued relief after 10 years. If surgery was offered in the late stages of

*References 3, 15, 16, 33, 43, 62, 87, and 102.

the disease, only 40% demonstrated improvement. The majority of the latter group had a progressive decline in their hearing.

The surgical technique is straightforward. After performance of a wide mastoidectomy, bone is removed from over the endolymphatic sac located in the posterior fossa dura just inferior to a line (Donaldson's line) drawn through the posterior semicircular canal where it is bisected by the horizontal semicircular canal (Fig 15–1). At this point the surgeon has the option of opening the sac and placing a drain or valve in it.

A recent modification of this technique introduced by Kartush (unpublished data) involves bony decompression not only of the posterior fossa dura and endolymphatic sac but also wide decompression of the sigmoid sinus. In conjunction, the sigmoid sinus size is reduced with the aid of bipolar cautery. Initial results have been promising, with 90% of patients demonstrating complete to substantial control of vertigo at one year.

Complications resulting from endolymphatic sac surgery are rare and occur in less than 2% of cases.[33] The risk of a neural hearing loss or a cerebrospinal fluid leak are slightly increased when the sac is opened and a valve or shunt is placed.

Revision sac surgery has been shown to be equally as effective as a primary endolymphatic sac procedure if symptoms recur.[45] Paparella and Sajjadih[84] have shown that, along with vertigo reduction, hearing gain can occur following a revision endolymphatic sac procedure.

Cochleosacculotomy

Schuknecht,[95] in 1982, introduced the concept of creating a fistula between the endolymphatic and perilymphatic spaces, thereby decompressing the endolymphatic compartment. The cochleosacculotomy procedure involves inserting a 4-mm hook through the round

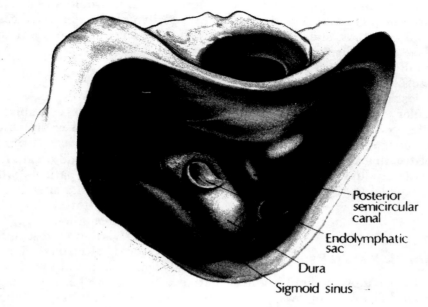

Posterior
semicircular
canal

Endolymphatic
sac

Dura

Sigmoid sinus

FIG 15–1.
Endolymphatic sac decompression. A wide mastoidectomy with bone removed from over the sigmoid sinus, posterior fossa dura, and endolymphatic sac is shown. Note position of the *endolymphatic sac* inferior to where the *posterior semicircular canal* is bisected by the horizontal semicircular canal. *(From Kartush JM, LaRouere MJ: Surgical Anatomy of the Ear. New York, Raven Press, in press. Used with permission.)*

window membrane and the osseous spiral lamina of the basal turn of the cochlea. The round window is then sealed. This procedure can be performed transcanal, under local anesthesia.

The procedure has been recommended for Meniere's disease. Because the surgery can be performed under local anesthesia, it can be done in the elderly and those who are poor surgical risks. Schuknecht and Bartley[98] reported that up to 72.6% of their patients obtained relief of vertigo, and 55% maintained hearing. Although considered a preservation procedure, it should not be performed in the sole hearing ear, as up to 45% of patients (11 of 90 in this study) develop a severe to profound sensorineural hearing loss in the operated ear. This operation has received little acceptance among otologic surgeons.

Microvascular Decompression of the Eighth Nerve Complex

Microvascular decompression of the eighth cranial nerve complex has been introduced by Janetta et al.[53] as a method to relieve disabling positional vertigo (DPV). Patients with DPV present with a constant sensation of being off balance that is associated with nausea. The diagnosis is usually made by history and abnormal auditory brain stem evoked response testing. A difference of 0.2 msec in the interwave interval of peaks I to III compared to those of the contralateral side or an interwave interval of peaks I to III that exceeds 2.3 msec is considered an indication of eighth cranial nerve compression.[52]

Following a retrosigmoid craniectomy, the eighth nerve complex is identified as it leaves the brain stem and enters the internal auditory canal. Vascular compression is reduced by inserting a small piece of Teflon felt between the nerve and a blood vessel which lies on the nerve.

Møller[75] reported the results of 41 patients undergoing microvascular decompression for DPV. Thirty patients became totally symptom free or had a marked improvement in symptoms. Two patients had a mild improvement in their symptoms, and nine experienced no relief. The author stated that all patients had a significant compression of the eighth cranial nerve by one or more vessels. One patient suffered a complete loss of hearing due to the microvascular decompression procedure. Møller concluded that microvascular decompression was an effective method of treating disabling positional vertigo, with gradual improvement of symptoms noted 4 to 12 months postoperatively.[75]

Perilymphatic Fistula Repair

A leak of perilymphatic fluid from either the round or oval windows, generally associated with an episode of barotrauma, can cause a variety of ear symptoms including sensorineural hearing loss and vertigo. Seltzer and McCabe[101] note that disequilibrium, with occasional spells of true vertigo, is the most common vestibular symptom pattern.

The technique of perilymphatic fistula repair involves an exploratory tympanotomy under local anesthesia. The oval and round windows are then observed. Patients are placed in the head down position and are asked to "bear-down" while the surgeon examines each window. Fascia, perichondrium, or fat, supported by gelfoam, is then used to seal each window.

Shelton and Simmons[105] reported that in patients in whom a perilymphatic fistula was observed, 64% had resolution of their major symptom. When no fistula was found, 44% demonstrated resolution of their major symptoms. Seltzer and McCabe[101] found that closure of a perilymphatic fistula improved vestibular symptoms in the majority of cases; however, auditory symptoms improved to a lesser degree.

The most difficult aspect of a perilymphatic fistula repair is the recognition of a true leak of perilymphatic fluid. To this end investigators are pursuing tests that would specifically identify perilymphatic fluid as compared with other body fluids or local anesthetics.[100]

Labyrinthectomy

A labyrinthectomy is an ablative procedure in which the sensory epithelium and distal nerve fibers are removed from the vestibular end organ. It is generally performed in patients with nonserviceable hearing (greater than 60 dB speech reception threshold and word recognition scores of less than 50%) and symptoms of vertigo or disequilibrium. In most cases, electronystagmography reveals hypofunction of the involved ear (that with a marked sensorineural hearing loss), although the vestibular response in the diseased ear may be normal or totally absent.

A labyrinthectomy can be performed by one or two approaches: transcanal or transmastoid. The transcanal labyrinthectomy, first described by Schuknecht in 1956,[94] involves removing the stapes and curettage of the vestibule. Armstrong,[6] in 1959, advocated removal of a portion of the promontory to allow for more complete removal of neural epithelium. Vertigo is controlled in over 90% of patients with a properly performed labyrinthectomy.

To allow for more complete removal of neural epithelium and distal nerve fibers, Pulec[88] described the transmastoid labyrinthectomy procedure in 1969. This technique involves a mastoidectomy with fenestration of the horizontal, posterior, and superior semicircular canals as well as the vestibule (Fig 15–2). Under direct vision, the ampullae of the three semicircular canals and maculae of the saccule and utricle can be completely removed. Graham and Kemink[34] reviewed their 5-year experience with this technique and noted a 93% success rate in controlling vertigo. As expected, all residual hearing is lost with this procedure. The complication rate following labyrinthectomy is low.

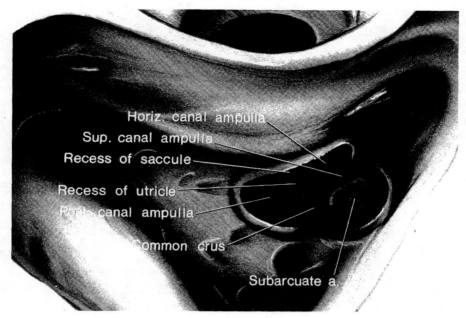

Horiz. canal ampulla
Sup. canal ampulla
Recess of saccule
Recess of utricle
Post. canal ampulla
Common crus
Subarcuate a.

FIG 15–2.
Transmastoid labyrinthectomy. Following a wide mastoidectomy, the *horizontal, superior,* and *posterior* semicircular canals are opened. The vestibule is also opened, exposing the *saccule* and *utricle.* Neuroepithelium is then removed from each structure under direct vision. *(From Kartush JM, LaRouere MJ: Surgical Anatomy of the Ear. New York, Raven Press, in press. Used with permission.)*

Vestibular Nerve Section

Vestibular nerve section has become the most accepted method of controlling medically refractive vertigo or disequilibrium caused by unilateral vestibular dysfunction in patients with serviceable hearing. In several studies,[14, 31, 70] regardless of the surgical approach, those patients with Meniere's disease fared better with respect to alleviation of vertigo than did non-Meniere's patients.

Currently, four surgical approaches are commonly used to perform a vestibular nerve section: middle cranial fossa, retrolabyrinthine, retrosigmoid, and translabyrinthine. All but the latter offer the opportunity for hearing preservation. Until 1961, vestibular nerve section was performed by the suboccipital route. In 1961, House[50] popularized the middle cranial fossa approach (Fig 15–3). This involves a temporal craniectomy with retraction of the temporal lobe medially, exposing the superior surface of the temporal bone. After opening of the internal auditory canal, the superior and inferior vestibular nerves are individually sectioned. Utilizing this approach, relief of vertigo was obtained in 85% to 99% of patients.[30, 107] The advantage of the middle cranial fossa approach over other surgical approaches used for vestibular nerve section is the ability to completely section all vestibular fibers prior to their becoming more intimately associated with cochlear fibers, as has been demonstrated in the cerebellopontine angle. The disadvantages of the middle cranial fossa technique stem from a greater risk of facial nerve injury and sensorineural hearing loss. The risk of neurologic complications (aphasia, seizures, and hemiparesis) may be higher with this approach.

In 1980, Silverstein and Norrell[106] introduced the retrolabyrinthine vestibular neurectomy. This allows direct access to the cerebellopontine angle (CPA). After a wide mastoidectomy is performed, bone is removed from over the sigmoid sinus and posterior fossa dura down to the posterior semicircular ca-

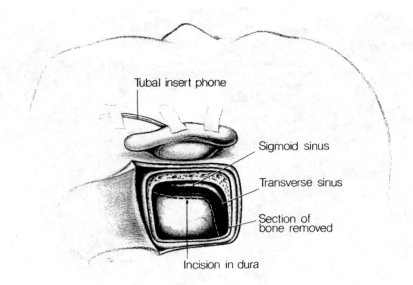

Tubal insert phone

Sigmoid sinus

Transverse sinus

Section of
bone removed

Incision in dura

FIG 15–3.
Middle cranial fossa approach. Following a temporal craniectomy the temporal lobe is retracted medially. The internal auditory canal is opened, exposing the inferior and *superior vestibular nerves.* The vestibular nerves are then divided. *(From Larouere MJ, Kartush JM: Facial nerve paralysis, in Meyerhoff WL, Rice D (eds): Otolaryngology—Head and Neck Surgery, vol 1. Philadelphia, WB Saunders, 1992. Used with permission.)*

nal. The dura is incised just inferior to the superior petrosal sinus, gaining exposure to the CPA. The eighth nerve complex is identified and the vestibular portion of the nerve, located on the tentorial side, is sectioned. Approximately 75% of nerves demonstrate a distinct cleavage plane between the cochlear and vestibular division.[108]

Results are excellent with the latter approach. In 1982, Silverstein and Novell[107] reported a 93% success rate in resolving or improving vertigo with no patients demonstrating a total neural hearing loss. The risk of facial nerve weakness compared to the middle cranial fossa approach was significantly reduced from 4% to 0%.[69] Drawbacks to the retrolabyrinthine approach include a 3% to 10% incidence of cerebrospinal fluid leakage, limited exposure of the neurovascular structures in the cerebellopontine angle, the risk of fallopian canal or posterior semicircular canal fenestration within the mastoid, and increased risk of limited exposure if the sigmoid sinus is ante-

rior, the jugular bulb is high, or the mastoid is sclerotic.[69]

Due to the limitations of the retrolabyrinthine approach several authors have advocated the retrosigmoid technique,[31, 108] for sectioning the vestibular nerve. This procedure involves exposing the sigmoid and lateral sinuses and performing a craniectomy posterior and inferior to these structures. The dura is cut in a curvilinear manner, exposing the cerebellum (Fig 15–4). Minimal retraction on the cerebellum results in wide exposure of the cerebellopontine angle (Fig 15–5). The vestibular nerve is then sectioned (Fig 15–6). The dura is closed tightly, markedly reducing the incidence of a cerebrospinal fluid leak.[56, 69]

Control of vertigo obtained after performing a retrosigmoid vestibular nerve section is similar to that obtained with the retrolabyrinthine approach (93% to 95%).[31] Disadvantages of the procedure involve the close association of cochlear and vestibular fibers in the cerebellopontine angle, as well as headaches.

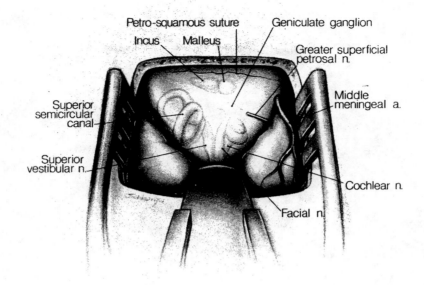

FIG 15–4.
Initial exposure for a retrosigmoid vestibular nerve section. After removal of a *bone plug* posterior to the *sigmoid sinus,* the posterior fossa dura is opened in a curvilinear manner. *(From Kartush JM, LaRouere MJ: Surgical Anatomy of the Ear. New York, Raven Press, in press. Used with permission.)*

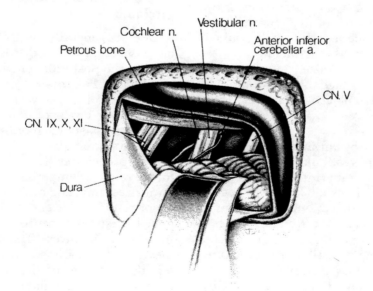

FIG 15–5.
Exposure during retrosigmoid vestibular nerve section. Mild posterior retraction on the cerebellum results in excellent exposure of the cochleovestibular nerve bundle. *(From Kartush JM, LaRouere MJ: Surgical Anatomy of the Ear. New York, Raven Press, in press. Used with permission.)*

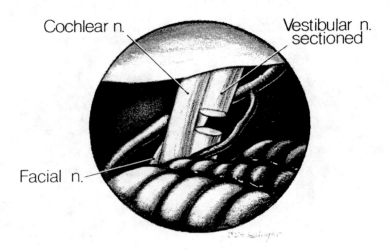

Cochlear n.

Vestibular n. sectioned

Facial n.

FIG 15–6.
Retrosigmoid vestibular nerve section. High magnification of the *cochlear* and *vestibular* nerves in the cerebellopontine angle. The vestibular nerve is sectioned, with visualization of the *facial nerve* below.

Headaches have nearly been eliminated with the use of two modifications introduced by Kartush et al.[56] Bicol, a soft, nonadherent collagenous material, is placed between the retractors and the cerebellum to minimize trauma, and the bone plug, obtained from the craniectomy site, is replaced after the dura is closed and covered with an abdominal fat graft.

The translabyrinthine approach for sectioning the vestibular nerve involves performing a labyrinthectomy, which exposes the internal auditory canal, with subsequent sectioning of the superior and inferior vestibular nerves.[89] This procedure, unlike other approaches for performing a vestibular neurectomy, involves total loss of hearing. In our experience, a complete transmastoid labyrinthectomy typically obviates the need for a translabyrinthine vestibular nerve section. Failure of the transmastoid labyrinthectomy to control vertigo results either from an incomplete procedure (retained neural epithelium) or from concurrent disease in the contralateral labyrinth or central nervous system.

Singular Neurectomy and Posterior Semicircular Canal Occlusion

BPPV is generally a self-limited disorder associated with a disease process involving the posterior semicircular canal ampullae.[99] Patients with BPPV are generally free of their vertiginous symptoms within 1 year of onset. Those with symptoms past 12 months appear to have intractable disease.

Two procedures have been advocated for the relief of symptoms of BPPV: singular neurectomy, and occlusion of the posterior semicircular canal. Gacek[28] introduced the singular neurectomy approach in 1974. It involves lifting a tympanomeatal flap by a transcanal approach. After identification of the round window membrane, the singular canal is found by drilling 1 to 2 mm deep to the inferior round window membrane in the posterior third of the round window niche. The nerve to the posterior ampullae is then avulsed with a hook. Relief of vertigo reportedly occurs in 91% to 97% of patients[29, 109] following this procedure. Drawbacks include a 6% to 8% incidence of sensorineural hearing loss when this procedure is performed by the most experienced surgeons.[29] The difficulty in adequately exposing the posterior ampullated nerve has led many otologic surgeons into performing a complete vestibular neurectomy for persistent BPPV.

Parnes and McClure[86] have introduced a transmastoid posterior semicircular canal occlusion procedure, effectively relieving intractable BPPV in two patients with severe hearing loss. Each patient demonstrated preserved lateral semicircular canal function. Both patients had a preoperative profound sensorineural hearing loss. The authors are examining the effect of this procedure in patients with serviceable hearing. After a mastoidectomy is completed, a small diamond burr is utilized to penetrate the posterior semicircular canal, impacting bone chips within the adjacent canal ends. A layer of fascia sealed with human fibrinogen glue is then placed on each canal end to secure occlusion.

Streptomycin Perfusion of the Labyrinth

A new surgical procedure introduced by Norris and co-workers in 1990[80] involves fenestration of the horizontal semicircular canal, creating a fistula between endolymph and perilymph, and applying streptomycin (125 µg) between the bony canal and membranous duct. Fifteen patients with Meniere's disease were treated in the initial study. According to the authors, all 15 enjoyed complete remission of their vertigo, and 7 of 8 patients treated with a 125 µg of streptomycin maintained their hearing. Although preliminary results are encouraging, further clinical trials will be needed to assess both short- and long-term vertigo control rates as well as hearing stability. A recent investigation by Monsell et al. (personal communication) involved a prospective multicenter study of 47 patients undergoing streptomycin application (25 µg) over a fenestration in the horizontal semicircular

canal. The authors demonstrated a high rate of hearing loss with this technique. Fifty-seven percent of their patients who had pure tone average worse than 40 dB preoperatively developed a severe to profound nerve hearing loss postoperatively.

CONCLUSION

Several medical approaches and surgical procedures are available for the control of vertigo. Essential to their use is a fundamental knowledge of the anatomy and physiology of the vestibular system and an understanding of the strengths and weaknesses of vestibular testing. With the development of newer modalities for vertigo control, prospective randomized studies will be helpful to assess the value of both new and old treatments that may relieve vertigo. The natural fluctuation of most types of vertigo, however makes an accurate study of treatment efficacy a challenging endeavor.

REFERENCES

1. Ad Hoc Committee on Classification of Headache: Classification of headache. *JAMA* 1962; 179:717–718.
2. Applebaum EL, Valvassori GE: Auditory and vestibular system findings in patients with vascular loops in the internal auditory canal. *Ann Otol Rhinol Laryngol* 1984; 92(suppl 112):63–69.
3. Arenberg IK: Results of endolymphatic sac to mastoid shunt surgery for Meniere's disease refractory to medical therapy. *Am J Otol* 1987; 8:335–344.
4. Arenberg IK, Ackley RS, Ferraro J, et al: ECOG results in perilymphatic fistula: Clinical and experimental studies. *Otolaryngol Head Neck Surg* 1988; 99:435–443.
5. Ariyasu L, Byl FM, Sprague MS, et al: The beneficial effect of methylprednisolone in acute vestibular vertigo. *Arch Otolaryngol Head Neck Surg* 1990; 116:700–703.
6. Armstrong BW: Transtympanic vestibulotomy for Meniere's disease. *Laryngoscope* 1959; 699:1071–1074.

7. Balkany T, Sires B, Arenberg I: Bilateral aspects of Meniere's disease. An underestimated clinical entity. *Otolaryngol Clin North Am* 1980; 13:603–609.

8. Baloh RW, Honrubia V, Jacobson K: Benign positional vertigo: Clinical and oculographic features in 240 cases. *Neurology* 1987; 37:371–378.

9. Barany R: Diagnose Von Krankheitserschernunggers in Berriche des Otolithenapparates. *Acta Otolaryngol* 1921; 2:434–437.

10. Barre JA: Le syndrome sympathique cervical posterieur. *Rev Neurol* 1926; 45:1246–1260.

11. Bernard C: Lecons sur La Physiologie et la pathologie du systeme nerveux. Paris, JB Bailliere, 1858.

12. Black FO: Vestibulospinal reflex function assessment upon moving platform posturography. *Am J Otol* 1985; 6:39–46.

13. Blayney AW, Colman BH: Dizziness in childhood. *Clin Otolaryngol* 1984; 9:77–85.

14. Boyce SE, Mischke RE, Goin DW: Hearing results and control of vertigo after retrolabyrinthine vestibular nerve section. *Laryngoscope* 1988; 98:257–261.

15. Brackmann DE, Nissen RL: Meniere's disease. Results of treatment with the endolymphatic subarachnoid shunt compared with the endolymphatic mastoid shunt. *Am J Otol* 1989; 8:275–282.

16. Bretlau P, Thompson J, Tos M, et al: Placebo effect in surgery for Meniere's disease; Nine year follow-up. *Am J Otol* 1989; 10:259–261.

17. Brookler KH, Rubin W: The dizzy patient: Etiologic treatment. *Otolaryngol Head Neck Surg* 1990; 103:6677–6680.

18. Brown JS: A ten year statistical follow-up of 245 consecutive cases of endolymphatic shunt and decompression with 328 consecutive cases of labyrinthectomy. *Laryngoscope* 1983; 93:1419–1424.

19. Cogan DG: Syndrome of nonsyphilitic interstitial keratitis with vestibuloauditory symptoms. A case with fatal aortitis. *Arch Ophthalmol* 1964; 71:172–175.

20. Dandy WE: Concerning the cause of trigeminal neuralysis. *Am J Surg* 1934; 24:447–455.

21. Dapsit CP, Linthicum FH: Diagnosis of perilymph fistula using ENG and impedience. *Laryngoscope* 1980; 90:217–223.

22. Davis LE, James CG, Fiver I, et al: Cytomegalovirus isolation from a human inner ear. *Ann Otol Rhinol Laryngol* 1979; 88:424–426.

23. Diamond S, Kudioros K, Stevens J, et al: Long-term study of propranolol in treatment of migraine. *Headache* 1982; 22:268–271.

24. Dix MR, Hallpike CS: The pathology, symptomatology and diagnosis of certain common disorders of the vestibular system. *Ann Otol Rhinol Laryngol* 1952; 61:987–1017.

25. Fox EJ, Balkany TJ, Arenberg IK: The Tulio phenomenon and perilymph fistula. Presented at the Annual Meeting of the American Neurotology Society, Denver, Colo, 1987.

26. Friberg U, Stahle J, Svedberg A: The natural course of Meniere's disease. *Acta Otolaryngol [Suppl]* 1984; 406:72.

27. Fujita S, Seidman MD, Shepard N: Atypical Meniere's disease: Perilymph fistula syndrome, in *Abstracts from 4th International Symposium of Meniere's Disease*, Boston, 1988.

28. Gacek RR: Transection of the posterior ampullae nerve for relief of benign paroxysmal positional vertigo. *Ann Otol Rhinol Laryngol* 1974; 83:596–605.

29. Gacek RR: Singular neurectomy update. *Ann Otol Rhinol Laryngol* 1982; 91:469–473.

30. Garcia-Ibanez E, Garcia-Ibanez JL: Middle fossa vestibular neurectomy: A report of 373 cases. *Otolaryngol Head Neck Surg* 1982; 90:778–782.

31. Glasscock ME, Thedinger BA, Cueva RA, et al: An analysis of the retrolabyrinthine vs. retrosigmoid vestibular nerve section. *Otolaryngol Head Neck Surg* 1991; 104:88–95.

32. Grad A, Baloh RW: Vertigo of vascular origin: Clinical and electronystmographic features in 84 cases. *Arch Neurol* 1989; 46:281–284.

33. Graham MD, Kemink JL: Surgical management of Meniere's disease with endolymphatic sac decompression by wide bony decompression of the posterior fossa dura: Technique and results. *Laryngoscope* 1984; 94:680–682.

34. Graham MD, Kemink JL: Transmastoid labyrinthectomy; Surgical management of vertigo in the non-serviceable hearing ear—a five year experience. *Am J Otol* 1984; 5:295–299.

35. Graham MD, Satafoff RT, Kemink JL: Titration streptomycin therapy for bilateral Meniere's disease: A preliminary report. *Otolaryngol Head Neck Surg* 1984; 92:440–446.

36. Grant JL, Martin R, Rhoton AL: Anatomical relationship of anterior inferior cerebellar artery and seventh and eighth cranial nerves. *Surg Forum* 1979; 30:429–431.

37. Grenman R: Involvement of the audiovestibular system in multiple sclerosis: An otoneurologic and audiologic study. *Acta Otolaryngol [Suppl]* 1985; 420:1–95.

38. Harker LA, Rassekh CH: Episodic vertigo in basilar artery migraine. *Otolaryngol Head Neck Surg* 1987; 96:239–250.

39. Harker LA, Rassekh CH: Migraine equivalent as a cause of episodic vertigo. *Laryngoscope* 1988; 98:160–164.

40. Hatch M, Tsai M, LaRouere MJ, et al: The effects of carbogen, carbon dioxide, and oxygen on noise-induced hearing loss. *Hear Res* (in press)

41. Havlik RJ, National Center for Health Statistics: *Aging in the Eighties: Impaired Senses for Sound and Light in Persons Age 65 and Over.* Preliminary data from the supplement on aging to the National Health Interview Surgery, United States. DHHS Pub No. (PHS) 86–1250. Advance Data from Vital and Health Statistics No. 125. January-June, 1984.

42. Haynes BF, Keiser-Kupfer MI, Mason P, et al: Cogan's syndrome studies in 13 patients, long-term follow-up and review of the literature. *Medicine* 1980; 59:426–441.

43. Hicks GW, Wright JW: Delayed endolymphatic hydrops: A review of 15 cases. *Laryngoscope* 1988; 98:845–848.

44. Hirata T, Sekitani T, Okinaka Y, et al: Serological study of vestibular neuronitis. *Acta Otolaryngol [Suppl].* 1989; 468:371–373.

45. Huang TS, Lin CC: Endolymphatic sac surgery for Meniere's disease: A composite study of 336 cases. *Laryngoscope* 1985; 95:1082–1086.

46. Hughes GB, Barner BP, Calabrese LH, et al: Clinical diagnosis of immune inner ear disease. *Laryngoscope* 1988; 98:251–253.

47. Hughes GB, Kinney SE, Barner BP: Autoimmune vestibular dysfunction: Preliminary report. *Laryngoscope* 1985; 95:893–897.

48. Grenman R: Involvement of the audiovestibular system in multiple sclerosis: An otoneurologic and audiologic study. *Arch Otolaryngol* 1988; 420:1–95.

49. Herrara, WG: Vestibular and other balance disorders in multiple sclerosis: Differential diagnosis of disequilibrium and topognostic localization. *Neurotol Clin* 1990; 8:407–420.

50. House WF: Surgical exposure of the internal auditory canal and its contents through the middle cranial fossa. *Laryngoscope* 1961; 71:1363–1395.

51. Hughes GB, Kinney SE, Barner BP, et al: Practical versus theoretical management of autoimmune inner ear disease. *Laryngoscope* 1984; 94:758–766.

52. Janetta PJ: The cause of hemifacial spasm: Definitive microsurgical treatment at the brainstem in 31 patients. *Trans Am Acad Ophthalmol Otolaryngol* 1975; 90:319–322.

53. Janetta PJ, Møller MB, Møller AR: Disabling positional vertigo (DPV). *N Engl J Med* 1984; 310:1700–1705.

54. Janetta PJ, Møller MB, Møller AR, et al: Neurosurgical treatment of vertigo by neurovascular decompression of the eighth nerve, *Clin Neurosurg* 1986; 33:645–665.

55. Johns M, Brackman DE, Kimmelman C, et al: Goals and mechanisms for training otolaryngologists in the area of geriatric medicine. *Otolaryngol Head Neck Surg* 1989; 100:262–265.

56. Kartush JM, LaRouere MJ, Graham MD: Modifications of the retrosigmoid technique. Abstract presented at the Middle Section of the Triologic Society, Tulsa, Oklahoma, 1990.

57. Kayan A, Hood J: Neuro-otological manifestation of migraine. *Brain* 1984; 107:1123–1142.

58. Kinney S: The metabolic evaluation in Meniere's disease. *Otolaryngol Head Neck Surg* 1980; 88:594–598.

59. Kitamura K, Toriyama M: Virus like particles in vestibular ganglion cells. *Arch Laryngol* 1985; 241:303–308.

60. Klockhoff I, Lindblum U, Stahle J: Diuretic treatment of Meniere's disease: Long-term results with chlorthalidone. *Arch Otolaryngol* 1974; 100:262.

61. Koch H, Smith MC: Office Based Ambulatory Care for Patients 75 Years and Over: National Ambulatory Medical Care Survey. 1980 and 1981. Advance Data from Vital and Health Statistics No. 110. DHHS Pub No. (PHS) 85–1250. National Center for Health Statistics. 1985.

62. LaRouere MJ, Graham MD: Wide bony decompression of the endolymphatic sac in the surgical management of Meniere's disease. *Operative Techniques Otol Head Neck Surg* 2:7–8.

63. Longridge MD, Barber HO: Bilateral paroxysmal positioning nystagmus. Presented at the 32nd Annual Meeting of the Canadian Otolaryngological Society, Quebec City, Quebec, 1978.

64. Luetje CM: Theoretical and practical implications for plasmapheresis in autoimmune inner ear disease. *Laryngoscope* 1989; 99:1137–1146.

65. McCabe BF: Autoimmune Sensorineural Hearing Loss. *Ann Otol Rhinol Laryngol* 1979; 88:585–589.

66. McCabe BF, Harker, LA: Vascular Loop as a Cause of Vertigo. *Ann Otol Rhinol Laryngol* 1983; 92:542–543.

67. McCabe BF, Sekitari T, Ryu JH: Drug effects on postlabyrinthectomy nystagmus. *Arch Otolaryngol* 1973; 98:310–313.

68. McDonald TJ, Vollertsen RS, Young BR: Cogan's syndrome: Audiovestibular involve-

ment and prognosis in 18 patients. *Laryngo-scope* 1985; 95:650–654.

69. McElveen JT, House JW, Hitselberger WE, et al: Retrolabyrinthine vestibular nerve section; A viable alternative to the middle fossa approach. *Otolaryngol Head Neck Surg* 1984; 92:136–140.

70. McElveen JT, Shelton C, Hitselberger WE, et al: Retrolabyrinthine vestibular neurectomy: A re-evaluation. *Laryngoscope* 1988; 98:502–506.

71. Melvill Jones G: Plasticity in the adult vestibulo-ocular reflex arc. *Philos Trans R Soc Lond [Biol]* 1977; 270:319–327.

72. Meniere P: Pathologie auriculaire maladies del'oreille interne offrant les symptomes de la congestion cerebrale apoplectiforme. *Gaz Med Paris* 1861; 16:88–89.

73. Miyamoto RT: Meniere's disease. *Indiana Med*, 1986, pp 961–965.

74. Mizukoshi K, Watanabe Y, Shujaku H, et al: Epidemiological studies on benign paroxysmal vertigo in Japan. *Acta Otolaryngol [Suppl]* 1988; 447:67–72.

75. Møller MB: Results of microvascular decompression of the VIIIth nerve as treatment of disabling positional vertigo. *Ann Otol Rhinol Laryngol* 1990; 99:724–729.

76. Mortiz W: Das Zervikale sympathicus Syndrom und seine Praktische Bedutung Zeischrr. *Laryngol Rhinol Otol* 1953; 32:270–283.

77. Noffsinger D, Olsen WO, Carhart R: Auditory and vestibular aberations in multiple sclerosis. *Acta Otolaryngol [Suppl]* 1972; 303:7–11.

78. Norre ME, DeWeerdt W: Treatment of vertigo based on habituation techniques and results of vestibular habituation training. *J Laryngol Otol* 1980; 94:971–977.

79. Norre ME, Stevens A: Cervical vertigo diagnostic and semilogical problems with special emphasis on cervical nystagmus. *Acta Otorhinolaryngol* 1987; 41:436–452.

80. Norris CH, Amedee RG, Risey JA, et al: Selective chemical vestibulectomy. *Am J Otol* 1990; 11:395–399.

81. Olesen J: Calcium antagonist in migraine and vertigo: Possible mechanisms of action and review of clinical trials. *Eur Neurol* 1990; 30(Suppl):21–34.

82. Oosterveld WJ: Betahistine dihydrochloride in the treatment of vertigo of peripheral vestibular origin. *J Laryngol Otol* 1984; 98:37.

83. Paines LS, Shimotakahara SG, Pelz D, et al: Vascular relationships of the vestibulocochlear nerve on magnetic resonance imaging. *Am J Otol* 1990; 11:278–281.

84. Paparella MM, Sajjadih H: Endolymphatic

sac revision for recurrent Meniere's disease. *Am J Otol* 1988; 9:441–447.

85. Parker W: Migraine and the vestibular system in childhood and adolescence. *Am J Otol* 1989; 10:364–371.

86. Parnes LS, McClure JA: Posterior semicircular canal occlusion for intractable benign paroxysmal positional vertigo. *Ann Otol Rhinol Laryngol* 1990; 99:330–334.

87. Portmann G: Saccus endolymphaticus and operations for drainage of same for relief of vertigo. *J Laryngol Otol* 1927; 42:809–927.

88. Pulec JL: The surgical treatment of vertigo. *Laryngoscope* 1969; 79:1783–1822.

89. Pulec JL: Translabyrinthine section of the VIIIth cranial nerve in Meniere's disease, in Pulec JL (ed): *Meniere's Disease.* Philadelphia, WB Saunders, 1978, pp 563–568.

90. Rahko T, Karma P: New clinical findings in vestibular neuronitis: High frequency audiometry hearing loss in the affected ear. *Laryngoscope* 1986; 96:198–199.

91. Rubbin W, Brookler KH: Etiologic diagnosis in neurotologic disease. *Otolaryngol Head Neck Surg*, 1990; 103:693–694.

92. Rubenstein R, Norman D, Schinder R, et al: Cerebellar infarction—a presentation of vertigo. *Laryngoscope* 1980; 90:505.

93. Schneider RC, Calhoun HD, Crosby EC: Vertigo and rotational movement in cortical and subcortical lesions. *J Neurol Sci* 1968; 6:493–516.

94. Schuknecht HF: Ablation therapy for the relief of Meniere's disease. *Laryngoscope* 1956; 66:859–870.

95. Schuknecht HF: Cochleosacculotomy for Meniere's disease: Theory, technique and results. *Laryngoscope* 1982; 92:853–858.

96. Schuknecht HF: Meniere's disease, pathogenesis and pathology. *Am J Otolaryngol* 1982; 3:349–352.

97. Schuknecht HF: The pathophysiology of Meniere's disease. *Am J Otolaryngol* 1984; 5:526–527.

98. Schuknecht HF, Bartley M: Cochlear endolymphatic shunt for Meniere's disease. *Am J Otol* 1985; 6:20–22.

99. Schuknecht HF, Ruby R: Cupulolithiasis. *Adv Otorhinolaryngol* 1973; 20:434–443.

100. Schweitzer VG, Woodson BT, Mawhinney TD, et al: Free amino acid analysis of guinea pig perilymph: A possible clinical assay for the PLF enigma. *Otolaryngol Head Neck Surg* 1990; 103:981–985.

101. Seltzer S, McCabe B: Perilymph fistula: The Iowa experience. *Laryngoscope* 1986; 94:37–49.

102. Shambaugh GE, Clemens JD, Arenberg IK: Endolymphatic duct and sac in Meniere's disease. *Arch Otolaryngol* 1969; 89:816–825.

103. Shambaugh GE, Glasscock ME: *Surgery of the Ear*, ed 3. Philadelphia, WB Saunders, 1980, p 578.

104. Shambaugh G Jr, Wiet R: (1980). The diagnosis and evaluation of allergic disorders with food intolerance in Meniere's disease. *Otolaryngol Clin North Am* 1980; 13:671–679.

105. Shelton C, Simmons FB: Perilymph fistula: The Stanford experience. *Ann Otol Rhinol Laryngol* 1988; 97:105–108.

106. Silverstein H, Norrell H: Retrolabyrinthine surgery: A direct approach to the cerebellopontine angle. *Otolaryngol Head Neck Surg* 1980; 88:462–469.

107. Silverstein H, Norrell H: Retrolabyrinthine vestibular neurectomy. *Otolaryngol Head Neck Surg* 1982; 90:778–782.

108. Silverstein H, Norrell H, Smouha E, et al: Combined retrolab retrosigmoid vestibular neurectomy: An evolution in approach. *Am J Otol* 1989; 10:166–169.

109. Silverstein H, White DW: Wide surgical exposure for singular neurectomy in the treatment of benign positional vertigo. *Laryngoscope* 1990; 100:701–706.

110. Singleton GT: Diagnosis and treatment of perilymph fistulas without hearing loss. *Otolaryngol Head Neck Surg* 1986; 94: 426–429.

111. Spencer J Jr: Hyperlipoproteinemia, hyperinsulinemia and Meniere's disease. *South Med J* 1981; 74:1194–1197.

112. Stahle J: Medical treatment of fluctuant hearing loss in Meniere's disease. *Am J Otolaryngol* 1984; 5:529–533.

113. Stahle J, Gerins J: Paroxysmal positional nystagmus: An electronystmographic and clinical study. *Ann Otol* 1965; 74:69–83.

114. Strome M, Topf P, Vernick DM: Hyperlipidemia in association with childhood sensorineural hearing loss. *Laryngoscope* 1988; 98:115–169.

115. Stupp H: Die Medikamentose Therapie der Meniereeschen Krankheit. *Arch Otorhinolaryngol* 1976; 212:375.

116. Tjernstrum O, Gasselbrunt M: Pressure chamber treatment in acute attacks of Meniere's disease, in Vosteen KH, et al. (eds): *Meniere's Disease.* Stuttgart, Georg Thieme, 1981; p 211.

117. Valvassori GE: Vertigo in vertebral-basilar insufficiency. *Revue Laryngol* 1985; 106:215–218.

118. Vollertsen RS: Vasculitis and Cogan's syndrome. *Rheumatic Dis Clin North Am* 1990; 16:433–439.

119. Waters WE, O'Conner PJ: Prevalence of migraine. *J Neurol Neurosurg Psychiatry* 1975; 38:613–616.

120. Weindruch R, Korper SP, Hadley E: The prevelance of disequilibrium and related disorders in older persons. *Ear Nose Throat J* 1989; 68:925–928.

121. Westmore GS, Pickard BH, Stern H: Isolation of mumps virus from the inner ear after sudden deafness. *Br Med J* 1979; 1:14–15.

122. Wolfson, RJ, Silverstein H, Marlowe FI, et al: Vertigo. *Clin Symp* 1981; 33:1–32.

123. Wouters L, Amery W, Towse G: Flunarizine in the treatment of vertigo. *J Laryngol Otol* 1983; 97:697–704.

124. Zee DS: Perspectives on the pharmacotherapy of vertigo. *Arch Otolaryngol* 1985; 111:609–611.

CHAPTER 16

Intraoperative Monitoring During Vestibular Surgery

James W. Hall III, Ph.D.
Mitchell K. Schwaber, M.D.

Within the past decade, auditory evoked responses have been increasingly applied in monitoring the functional integrity of the cochlea, eighth cranial nerve, and auditory brain stem during surgical procedures. Although various surgical procedures place these auditory structures at risk, posterior fossa surgery is associated with considerably greater risk of injury. The primary objective of monitoring intraoperatively during vestibular surgery is to preserve auditory function. Two auditory evoked responses—electrocochleography (ECochG) and the auditory brain stem response (ABR)—are typically applied intraoperatively to meet this objective. Most of our discussion, therefore, focuses on the application of ECochG and ABR in monitoring cochlear and eighth nerve integrity during vestibular surgery. A secondary and somewhat controversial monitoring goal is to document, by means of intraoperative ECochG data, the effect of the surgical procedure on vestibular system physiology. Whether this goal is met consistently is not yet clear; however, we discuss the issue and present original intraoperative ECochG data in support of our viewpoint. Finally, it is in some cases appropriate to also monitor facial nerve integrity intraoperatively. Rationale and protocols for intraoperative facial nerve monitoring during vestibular surgery are also included in the chapter.

RATIONALE

Surgery

We perform intraoperative auditory monitoring during suboccipital vestibular nerve section, microvascular decompression of the cochleovestibular nerve, endolymphatic sac decompression, and labyrinthotomy with streptomycin infusion (LSI). For suboccipital procedures, auditory evoked potential monitoring provides information regarding excessive retraction of the cochleovestibular nerve or excessive manipulation of the cochlear nerve during the procedure. For endolymphatic sac decompression and LSI, we obtain the auditory evoked potentials to document any changes of the summating potential. It has been theorized, not proved, that changes in the summating potential reflect changes in the fluid dynamics in the inner ear. However, at this writing, we have not been able to confirm this theory. As new vestibular surgical procedures evolve, our technique of monitoring can be applied. One such procedure is transmastoid posterior semicircular canal occlusion for benign paroxysmal positional vertigo (BPPV). Though we have not performed this procedure yet, we anticipate doing so in the near future.

Providing audiologic coverage for intraoperative monitoring requires planning and coordination. We try to do all of our neurotologic surgical procedures on the same specific day of the week (Wednesday), a policy that allows the audiology service to coordinate personnel. This policy has also worked well with the neurosurgical service. At the time the surgical case is scheduled, the audiology service is notified of the type of surgery, the projected monitoring needs, the date, and the time. Prior to the patient being brought into the operating room, it is the responsibility of the surgeon and the audiologist to inform the anesthesiologist that the patient is going to be monitored. At this time, we discuss our specific needs and which agents might interfere. For ECochG monitoring, we have no prerequisites other than maintenance of body temperature, oxygen saturation, and other physiologic parameters. For simultaneous facial nerve monitoring, we ask the anesthesiologist to avoid the use of muscle relaxant agents. This information is discussed in private to avoid any potential embarrassment which might arise if it were discussed in front of the patient.

Use of Evoked Responses

Evidence has accumulated over the past 10 years that evoked responses, in general, can provide an early indicator of changes in neurophysiologic status of the peripheral and central nervous system during surgery. These changes may be due to a variety of physiologic and surgical factors, including hypotension, hypoxia, and either compression or retraction of cranial nerves or brain tissue. Early detection of a significant alteration in neurophysiologic status can potentially lead to effective medical or surgical correction of the problem, with reversal of the pathophysiologic process.

In monitoring with auditory evoked responses, the integrity of the cochlea is essential. If serious cochlear impairment develops intraoperatively, audi-tory evoked responses will be markedly altered or even abolished. Surgery-related compromise of blood supply to the cochlea produces "cochlear ischemia" and sensory hearing impairment (Table 16–1). Obvious damage to the blood vessels is not necessary to produce cochlear deficit. Manipulation of labyrinthine blood vessels may result in vasospasm and subsequent interruption of blood supply to the cochlea and eighth cranial nerve. The relationship between blood supply and cochlear function has been appreciated for over 30 years. Perlman and workers[8] showed in experiments with animals that the cochlea could survive up to 5 minutes of interruption in blood supply. The *cochlear microphonic* (CM) and *action potential* (AP) (see Response Analysis, later in this chapter) disappeared within 30 seconds, but returned after blood supply was restored. Other mechanisms for cochlear damage resulting from surgery include fenestration of the labyrinth and disruption of cochlear nerve fibers.

Maintenance of integrity of the auditory portions of the eighth cranial nerve intraoperatively is, of course, essential for postoperative preservation of hearing. As summarized in Table 16–1, damage to the auditory portion of the eighth nerve may result from direct trauma or from secondary mechanisms, such as interruption of blood supply. At this point, it is appropriate to make an important distinction in the objectives of intraoperative monitoring with auditory evoked responses among types of neurotologic surgery. Vestibular neurectomy, by definition, involves sectioning of the vestibular branch of the eighth nerve. The goal of monitoring is to assure that the auditory branch and the facial nerve remain intact. In contrast, with other posterior fossa surgeries, such as tumor removal, the objective is to prevent intraoperative damage to the entire eighth cranial nerve (vestibular and auditory portions) and to the facial nerve.

TABLE 16–1.

Possible Factors in the Interpretation of Intraoperative Electrocochleography and Auditory Brain Stem Response Findings During Vestibular Surgery*

Type and Site	Factor
Physiologic	
General	Systemic body temperature
	Focal body temperature
	Effect of anesthetic agents
	Effect of chemical paralysis (facial nerve only)
Outer ear	Severely retracted pinna with excessive bending of insert ear tube
Middle ear	Blood and irrigation fluid
	Ossicular chain disruption
Inner ear	Effect of drilling
	Direct labyrinthine damage
	Interruption in blood supply
Eighth nerve	Traction
	Stretching
	Compression
	Ischemia secondary to interruption of blood supply
	Partial or complete severing of cochlear fibers
Technical	
Electrical artifact	Bipolar electrocautery
	Bovie
	Electric drill
	Surgical microscope
	Radiographic viewing box
	Other operating room electrical devices
Evoked response system	Electrode placement stability
	Earphone placement
	Patent insert earphone tube
	Distance between transducer and electrode leads
	Distance between electrode leads and electrical devices (see other items in this table) and their power cables

*Adapted from Hall JW III: Handbook of Auditory Evoked Responses. Needham, Mass, Allyn & Bacon, 1992.

SURGICAL TECHNIQUES

Most inner ear surgical procedures are performed through a transmastoid approach. These include endolymphatic sac surgery, labyrinthectomy, LSI, and posterior semicircular canal occlusion. During these procedures, a general postauricular incision is made, and the musculoperiosteum is incised to provide exposure of the mastoid. A simple mastoidectomy is performed, and the following landmarks identified: tegmen plate, sigmoid sinus, digastric ridge, antrum, short process of the incus, and horizontal semicircular canal. At this point, the surgeon stops all drilling, and auditory evoked potentials are obtained. In most cases, we then identify the location and course of the vertical segment of the facial nerve.

For an *endolymphatic sac decompression*, we then use a combination of cutting and drilling with diamond burrs to expose the posterior fossa dura and the sigmoid sinus. We obtain auditory evoked potentials before and after actually removing the last remnant of bone overlying the sac. Any changes are noted and are recorded in the operative notes. For LSI, we use diamond burrs to expose the endosteal membrane of the horizontal semicircular canal. The endosteal membrane is opened carefully, and auditory evoked potentials are recorded before and after infusion of streptomycin. We have not used ECochG data to determine if the endolymphatic membrane should be penetrated during the procedure.

We choose to perform *vestibular neurectomy* and *microvascular decompression of the cochleovestibular nerve* through a suboccipital approach. We place the patient head in Mayfield pinions and position the patient so that the subocciput is uppermost in the incision. A C-shaped incision is made about four fingerbreadths behind the postauricular crease, and a skin flap is elevated. The musculoperiosteum is incised into a trifurcated flap, based superiorly on the temporalis muscle, inferoposteriorly on the splenius capitis and obliquus muscles, and enteroinferiorly on the mastoid periosteum. As bone removal begins, the anesthesiologist administers mannitol, 1 g/kg body weight, to dehydrate the brain. A circular plate of suboccipital bone is removed, and the dura is opened using a cruciate incision. The cerebellum is initially retracted posterosuperiorly to allow the basilar cistern to be opened and cerebrospinal fluid to be drained off. The cerebellopontine angle is then exposed, and the various cranial nerves identified. After the Wiet retractor is positioned, the audiologist obtains auditory evoked potentials to be certain that there is no excessive retraction of the cerebellum or the cochleovestibular nerve.

For *microvascular decompression,* we systematically elevate all of the various arteries and veins off of the cochleovestibular nerve. This includes the lysis of arachnoidal adhesion as well as the dissection of vessels on the anterior side of the cochleovestibular nerve. Small pledgets of cardiac felt are then placed to prevent readhesion of the vessels. For vestibular neurectomy, the cleavage plane is developed between the cochlear and the vestibular nerves. The superior half of the nerve represents most of the vestibular fibers. The vestibular fibers are cut, taking great care to avoid injuring the facial nerve and any nearby vessels. During the microvascular decompression procedures the audiologist obtains continuous recordings of the auditory evoked potentials. If a change occurs, the surgeon is immediately notified. The surgeon then takes appropriate action based on the perceived problem.

EVOKED RESPONSE MONITORING TECHNIQUES

Background

Intraoperative monitoring can be extremely challenging. The test environment typically contains multiple sources of electrical activity, which may interfere with evoked response measurement. The surgical protocol limits ready access to the patient. In addition, the patient's status is not always stable. In fact, momentary alterations in neurophysiologic status, and therefore evoked response patterns, are commonplace. These neurophysiologic alterations may result from surgical manipulations, from anesthetic agents, and from changes in physiologic parameters (such as body temperature and blood pressure). The challenge is to differentiate as quickly as possible between causes of auditory evoked response or the facial nerve response alterations related to surgery versus all other causes. This evoked response interpretation may seriously influence surgical decisions and, ultimately, patient outcome. Whether a patient's hearing or facial nerve integrity is preserved can depend to a large extent on prompt and accurate interpretation of intraoperative evoked response findings.

The most common cause of evoked response alterations, and the one of primary interest intraoperatively, is mechanically induced disruption of auditory system or seventh cranial nerve function (see Table 16–1). Naturally, these alterations will be detected only during the intraoperative period when auditory or facial nerve structures are being manipulated. Other intraoperative events, such as saline irrigation within the surgical field, may also produce neurophysiologic changes due, for example, to reduced focal temperature. In contrast, other auditory evoked response changes due to systemic factors (such as hypothermia or hypotension) can occur, theoretically, at any time during surgery, from induction of anesthesia to closing of the incision. It is advisable, then, for the tester to be informed of the surgeon's activities throughout the procedure and to remain especially vigilant during manipulations such as retraction of structures (for example, the cerebellum), decompression of the endolymphatic sac, or sectioning of the vestibular portion of the eighth cranial nerve.

Response Analysis

Electrocochleography

Although recent articles have described the application of automated analysis techniques in intensive care unit and operating room neurophysiologic monitoring,[2] manual calculations of sensory evoked response latency and amplitude remain the conventional analysis approach at this time.[3] The ECochG waveform consists of two or three major components (Fig 16–1), depending on certain stimulus parameters. With single polarity (rarefaction or condensation) stimuli, the CM, an oscillating waveform, is observed from stimulus onset until the appearance of the AP. The CM is generated by hair cells. The *summating potential* (SP) takes the form of either a distinct peak less than 1 msec before the AP, and usually less than half as large as the AP, or as a hump on the initial slope of the AP component. The precise generator

of the SP is not known, but it is thought to be associated with distortion products in cochlear activation. The AP is actually an average of compound action potentials arising from distal eighth nerve fibers (as they leave the cochlea). The AP is sometimes referred to as the "N1" component because with it appears the initial negative peak in the ECochG waveform, often recorded with the traditional test protocol. The AP or N1 component is equivalent to ABR wave I.

The CM is not routinely analyzed in clinical ECochG applications. In fact, stimulus parameters are usually manipulated so as to minimize detection of the CM. The CM may have value, however, as a general measure of cochlear integrity and, specifically, of outer hair cell integrity. It is likely that CM does not permit more precise characterization of cochlear status along the basilar membrane (for example, basal versus apical), even with tone burst stimulation. At high stimulus intensity levels, activation of the basal region of the cochlea probably predominates in the genera-

ECochG

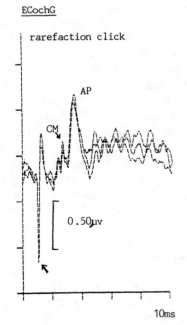

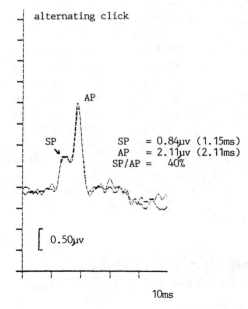

FIG 16–1.
Characteristic electrocochleography *(ECochG)* waveform for single polarity *(rarefaction)* and alternating polarity *(click)* stimuli. Major components are the cochlear microphonic *(CM)*, summating potential *(SP)*, and action potential *(AP)*. A prestimulus baseline was employed.

tion of the CM. Analysis of the CM is limited, for the most part, to simply a determination of its presence or absence.

A common ECochG analysis approach is calculation of SP and AP amplitude (in microvolts) from a common baseline, and then computation of an *SP/AP amplitude ratio*.[3] An estimate of baseline is made somewhere in the waveform preceding both the SP peak and the AP. Then, the amplitude from this baseline to the SP peak and to the AP peak is determined, and the SP/AP quotient computed. If, for example, SP amplitude is 0.60 μV and AP amplitude is 1.50 μV, then the SP/AP ratio is 0.40 or 40%. One major problem in this process is confident estimation of a baseline value. The high-pass filter setting for ECochG is typically as low as 10 Hz, in order to facilitate detection of the SP, which is considered a direct current potential. This filter setting, however, often results in considerable baseline drift and difficulty in determining the most representative baseline value. We deal with this problem by including a prestimulus baseline period in the ECochG analysis time. We also routinely collect at least three separate ECochG averages for the test ear. After verifying response replicability (the major components are present consistently across waveforms), we digitally add the separate waveforms and calculate SP and AP amplitude, and the SP/AP ratio, from the summed (composite) waveform. The same technique is always used for each ear.

In analyzing ECochG data, one must appreciate factors that can differentially influence the SP versus AP. Aside from polarity (noted above), electrode site, stimulus intensity, and stimulus rate probably have the most pronounced effects on the SP/AP ratio. As the recording electrode is moved closer to the cochlea, amplitude increases for the SP and for the AP, but the increase is relatively greater for the AP. Consequently, the SP/AP ratio invariably become smaller when recorded closer to the cochlea. For example, the upper limit for

normal SP/AP ratio is 50% for an ear canal (TIPtrode) electrode versus 30% for a promontory electrode. The practical implications of this phenomenon are significant for clinical ECochG measurement and interpretation, particularly if various electrode types and sites are used. This is not a factor, of course, when recording ECochG intraoperatively with a single electrode site. An SP is characteristically not detected for stimulus intensity levels of less than 55 to 60 dB sound pressure level. The most stable SP/AP ratio is found at very high stimulus intensity levels. With increasing stimulus rates (for example, from a slow rate of 7.1/sec to a rapid rate of more than 100/sec), AP amplitude will decrease whereas SP amplitude shows little change. The result is a progressive increase in the SP/AP ratio with increasing rate. Thus, rate should be held constant intraoperatively for confident SP/AP interpretation. Finally, it is important to note that there is some controversy surrounding the significance of the SP as typically recorded with alternating polarity stimuli. Some investigators[6] have recently expressed concern that the peak recorded under this test condition is actually not the SP but, rather, a remnant of the CM that is not completely canceled out in the averaging process.

Two final ECochG analysis parameters are AP latency and amplitude. Latency is usually calculated as the time (in milliseconds) between stimulus onset and AP peak. Amplitude (in microvolts) is generally calculated either from a preceding baseline value to AP peak, or from AP peak to the immediately following trough. Another analysis parameter described in early ECochG studies but rarely reported now is a measure of the time in milliseconds from the onset of the SP to the AP return to baseline (SP plus AP width).

Auditory Brain Stem Response

Analysis of ABR commonly consists of the calculation of absolute latency values for major components (I, III, and

V), and corresponding relative or inter-wave latency values (I to III, III to V, and I to V), all in milliseconds (Fig 16–2). Absolute amplitude for waves I and V, and the wave V/I amplitude ratio, are also sometimes analyzed clinically. Latency is defined as the time in milliseconds between stimulus onset and the peak of wave I and wave III. For wave V, some clinicians calculate latency on the basis of the peak, whereas others make the calculation based on the shoulder of the downward slope of wave V. Amplitude of ABR waves I and V is typically calculated from the peak to the following trough. Clinical experience, and statistical analysis, have shown that ABR amplitude is far more variable than ABR latency. The wave V/I amplitude ratio is often calculated to minimize the effect of this variability on amplitude analysis within subjects. In the clinic, normative latency and amplitude statistics are essential for meaningful ABR analysis for a given patient. This is not a major issue, however, in the operating room, where interpretation is based largely on analysis of postbaseline changes in ABR latency or amplitude over time.

Measurement Parameters

Stimulus and acquisition parameters employed in intraoperative monitoring with auditory evoked responses, and their respective rationales, are summarized in Table 16–2. The overall objective in the selection of these parameters is to optimize neurophysiologic recording of the pertinent auditory system in the operating room environment. Specifically, the goal is to rapidly detect robust and reliable responses from the cochlea, the eighth cranial nerve, and auditory regions of the brain stem, while minimizing physiologic and electrical artifact. A flexible measurement technique is essential for consistently successful intraoperative evoked response recordings. Test conditions and physiologic status invariably changes, both from one patient to

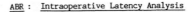

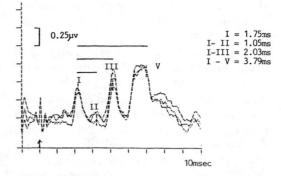

FIG 16–2.
Auditory brain stem response *(ABR)* waveform for high-intensity click stimuli showing major wave components *(I, III,* and *V)* and corresponding interwave latency values monitored intraoperatively *(horizontal lines, I–II, I–III, and I–V)*. A prestimulus baseline *(arrow)* was employed.

the next and within a single patient during surgery. It is often necessary to modify the test protocol promptly in response to these changes. In short, the only "correct" test protocol is the one that produces optimal evoked response results for a particular patient under test conditions encountered at the time of the monitoring.

A detailed discussion of the principles underlying the selection of the measurement parameters listed in Table 16–2 is beyond the scope of this chapter. The reader is referred to a recent text[3] for this invaluable background information. Several rather straightforward points should, however, be kept in mind. First, the closer the recording electrodes are to the anatomic region of interest, the larger the response recorded. For example, if the region of interest is the cochlea, then the promontory is the preferred recording site. Any other electrode site (for example, ear canal or ear lobe) is suboptimal. Our simplified promontory recorded technique for ECochG[11] is described in the following section. Second, selection of some test parameters can be made only at the time of monitoring. Stimulus polarity is a parameter that illustrates this point. Alternating polarity clicks are often used in recording ECochG clinically and in the operating room. That is, a response is averaged from a comparable number of rarefaction (negative) polarity and condensation (positive) polarity clicks, each polarity presented in an alternating fashion. Some patients, however, will show little or no ECochG for alternating polarity stimuli, yet produce a clear and reliable response with a single polarity (either rarefaction or condensation). Again, the overriding practical principle is to employ whatever test strategy works for a given patient at a given time during surgery. While intraoperative alterations in test protocol are often essential to obtain high-quality data, unnecessary deviations from the customary test protocol should be avoided because it is possible that they will produce evoked response changes that

are mistaken as evidence of impending damage to the auditory system.

In summary, each clinician is likely to develop a test strategy that is best suited for his/her intraoperative monitoring needs, objectives, and measurement conditions. Nevertheless, the overall goal during intraoperative monitoring with auditory evoked responses invariably remains the same regardless of the factors just noted: to record a response with all major waves clearly, reliably, and quickly throughout surgery.

A Simplified Transtympanic Electrocochleography Approach

A sterile stainless steel subdermal needle electrode (Nicolet Biomedical In-

TABLE 16–2.

Guidelines for Intraoperative Electrocochleography (ECochG)/Auditory Brain Stem Response (ABR) Test Protocol*

Parameter	Suggestion	Rationale/Comment
Stimulus		
Transducer	ER-3A	Permits TIPtrode usage, secures transtympanic electrode placement; feasible in operating room (OR) with otologic operations, does not invade surgical field or obstruct the surgical procedure
Type	Click	Produces robust response, but only evaluates basal turn of cochlea; tone bursts can be used
Duration	0.1 ms	For this onset response; an extended duration tone burst useful in summation potential (SP) delineation; 2-1-2 cycle duration for tone bursts
Polarity	Alternating	ECochG: Cancels out cochlear microphonic (CM); single polarity used for CM detection
	Rarefaction	ABR: Usually enhances waveform definition, but manipulate polarity if response is not optimal
Rate	7.1/sec	Slow rate enhances N1 action potential (AP) component; a very rapid rate (e.g., >91/sec) is useful for SP delineation; modifying rate slightly may reduce some types of electrical interference; rate of 21.1/sec is appropriate if a robust AP (wave I) is present
Intensity	70 to 95 dB	Produces robust response (normally there is no ECochG SP for intensities below about 50 dB HL); intensity is decreased to estimate sensorineural hearing threshold levels
Masking	None	Masking is never necessary for ECochG (a detectable AP response is always from the test ear); very rarely required for ABR (only with markedly delayed wave V latency and absent wave I)
Presentation		
Ear	Monaural	
Mode	Air conduction	Bone conduction ECochG and ABR are possible, but not typically required in the OR

(Continued.)

TABLE 16–2   (cont.)

Parameter	Suggestion	Rationale/Comment
Acquisition		
Electrodes		
Types	Needles	Sterile stainless steel, subdermal-type needle electrodes are used exclusively for ECochG and ABR recording in the OR, including promontory site
Array (options ranked)		
1	Fz - prom[†]	Noninverting electrode (Fz) is at upper forehead, approximately at the hairline; technically at a point midway between vertex and nasion; this array typically yields a response of large amplitude (e.g. 4 to 20μV)
2	Fz - IEAC	For example, with TIPtrode in the ipsilateral external ear canal (IEAC); noninvasive (no advantage in OR), but amplitude rarely exceeds 0.6μV
3	AC - prom[†]	Customary ECochG electrode array; yields response of large amplitude and sometimes reduced electrical artifact interference
	Ground = Fpz	Low forehead (Fpz) ground electrode is convenient and is used for both ECochG and ABR
Impedance	<5 to 10 kΩ	Except for promontory electrode, impedance should be less than 5 kiloohms (kΩ); for promontory electrode, impedance should be less than 10 kΩ
Filter	10–1,500 Hz	Encompasses response frequencies; lower high pass cutoff may be desirable for SP definition
	Notch	Not recommended, may introduce response distortion
Amplification	×75,000	Adequate for large ECochG response
Analysis time	5, 10, or 15 msec	Shorter time for ECochG and longer time for ABR or combined ECochG/ABR recording
Sweeps	<50–> 1,500	Often less than 50 sweeps are needed with promontory electrode; over 1,500 for EAC electrode

*Adapted from Hall JW III: Handbook of Auditory Evoked Responses. Needham, Mass, Allyn & Bacon, 1992
[†]prom = promontory; AC = contralateral earlobe.

struments) is placed transtympanically onto the promontory.[11] The needle has a 12-mm shank and a 0.4-mm diameter, a 1-m wire, and a standard pin (Fig 16–3). In the operating room, all recordings (for example, from forehead and earlobe electrode sites) are also made with this type of electrode. The patient is under general anesthesia at this point in the procedure. The promontory electrode is placed by the otologist under an operating room microscope. The insulated portion of the sterile subdermal needle electrode (between the shank and the wire) is grasped with bayonet forceps, and the electrode is directed down the external auditory canal. The needle is then inserted through the inferior-posterior portion of the tympanic membrane to rest on the promontory. After transtympanic electrode placement, the electrode lead, which extends from just lateral to the tympanic membrane, is secured temporarily by hand against the wall of the ear canal. The otologist then takes a compressed gold foil foam ear insert or TIPtrode and places it within the ear canal in the customary fashion. The electrode and the foam insert or TIPtrode can be sterilized for intraoperative ECochG. Both the promontory electrode lead and transducer tube are then secured with surgical tape to the patient's neck or chest. At the end of closing, the ear phone and electrode system are removed by simply pulling them gently out of the canal. The foam insert or TIP-

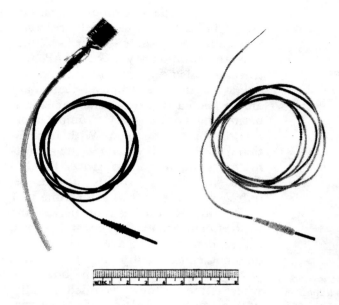

FIG 16–3.
Subdermal stainless steel needle electrode *(right)* and gold-coated foam insert (TIPtrode) *(left)* used in electrocochleography recordings intraoperatively as described by Schwaber & Hall [6]. Acoustic tubing connects insert ear cushion to an ER-3A transducer box (not shown).

trode is discarded and the needle electrode is sent for gas sterilization. The entire promontory electrode placement procedure requires less than 1 minute in the operating room. To date, no promontory electrode placed with this technique has become dislodged during intraoperative monitoring. Furthermore, there have been no known medical complications or tympanic membrane or middle ear damage arising from promontory needle placement.

Combined ECochG, ABR, and Direct Eighth Nerve Recording

The conventional ECochG and ABR recording techniques are still important for intraoperative monitoring during neurotologic surgery.[4] The main disadvantages of the technique have already been noted. Because amplitude of wave V is relatively small, as recorded with the far field electrode array, the response often must be averaged from as many as 1,000 or more stimuli in order to obtain an adequate signal-to-noise ratio. Whereas a clear response with stable latency throughout surgery is generally considered evidence of auditory integrity, interpretation of an alteration

or loss of the response is less straightforward.

A three channel measurement technique combining promontory ECochG, conventional ABR, and direct eighth nerve recordings is therefore sometimes preferable.[3] There is substantial clinical evidence that combined ECochG, ABR, and eighth nerve recording is an effective intraoperative monitoring technique for preservation of hearing. Near-field auditory evoked response recordings, by definition, produce relatively large amplitude responses. The near-field ECochG detected with a promontory electrode, therefore, provides the major clinical advantage of a large response, namely, a very favorable signal-to-noise ratio. A clear ECochG AP wave (ABR wave I) is observed with minimal signal averaging, as depicted in Figure 16–4. In most cases, AP amplitude is on the order of 5 to 10 μV with a promontory electrode, as compared to less than 0.5 μV with an ear canal electrode type (such as the TIPtrode). Furthermore, with the promontory electrode site a distinct AP is typically recorded, even from patients with severe [60 to 75 dB hearing level (HL)] high-frequency sensorineural hearing impairment, at max-

Intraoperative ABR/ECochG

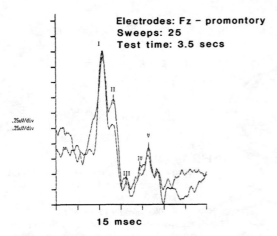

Electrodes: Fz – promontory
Sweeps: 25
Test time: 3.5 secs

.25uV/div
.25uV/div

15 msec

FIG 16–4.
An ECochG/ABR waveform recorded intraoperatively with the simplified transtympanic electrode technique. All major components were reliably recorded with only 25 sweeps and total test time of 7 seconds.

imum stimulus intensity levels. In contrast, a reliable AP is rarely observed from patients with high-frequency sensorineural hearing impairment greater than approximately 35 to 40 dB HL with ear canal electrode designs (Fig 16–5).

A secondary and related advantage is that a wave I or AP component may be recorded with the near-field transtympanic technique when no response can be detected with surface electrodes, including ear canal types. One must keep in mind, however, that presence of an ECochG AP component, in isolation, appears to be an insufficient intraoperative measure of auditory function. Although disappearance of the component must be considered strong evidence of cochlear deficit, preservation of the AP component intraoperatively does not necessarily imply auditory integrity. Even complete sectioning of the eighth nerve resulting in profound hearing impairment does not invariably eliminate the ECochG AP, provided cochlear blood supply remains intact.[9, 10, 13]

Recording a response directly from the eighth cranial nerve as it exits the internal auditory canal or enters the brain stem offers similar advantages.[7, 12] In fact, this near-field response may be larger by up to four or five times than the promontory ECochG AP and, therefore, also requires little or no signal averaging. Electrophysiologic data are collected almost instantaneously, permitting continuously prompt information for the surgeon. With conventional ABR measurement in the operating room, signal averaging over 1,000 to 2,000 stimulus repetitions may be required with a data collection time of 1 to 2 minutes. During this period the ABR/ECochG may not be stable but, rather, dynamic. The averaged response does not, consequently, reflect the status of the auditory system at any one time, whereas the response recorded directly, with at most several seconds of averaging, is essentially time specific. A second and very important advantage of the direct eighth nerve recording is site specificity. Presumably, the technique provides information on status of the proximal portion of the nerve, between the porus of the internal auditory canal and the root entry zone near the brain stem. A major disadvantage of the technique is that an electrode cannot be placed directly on the nerve until the nerve is exposed, and then it often must be removed for periods of time during surgery so as not to interfere with dissection of tumor, transection of the vestibular portion of the nerve, or other manipulations. A fine silver wire with a cotton wick at the end is less obtrusive.

Criteria for Intraoperative ABR/ECochG Alterations

There are few published guidelines for interpreting the significance of intraoperative changes in auditory evoked response findings.[3] Selected response parameters that may be analyzed intraoperatively are displayed in Table 16–3. In interpretation of auditory evoked response data intraoperatively, regardless of the parameters analyzed or the criteria for abnormality used, it is assumed

Intraoperative ABR/ECochG

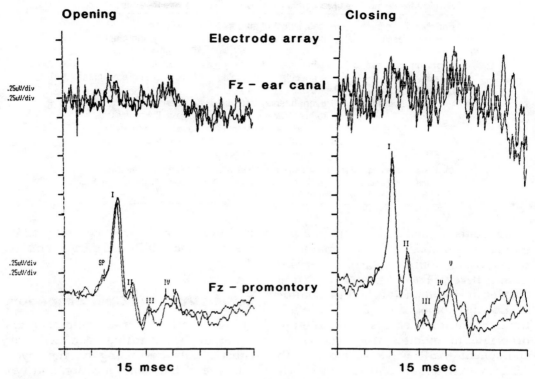

Opening   **Closing**

Electrode array

Fz – ear canal

Fz – promontory

.25uV/div
.25uV/div

.25uV/div
.25uV/div

15 msec   15 msec

FIG 16–5.
Comparison of ECochG/ABR waveforms recorded intraoperatively with ear canal (TIPtrode) versus transtympanic promontory electrode. Note considerably larger amplitude and higher quality for waveforms recorded from the promontory electrode.

that potential nonsurgical causes of evoked response changes are first ruled out. Examples of these nonsurgical causes would include physiologic fluctuations (such as body temperature or blood pressure), equipment problems (such as electrode or transducer slippage), modifications in measurement parameters, and effects of anesthesia. We should point out here that there is a strong argument against reliance on only wave V absolute latency, or amplitude in intraoperative evoked response monitoring. Absolute wave V latency or amplitude reflects both central *and* peripheral (including middle ear and cochlear) auditory functioning, whereas interwave intervals (for example, wave I to II, I to III, or I to V latencies) predominantly reflect integrity of the eighth cranial nerve through the auditory brain stem. A re-

duction in stimulus intensity level, for example, due to slippage of an insert earphone during surgery, would be likely to affect the amplitude and latency of wave V but not the wave I to III or I to V latency interval, assuming a clear wave I remained present. The importance of recording a distinct wave I (ECochG AP component) is clear from this discussion. Patients with hearing sensitivity deficits, particularly in the high-frequency region, may not have a detectable wave I with extratympanic recording electrode techniques. As noted previously, however, a clear wave I can be recorded from most patients with a transtympanic electrode approach.

Optimally, one should record an evoked response component from the structure that is being operated on, and also from

TABLE 16–3.

Summary of Intraoperative Monitoring During Vestibular Surgery

Surgical Procedure	Monitoring Objective	Analysis Parameters*
Endolymphatic sac decompression	Assess effect of surgery on cochlear functioning	SP/AP ratio[†] AP latency and amplitude AP threshold
Endolymphatic sac shunt	Assess effect of surgery on cochlear functioning	SP/AP ratio AP latency and amplitude
Labyrinthectomy	None	
Vestibular neurectomy	Prevent hearing loss due to cochlear nerve damage or compromise of cochlear blood supply	AP latency and amplitude Wave I–II latency Wave I–III latency Wave I–V latency

*Analysis criteria and guidelines for response interpretation are provided in the text.
†SP, summating potential; AP, action potential; electrocochleography AP and auditory brain stem response wave I are equivalent components

components immediately distal (peripheral to) and immediately proximal (central to) the anatomic region of surgery intraoperatively. For surgery putting the cochlea at risk, then, it is best to monitor all ECochG components (CM, SP, AP). If the eighth cranial nerve is at risk, it is appropriate to monitor the ECochG AP component (ABR wave I), along with ABR waves II, and III, and the wave I to II and I to III intervals. When the auditory brain stem is also at risk, all ABR components, including wave V, should be monitored. Perhaps the best approach for rapidly and consistently obtaining this information is the two or three channel measurement of ECochG/ABR, described above, with electrodes located on the promontory, the forehead, and, on occasion, directly on the eighth nerve as it enters the brain stem.

It is important to emphasize that latency and amplitude of ABR wave I (ECochG AP) is *not* sensitive to proximal eighth cranial nerve or auditory brain stem dysfunction. There are repeated accounts of brain stem dysfunction or inactivity and marked eighth nerve dysfunction, including complete transection of the nerve, in the presence of a consistently recorded and normal appearing wave I or AP component.[3, 5, 9] Hearing in these cases is, of course, entirely lost. In time, there is apparently retrograde degeneration of cochlear functioning, or delayed vascular disturbance, and the ABR wave I (ECochG AP) also disappears.

Setting Up in the Operating Room

The location of the equipment and tester in the operating room will vary substantially depending on the layout and size of the room, location and type of other equipment in the room, the other personnel involved in the case, and even the patient's surgical position.[3] The clinician is advised to visit an operating room in advance in order to develop a plan for equipment set up. Then, once the patient has been brought to the operating room this plan can be discussed with the surgeon(s), head operating room nurse or technician, and the anesthesiologist. Features of a satisfactory equipment arrangement are, minimally, access to an appropriate electrical outlet; proximity to the patient and surgeon; location away from possible sources of electrical interference; and location of equipment, tester, and evoked response electrode and stimulus cables away from main traffic areas. Convenient location of the electrode box, a distance away from the surgeons whenever possible, is particularly important to facilitate access to electrode leads in the event that changes are required during surgery. A remote electrode box location also may allow the clinician to disconnect electrodes from the equipment during or at the end of monitoring to move equipment or turn equipment power off. It may be necessary to set up evoked response equipment only after the operating table and patient have been moved into position for surgery and essential surgical equipment (such as microscope, coagulator, laser, or TV monitor) are in place. Finally, the clinician should insist on having access to a stool or small chair during monitoring.

The operating room typically contains multiple sources of electrical activity that may interfere with auditory evoked response measurements, including the monopolar and bipolar cauteries, surgical lasers, microscopes, and even the electrocardiographic leads. Another electrical interference is the "twitch monitor," the electrical stimulator that anesthesiologists place on the wrist of the patient to determine the status of neuromuscular blockade. Even if electrical artifacts can be eliminated, the operating room is a very noisy environment, and it is extremely difficult, if not impossible, to monitor auditory evoked potentials while the surgical drill is being used. Each of these factors must be taken into account during the monitoring process. The best way to deal with artifacts during surgery is to anticipate them before the procedure begins. The electrode wires, the boxes in which they are plugged, and the cables leading to the monitors should be isolated from other electrical cables as much as practical. To prevent electrodes from being pulled out inadvertently, we tape our electrodes and cables into the desired position. We use subdermal needle electrodes for all intraoperative monitoring procedures, this provides a somewhat secure placement of the electrodes as well as low electrode impedance (3.0 KΩ). Also, needle electrodes significantly improve the signal-to-noise ratio for recording bioelectric potentials.

The location of the monitoring equip-ment depends primarily on which ear is to be operated. In either case, the monitors are located near the foot of the patient, so that the various electrode boxes are placed near the head and the cords run toward the foot of the patient. Immediately after the induction of general anesthesia, the cords and electrodes are placed. One of the inherent difficulties of intraoperative monitoring is the need to have the various monitoring electrodes and the sound tube immediately adjacent to a sterile field. Maintenance of a sterile field during surgery is essential, and this can be accomplished in several different ways. One technique that we have used is to have the electrodes, the ear plug, and the sound tube gas sterilized so that it can be placed by the surgeon after the field has been made ready. Alternatively, the electrodes and sound tube can be placed prior to preparing the patient. The electrodes are then covered with a topical antiseptic solution (Betadine). The ear plug, sound tube, and the electrodes are draped out of the sterile field by using a plastic drape impregnated with topical antiseptic (Betadine). The surgeon then must make certain that this portion of the field is not violated during the procedure. While the surgeon is scrubbing in preparation for the operation, the audiologist obtains baseline values for the various parameters being monitored.

Steps in Monitoring

The most important step during monitoring is to *trend* evoked response findings. This is particularly important for auditory evoked responses, as opposed to facial nerve findings. Trending is the display of responses as a function of time. One approach is to display a representative baseline averaged waveform at the top of the evoked response system oscilloscope (screen) and then to also display the waveform being averaged (monitored) just below. One cursor is placed on a peak of interest (for example, ABR wave V) in the baseline waveform and the other cursor is placed on this same peak in the ongoing average. The latency difference can then be continuously calculated. Amplitude values can be similarly calculated periodically during surgery. As surgery proceeds, representative waveforms recorded at certain surgical events are displayed on the screen, along with the baseline and ongoing averaged waveform. To facilitate accurate analysis of evoked response waveforms, especially calculation of amplitude, it is important to display all waveforms with the same gain setting. Use of an automatic gain setting option often presents a very misleading display of waveforms because amplitudes displayed for each waveform are adjusted to be equivalent by the equipment. With automatic gain adjustment, substantial differences between waveforms, and changes in the amplitude among the waveforms over time, can easily go undetected.

INTRAOPERATIVE EVOKED RESPONSE APPLICATIONS

Endolymphatic Sac Decompression and Shunt Insertion

Rationale

Whether improvements in ECochG data from presurgical to postsurgical assessment are actually due to the operation, or due instead to coincidental fluctuations associated with Meniere's disease, is the topic of debate. In 1989, Arenberg and co-workers[1] described the use of ECochG during endolymphatic sac surgery. Specifically, their objective was "to continually monitor the electrophysiologic parameters of the SP/AP ratio to document the changes effected by any mechanical or neural manipulation of the auditory system during nondestructive inner ear surgery."[1, p2] These investigators compared the SP/AP ratio at closing versus *surgical* baseline and considered a decrease of 15% or more (assuming an initial SP/AP ratio of at

least 40%) evidence of a significant intraoperative change. Their preliminary findings appeared to show that when the inner ear with endolymphatic hydrops was decompressed, clear reductions in the SP/AP ratio occurred rapidly (often in less than 30 seconds).

Based on these findings, the authors concluded that

if "hydropic labyrinth is decompressed, but there is no change from abnormal, stable baseline ECochG, the inner ear can be reapproached to try and decompress the hydropic system from a different incision . . . if after due diligence, a nondestructive approach to the hydropic ear is not successful, according to changes in ECochG parameters, then the surgeon can proceed during the same surgery to a destructive procedure, either a labyrinthectomy or a vestibular nerve section. . ."[1, p6]

Inspired by these promising preliminary findings, we have recorded ECochG intraoperatively from a series of patients with Meniere's disease undergoing an endolymphatic sac decompression or shunt procedure. Our primary objective was to apply ECochG in surgical decision-making. Specifically we were interested in determining whether decompression produced a change in cochlear status or, if ECochG remained unchanged, whether the operation should include the shunt procedure. A secondary objective was to assure cochlear integrity intraoperatively, at least through closing. Each of these monitoring goals is illustrated with a case report in the following sections.

Technique

Electrocochleography is recorded with measurement parameters, and the simplified promontory electrode approach, described previously in the chapter. Briefly, a noninverting (needle) electrode is placed on either the high forehead (Fz) or the nontest ear lobe. The inverting electrode is a transtympanic needle on the promontory of the operated ear. A ground (also needle) electrode is typically located on the low forehead (Fpz). The ECochG is continuously monitored with a high-intensity stimulus (90 or 95 dB HL), although ECochG threshold (lowest intensity level producing a reliable AP) is routinely determined at baseline (opening) and closing. The stimulus is almost always an alternating polarity click. Single polarity (rarefaction or condensation) click stimuli and tone burst stimuli are occasionally employed in addition to the clicks if there are indications that the click-evoked response is suboptimal. With the promontory electrode, reliable SP and AP components are typically detected with as few as 50 to 100 stimulus repetitions, or even less in patients with reasonably good hearing sensitivity.

Analysis parameters continuously calculated and trended from moment to moment include AP latency and amplitude, and the SP/AP amplitude ratio. As a rule, these calculations are made on two or three sequentially recorded waveforms recorded over a period of approximately 1 minute, rather than from a single averaged response. By analyzing data for summed waveforms, the possible effects of irrelevant perturbations in SP and AP amplitude are minimized. Based on our intraoperative ECochG statistics on normal variability (in patients not undergoing endolymphatic decompression, as summarized earlier in the chapter), we view a consistent change in the SP/AP ratio of greater than 10% as evidence of altered cochlear status. In this analysis, it is important to first rule out the possible influence on SP/AP data of spurious factors, especially temporal bone drilling. This point is discussed in greater detail in the next section.

During the entire monitoring process, care is taken to document pertinent anethestic maneuvers (such as administration of drugs) and surgical events, such as temporal bone drilling, thinning of the bone over the endolymphatic sac, sac decompression, and shunt insertion (see waveforms displayed in Figure 16–7, Case 1, in the following section). Although analyzed on-line, all ECochG data are also stored on computer disk. A report of intraoperative findings is prepared during closing and inserted immediately into the patient's medical record. The surgeon also dictates a description of monitoring findings in the operative report.

Case 1

The patient was a 40-year-old man with a 4-month history of dizziness which was initiated with a change in head position. During episodes of severe dizziness he was unable to walk or drive a car. He had tinnitus and fullness in the left ear and bilateral progression of hearing loss. The patient denied noise exposure. Magnetic resonance images of the head were normal. Serial audiograms (Fig 16–6) confirmed a high-frequency sensorineural pattern, although the degree of loss on the left fluctuated. The patient's ABR waveforms were normal and bilaterally symmetrical for click and 1,000 Hz tone burst stimuli at the conventional rate (21.1/sec), but there was no clear wave V on the left ear at a rapid click rate (91.1/sec). Electronystagmographic abnormalities (left unilateral weakness, right-beating nystagmus, and direction fixed positional nystagmus) were consistent with a left peripheral site of lesion.

The patient underwent endolymphatic sac decompression and shunt on the left side for Meniere's disease. Auditory status was monitored intraoperatively by a combined ECochG/ABR technique. As shown in Figure 16–7, there was a clear and reliable response before, during, and after endolymphatic sac decompression. Following exposure of the sac, latency of the ECochG AP component (ABR wave I) became abnormally prolonged in association with fluid (saline irrigation) in the middle ear space. When the fluid was suctioned, latency returned to baseline values. The SP/AP ratio was 12% at baseline, but increased to 83% at sac exposure and remained abnormally high (85%) with insertion of the shunt and even at closing (41%). Monitoring provided evidence of cochlear functioning at the conclusion of surgery. Rather than showing normalization with surgical therapy, the SP/AP ratio actually increased from being within normal limits to abnormally large during the course of the procedure.

After surgery the patient was treated with

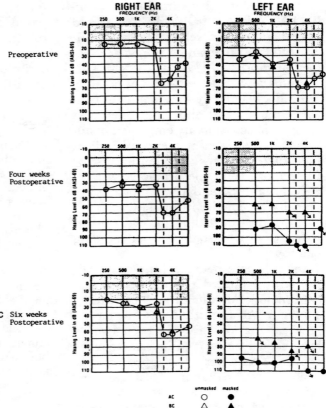

FIG 16–6.
Preoperative and postoperative audiometric findings for an adult man with Meniere's disease who underwent a left endolymphatic sac decompression and shunt procedure (Case 1). Hearing decreased after surgery. Intraoperative ECochG/ABR findings for this patient are shown in Figure 16–7.

intravenous antibiotics and discharged with a prescription of antibiotics. Within the first week following surgery, the patient did well. He then developed fluctuant hearing loss, more severe than preoperatively, which progressed. Treatment with steroids produced some transient improvement in hearing, but when the severe hearing loss persisted an adverse reaction to the Silastic endolymphatic shunt material was considered. A second operation was done to remove the shunt. Large amounts of cholesterol granuloma and fibrous reaction was noted throughout the mastoid and removed. Hearing evaluation after the second surgery continued to show a severe to profound loss (see Fig 16–6).

As noted earlier, there are published claims that ECochG can be used to assess the effectiveness of surgical therapy for endolymphatic hydrops. That is, reduction in an abnormally enlarged SP/AP ratio with sac decompression and/or insertion of a shunt, is evidence that

the cochlear pathophysiology has been successfully treated. This case, however, illustrates a trend which the authors have observed intraoperatively during inner ear surgery. The SP/AP ratio may actually become enlarged as the operation progresses, perhaps secondary to manipulation and minor trauma of the cochlea (for example, due to drilling), and remain abnormally enlarged at the conclusion of surgery. Unfortunately, this ECochG trend may be an early neurophysiologic indicator of postoperative deterioration in cochlear function. In any event, with this case the presence of a reliable and normal appearing ECochG/ABR at the conclusion of inner ear surgery confirmed cochlear integrity. This was, in retrospect, an important finding, as the patient's hearing worsened markedly at some point during the interval from surgery to 1 week later. Without intraoperative AER evidence of a func-

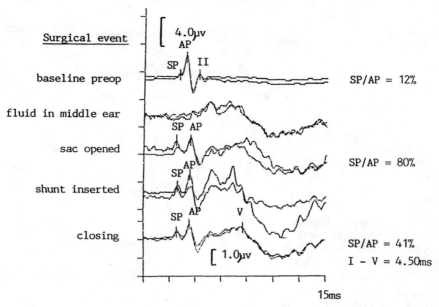

FIG 16–7.
Electrocochleographic waveforms recorded intraoperatively from a young adult man during endolymphatic sac decompression/shunt procedure (Case 1). The SP amplitude increased during the procedure. A reliable response was noted at closing.

tional cochlea, it would have been impossible to rule out surgery-related damage.

Case 2

The patient was a 36-year-old woman with the chief complaint of severe incapacitating vertigo. Initially, her hearing was normal. One month after the onset of vertigo, repeat hearing assessment at another facility showed a low-frequency sensorineural hearing loss on the right ear. The patient then also noted tinnitus on the right side. The patient was referred to the Vanderbilt University Medical Center. Another audiogram revealed further hearing loss on the right ear and normal hearing on the left ear. Middle ear function was normal bilaterally. Acoustic reflexes were present at expected normal levels. Word recognition was excellent. The pattern of audiometric findings and history were consistent with Meniere's disease. Auditory brain stem response was reliably recorded, showing absolute and interwave latency values within normal limits bilaterally. Retrocochlear auditory dysfunction was ruled out. On ECochG assessment, a reliable SP and AP were re-

corded in three replicated waveforms for both ears. The SP/AP ratio was 35% on the left ear and 57% on the right ear. This pattern was compatible with Meniere's disease of the right ear.

The patient was initially managed medically, with diazide, antivert, and a low salt diet. She also eliminated caffeine from her diet. Her episodic but incapacitating vertigo persisted. She underwent an endolymphatic sac decompression with shunt insertion. Promontory recorded ECochG was monitored during exposure, opening of the endolymphatic sac, and insertion of a sac-to-mastoid shunt. As seen in Figure 16–8, a reliable response was detected throughout the case. The SP/AP ratio was 44% at the start of surgery. A value of over 30% is considered abnormal with the promontory electrode technique. During sac decompression and shunt insertion, and over a 15-minute period during closing, the SP/AP ratio remained in the 33% to 40% range. Comparison of ECochG for a 40-dB click stimulus intensity level before and after surgery showed no alteration in latency or amplitude. In this patient, intraoperative ECochG documented cochlear integrity during surgery but showed no

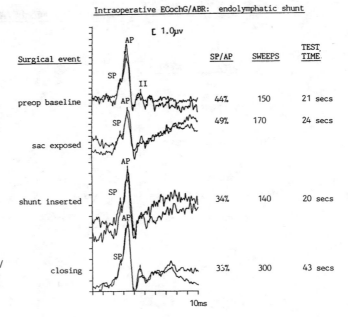

Intraoperative ECochG/ABR: endolymphatic shunt

Surgical event	SP/AP	SWEEPS	TEST TIME
preop baseline	44%	150	21 secs
sac exposed	49%	170	24 secs
shunt inserted	34%	140	20 secs
closing	33%	300	43 secs

FIG 16–8.
ECochG waveforms recorded intraoperatively from young adult female during endolymphatic sac decompression/shunt procedure (Case 2). The SP/AP amplitude relation showed no systematic decrease during decompression.

conclusive evidence of a change in cochlear pathophysiology. A report of intraoperative ECochG findings was prepared on the evoked response system computer, printed, and placed in the patient's medical record during closing.

Vestibular Neurectomy

Rationale

There are numerous reports describing the application of auditory evoked responses, particularly ABR, in monitoring eighth cranial nerve status during vestibular neurectomy.[3, 4, 10] The main goal of monitoring is continuous documentation of the integrity of the auditory portion of the eighth nerve, particularly as the vestibular portion is purposefully severed. However, monitoring also permits early detection of possible auditory dysfunction secondary to manipulation of the nerve or blood vessels serving the nerve or the cochlea. Because the focus of intraoperative concern is the eighth cranial nerve between the porus of the internal auditory canal and the brain stem, it is most effective to monitor auditory evoked response components arising both distal and proximal to this region.

Technique

We have found that a combined ECochG/ABR approach is well suited for this monitoring objective (see Table 16–2). The ECochG AP component (recorded as described earlier) provides a robust distal eighth nerve marker. Both ECochG and ABR recordings yield a wave II (N2) component which, presumably, arises from proximal eighth nerve. However, the wave II is not always clearly observed. In such cases, the ABR wave III serves as the proximal marker and the AP (wave I) to wave III latency interval is monitored closely (see Table 16–3). The wave I to III interval is preferable to the wave I to V interval for early and confident detection of eighth cranial nerve trauma. Wave V is less site specific than wave III in this context. That is, a change in wave V (latency or amplitude) may reflect brain stem dysfunction, rather than eighth nerve dysfunction. This might result, for example, from retraction of the cerebellum as the eighth nerve is properly exposed. Naturally, as we are also interested in early detection of possible brain stem dysfunction, the wave V component (and the wave III to V latency interval) is typically monitored as well. Measurement parameters are manipulated so that each of these

ECochG/ABR components is large in amplitude and reliably recorded with the least number of stimulus repetitions (least test time). There are no "standardized" absolute or interwave latency criteria for intraoperative interpretation of ECochG/ABR findings. Assuming the presence of a reliable AP (wave I) and wave III, the surgeon is warned of a change in the interwave latency of greater than 0.5 msec. A wave I to III increase of greater than 1 msec is considered a serious sign of danger (potentially reversible) to the eighth nerve. Persistent loss of wave III (and wave V) is viewed as evidence of total eighth nerve dysfunction.

Case 3

The patient was a 28-year-old woman with a 3-year history of recurrent vertigo, fluctu-

ant hearing loss, and fullness of the left ear. Within the past 2 to 3 months, the episodes had become immobilizing. Otoscopic examination was unremarkable. Magnetic resonance imaging was negative for retrocochlear disease. Audiometry showed a low-frequency, sensorineural hearing loss (Fig 16–9). Clinical ECochG recordings revealed a normal SP/AP ratio on the right ear but an enlarged SP/AP ratio on the left ear. A left suboccipital vestibular nerve section was scheduled.

Monitoring was carried out with a combined ECochG/ABR technique using a promontory inverting electrode. Waveforms recorded at selected intraoperative events are displayed in Figure 16–10. There was a clear AP (wave I), and waves II through V were clear. No changes in absolute or interwave latency values, or response amplitude, were observed from baseline measurements through nerve sectioning to closing. Interwave latencies were consistently within normal limits. Thus, intraoperative ECochG/ABR confirmed cochlear and eighth nerve

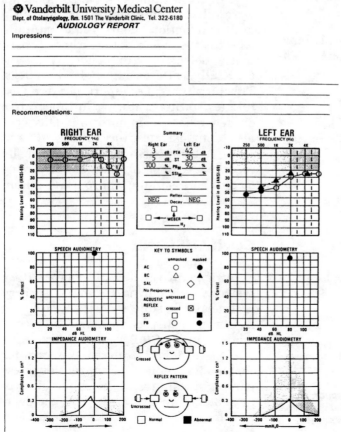

FIG 16–9.
Audiometric findings for a young adult woman with left-side Meniere's disease prior to vestibular neurectomy (Case 3).

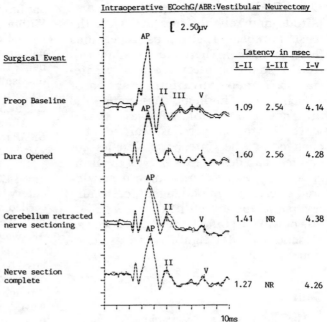

Intraoperative ECochG/ABR: Vestibular Neurectomy

[2.50μv

Surgical Event		Latency in msec		
		I-II	I-III	I-V
Preop Baseline		1.09	2.54	4.14
Dura Opened		1.60	2.56	4.28
Cerebellum retracted nerve sectioning		1.41	NR	4.38
Nerve section complete		1.27	NR	4.26

10ms

FIG 16–10.
The ECochG/ABR waveforms recorded from a young adult woman during vestibular neurectomy (Case 3). Interwave latency values were consistently within normal limits and showed no change before, during, and after sectioning of the vestibular nerve.

integrity during vestibular neurectomy. Hearing was unchanged at postoperative assessments.

As illustrated in Figure 16–11, however, stimulus polarity may exert a defi-

Intraoperative ECochG/ABR

[0.25μv

Stimulus polarity

alternating clicks

condensation clicks

I   II

V

rarefaction clicks

15ms

FIG 16–11.
Effect of stimulus polarity on the morphology of ECochG/ABR waveforms recorded intraoperatively from a patient during opening prior to vestibular neurectomy. A clear and reliable response was present for rarefaction polarity clicks. Morphology was poor with condensation polarity clicks, and no reliable wave components were apparent for the alternating polarity stimulus condition.

nite influence on waveform morphology. In this example, wave components were reliably observed intraoperatively with rarefaction polarity click stimuli, whereas they were not clearly or consistently detected with condensation or, especially, alternating polarity clicks. This highlights the importance of a flexible test protocol during intraoperative evoked response monitoring. This case also demonstrates the robust AP and wave II components that are typically recorded with a promontory inverting electrode, assuming appropriate stimulus parameters.

CONCLUSIONS

Intraoperative monitoring of auditory system status during vestibular surgery is clinically feasible and useful. Although it is technically challenging to record quality ECochG/ABR data intraoperatively, we demonstrate in this chapter that modification of the conventional test paradigm can result in rapid electrophysiologic measurement of cochlear, eighth nerve, and auditory brain stem function.

Vestibular neurectomy endangers the auditory portion of eighth cranial nerve. A combined ECochG/ABR monitoring approach can provide the surgeon with moment-to-moment information on nerve integrity, and also verify adequate cochlear function when blood supply to the sensory apparatus is at risk. The role of intraoperative monitoring during other surgical therapies for vestibular disorder, such as endolyphatic sac surgery and labyrinthectomy with streptomycin infusion, is less established. The relationship between intraoperative evoked response findings and both cochlear function intraoperatively and long-term vestibular outcome is not yet adequately defined. However, it is likely that evoked response applications during vestibular surgery will continue to develop as new surgical techniques are introduced and as our intraoperative experience with ECochG and ABR accumulates.

Acknowledgments

This work was supported in part by a Vanderbilt University Research Council Grant awarded to Dr. Hall. Timothy Trine, M.S., assisted in data analysis.

REFERENCES

1. Arenberg IK, Gibson WPR, Bohlen HKH, et al: An overview of diagnostic and intraoperative electrocochleography for inner ear disease. *Insights Otolaryngol* 1989; 4:1–6.

2. Bertrand O, Garcia-Larrea L, Artru F, et al: Brain-stem monitoring. I: A system for high-rate sequential BAEP recording and feature extraction. *Electroencephalogr Clin Neurophysiol* 1987; 68:433–445.

3. Hall JW III: *Handbook of Auditory Evoked Responses*. Needham, Mass, Allyn & Bacon, 1992.

4. Kileny PR, Niparko JK, Shepard NT, et al: Neurophysiologic intraoperative monitoring: I. Auditory function. *Am J Otol* 1988; 9:17–24.

5. Levine RA, Ojemann RG, Montgomery WW, et al: Monitoring auditory evoked potentials during acoustic neuroma surgery: Insights into the mechanism of hearing loss. *Ann Otol Rhinol Laryngol* 1984; 93:116–123.

6. Margolis RH, Levine SC, Fournier EM, et al: Extratympanic electrocochleography: Abnormal response patterns. *Audiol Today* 1991; 3:39.

7. Moller AR, Jannetta P: Monitoring auditory functions during cranial microvascular decompression operations by direct recording from the eighth nerve. *J Neurosurg* 1983; 59:493–499.

8. Perlman H, Kimura R, Fernandez C: (1959). Experiments on temporary obstruction of the internal auditory artery. *Laryngoscope* 1959; 69:591–613.

9. Ruben R, Hudson W, Chiong A: Anatomical and physiological effects of chronic section of eighth nerve in cat. *Acta Otolaryngol* 1963; 55:473–484.

10. Ruth RA, Lambert PR, Ferraro JA: Electrocochleography: Methods and clinical applications. *Am J Otol* 1988; 9:1–11.

11. Schwaber MK, Hall JW III: A simplified technique for transtympanic electrocochleography. *Am J Otol* 1990; 11:260–265.

12. Silverstein H, McDaniel A, Norrell H, et al: Hearing preservation after acoustic neuroma surgery with intraoperative direct eighth cranial nerve monitoring. II: A classification of results. *Otolaryngol Head Neck Surg* 1986; 95:285–291.

13. Silverstein H, Wazen J, Norrell H, et al: Retrolabyrinthine vestibular neurectomy with simultaneous monitoring of VIIIth nerve action potentials and electrocochleography. *Am J Otol* 1984; 5:552–555.

CHAPTER 17

Balance Handicap Assessment

Craig W. Newman, Ph.D.
Gary P. Jacobson, Ph.D.

Dizziness or unsteadiness can be debilitating to an individual if it limits his or her ability to perform the normal activities of everyday life. While obtaining case history information from a patient suffering from a balance disorder, it is not uncommon for clinicians to hear complaints such as, "I'm afraid to drive because of my dizziness," or "It is difficult to walk by myself because of my unsteadiness." Clinical efforts in relation to these problems have been directed traditionally toward determining the site and laterality of vestibular system disease through the application of electronystagmography (ENG). More recently, additional techniques have been incorporated into the clinician's vestibulometric test battery to provide greater insight into the "balance system." The procedures which supplement the conventional ENG examination include rotary chair testing (see Chapters 10 and 11) and computerized dynamic posturography (see Chapters 13 and 14).

In contrast to the amount of clinical and research effort devoted toward determining the physiologic origins of a balance system disorder, little attention has focused on quantifying the physical and psychosocial consequences associated with severe or recurring equilibrium problems. Moreover, quantifying the sequelae of balance system disease may have important ramifications to the clinician regarding patient management and the documentation of treatment outcome.

This chapter focuses on the assessment of balance function handicap by exploring two major questions. First, why evaluate balance function handicap? Second, what tools are available for meeting the need? In order to answer these primary questions, five related areas are addressed. First, definitions of balance function handicap and balance function impairment will be provided. Second, cross-discipline scales for measuring a number of different physical and psychosocial domains are summarized. Third, instruments developed specifically for assessing functional outcome following intervention efforts (medical, surgical, rehabilitative) for dizziness/unsteadiness are discussed. Fourth, the clinical usefulness of a self-assessment balance function handicap scale is illustrated through case history examples. Fifth, future research needs are suggested.

BACKGROUND

Definitions

The terms *impairment* and *handicap* are often misused by students, practicing clinicians, and researchers alike. Because an important distinction exists between these two concepts, the following section presents operational definitions for *balance function impairment* and *balance function handicap*.

Balance Function Impairment

The World Health Organization[43] broadly defines *impairment* as any loss or abnormality of psychological, physiological, or anatomical structure or function. In this context, balance function impairment may be considered an abnormality in any of the three interdependent sensory systems required for individuals to maintain stability, including vision, proprioception (the gravity-sensing apparatus located in the muscles, tendons, and joints), and the vestibular system. Balance system impairment is usually measured through vestibulometric and/or posturographic tests. For example, a calculation derived from measuring the slow-phase velocity of nystagmus resulting from bithermal caloric irrigations can serve to quantify the symmetry of the peripheral vestibular response. Thus, a patient can be described as having, for example, a 30% unilateral weakness on the right side, suggesting a significant asymmetry in tonic peripheral vestibular input.

Balance Function Handicap

Generally speaking, *handicap* refers to a disadvantage for a given individual, resulting from an impairment that limits or prevents the fulfillment of a role that is normal.[43] Accordingly, balance function handicap occurs when a balance impairment is severe enough to affect an individual's physical function (for example, one is unable to stand up quickly) and/or psychosocial function (for example, fear of driving due to episodic dizziness). Unlike balance function impairment, balance function handicap may be more difficult to quantify. An individual's response to a balance function impairment is multifaceted and is probably determined by a number of factors including personality, age, occupational status, psychosocial adjustment, and general physical health.

Many clinicians have developed their own dizziness questionnaires or use those previously published[6] in an attempt to qualitatively document a patient's dizziness complaint. The typical areas covered in the history of a patient complaining of balance problems include the following: character of the dizziness (vertigo, unsteadiness, giddiness); time course of dizziness (single episode, recurrent episode, continuous); precipitating factors (head movement, position changes, sneezing, excessively loud noises); associated symptoms (nausea and vomiting, blurred vision and oscillopsia, auditory symptoms, brain stem symptoms); family history; and predisposing factors (infectious disease, trauma surgery, vascular disease, metabolic disease, developmental disorders, drugs).[2,3] Although these data are important in the clinical decision-making process, it is noteworthy that the impact such clinical features have on the patient's psychosocial well-being or quality of life is not explored.

The Need to Assess Handicap

One of the most difficult problems faced by medical and nonmedical professionals is that of determining the effectiveness of medical, surgical, and rehabilitative treatment. A number of methods have been advocated in attempts to measure the benefit of health care on the quality of life.[10] The issue of documenting therapeutic outcome is important in that it affects patients, payors, and providers.

The application of self-report measures is one approach for measuring outcome which has gained recognition in the health care field.[10] The usefulness of handicap assessment in the clinical setting assumes that the magnitude of success or failure of a treatment protocol is determined by the subjective reaction of the patient. For example, successful treatment of a balance system disorder (through pharmacologic management, vestibular nerve section, endolymphatic sac decompression, Cawthorne exercises) should relieve the symptoms of dizziness and/or unsteadiness. Accordingly, a patient's response to treatment should be reflected by a reduction in self-perceived handicap. On the other hand, self-perceived handicap should not change if the treatment approach was unsuccessful. Therefore, the assessment of balance function handicap before and after treatment protocols may help quantify the outcome of therapeutic strategies. In this way, it may be possible to determine the benefits derived from a particular intervention approach by quantifying an individual's physical and psychosocial behavior. Moreover, because the quality of services is indirectly evaluated with self-report tools, these measurement instruments may be ideal for use as quality indicators for external accrediting agencies such as the Joint Commission on Accreditation of Healthcare Organizations.

A number of important questions surround any attempts to measure the impact of medical, surgical, or rehabilitative treatment on the quality of life. These issues involve psychometric factors such as reliability and validity of the measuring instrument. That is, if a scale is to assess change over time or measure benefits derived from a particular treatment, it must possess good test-retest reliability. Clinicians must be confident that score differences are due to treatment per se, and not to measurement error.[8] Further, it may be important to know the mode of administration (for example, face-to-face or paper-pencil) of the self-assessment scale, in that the administration approach taken could affect test-retest reliability.[29, 41] The validity of a scale must be examined to ensure that the instrument measures what it purports to measure. Moreover, one must question whether a patient's subjective opinions about well being can be treated objectively as direct pathophysiologic observations and electrophysiogic data.

Cross-Discipline Assessment Tools

The availability of a wide range of scales that allow one to examine a number of domains attests to the usefulness of self-report measures. Over the years, a number of self-assessment scales have been developed and employed by clinicians and researchers in order to document physical health status,[23, 34] anxiety and depression,[25, 39, 44] personality,[13, 20] happiness or well-being,[26] and the ability to cope with activities of daily living.[19] In addition to measuring single domains with self-assessment scales, multidimensional assessment batteries have been developed which provide a more global assessment of an individual's functional status.[12, 14, 33] For example, The Sickness Impact Profile (SIP) is a 136-item standardized questionnaire grouped into 12 subscales: ambulation, mobility, body care/movement, social interaction, communication, alertness, emotional, sleep/rest, eating, work, home management, and recreation/pastimes.[4, 5, 12]

It is apparent that a wide spectrum of instruments have been developed which probe a variety of physical, mental, and social realms. In general, the applications of these scales have been limited to (1) obtaining information concerning the degree and type of illness or dysfunction experienced by an individual; and (2) determining functional health capacities based on how restricted a given individual is in his activities because of their physical condition.[11] By examining a number of the extravestibulometric/postural variables associated with the above-mentioned scales, clinicians may gain insight into a patient's emotional and psychosocial response to balance system disease not explained solely by ENG, rotational testing, and/or computerized dynamic posturographic examinations. For the most part, self-report measures employed by psychologists, geron-tologists, nurses, social workers, and physicians have not been used for docu-menting treatment outcome, but rather as questionnaires for structuring and standardizing the clinical interview.

In contrast, audiologists have taken advantage of handicap scales by using them to monitor the impact of audiolog-ic/otologic intervention efforts. Insight into hearing and tinnitus handicap is important, in that many patients suffer-ing with dizziness also have auditory complaints as well (for example, Me-niere's disease). Following are examples of the application of auditory handicap assessment in the audiologic/otologic setting.

Hearing Handicap

A variety of self-report hearing handi-cap inventories have been developed which probe the communication and psychosocial handicap that accompany a hearing loss. The audiologic literature is replete with studies employing self-assessment hearing handicap scales as criterion indicators against which to judge hearing aid benefit. In general, these investigations have demonstrated a reduction in self-perceived emotional and social-situational handicaps follow-ing a period of hearing aid use,[9, 21, 28, 30] indicating that benefit was provided by the amplification device. It has been sug-gested by a number of authors[30, 35, 40] that data obtained from hearing handi-cap inventories provide information re-garding communication function that cannot be derived or predicted from the conventional audiometric evaluation (pure-tone and speech audiometry).

Tinnitus Handicap

Several tinnitus handicap scales have been developed in an attempt to validate the efficiency of different tinnitus treat-ment approaches.[18, 38, 42] For example, Sweetow et al.[38] developed the Tinnitus Severity Scale (TSS) to be used as a base-line measure from which therapeutic progress could be compared. They rec-ommended that the TSS should be given once per month after the initial adminis-tration, for as long as active therapeutic management (such as tinnitus maskers, biofeedback, drug treatment, cognitive-behavioral therapy) continues. In this way, it would be possible to monitor the benefit derived from any one particular therapeutic approach over specific time intervals.

QUANTIFYING OUTCOME FOR THE TREATMENT OF BALANCE IMPAIRMENT

Quantifying the outcome of medical, surgical, and rehabilitative treatment of the dizzy patient is especially difficult. For example, caloric testing is ineffective in measuring the effects of treatment. That is, a unilateral weakness docu-mented during the pretreatment exami-nation is usually present on reexamina-tion after treatment has stopped. Al-though pretreatment and posttreatment rotational and posturographic testing may provide information concerning the process of central vestibular compensa-tion, these latter diagnostic techniques do not quantify the handicapping effects imposed by vestibular/postural control maintenance system disease. Accord-ingly, conventional diagnostic testing procedures do not measure the effects of specific treatment protocols on the way patients function in everyday life.

Methods designed to evaluate the effi-cacy of treatment protocols for dizziness and unsteadiness have been limited. The following will summarize three specific techniques, each developed in an at-tempt to document treatment outcome. Each method attempts to quantify out-come based on the functional capabili-ties of the patient.

Formula Method

In 1985, the Committee on Hearing and Equilibrium of the American Acad-emy of Ophthalmology and Otolaryngology proposed a revised method for reporting the results of treatment for Meniere's disease.[7] A report issued by the AAO-HNS indicated that the medical and surgical treatment employed to control vestibular symptoms (vertigo) may decrease the frequency of the symptoms but may not completely eliminate the presence of definitive spells. Accordingly, a formula, resulting in a single numerical value, was suggested to express the change in definitive spells following medical or surgical intervention.

Formula Calculation

The formula expressing the effect of treatment is calculated in the following manner. The average number of dizzy spells a patient experiences per month, 24 months after the initiation of treatment, is divided by the average number of spells per month, 6 months prior to treatment. If the observed period of time prior to treatment is less than 6 months, the denominator is the average number of definitive spells for the period of observation (and should be specified). This quantity, multiplied by 100, will result in a single value reflecting the effects of treatment on the vertiginous spells.

Scoring

The resultant value is placed into one of the following five categories representing the degree of change in definitive spells of vertigo after treatment: 0 = complete control of definitive spells; 1 to 40 = substantial control of definitive spells; 41 to 80 = limited control of definitive spells; 81 to 120 = insignificant control of definitive spells; over 120 = worse (poorer) control of definitive spells.

Strengths and Weaknesses

The major strength of this approach is that the calculation is easy to perform and may provide the managing physician information regarding the overall success or failure of treatment. It is note-worthy that the importance of quantifying the effects of treatment of dizziness, based on a patient's functional status (at least in terms of controlling dizzy spells), was recognized by the AAO-HHS. However, a definition of what constitutes a definitive spell was not provided by the report. Further, the validity of the value derived from the formula relies on the patient's ability to count accurately the number of spells experienced. Although this formula takes into account the frequency of dizziness attacks, it does not attempt to evaluate the impact of dizziness on the way a patient functions from day-to-day, and therefore, is not a true measure of balance function handicap. This method has been criticized recently in that quantifying specific aspects of balance handicap may be a more useful and meaningful way of validating treatment outcome.[16] The latter authors illustrated their point through the following example. Patients who have experienced only a few attacks of violent vertigo may be sufficiently alarmed to the extent of restricting their activities (such as quitting their occupations or avoiding certain social situations), so as not to be vulnerable should another attack of vertigo occur. Therefore, a simple value representing the changes in the number of definite dizziness episodes may not provide an accurate picture of a patient's ability to resume his or her premorbid vocational and/or avocational activities.

Subjective Disability and Symptom Measure

Vestibular rehabilitation programs employing a variety of exercise approaches are gaining recognition as viable methods in the management of patients with persistent symptoms of imbalance (see Chapter 18). Vestibular rehabilitation strategies help facilitate central nervous system compensation following labyrinthine disease. The underlying physiologic mechanisms associated with compensation have been attributed to vestibular adaptation, sensory substitution, and rebalancing of tonic activity in central vestibular centers.[1, 22, 32, 36] Studies reporting changes in postural stability or the reduction of dizziness/unsteadiness have employed primarily qualitative (anecdotal) measures of outcome rather than quantitative techniques.[15, 22, 31]

Recently, Shepard et al.[37] developed two measures of overall therapy performance in order to quantify the success rate of their management program. These focused on (1) reducing or eliminating motion-provoked and/or positional sensitivity; and (2) the correction of functional deficits of balance and gait. They referred to their first outcome measure as the Subjective Disability Scale (SDS), administered in a pretherapy and posttherapy paradigm. The second measure is a posttherapy symptom score.

Scoring

The pretherapy and posttherapy disability score is determined by the clinician using the classification scheme outlined in Table 17–1. The authors indicated that for patients who are either retired or students, the word "work" in the classification scheme refers to the patient's ability to perform household chores or academic activities, respectively. The posttherapy symptom score is based on a comparison between a patient's symptoms at the completion of therapy and prior to the initiation of the program. The posttherapy scoring system is displayed in Table 17–2. It is recommended[37] that the SDS and the symptom scale be used in conjunction with each other. Further, they indicated that improvements in the SDS do not always coincide with a reduction in symptoms.

Reliability and Validity

Shepard et al.[37] assessed the reliability of the SDS on a sample of 98 adults (mean age, 53 years; standard deviation, 15 years) with a wide range of balance disorders. All subjects had symptoms for greater than 6 months. Assignment

TABLE 17–1.

Scoring Classification System for the Disability Rating Scale*

Score	Description
0	No disability; negligible symptoms
1	No disability; bothersome symptoms
2	Mild disability; performs usual work duties, but symptoms interfere with outside activities
3	Moderate disability; symptoms disrupt performance of both usual work duties and outside activities
4	Recent severe disability; on medical leave or had to change jobs because of symptoms
5	Long-term severe disability; unable to work for > 1 yr or established permanent disability with compensation payments

*Adapted from Shepard NT, Telian SA, Smith-Wheelock M: Neurol Clin 1990; 8:459–475.

of the disability score was performed by at least two of the three investigators. Inter-judge reliability of assigning a disability score was in agreement in 94 out of 98 cases (96%); however, test-retest reliability of the SDS was not measured.

Shepard and his co-workers[37] demonstrated statistically significant ($p < .0001$) lower mean disability scores following rehabilitation. Using the posttherapy symptom scores, 87% of the patients experienced some reduction in symptoms as a result of therapy, with 31% indicating complete absence of

TABLE 17–2.

Post-therapy Scoring Classification*

Score	Description
0	No symptoms remaining at the end of therapy
1	Marked improvement in symptoms, mild symptoms remaining
2	Mild improvement, definite persistent symptoms remaining
3	No change in symptoms relative to pre-therapy period
4	Symptoms worsened with therapy activities on a persistent basis relative to pre-therapy period

*Adapted from Shepard NT, Telian SA, Smith-Wheelock M: Neurol Clin 1990; 8:459–475.

symptoms. These findings attest to the construct validity of the measures.

Strengths and Weaknesses

The SDS attempts to assess the functional deficits of patients suffering from dizziness or unsteadiness. Taken together, the SDS and the symptom scale provide a two-dimensional approach for assessing therapy outcome. The evaluation is quick to perform; however, the authors did not provide a quantitative method for categorizing "marked improvement" or "mild improvement" for symptom scoring. Further, the SDS is narrow in scope, focusing solely on work duties and other "outside activities." Because scale scores are assigned by the clinician, insight into self-perceived (patient-perceived) balance handicap is not provided.

Dizziness Handicap Inventory

Rationale for Development

The Dizziness Handicap Inventory (DHI) was developed by Jacobson and Newman[16] in response to the lack of instruments designed to identify specific functional, emotional, or physical problems associated with an individual's reaction to balance function impairment. The authors indicated that the results of ENG and rotational examinations have little to do *with*, and are not predictive *of*, how a patient interacts with his or her environment after leaving the physician's office. The DHI was developed in an attempt to help alleviate this problem. The DHI assesses the patient's perception of the effects of their balance impairment and the functional and emotional adjustment of individuals suffering from dizziness or unsteadiness. Further, the scale probes the physical limitations imposed on an individual as a consequence of his or her balance problem.

Scoring, Response System, and Administration

The DHI is a 25-item self-assessment inventory composed of a 9-item func-

tional subscale, 9-item emotional subscale, and a 7-item physical subscale (Table 17–3 is a complete listing of all questions). The patient responds to each question with either a "yes," "no," or "sometimes." A "yes" response is awarded 4 points, a "sometimes" 2 points, and a "no" 0 points. Scores on the total scale range from 0, suggesting no perceived handicap, to 100, indicating significant perceived balance handicap.

Reliability and Validity

Cronbach's alpha coefficient was employed to measure reliability of the DHI based on internal consistency. The final version of the DHI was administered to 106 consecutive patients undergoing vestibulometric tests and yielded good internal consistency for the total (alpha = .89), functional (alpha = .85), emotional (alpha = .72) and physical (alpha = .78) scales. The test-retest reliability of the DHI, based on Pearson product-moment correlations, was excellent (total scale, r = .97). The standard error (SE) of measurement and the SE of the difference between two administrations of the DHI was calculated. The SE associated with a face-to-face administration of the DHI was 6.2, suggesting that pre-treatment and post-treatment scores would have to differ by at least 18 points (95% critical difference for a true change) before intervention efforts could be said to have effected a significant change in a patient's self-perceived balance handicap.

The DHI has both content and criterion validity. The fact that the final items selected to compose the DHI were developed empirically from case-history reports of patients with dizziness attests to the scale's content validity. The criterion validity of the DHI is based on a study conducted by Jacobson and his colleagues[17] in which relationships between components of the balance function examination (ENG, rotational testing, and posturography) and DHI scores were explored. Based on the observations of 367 patients seen consecutively

TABLE 17–3.

Items Comprising the Dizziness Handicap Inventory*

P1.[†]	Does looking up increase your problem?
E2.[†]	Because of your problem do you feel frustrated?
F3.[†]	Because of your problem do you restrict your travel for business or recreation?
P4.	Does walking down the aisle of a supermarket increase your problem?
F5.	Because of your problems do you have difficulty getting into or out of bed?
F6.	Does your problem significantly restrict your participation in social activities such as going out to dinner, movies, dancing, or parties?
F7.	Because of your problem do you have difficulty reading?
P8.	Does performing more ambitious activities like sports, dancing, and household chores such as sweeping or putting dishes away increase your problem?
E9.	Because of your problems are you afraid to leave your home without having someone accompany you?
E10.	Because of your problem have you been embarrassed in front of others?
P11.	Do quick movements of your head increase your problem?
F12.	Because of your problem do you avoid heights?
P13.	Does turning over in bed increase your problem?
F14.	Because of your problem is it difficult for you to do strenuous housework or yardwork?
E15.	Because of your problem are you afraid people may think you are intoxicated?
F16.	Because of your problem is it difficult for you to go for a walk by yourself?
P17.	Does walking down a sidewalk increase your problem?
E18.	Because of your problem is it difficult for you to concentrate?
F19.	Because of your problem is it difficult for you to walk around your house in the dark?
E20.	Because of your problem are you afraid to stay home alone?
E21.	Because of your problem do you feel handicapped?
E22.	Has your problem placed stress on your relationships with members of your family or friends?
E23.	Because of your problem are you depressed?
F24.	Does you problem interfere with your job or household responsibilities?
P25.	Does bending over increase your problem?

*Adapted from Jacobson GP, Newman CW, Hunter L, et al: J Am Acad Audiol 1991; 2:253–260.

†"P" denotes physical subscale items, "E" denotes emotional subscale items, and "F" denotes functional subscale items.

for balance function evaluations, the largest proportion of significant correlations existed between the DHI and the Sensory Organization Tests (SOT) of platform posturography. Significant negative correlations between the DHI total, functional, and emotional scales and conditions 2 (absent vision/fixed support), 3 (sway-referenced vision/fixed support), 4 (normal vision/sway-referenced support), 5 (absent vision/sway-referenced support), and 6 (sway-referenced vision/sway-referenced support) on the SOT were observed. Thus, diffi-culties in maintaining balance as identified through platform posturography were associated with higher DHI scores (greater perceived balance function handicap). Accordingly, as various sensory inputs to the patient were systematically removed (such as loss of vision by closing the eyes), attenuated (attenuating proprioceptive information by sway-referencing the platform) or distorted (distortion of vision by sway-referencing the surround) postural stability decreased and self-perceived balance function handicap increased. Therefore, the criterion validity of the DHI was demonstrated using platform posturography (SOT) as the external criterion indicator.

Strengths and Weaknesses

The DHI is reliable, requires little clinical time to administer, and is easy to score. In view of the high test-retest reliability and low standard error of measurement, changes in handicap scores following therapeutic intervention probably reflects the treatment per se, rather than variability inherent to the measuring instrument. Further, the DHI could be used to identify specific functional, emotional, or physical problems associated with vestibular system disease. Responses to individual items on the DHI may provide a basis for making referrals to other professionals. For example, if the patient has difficulty walking (item 16) and is afraid to leave home without being accompanied by someone else (item 9), referral to a physical therapist may be appropriate. The need for family counseling may be signaled by an affirmative response by the patient to an item such as "Has your problem placed stress on your relationships with members of your family or friends?" The DHI is the only available self-assessment balance handicap scale which explores the physical and psychosocial impact of balance system disease and maintains psychometric adequacy. The single form of the scale may limit its use. Further, the construct validity should be examined more carefully by means of a well-controlled intervention study.

CASE STUDIES

The following two brief case studies demonstrate the application of the self-assessment technique. The DHI was chosen to illustrate the usefulness of administering a scale in a pretreatment and post-treatment format.

Case 1

The first patient is a 33-year-old man with a history of intractable vertigo who was treated for dizziness and did not derive significant improvement from the treatment as measured by the DHI. A summary of the test results on this patient is shown in Table 17–4. The first balance function test was administered on November 11, 1990. The results of the balance function examination demonstrated a 30% unilateral weakness on the right side. Rotational test results were normal at this time. Therefore, this patient demonstrated evidence of compensated peripheral vestibular system disease on the right side. A DHI was administered at this time. The total score was 32 points. The patient was taken to surgery on April 18, 1991, for a streptomycin infusion procedure (chemical ablation of vestibular end organ). The patient was reevaluated on June 13, 1991 (2 months following the operation). At this time the patient demonstrated a 100% unilateral weakness on caloric testing and also demonstrated a significant rotational asymmetry to the right side (the treated ear).

These findings suggested that the surgical procedure succeeded in destroying the vestibular receptors, but this deficit was not compensated for by the central vestibular system at the time of retest. The total DHI score at retest was 20 points. This represented an improvement over the preoperative DHI. However, the net difference between the pre- and posttreatment scores did not exceed 18 points, which is the critical difference before a change can be said to be statistically significant. It is likely that the lack of significant improvement in the total DHI score occurred due to the fact that the unilateral total deficit had not been completely compensated for by the central vestibular system.

Case 2

The second patient is a 68-year-old woman with intractable vertigo who derived significant benefit from surgical treatment as indicated by DHI measures. A summary of the test results from this patient is shown in Table 17–5. A preoperative balance function test was performed on March 27, 1990.

TABLE 17–4.

Summary of Presurgical and Postsurgical Balance Function Test and Dizziness Handicap Inventory (DHI) Values for Case 1.

Status	Caloric Test*	Rotation	DHI (Total Score)
Presurgery	30% UW, rt.	Normal	32 points
Postsurgery	100% UW, rt.	Asymmetric, rt.	20 points

*UW, unilateral weakness; rt, right side.

The results of caloric testing showed a 42% unilateral weakness on the right side. Rotational testing demonstrated a significant asymmetry to the right, which supported the presence of an uncompensated peripheral vestibular system disorder on the right. A DHI was administered on this date. The total score was 70 points, suggesting significant self-perceived dizziness handicap. A streptomycin infusion procedure was performed on April 5, 1990. The patient was reevaluated on June 20, 1990 (approximately 2 months postoperatively). On this date, caloric testing showed an 84% unilateral weakness. Rotational testing and SOT (on the Equitest–computerized dynamic posturography system) test results were normal.

These findings suggested that the central vestibular system had compensated for the surgical destructive procedure. A second DHI was administered and the total score was 28 points. This represented a statistically significant improvement in self-perceived dizziness handicap.

CONCLUSIONS AND RESEARCH NEEDS

A major goal of medical, surgical, and rehabilitative intervention with patients suffering from dizziness or unsteadiness is to help them overcome the physical discomforts and psychosocial consequences associated with balance system disease. The addition of a psychometrically adequate balance handicap measure to the clinician's test battery may (1) help substantiate a patient's balance complaint not readily apparent by results of conventional vestibulometric testing, (2) facilitate decisions regarding candidacy for vestibular rehabilitation, (3) assist in the counseling process, and (4) serve as a criterion measure in documenting the effects of medical, surgical, or rehabilitative intervention. This final point needs to be emphasized. Now it is possible to quantify the outcome of medical, surgical, or rehabilitative intervention based on the patient's subjective assessment of their functional capabilities.

The following research needs may help broaden our understanding of balance function handicap and its place in the overall assessment of the dizzy patient.

1. The use of the formula approach proposed by the AAO-HNS for evaluation of therapy for Meniere's disease, combined with a clinician rating scale and a self-assessment inventory, would help evaluate the efficacy of treatment from different perspectives.

2. A multivariate examination of

TABLE 17–5.

Summary of Presurgical and Postsurgical Balance Function Test and Dizziness Handicap Inventory (DHI) Values for Case 2.

Status	Caloric Test*	Rotation	DHI (Total Score)
Presurgery	42% UW, rt.	Asymmetric, rt.	70 points
Postsurgery	84% UW, rt.	Normal	28 points

*UW, unilateral weakness; rt, right.

nonvestibulometric/nonpostural control factors (such as general health, depression, personality) and vestibulometric/postural control variables (such as calorics, rotary chair asymmetry, posturography) may provide greater insight into the concept of balance function handicap.

3. The value of using self-assessment scales to monitor the long-term effects of treatment requires further attention. The application of self-assessment tools over selected time intervals following intervention would be an important avenue of study. The optimal time interval necessary to measure benefit derived from treatment is, at present, undefined.

REFERENCES

1. Allum JHJ, Yamane M, Pfaltz CR: Long-term modifications of vertical and horizontal vestibulo-ocular reflex dynamics in man. *Acta Otolaryngol* 1988; 105:328–337.

2. Baloh RW, Honrubia V: *Clinical Neurophysiology of the Vestibular System.* Philadelphia; F.A. Davis, 1979.

3. Baloh RW, Honrubia V: *Clinical Neurophysiology of the Vestibular System.* Philadelphia; F.A. Davis, 1990.

4. Bergner M, Bobbitt RA, Carter WB, et al: The Sickness Impact Profile: Developments and final revision of a health status measure. *Med Care* 1981; 19:787–805.

5. Bergner M, Bobbitt RA, Pollard WE, et al: The Sickness Impact Profile: Validation of a health status measure. *Med Care* 1976; 14:57–67.

6. Busis SN: Diagnostic evaluation of the patient presenting with vertigo. *Otolaryngol Clin North Am* 1973; 6:3–23.

7. Committee on Hearing and Equilibrium of the American Academy of Ophthalmology and Otolaryngology. *Meniere's Disease: Criteria for Diagnosis and Evaluation of Therapy for Reporting.* AAO-HNS Bull. July 6–7, 1985.

8. Demorest ME, Walden BE: Psychometric principles in the selection, interpretation, and evaluation of communication self-assessment inventories. *J Speech Hear Disord* 1984; 49:226–240.

9. Dempsey J: The Hearing Performance Inventory as a tool in fitting hearing aids. *J Acad Rehabil Audiol* 1986;19:116–125.

10. Ellwood PM: Outcomes management—a technology of patient experience. *New Engl J Med* 1988; 318:1549–1556.

11. Gallagher D, Thompson WE, Levy SM: Clinical psychological assessment of older adults, in Poon LW (ed): *Aging in the 1980s—Psychological Issues.* Washington DC, American Psychological Association, 1980, pp 19–40.

12. Gilson BS, Gilson JS, Bergner M, et al: The Sickness Impact Profile: Development of an outcome measure of health care. *Am J Public Health* 1975; 65:1304–1310.

13. Guilford JP, Zimmerman WS: *The Guilford-Zimmerman Temperament Survey: Manual of Instruction and Interpretation.* Beverly Hills, Calif, Sheridan House, 1949.

14. Gurland B, Fleiss J, Cooper J, et al: The Comprehensive Assessment and Referral Evaluation (CARE)—rationale, development, and reliability. *Int J Aging Human Dev* 1977; 8:9–42.

15. Herdman SJ: Exercise strategies for vestibular disorders. *Ear Nose Throat J* 1989; 68:961–964.

16. Jacobson GP, Newman CW: The development of the Dizziness Handicap Inventory. *Arch Otolaryngol Head Neck Surg* 1990; 116:424–427.

17. Jacobson GP, Newman CW, Hunter L, et al: Balance function test correlates of the Dizziness Handicap Inventory. *J Am Acad Audiology* 1991; 2:253–260.

18. Kuk F, Tyler R, Russell D, et al:The psychometric properties of a tinnitus handicap questionnaire. *Ear Hear* 1990; 21:434–445.

19. Lawton MP, Brody EM: Assessment of older people: Self-maintaining and instrumental activities of daily living. *Gerontologist* 1969; 9:179–188.

20. Lawton MP, Whelihan WM, Belsky JK: Personality tests and their uses with older adults, in Birren J (ed): *Handbook of Mental Health and Aging.* Englewood Cliffs, NJ, Prentice-Hall, 1980; pp 537–553.

21. Malinoff R, Weinstein B: Measurement of hearing aid benefit in the elderly. *Ear Hear* 1989; 10:354–356.

22. Maoli C, Precht W: On the role of vestibulo-ocular reflex plasticity in recovery after unilateral peripheral vestibular lesions. *Exp Brain Res* 1985; 59:267–272.

23. Markides KS, Martin HW: Predicting self-related health among the aged. *Res Aging* 1979; 1:97–112.

24. McCabe BF: Labyrinthine exercises in the treatment of diseases characterized by vertigo: Their physiologic basis and methodology. *Laryngoscope* 1970; 80:1429–1433.

25. McNair DM, Lorr M, Droppleman LF: *Profile of Mood States: Manual.* San Diego, Calif, Educational and Industrial Testing Service, 1971.

26. Neugarten BL, Havighurst RJ, Tobin SS: The measurement of life satisfaction. *J Gerontol* 1961; 16:134–143.

27. Newman CW, Jacobson GP, Hug GA, et al: Practical method for quantifying hearing aid benefit in older adults. *J Am Acad Audiol* 1991; 2:70–75.

28. Newman CW, Weinstein BE: The Hearing Handicap Inventory for the Elderly as a measure of hearing aid benefit. *Ear Hear* 1988; 9:81–85.

29. Newman CW, Weinstein BE: Test-retest reliability of the Hearing Handicap Inventory for the Elderly using two administration approaches. *Ear Hear* 1989; 10:190–191.

30. Newman CW, Weinstein BE, Jacobson GP, et al: The Hearing Handicap Inventory for Adults: Psychometric adequacy and audiometric correlates. *Ear Hear* 1990; 11:430–433.

31. Norre ME, DeWeerdt W: Treatment of vertigo based on habituation. *J Laryngol Otol* 1980; 94:971–977.

32. Paige DG: Nonlinearity and asymmetry in the human vestibulo-ocular reflex. *Acta Otolaryngol* 1989; 108:1–8.

33. Pfeiffer E: *Multidimensional Functional Assessment: The OARS Methodology.* Center of the Study of Aging and Human Development. Durham, NC, Duke University, 1976.

34. Rosow I, Breslau N: A Guttman health scale for the aged. *J Gerontol* 1966; 21:556–559.

35. Schow RL, Gatehouse S: Fundamental issues in self-assessment of hearing. *Ear Hear* 1990; 11(suppl):65–165.

36. Segal BN, Katsarkas A: Long-term deficits of goal-directed vestibulo-ocular function following total unilateral loss of peripheral vestibular function. *Acta Otolaryngol* 1988; 106:102–110.

37. Shepard NT, Telian SA, Smith-Wheelock M: Habituation and balance retraining therapy. *Neuro Clin* 1990; 8:459–475.

38. Sweetow RW, Levy MC: Diagnostic and therapeutic tinnitus severity scaling. *Tinnitus Today—J Am Tinnitus Assoc* 1989; 14:4–8.

39. Taylor J: A personality scale of manifest anxiety. *J Abnorm Soc Psych* 48:285–290.

40. Weinstein BE: A review of hearing handicap scales. *Audiology* 1984; 9:91–109.

41. Weinstein BE, Spitzer JB, Ventry IM: Test-retest reliability of the Hearing Handicap Inventory for the Elderly. *Ear Hear* 1986; 7:295–299.

42. Wilson WH, Henry J, Bowen M, et al: Tinnitus Reaction Questionnaire: Psychometric properties of a measure of distress associated with tinnitus. *J Speech Hear Res* 1991; 34:197–201.

43. World Health Organization: International classification of impairments, disabilities and handicaps: A manual of classification relating to the consequences of disease. Geneva World Health Organization, 1980, pp 25–43.

44. Zung WWK: A rating instrument for anxiety disorders. *Psychosomatics* 1971; 12:371–379.

CHAPTER 18

Balance Rehabilitation: Background, Techniques, and Usefulness

Susan J. Herdman, Ph.D., P.T.

The use of exercises has been advocated as an important intervention strategy in the rehabilitation of vestibular patients for many years. Exercises were introduced as a treatment for vertigo and disequilibrium in patients with peripheral vestibular disorders in the 1940s.[12] Cawthorne, an otolaryngologist in England, recognized that the patient who moved his head improved faster than did the patient who restricted his head movements. He asked Cooksey, a physiotherapist, to develop a series of exercises that would encourage patients to move their heads through progressively more difficult tasks (Table 18–1). The goal of these exercises was to improve the patient's overall function. The exercises used today are based on Cawthorne and Cooksey's concept that to facilitate recovery after a vestibular lesion, the patient must be encouraged to move. The purpose of this chapter is to describe several exercise approaches that are used in the treatment of the problems associated with vestibular hypofunction. Certain types of vestibular disorders, such as positional vertigo, Meniere's disease, fistula, and complete bilateral vestibular loss, will not be discussed here because they present different problems.

NORMAL VESTIBULAR FUNCTION

To understand the effect of unilateral vestibular deficits on function, it is important to understand how the normal vestibular system works. It is not the intent of this chapter to review extensively vestibular physiology and anatomy, but some general concepts need to be emphasized. First, head movement and head position are detected by different receptors in the vestibular apparatus. The receptors in the semicircular canals respond to angular acceleration, while the receptors in the utricle and saccule respond to linear acceleration and the pull of gravity. The orientation of the three canals enables detection of head movement in all planes. The receptors in each canal respond best to movement in the plane of that canal. The utricle and the saccule are oriented such that the utricle responds best to movement along the horizontal plane and the saccule responds best to movement along the vertical plane.

When the head is stationary, vestibular neurons fire at a tonic or resting level. Movement of the head modulates this resting firing rate. For example, if the head is turned to the right, the right

TABLE 18–1.

Cawthorne-Cooksey Exercises*

I. *In bed*
  A. Eye movements, at first slow, then quick
    1. Up and down
    2. From side to side
    3. Focusing on finger moving from 3 feet to 1 foot away from face
  B. Head movements at first slow, then quick; later with eyes closed
    1. Bending forward and backward
    2. Turning from side to side
II. *Sitting (in class)*
  A. IA and IB, as above
  B. Shoulder shrugging and circling
  C. Bending forward and picking up objects from the ground
III. *Standing (in class)*
  A. IA, IB, and IIC, as above
  B. Changing from sitting to standing position with eyes open and shut
  C. Throwing a small ball from hand to hand (above eye level)
  D. Throwing ball from hand to hand under knee
  E. Change from sitting to standing and turning round in between
IV. *Moving about (in class)*
  A. Circle round center person who will throw a large ball and to whom it will be returned
  B. Walk across room with eyes open and then closed
  C. Walk up and down slope with eyes open and then closed
  D. Walk up and down steps with eyes open and then closed
  E. Any game involving stooping and stretching and aiming such as skittles, bowls, or basketball
Diligence and perseverance are required but the earlier and more regularly the exercise regime is carried out, the faster and more complete will be the return to normal activity.

*Adapted from Dix MR: Acta Otorhinolaryngol 1979; 33:370–384.

horizontal canal is stimulated and the receptors in the left horizontal canal are inhibited. In the vestibular nucleus, there is an increase in the firing of the type I neurons ipsilaterally and a decrease in firing of the type I neurons contralaterally. This push-pull relationship is further supported by the commissural inhibitory system (Fig 18–1). A similar push-pull relationship exists for the otoliths. It is important to remember that with progressively higher head acceleration, the firing rate of the neurons on the contralateral side will gradually decrease to zero.

The signals from the neurons in the semicircular canals generate a compensatory eye movement called the vestibulo-ocular reflex (VOR). The VOR holds the eye stationary in space during head movements. If the head moves at 30°/sec to the left, the VOR produces a 30°/sec slow-phase eye movement to the right. This enables the image of a viewed object to remain on the fovea of the retina, the area of greatest visual acuity, during head movements. Some of the signals from the canals are also used to produce the appropriate postural responses during head movements.

The signals from the receptors in the otoliths are used to generate compensatory postural responses. The vestibulospinal reflex (VSR) produces appropriate muscle activation in the axial and extremity muscles to maintain postural stability during head movements. The contribution of the otoliths to gaze stability is small. The tonic otolith input is used to hold the eyes in a level, horizontal plane within the orbit. The otolith input also produces the small, counterrolling of the eye that occurs during head tilt.

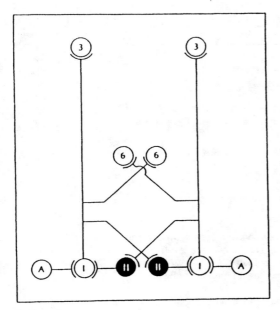

FIG 18–1.
Schematic drawing of projections from type I *(open circles)* and type II *(closed circles)* neurons of vestibular nuclei. Type I neurons are facilitory and project to the abducens nucleus *(6)* and through interneurons (not shown) to the oculomotor nucleus *(3)*. A collateral from the type I neuron facilitates the contralateral type II neuron, which is inhibitory. (Note vestibular labyrinth is denoted by letter A.) (From Halmagyi GM, Curthgoys IS, Gibson WPR: Vestibular neurectomy and the management of vertigo. *Curr Opinion Neurol Neurosurg* 1988; 1:879–889. Used with permission.)

DEFICITS PRODUCED BY VESTIBULAR LESIONS

Patients with unilateral vestibular lesions complain of vertigo (the sense that they or the world are rotating), nausea, and disequilibrium (the sense of being off-balance). These symptoms reflect both the abnormal vestibular signal and the interaction of the abnormal vestibular signal with normal visual and somatosensory information.[6] This perhaps explains why patients with acute vestibular lesions often prefer to lie with their head still, reducing the vestibular signals, and with their eyes closed, reducing the visual-vestibular conflict.

The effects of unilateral vestibular lesions on function can be described by considering changes that occur in the VOR and the VSR. Unilateral vestibular lesions have an effect on both tonic and dynamic vestibular responses.

Tonic Disturbances

The disruption of *tonic vestibulo-ocular responses* results in spontaneous nystagmus and a skew deviation. When the head is stationary, there is a balance of the tonic firing of the neurons in the vestibular nuclei. Removal of the input from the semicircular canals unilaterally results in a relative imbalance in the inputs between the two sides. The loss of the signal from the semicircular canals on one side causes the generation of a slow-phase eye movement toward the side of the deficit (away from the intact side). This slow-phase eye movement is interrupted by a quick phase in the opposite direction which resets the eye position. Typically the fast-phase eye movement is toward the intact side regardless of the position of the eye in the orbit. The amplitude and velocity of slow-phase eye movements will vary with changes in the position of the eye in the orbit. Removal of the input from the utricle on one side results in a skew deviation. The eye on the side of the lesion drops in the orbit, causing a vertical diplopia.[18]

Disruption of the *tonic-vestibulo-spinal responses* results in an asymmetry in electromyographic activity in the lower extremities while the patient is standing,[1] a shift in the center of gravity toward the side of the lesion,[48] and a postural asymmetry which can be detected clinically.[19] The asymmetry in the vestibulo-spinal responses are readily suppressed by visual cues.[1]

Dynamic Disturbances

The disturbance of the *dynamic vestibulo-ocular response* is characterized by a decrease in the gain of the system during head movements. Gain is a measure of the relationship of the output of the system to the input of the system, in this case slow-phase eye velocity (output) to head velocity (input). In the healthy individual, when the head moves at a certain velocity, the eye movement generated in the opposite direction will have the same or close to same velocity and the gain of the system (output/input) will approach "1." In patients with acute, unilateral vestibular deficits, the gain of the system is decreased by as much as 75% for head movements toward the side of the lesion and by 50% for head movements away from the side of the lesion.[2]

The disturbance of the *dynamic vestibulo-spinal response* is characterized by a gait ataxia. Patients ambulate with a widened base of support with frequent side-stepping and a tendency to drift from one side to another while ambulating. They also tend to decrease their trunk and head rotation in an attempt to improve stability. This is probably because head movement results in an asymmetric vestibular signal that increases their sense of disequilibrium and the ataxia.

RECOVERY FROM VESTIBULAR DEFICITS

There are several mechanisms involved in the recovery of function following unilateral vestibular lesions. These include spontaneous recovery, adaptation or plasticity of the remaining vestibular system, and the substitution of alternative strategies for the lost function.

Spontaneous Recovery

The disturbances of static vestibular function (nystagmus, skew deviation, and postural asymmetries in stance) all seem to recover spontaneously. The timing of the disappearance of these symptoms parallels the recovery of the resting firing rate of the vestibular neurons.[51] Although visual cues can also be used to suppress spontaneous nystagmus and the postural asymmetry, several studies have demonstrated that recovery of spontaneous nystagmus is not dependent on visual inputs per se.[13] Nystagmus decreases at the same rate in animals kept in the dark immediately after unilateral labyrinthectomy as in animals kept in a lighted environment.

Vestibular Adaptation

The mechanism behind the recovery of the dynamic vestibulo-ocular responses is at least in part the adaptive capability of the vestibular system, that is its ability to make long-term changes in the neuronal response to input. Allum et al.[2] and Paige[40] report that VOR gain during triangular or sinusoidal stimulation improves with time after unilateral vestibular loss in humans and is within normal limits in 1 to 3 months. It is not clear whether VOR gain during head movements that are more physiologic, such as quick head thrusts, recover, however.[17]

The adaptive capability of the vestibular system is important during development and maturation and in response to disease and injury. The potential for adaptation can be used in patients with vestibular hypofunction as a mechanism to induce recovery. The signal for inducing adaptation is the movement of an image across the retina (retinal slip) while you are trying to keep the image in focus.[36] This creates an error signal which the brain attempts to minimize by increasing the gain of the VOR. Wearing reversing prisms or magnifying glasses, for example, increases retinal slip and will induce a change in the gain of the system.[10, 23]

Recovery from the dynamic disturbances of vestibular function seem to require both visual inputs and movement of the body and head.[9, 22, 34] Several studies have shown that the gain of the vestibulo-ocular response does not recover if cats or monkeys are kept in the dark following unilateral labyrinthectomy.[9, 13] Once the animals are returned to a lighted environment, recovery begins. Furthermore, if animals are prevented from moving after unilateral vestibular nerve section, there is a delay in the onset of the recovery of locomotor function and the rate of recovery is prolonged[29] (Fig 18–2).

Recovery from the dynamic disturbances in postural stability may be due to an improvement in the VSR. Black et al.[5] found that in the acute stage following unilateral vestibular loss, patients were unable to maintain their balance on tests in which they were forced to rely on vestibular cues alone. With time, however, they recovered their ability to maintain balance on these tests, suggesting an improved ability to use vestibular cues.

Substitution

A third mechanism of recovery is the substitution of alternative strategies for the lost function. Recovery of gaze stability in patients with unilateral vestibular loss may be due to the enhancement of the cervico-ocular reflex.[7, 26] During low-frequency, brief head movements, sensory inputs from neck muscles and joint facets act to produce a slow-phase eye movement that complements the VOR. This response is potentiated in patients with bilateral vestibular loss, and Maoli and Precht[33] suggest that neck proprioceptive inputs have increased influence on gaze stability after unilateral vestibular loss. Another strategy would be the substitution of saccadic eye movements to regain the visual target.[46] Saccadic eye movements are not a particularly useful alternative for a poor VOR because patients still would not be able to see the target clearly during head movements.

Recovery of postural stability also may be due to the substitution of alternative strategies for the lost function. Patients learn, for instance, to rely more on visual cues for balance than on

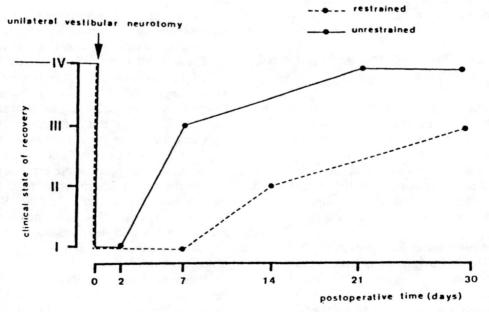

FIG 18–2.
Effect of restricting mobility on rate of recovery following unilateral transection of vestibular nerve. Baboons that were restrained after unilateral vestibular nerve section had a delayed onset of recovery and a more prolonged recovery than those animals that were allowed free movement. (From Lacour M, Roll JP, Appaix M: Modifications and development of spinal reflexes in the alert baboon *(papio papio)* following an unilateral vestibular neurectomy. *Brain Res* 1976; 113:255–269. Used with permission.)

vestibular cues and therefore become less stable when visual cues are removed.[37, 48] Black et al.[5] showed that, for at least one patient in the acute stage following resection of acoustic neuroma, there was a decrease in postural stability when proprioceptive cues from the feet and ankles were distorted, suggesting that this patient had substituted the use of somatosensory cues for vestibular cues.

Although the substitution of visual or somatosensory cues strategy may provide sufficient information for postural stability, the patient will be at a disadvantage if trying to walk when those cues are not available such as in a dimly lighted environment. At its extreme, some patients may modify their behavior to avoid situations where visual or somatosensory cues are diminished such as going out at night.

Another undesirable strategy would be that patients might opt to restrict head movements. This also would not be a particularly successful way to improve gaze or postural stability. Ultimately it would limit everyday activities and still would not provide a mechanism for seeing clearly or for maintaining balance during head movements.

To summarize, human beings use a variety of strategies, which may differ from patient to patient, to try to improve gaze and postural stability following unilateral vestibular loss (UVL). These strategies would be only partially successful in substituting for decreased vestibular responses. The most effective mechanism for improving gaze and postural stability during head movements would be to increase VOR gain.

EXERCISE PARADIGMS

Although studies in animals support the concepts that visuo-motor experience facilitates the rate of recovery and improves the final level of recovery following vestibular dysfunction,[9, 22, 34] only anecdotal evidence supports the use of exercises in human beings as a mechanism for improving recovery.[12, 20, 21, 35, 47, 52] Studies that have reported changes in postural stability or reduction of vertigo and disequilibrium after vestibular exercises either measured change subjectively rather than quantitatively, or did not compare the treated group with a control group.[38, 39, 48, 49] Without a control group of some type, it is not clear whether the same recovery might have occurred spontaneously. Thus, the efficacy of the exercise treatments is still unknown in human beings with vestibular lesions, although this treatment approach looks very promising.

Exercise Approaches

Several different exercise approaches are advocated for the treatment of patients with vestibular hypofunction. The common element in all vestibular exercises is the requirement of head movement. The Cawthorne-Cooksey exercises (see Table 18–1) are designed to take the patient through a series of exercises that slowly require more and more movement. Notice that there is a progression from performing exercises in sitting to performing exercises while standing, and then finally while walking.[12] Norre recommends identifying which movements induce the symptoms of either vertigo or disequilibrium in the patient[37] (Table 18–2). These movements then become the basis for the exercises used with that patient. He suggests that changes in the number of maneuvers that provoke dizziness in the patient can also be used as criteria for determining if the patient is improving. In one study, he notes that patients who were untreated, who performed the exercise movements slowly, or who refused to do the exercises because the movements made them dizzy, did not improve.[38]

The exercises used in our vestibular rehabilitation program are based on the

TABLE 18–2.

Vestibular habituation training*

Task	Vertigo Typ/at†	Intensity	Neuroveget	Duration	Score
1. Sitting, moves to supine					
2. Supine, moves to left side					
3. Supine, to right side					
4. Supine, to sitting					
5. Standing—turning to right					
6. Standing—turning to left					
7. Sitting—nose to left knee					
8. Sitting—nose to right knee					
9. Sitting, turning head counterclockwise					
10. Sitting, turning head clockwise					
11. Sitting, bending forward					
12. Sitting, moves to erect					
13. Sitting, head moves fore-aft					
14. Left Hallpike					
15. Moves to sitting					
16. Right Hallpike					
17. Moves to sitting					
18. Supine, head hanging					
19. Moves to sitting					
				Total:	

*Adapted from Norre ME, Beckers A: Otolaryngol Head Neck Surg 1989; 101:14–19.
†Typ/at = typical or atypical rotary nystagmus.

Cawthorne-Cooksey regime but have been modified to reflect the mechanisms of vestibular adaptation (Table 18–3).[21, 52] As mentioned, the best stimulus to improve gaze stability is one which results in an error-signal that the central nervous system attempts to reduce by modifying the gain of the vestibular system. Although movement of the visual world (optokinetic stimuli) can increase the gain of the vestibular system, the best stimuli appear to be those which also incorporate head movements.[8]

The best stimuli to improve postural stability are those which incorporate movement.[22, 29, 34] Again, this results in an error signal which the brain attempts to correct. Exercises should be designed to enhance vestibular adaptation as well as facilitate the use of visual and somatosensory cues for balance (Table 18–4).[21]

One difference between the original Cawthorne-Cooksey exercises and those proposed here is that we no longer include an exercise that involves movement of the eyes only (see Table 18–1,IA). Rather, all of the exercises emphasize head movement in order to stimulate that vestibular system. Furthermore, some of the exercises in the Cawthorne-Cooksey regime and in Norre's approach would not be appropriate for certain surgery patients during the period when bending over is restricted because of the possibility of cerebrospinal fluid leak.

TABLE 18–3.

Exercises to Improve Gaze Stability

Acute stage (also used with chronic, uncompensated patients)*
  A business card or other target with words on it (foveal target) is taped on the wall in front of the patient so
    he can read it. The patient moves his head gently back and forth horizontally for 1 minute while keeping
    the words in focus
  This exercise is repeated moving the head vertically for 1 minute
  Depending on whether this induces any nausea, the exercise is then repeated using a large pattern such as
    a checkerboard (full-field stimulus), moving the head horizontally
  The exercise with the checkerboard is then repeated moving the head vertically
Subacute stage†
  The patient holds a business card in front of him so that he can read it. He moves the card and his head
    back and forth horizontally in *opposite* directions keeping the words in focus for 1 minute without stopping
  This is repeated with vertical head movements and with a large, full-field stimulus

---

*The patient should repeat each exercise at least three times a day. The duration of each of the exercises is extended gradually
from 1 to 2 minutes. Patients should be cautioned that the exercises may make them feel dizzy or even nauseated but that they
should try to persist for the full 1 to 2 minutes of the exercise, resting between exercises.
†The duration is gradually extended from 1 to 2 minutes. The patient should repeat each exercise at least three times each day.

GUIDELINES FOR DEVELOPING EXERCISES

The starting point in developing an exercise program for patients with vestibular deficits is the assessment of the patient (Table 18–5). Evaluation of the patient must take into consideration not only vestibular system function but also visual, somatosensory, motor, and biomechanical factors. The complete clinical examination may take a full hour or more. Other tests such as caloric, rotary chair, and posturography are also im-

TABLE 18–4.

Exercises to Improve Postural Stability*

The patient stands with his feet as close together as possible, with both hands or one hand helping maintain
  balance by touching a wall if needed. He then turns his head to the right and to the left horizontally while
  looking straight ahead at the wall for 1 minute without stopping. The patient takes his hand or hands off the
  wall for longer and longer periods of time while maintaining balance. The patient then tries moving his feet
  even closer together
The patient walks, with someone to assist him if needed, as often as possible (acute disorders)
The patient begins to practice turning his head while walking. This will make the patient less stable, so the
  patient should stay near a wall as he walks
The patient stands with his feet shoulder width apart with eyes *open*, looking straight ahead at a target on the
  wall. He progressively narrows his base of support from feet apart to feet together to a semi heel-to-toe
  position. The exercise is performed first with arms outstretched, then with arms close to the body and then
  with arms folded across the chest. Each position is held for 15 seconds before the patient does the next most
  difficult exercise. The patient practices for a total of 5 to 15 minutes
The patient stands with his feet shoulder width apart, with eyes open, looking straight ahead at a target on the
  wall. He progressively narrows his base of support from feet apart to feet together to a semi heel-to-toe
  position. The exercise is performed with eyes *closed*, at first intermittently and then for longer and longer
  periods of time. The exercise is performed first with arms outstretched, then with arms close to the body and
  then with arms folded across the chest. Each position is held for 15 seconds, and then the patient tries the
  next position. The patient practices for a total of 5 to 15 minutes
The patient practices standing on a cushioned surface. Progressively more difficult tasks might be a hard floor
  (linoleum, wood), thin carpet, shag carpet, thin pillow, or sofa cushion. Graded density foam can also be
  purchased
The patient practices turning around while he walks, at first making a large circle but gradually making smaller
  and smaller turns. The patient must be sure to turn in both directions

---

*There are many different balance exercises that can be used. These exercises are devised to incorporate head movement
(vestibular stimulation) or to foster the use of different sensory cues for balance.

TABLE 18–5.

Patient Assessment Prior to Beginning Exercise Regimen

Oculomotor examination
  In room light: extraocular movements, pursuit, saccades, spontaneous nystagmus, gaze-evoked nystagmus,
    VOR cancellation (VORc), VOR to slow and rapid (Halmagyi maneuver) head thrusts, visual acuity test
    with head stationary and during gentle oscillation of the head
  With Frenzel's lenses: Spontaneous and gaze-evoked nystagmus, head-shaking nystagmus, tragal–pressure
    induced nystagmus, hyperventilation-induced nystagmus, positional nystagmus
Sensation
  Proprioception, light touch, vibration, kinesthesia, pain quantified tests: vibration threshold, tuning-fork test
Coordination: upper and lower extremities
  Optic ataxia/past pointing, rebound, diadokokinesia, heel to shin, postural fixation
Range of Motion: (note whether active or passive)
  Upper extremity, lower extremity, neck (rotation, extension, flexion, lateral flexion)
Strength (gross)
  Grip: Upper extremity; lower extremity; trunk
Sitting Balance: passive/active
  Anterior/posterior and laterally
    Weight shift
    Head righting
    Equilibrium reactions: upper extremity, lower extremity
    Trunk recovers vertical
Static balance: (normal values by age; perform with eyes open and eyes closed)
  Romberg
  Sharpened Romberg
  Single leg stance
  Standing on foam surface
Dynamic balance (self-initiated movements)
  Fukuda's stepping test
Ambulation
  Normal gait
  Tandem walk
  Walk while turning head

portant. The caloric and rotary chair tests measure the vestibulo-ocular system. Posturography assesses the patient's ability to maintain balance using different sensory cues.

Once the patient's problems have been identified, an exercise program can be developed. The following points should be taken into consideration when developing exercises to enhance vestibular adaptation and when anticipating recovery in patients.

1. Adaptation is frequency dependent.[16, 31] That is, if you adapt the system at a specific frequency, gain will increase most at that frequency. Normal movement requires a wide range of frequencies of head movement. Therefore, the patient must perform the head movement exercises at many different frequencies for optimal effects.

2. Adaptation takes time. Most studies on vestibular adaptation have used paradigms in which the stimulus is present for long periods of time.[11, 25] This is clearly not appropriate for patients, especially for those with acute lesions. More recent studies have suggested that vestibular adaptation can be induced with periods of stimulation as brief as 1 to 2 minutes.[8, 43] The brain, however, clearly needs time to reduce the error signal produced by the mismatch of head movement and retinal slip. During that period of time, the patient may experience an increase in his or her symptoms but must be encouraged to continue to perform the exercise without stopping.

3. Vestibular adaptation is affected by voluntary motor control.[3, 14, 24] For example, VOR gain can be increased even in the dark if the subject simply

imagines that he or she is looking at a stationary target on the wall. Furthermore, exercises should always be performed at the limit of the patient's ability. Thus the patient must concentrate on the task.

4. Adaptation of the vestibulo-ocular system is context specific and therefore, for optimal recovery, exercises must stress the system in different ways.[8] Exercises should combine vestibular, optokinetic, and somatosensory cues as well as the possibility of central pre-programming to improve gaze stability. This reflects the normal interactions of the vestibular system with other sensory and motor systems.

5. As mentioned, recovery may be delayed or possibly prevented if the patient restricts head movement or if visual inputs are minimized.[9, 13, 29] Another factor that may delay recovery or even limit the final level of recovery may be the use of vestibular suppressant drugs.[52]

6. The presence of other disorders affecting the peripheral or central nervous systems can affect recovery. Lesions in the central nervous system may affect structures that are involved in vestibular adaptation, such as the vestibular nuclei and cerebellum[15, 30] or structures involved in the substitution of alternative strategies, such as using visual or somatosensory cues for balance.

7. Age-related changes in the vestibular, visual, and somatosensory systems may affect the rate of recovery and the final level of recovery of patients in several ways.* First, the adaptive capability of the vestibular system is somewhat reduced in the older patient.[41] Second, the loss of more than one sensory cue has a significant impact on postural stability. An individual has good stability with eyes closed (loss of one sensory cue) but not with eyes closed and a vestibular lesion. Third, diminished visual and somatosensory cues may affect the

*References 4, 27, 28, 32, 41, 42, 44, 45, and 50.

useful substitution of alternative strategies to improve postural stability.

MANAGEMENT

Acute Vestibular Deficits: Support for Early Intervention

There is evidence that the vestibular system can be modified during the acute stage after unilateral vestibular lesions. Studies have noted a delay in the recovery of the VOR in cats and monkeys deprived of vision immediately after labyrinthectomy.[9, 13] Furthermore, the initiation of the recovery of postural responses is delayed and the course of recovery is prolonged when motor activity is restricted in baboons after vestibular nerve section in comparison to recovery in restrained animals.[29] Finally, it has been shown that VOR adaptation can be induced in unilateral labyrinthectomized cats as early as the third day after surgery.[33]

There is also some evidence that the vestibular system in human beings can be adapted during the acute stage after unilateral vestibular loss. Pfaltz[43] found that optokinetic stimulation increased VOR gain in patients with unilateral vestibular loss compared to untreated patients. Pfaltz's study is particularly significant because he showed that even brief periods of stimulation can produce VOR gain changes. This would be particularly useful in the treatment of patients with acute vestibular lesions. Prolonged stimulation of the vestibular system is not feasible in the acute stage following unilateral vestibular loss in human beings because of the vertigo, nausea, and vomiting that are usually induced with head movement.

During the initial stage after a unilateral vestibular lesion, patients often complain of severe vertigo and are usually nauseated and vomiting. Any head movement makes these symptoms worse, and patients will prefer to lie quietly, often in a darkened room or with eyes closed. At this stage, patients may also be taking medications to suppress these vegetative responses and may be receiving intravenous fluid replacement. After a few days, however, these symptoms should resolve and spontaneous nystagmus and the skew deviation should be decreasing as the resting state of the vestibular neurons recovers. Good visual inputs and head movement should be encouraged as soon as possible after the onset of the vestibular loss. Patients can begin exercises to facilitate adaptation of the vestibular system 2 or 3 days after the onset of the deficit. Initially, an exercise might be performed for only 1 minute with a period of rest in between each exercise. Increased vertigo or disequilibrium is not a reason to stop the exercises; vomiting is. Most of the recovery from the vertigo and nausea will occur within a few days. Because VOR gain in the acute stage after UVL is poor (0.25 to 0.5), relatively slow head velocities and low frequencies should be used, and the patient should be instructed to keep the visual target in focus at all times. Recovery of postural stability will occur more gradually, over the course of weeks to even several months. Patients should be walking independently, albeit with a widened base of support, within 1 week.

Management of Chronic Vestibular Deficits

Although patients with chronic vestibular deficits often do not have vertigo, nausea, and vomiting (the exception being those patients with episodic vestibular disorders such as Meniere's disease), they frequently have limited their movements, or at least their head movements, in an attempt to avoid precipitating any symptoms. Head movements must be encouraged in these patients. These patients may complain that they feel worse rather than better as they perform the exercises. This is be-

cause they are stressing the vestibular system by performing head movements that they had been avoiding. It is reasonable to expect improved function within 6 weeks in patients who are compliant about doing their exercises but, anecdotal evidence suggests that, the longer the problem has existed, the longer it may take to see improved function.

In summary, patients with incomplete loss of vestibular function can be expected to recover from the vertigo and/or disequilibrium they first experience. Studies in animals and anecdotal evidence in human beings suggests that exercises facilitate recovery of vestibular system function. Also, there is evidence that early intervention is important in optimizing recovery. Restricting movement or preventing visual inputs delays the onset of recovery and may limit the final level of recovery. Several exercise approaches have been developed for patients with vestibular hypofunction. The common element of all exercise programs is that they encourage head movement.

Case 1

The patient is a 67-year-old man who reported that in the early 1970s he experienced an episode of disequilibrium in which he felt as if he were suddenly pushed in one direction and then was rocking back and forth. The disequilibrium persisted for 1 year but was intermittent. Approximately 18 months ago, he again experienced some disequilibrium which was associated with left upper extremity weakness. At this time, he complained that he felt off-balance when standing or walking but not when sitting or lying down. His balance is worse when walking in the dark or in a busy visual environment such as in a grocery store. He denies falls or stumbling. Past medical history is significant for bilateral knee replacements secondary to arthritic changes. He denies diabetes, heart disease, or hypertension. He is on no medications except aspirin. He drinks only socially and stopped smoking 15 years ago.

Hearing tests show a bilateral sensorineural high frequency hearing loss (30 to 40 dB at 3,000 to 8,000 Hz). Electronystagmography showed a spontaneous, left-beating nystagmus in the dark. There was no gaze-evoked nystagmus. Left-beating nystagmus was present with the patient supine, with the head turned left, and with left side-lying. Caloric tests showed a unilateral weakness on the right (45% decrease).

Physical therapy assessment showed normal *strength* in upper and lower extremities bilaterally. *Neck range of motion* was decreased on lateral flexion to the right, neck flexion to the right, and neck rotation to the right. Examination of *eye movements* showed normal pursuit, saccades, VOR cancellation, and VOR to slow head movements. Under Frenzel's lenses, there was no spontaneous or gaze-evoked nystagmus, no head-shaking induced nystagmus to either horizontal or vertical head movements, no tragal-pressure induced nystagmus, and no positional induced nystagmus. Assessment of *balance* showed a positive Romberg on the first eyes closed trial. Sharpened Romberg could be maintained for 30 seconds with eyes open (normal) but for only 4 seconds with eyes closed (abnormal). Fukuda's stepping test resulted in a 14-inch forward progression with no turn with eyes open (normal) and in a 27-inch forward progression with a 45° turn to the right with eyes closed (abnormal). Considerable left upper extremity drift was noted with eyes closed. *Gait* was slightly wide-based, with decreased rotation through the trunk and neck. The patient complained of increased disequilibrium when asked to walk and turn his head at the same time. Quantitative *vibration* threshold testing showed elevated thresholds bilaterally in the feet. *Posturography* tests showed normal ability to use visual, vestibular, and somatosensory cues for balance. Automatic postural responses were normal except for delayed onset of force development to sudden translations of the support surface. Patient had normal short-, middle- and long-latency responses as measured by electromyography using surface electrodes.

The caloric test clearly shows a unilateral vestibular deficit, probably peripheral. At the time of the physical therapy assessment, the patient appeared to have a normal VOR on clinical examination but still complained of disequilibrium. Recovery of balance for this patient is complicated by the decreased sensation in feet and by the mild left hemiparesis indicated by left upper extremity drift during Fukuda's stepping test.

The patient was placed on an exercise program designed to enhance the adaptation of his vestibular system and to improve his balance. These exercises consist of head movements while focusing on foveal and full-field stimuli at close and distance viewing (see Table 18–3). He was to perform the exercises in both sitting and standing positions, three times a day. *On follow-up* visit, the patient reported that he was doing much better and had a significant decrease in his sense of disequilibrium. He was able to perform his vestibular adaptation exercises standing with his feet in a semitandem position and was given additional exercises requiring him to turn his head while ambulating. The patient was to continue with the exercises for another 2 weeks, at which time he would be reevaluated.

Case 2

The patient is a 71-year-old man with a history of chronic otitis media and mastoiditis, tympanic perforation, and cholesteatoma of the left ear. The patient reported that approximately 20 years ago he had an episode of vertigo with nausea and emesis that lasted for several days. Since that time, whenever he has had a cold, the vertigo reoccurred. He also reported that when he pressed his left ear while cleaning it and when he sneezed or coughed, he felt as if his head were pulled briefly to the left. Computed tomography showed a large cholesteatoma which filled the left mastoid and which had resulted in a bony fistula of the horizontal semicircular canal. Pure-tone audiometry revealed a moderate mixed hearing loss on the left side.

The patient underwent a left mastoidectomy with tympanoplasty and meatoplasty, and the cholesteatoma was successfully removed. During the surgery a 2-mm bony fistula exposing the horizontal semicircular canal was visualized. The fistula was covered with a fascia graft. After the surgery the patient had nystagmus and dizziness but denied any true vertigo. He complained of disequilibrium when walking. One month later he still had complaints of balance problems and was referred for physical therapy. Although the patient did not have a caloric test or rotary chair test, the impression was that the patient had a vestibular deficit secondary to the bony fistula from the cholesteatoma. This was based on the nystagmus noted immediately after surgery and on his present complaints of disequilibrium.

At the time when the patient was first referred for physical therapy, he noted that his balance was worse in the morning when he first got up and was worse when he was walking outside the house as opposed to inside. He stated that he frequently side-stepped but he denied stumbling or falls. The patient was particularly concerned about his balance because in the summer he operated chartered deep sea fishing boats. Significant findings on assessment included (1) positive Romberg (sharpened Romberg and tandem walking tests were not performed), (2) tendency to walk with a widened base of support and with exaggerated internal rotation of the left lower extremity during the stance phase (he had decreased arm swing on the right and tended to carry his right arm in a flexed posture; a slight tremor was noted in his right hand during ambulation), and (3) normal vibration thresholds bilaterally in his feet at quantitative vibration threshold testing.

The goals for this patient were to improve his static and dynamic balance to within normal limits for his age and to decrease his sense of imbalance when moving. The exercises he was taught were designed to improve his balance by enhancing vestibular adaptation and through the substitution of visual and somatosensory cues. The patient was given exercises designed to increase the gain of his vestibular system (see Table 18–3). He was to perform these exercises while standing to help improve his postural stability. He was instructed to move his head during the exercises as quickly as he could as long as he kept the visual target in focus. In addition, he was given exercises designed to improve his balance by manipulating which sensory cues he had available for balance (see Table 18–4). He was to perform the exercises two or three times daily and was scheduled for a follow-up visit in 2 weeks. On follow-up, he reported that his balance was slightly improved subjectively, but no change was noted on testing. He re-

ported that when performing his exercises, he would stop his head movements as soon as he became dizzy (approximately 15 seconds). Because vestibular adaptation requires a more prolonged vestibular signal, he was encouraged to continue with the head movements for 1 to 2 minutes and to work through the feeling of dizziness. In addition, it was suggested to the patient that he should practice his balance exercises while on his boat. That would enable him to determine if the movement of the boat and of the visual environment (sunlight on water) would adversely affect his balance. Because he was to return to that working environment, it would be a good exercise. The patient was scheduled for follow-up in a few weeks but did not return for 1 month. At that time he reported that his balance was significantly improved, although he was having "good days and bad days." He had returned to many of his normal activities and was painting his boat in preparation for the summer fishing season. He no longer had complaints of dizziness. Assessment showed that his Romberg was now normal and he no longer side-stepped when walking. The patient was discharged from therapy significantly improved.

REFERENCES

1. Allum JHJ, Pfaltz CR: Postural control in man following acute unilateral peripheral vestibular deficit, in Igarashi M, Black O, (eds): *Vestibular and Visual Control on Posture and Locomotor Equilibrium.* Basel, S Karger, 1985, pp 315–321.

2. Allum JHJ, Yamane M, Pfaltz CR: Long-term modifications of vertical and horizontal vestibulo-ocular reflex dynamics in man. *Acta Otolaryngol* 1988; 105:328–337.

3. Baloh RW, Lyerly K, Yee RE, et al: Voluntary control of the human vestibulo-ocular reflex. *Acta Otolayrngol* 1984; 97:1–6.

4. Bergstrom B: Morphology of the vestibular nerve. II: The number of myelinated vestibular nerve fibers in man at various ages. *Acta Otolaryngol* 1973; 76:173–179.

5. Black FO, Shupert CL, Peterka RJ; et al: Effects of unilateral loss of vestibular function on the vestibulo-ocular reflex and postural control. *Ann Otol Rhinol Laryngol* 1989; 98:884–889.

6. Brandt T, Daroff RB: The multisensory physiological and pathological vertigo syndromes. *Ann Neurol* 1980; 7:195–203.

7. Bronstein AM, Hood JD: The cervico-ocular reflex in normal subjects and patients with absent vestibular function. *Brain Res* 1986; 373:339–408.

8. Collewijn H, Martins AJ, Steinman RM: Compensatory eye movements during active and passive head movements: Fast adaptation to changes in visual magnification. *J. Physiol* 1983; 340:259–286.

9. Courjon JH, Jeannerod M, Ossuzio I, et al: The role of vision on compensation of vestibulo ocular reflex after hemilabyrinthectomy in the cat. *Exp Brain Res* 1977; 28:235–248.

10. Davies P, Jones GM: An adaptive neural model compatible with plastic changes induced in the human vestibulo-ocular reflex by prolonged optical reversal of vision. *Brain Res* 1976; 103:546–550.

11. Demer JL, Porter FI, Goldberg J, et al: Adaptation to telescopic spectacles: Vestibulo-ocular reflex plasticity. *Investi Ophthalmol Vis Sci* 1989; 30:159–170.

12. Dix MR: The rationale and technique of head exercises in the treatment of vertigo. *Acta Oto rhino Laryngol B* 1979; 33:370–384.

13. Fetter M, Zee DS: Recovery from unilateral labyrinthectomy in Rhesus monkeys. *J Neurophysiol* 1988; 59:370–393.

14. Furst EJ, Goldberg J, Jenkins HA: Voluntary modification of the rotatory-induced vestibulo-ocular reflex by fixating imaginary targets. *Acta Otolaryngol* 1987; 103:131–140.

15. Galiana HL, Flohr H, Jones GM: A reevaluation of intervestibular nuclear coupling: Its role in vestibular compensation. *J Neurophysiol* 1984; 51:242–259.

16. Goodaux E, Halleux J, Gobert C: Adaptive change of the vestibulo-ocular reflex in the cat: The effects of a long-term frequency-selective procedure. *Exp Brain Res* 1983; 49:28–34.

17. Halmagyi GM, Curthoys IS, Cremer PD, et al: The human horizontal vestibular-ocular reflex in response to high-acceleration stimulation before and after unilateral vestibular neurectomy. *Exp Brain Res* 1990; 81:479–490.

18. Halmagyi GM, Curthoys IS, Dai MJ: Diagnosis of unilateral otolith hypofunction. *Diagn Neurotology* 1990; 8:313–329.

19. Halmagyi GM, Curthoys IS, Gibson WPR: Vestibular neurectomy and the management of vertigo. Opinion in *Neurol Neurosurg* 1988; 1:879–889.

20. Herdman SJ: Exercise strategies for vestibular disorders. *Ear, Nose Throat J* 1989; 68:961–964.

21. Herdman SJ: Assessment and treatment of balance disorders in the vestibular-deficient patient; in Duncan P (ed): *Balance, Proceedings of the American Physical Therapy Association Forum*. Nashville, Tenn, APTA, 1990, pp 87–94.

22. Igarashi M, Levy JK, O-Uchi T, et al: Further study of physical exercise and locomotor balance compensation after unilateral labyrinthectomy in squirrel monkeys. *Acta Otolaryngol* 1981; 92:101–105.

23. Istl-Lenz Y, Hyden D, Schwarz DWF: Response of the human vestibulo-ocular reflex following long-term 2× magnified visual input. *Exp Brain Res* 1985; 75:448–455.

24. Jones GM, Berthoz A, Segal B: Adaptive modification of the vestibulo-ocular reflex by mental effort in darkness. *Exp Brain Res* 1984; 56:149–153.

25. Jones GM, Guitton D, Berthoz A: Changing patterns of eye-head coordination during 6 h of optically reversed vision. *Exp Brain Res* 1988; 69:531–544.

26. Kasai T, Zee DS: Eye-head coordination in labyrinthine-defective human beings. *Brain Res* 1978; 144:123–141.

27. Kenshalo DR: Age changes in touch, vibration, temperature, kinesthesis and pain sensitivity, in Birren JE, Schaie KW (eds): *Handbook of the Psychology of Aging*. New York, Van Nostrand Reinhold, 1977.

28. Kosnik W, Winslow L, Kline D, et al: Visual changes in daily life throughout adulthood. *J Gerontol Psychol Sci* 1988; 43:63–70.

29. Lacour M, Roll JP, Appaix M: Modifications and development of spinal reflexes in the alert baboon (papio papio) following a unilateral vestibular neurectomy. *Brain Res* 1976; 113:255–269.

30. Lisberger SG: Role of the cerebellum during motor learning in the vestibulo-ocular reflex. *Trends Neurosci* 1982; 3:437–441.

31. Lisberger SG, Miles FA, Optican LM: Frequency-selective adaptation: evidence for channels in the vestibulo-ocular reflex. *J Neurosci* 1983; 3:1234–1244.

32. MacLennan S: Vibration sense, proprioception, and ankle reflexes in old age. *J Clin Exp Gerontol* 1980; 2:159–171.

33. Maoli C, Precht W: On the role of vestibulo-ocular reflex plasticity in recovery after unilateral peripheral vestibular lesions. *Exp Brain Res* 1985; 59:267–272.

34. Mathog RH, Peppard SB: Exercise and recovery from vestibular injury. *Am J Otolaryngol* 1982; 3:387–407.

35. McCabe BF: Labyrinthine exercises in the treatment of diseases characterized by vertigo: Their physiologic basis and methodology. *Laryngoscope* 1970; 80:1429–1433.

36. Miles FA, Eighmy BB: Long-term adaptive changes in primate vestibuloocular reflex. I: Behavioral observations. *J Neurophysiol* 1980; 43:1406–1425.

37. Norre ME, Beckers A: Vestibular habituation training: Exercise treatment for vertigo based upon the habituation effect. *Otolaryngol Head Neck Surg* 1989; 101:14–19.

38. Norre ME, DeWeerdt W: Treatment of vertigo based on habituation. *Laryngol Otol* 1980; 94:971–977.

39. Norre ME, Forrez G, Beckers A: Vestibulospinal findings in two syndromes with spontaneous vertigo attacks. *Ann Otol Rhinol Laryngol* 1989; 98:191–195.

40. Paige GD: Nonlinearity and asymmetry in the human vestibulo-ocular reflex. *Acta Otolaryngol* 1989; 108:1–8.

41. Paige GD: Vestibulo-ocular reflex (VOR) and adaptive plasticity with aging. *Soc Neurosci Abstr* 1989; 15:515.

42. Perret E, Regli F: Age and the perceptual threshold for vibratory stimuli. *Eur Neurol* 1970; 4:65–76.

43. Pfaltz CR: Vestibular compensation. *Acta Otolaryngol* 1983; 95:402–406.

44. Richter E: Quantitative study of human scarpa's ganglion and vestibular sensory epithelium. *Acta Otolaryngol* 1980: 90:199–208.

45. Rosenhall U: Degenerative patterns in the degenerating human vestibular neuro-epithelia. *Acta Otolaryngol* 1973; 76:208–220.

46. Segal BN, Katsarkas A: Long-term deficits of goal-directed vestibulo-ocular function following total unilateral loss of peripheral vestibular function. *Acta Otolaryngol* 1988; 106:102–110.

47. Shumway-Cook A, Horak FB: Vestibular rehabilitation: An exercise approach to managing symptoms of vestibular dysfunction. *Semin Hear* 1989; 10:196–209.

48. Takemori S, Ida M, Umezu H: Vestibular training after sudden loss of vestibular functions. *ORL J Otorhinolaryngol Relat Spec* 1985; 47:76–83.

49. Tangeman PT, Wheeler J: Inner ear concussion syndrome: Vestibular implications and physical therapy treatment. *Top Acute Care Trauma Rehabil* 1986; 1:72–83.

50. Wall C, Black FO, Hunt AE: Effects of age, sex and stimulus parameters upon vestibulo-ocular responses to sinusoidal rotation. *Acta Otolaryngol* 1984; 98:270–278.

51. Yagi T, Markham CH: Neural correlates of compensation after hemilabyrinthectomy. *Exp Neurol* 1984; 84:98–108.

52. Zee D: Vertigo, in *Current Therapy in Neurological Disease*. Ontario, BC, Decker, 1985; pp 8–13.

53. Zee D: The management of patients with vestibular disorders, in Barber HO, Sharpe JA (eds): *Vestibular Disorders*. Chicago, Mosby-Year Book, 1988, pp 254–274.

CHAPTER 19

Vestibular Evoked Potentials*

Josef Elidan, M.D.
Haim Sohmer, Ph.D.

Vestibular evoked potentials (VsEPs) are a series of electrical waves that are generated by the vestibular pathways in response to electrical or mechanical stimuli, and can be recorded by means of surface electrodes.

During recent years, it was shown, first in this laboratory and later in a few other studies, that the vestibular end organ and pathways can respond to short and intense angular acceleration stimuli, and that the response can be recorded by skin electrodes as evoked potentials. This finding was a major change in the concept of the physiology of the vestibular end organ. According to the simple torsion pendulum model, the sensitivity relative to head angular acceleration of the vestibular afferents innervating the semicircular canals (SCCs) in response to angular rotations should decrease at a rate of about 1 log unit per decade of frequency increase between 0.015 and 48 Hz, and theoretically at twice this rate for higher frequencies.[43] This decline in gain was observed by several authors, recording from both the first and the second order neurons.[31, 38] Thus, the gain of the vestibular neurons to a stimulus of very high frequency, equivalent to the acceleration impulses used in our technique, would be extremely low, so that induc-

tion of VsEPs to acceleration impulses was considered impractical.

This chapter describes the technical details of our method for induction and recording of VsEPs to acceleration impulses, the data which were collected in experimental animals, and the implementation of the method in humans which is now in progress. In addition, the literature will be reviewed with regard to other efforts to induce and record VsEPs in animals and in humans and to vestibular potentials evoked by natural and by electrical stimulation.

VESTIBULAR EVOKED POTENTIALS IN EXPERIMENTAL ANIMALS

Responses to Electrical Stimulation

Near-Field Recorded Potentials

Stimulation of the vestibular nerve in the cat by short electrical pulses evoked a series of field potentials, recorded by gross electrodes in the vicinity of the vestibular nuclei in the brain stem.[34] This response consisted of three components: (1) an initial positive-negative complex that indicates the arrival of current in the primary vestibular fibers; (2) a negative wave (N1) with a latency of less than 1 msec, and (3) a second negative wave (N2) with a latency of

*This research was supported in part by grant 89-00191 from the United States–Israel Binational Science Foundation, Jerusalem, Israel.

about 2.5 msec. Recordings by micro-electrodes of the activity of second order vestibular neurons in response to the same electrical stimuli has shown that some neurons are activated with a short latency—0.5 to 1.0 msec (corresponding to the timing of the N1 wave)—suggesting that they receive monosynaptic input. These neurons have low, irregular spontaneous firing rates and high sensitivity and are termed the "kinetic" neurons.[37] Other neurons, with higher and regular spontaneous activity and lower sensitivity (the "tonic" neurons), are activated after a delay of about 2.5 msec (corresponding to the N2 wave), although some of these neurons are activated with a latency of as long as 8 msec.[37] The "tonic" neurons are activated, probably, through multisynaptic connections in the brain stem.

Far-Field Recorded Potential

Schmidt[36] described a method to induce and record short latency (less than 10 msec) vestibular evoked potentials in the cat using short electrical stimuli (1 msec duration, 2 mA) delivered by an electrode placed in the external auditory canal. The evoked potential consisted of two negative waves, about 200 nV in amplitude, with latencies of 1.3 and 3 msec, followed by much smaller positive potentials (20 to 30 nV). Paralysis of the animals did not affect the potentials with regard to latencies and amplitudes. However, hypoxia for a short period caused marked reduction in the amplitude of the waves. Excision of the vestibular nerves caused disappearance of the evoked potentials. Based on these experiments, Schmidt attributed the two major negative waves to the vestibular nerve and the vestibular nucleus in the brain stem.

The drawbacks of this method are obvious. An electrical stimulus delivered in the external canal might stimulate multiple neural structures in addition to the vestibular system, for example, the cochlear pathways, the somatosensory system, and the facial nerve tracts.

Moreover, even for the vestibular system, the site of excitation is not clear. The electrical pulses stimulate, probably, the vestibular nerve, bypassing the end organ.

RESPONSES TO ACCELERATION STIMULI

Short Latency VsEPs to Angular Acceleration Impulses

A method for natural stimulation of short latency vestibular evoked potentials and their recording by skin electrodes has been developed by our group over the past decade (patent pending). The characteristics of these evoked potentials, their neural sources, and the effect of various drugs and conditions on the VsEPs were investigated extensively in various experimental animals,[9–11, 13, 14, 16–19] but most of the data were collected in cats.

For this technique, the animals are intubated and placed in an upright position in a special stimulation drum which in its present version is capable of producing clockwise (CW) or counterclockwise (CCW) impulsive angular acceleration stimuli, with a rise time of 1.5 to 3 msec and variable peak amplitude between 1,000° to 30,000°/sec.[9] The acceleration stimuli are transmitted to the animal's head by a head holder, which grips the head by means of the orbital rims and the hard palate. With this apparatus, the acceleration impulses have a rise-time of 2 to 3 msec. The acceleration can be measured directly on the animal's head by a linear accelerometer but is usually connected to the shaft of the head holder. In most of the experiments, the head is held in the position presumed to cause maximal stimulation of the lateral SCCs: 20° to 25° flexion with respect to the horizontal plane.[1] In some experiments, however, usually after unilateral labyrinthectomy, the vertical SCCs were tested by tilting the head to the appropriate position.[9]

The electrical activity is differentially

recorded by needle electrodes attached to one pinna and vertex, with the other pinna serving as ground. The response to 256 acceleration stimuli are amplified 10,000 times, filtered (300 Hz to 3 KHz), averaged by a computer, displayed vertex positive upward, and recorded by an X-Y plotter. The electrical pulse that drives the motor producing the mechanical stimuli also triggers the averager. Thus the initiation of acceleration of the cat's head occurs after a delay of about 2 msec with respect to the electrical pulse, which is synchronous with the onset of the trace.[9, 19] Recordings from the round window were performed by needle electrodes attached to the adjacent mucosa.

Characteristics of Response

The VsEPs in a normal cat consisted of five to eight waves, several microvolts in amplitude, during the first 10 msec after the start of the trace (Fig 19–1,A). Each wave was 0.6 to 1.5 msec in duration. The latency of the first wave (P1: vertex positive) was about 2 msec with respect to the start of head acceleration (3.8 to 4.5 msec from the beginning of the trace) when high acceleration stimuli ($\geq$20,000°/sec^2) are used (Fig 19–1,E). The first two waves, P1 and P2, were the most consistent ones, having a high degree of inter-test repeatability. The other waves, which appear consecutively with interpeak intervals of 0.5 to 1.5 msec, were less consistent and sometimes changed with changes in the animal's condition and level of anesthesia.[9, 16, 19]

Quite often the earlier, presumably neurogenic, waves were followed by waves of large amplitude and longer duration with latencies of 8 to 15 msec. These waves have been shown to be of myogenic origin, since they disappeared after paralysis of the animal by administration of succinylcholine (with artificial respiration), whereas the earlier neurogenic waves were not affected.[19] In the intact animal, the VsEPs were similar whether CW or CCW rotational stim-

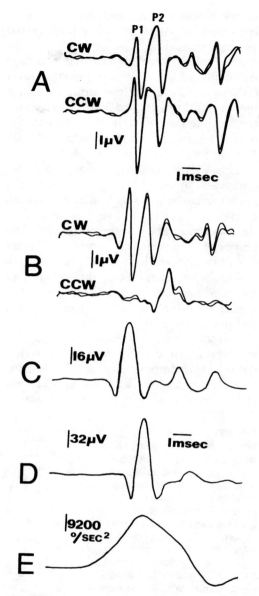

FIG 19–1.
A, vestibular evoked potentials (VsEPs) of the cat, in response to clockwise *(CW)* and counterclockwise *(CCW)* acceleration impulses, recorded by right pinna and vertex electrodes. Each trace is composed of two consecutive recordings. **B,** the VsEPs after left labyrinthectomy. Note the typical pattern of excitation *(CW)* versus inhibition *(CCW)* (see text). **C** and **D,** potentials recorded from the right vestibular nerve and nucleus, respectively. **E,** the acceleration waveform. *(From Elidan J, Langhofer L, Honrubia V: The neural generators of the vestibular evoked response.* Brain Res *1987; 423:385–390. Used by permission.)*

uli were used, and whether they were recorded by right or left pinna versus vertex electrodes.

The VsEPs were not affected by white noise masking of 80 dB hearing level (HL) applied close to the animal's ear. It was possible to record VsEPs and auditory evoked potentials simultaneously, and it seems that there was no interaction between the two responses.[9]

The VsEPs, however, were partially "masked" by ice water irrigation of the cat's ear canal for 3 to 5 minutes, which caused a decrease in amplitude and an increase in latency of the response.[9] The response disappeared completely after the animal's death.

Cerebellectomy, sectioning of the spinal cord above C1 nerve roots, or decerebration rostral to the superior colliculi did not significantly affect the VsEPs.

Bilateral labyrinthectomy or excision of the eighth cranial nerves caused a complete disappearance of the VsEPs. Unilateral labyrinthectomy or excision of the vestibular nerve caused an asymmetric response. The P1 and P2 waves were prominent with excitatory (ipsilateral) rotational stimulation of the remaining inner ear in the horizontal plane (CW for the right ear, CCW for the left ear) while with inhibitory (contralateral) rotational stimuli were either absent or replaced by a small downward deflection at the same latency (see Fig 19–1,B); the first upper peak appears at a longer latency (about 6 msec).

In unilateral labyrinthectomized animals, not only the horizontal canals but each of the vertical SCCs of the remaining inner ear can be tested separately by positioning the extended head at the appropriate angle (Fig 19–2). In these cases the results of the tests were in accordance with Ewald's laws of SCC excitation versus inhibition.[9, 16, 19]

The threshold of the VsEPs was determined to be between 1,000° and 1,500°/sec.[2] Increasing the stimulus intensity above threshold caused a decrease in latencies in exponential fashion and increase in the amplitude of P1, P2, and

FIG 19–2.
Vestibular evoked potentials recorded by left pinna and vertex electrodes after right labyrinthectomy and positioning of the cat's head for maximal stimulation of the left posterior semicircular canal (CW stimuli are excitatory in this position). *(From Elidan J, Langhofer L, Honrubia V: Recording of short-latency vestibular evoked potentials induced by acceleration impulses in experimental animals: Current status of the method and its applications. Electroencephalogr Clin. Neurophysiol 1987; 68:58–69. Used with kind permission from Elsevier Science Ireland Ltd., Bay 15K, Shannon Industrial Estate, Co. Clare, Ireland)*

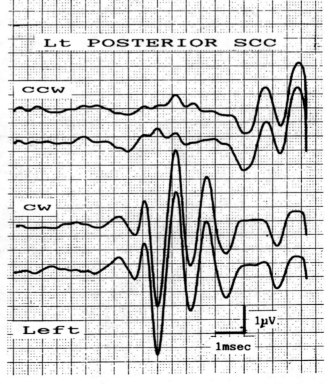

other waves. The amplitude of P1 wave changed in a relatively narrow dynamic range: between 1,000° and 10,000°/sec² (20 dB) (Fig 19–3).

Neural Origins of the Vestibular Evoked Potential

Many experiments were conducted to elucidate the neural sources of the VsEPs. Lidocaine (4%) applied to the perilymph through the oval window of the remaining inner ear of unilateral labyrinthectomized cats caused the abolishment of the neural waves in a few minutes, with full recovery later on (Fig 19–4). Similar results were obtained by injection of lidocaine into the eighth cranial nerve in the cerebellopontine angle, but in this case a series of smaller waves with shorter latency and longer duration could be recorded by a round window electrode, whose polarity reversed with the direction of the angular acceleration (Fig 19–5). Their amplitude was markedly decreased by anoxia, and they disappeared following labyrinthectomy of the remaining side. We believe that these waves represent microphonic and/or generator potentials, generated by the hair cells and the postsynaptic afferent terminals in the vestibular labyrinth.[40, 42]

Comparisons were made between the surface recorded VsEPs and those obtained by differential bipolar recording from various intracranial sites (see Fig 19–1,C and D). Recording from the vestibular nerve in response to excitatory acceleration impulses usually showed a prominent wave (20 to 120 μV) with a latency similar to that of the first wave (P1) of the surface recorded potential.[9, 19] Similar recordings from the vestibular nucleus showed waves with latencies similar to that of the second and third waves of the surface recorded VsEPs. Recordings from more rostral locations in the vicinity of the third, fourth, and sixth cranial nerve nuclei revealed potentials with longer latency.

In order to verify that the vestibular end organ and pathways can indeed re-

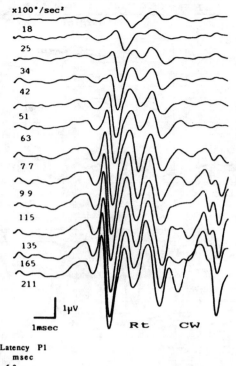

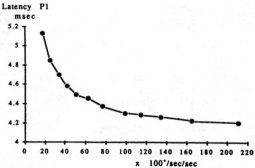

FIG 19–3.
Intensity function of the short latency VsEPs after right labyrinthectomy and with CCW acceleration impulses in the cat. The exponential curve shows the latency of P1 as a function of the acceleration, in degrees per sec.². *(From Elidan J, Langhofer L, Honrubia V: Recording of short-latency vestibular evoked potentials induced by acceleration impulses in experimental animals: Current status of the method and its applications.* Electroencephalogr Clin Neurophysiol *1987; 68:58–69. Used with kind permission from Elsevier Science Ireland Ltd.)*

spond to brief acceleration impulses, the activity of second order vestibular neurons was recorded extracellularly by tungsten microelectrodes, applying the same acceleration stimuli used for the induction of the surface recorded VsEPs (usually 8,000°/sec²). In addition, the responses of these neurons to sinusoidal

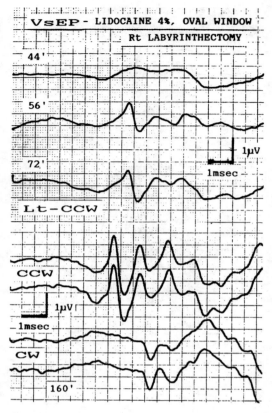

FIG 19–4.

The effect of application of 4% lidocain into the perilymph of the left ear of the cat after right labyrinthectomy. The VsEPs disappeared in 5 minutes, and reappeared gradually after about an hour. After 160 minutes the VsEPs were completely recovered and showed the typical pattern of right labyrinthectomy. *(From Elidan J, Langhofer L, Honrubia V: (1987) Recording of short-latency vestibular evoked potentials induced by acceleration impulses in experimental animals: Current status of the method and its applications.* Electroencephalogr Clin Neurophysiol *1987; 68:58–69. Used with kind permission from Elsevier Science Ireland Ltd.)*

quired intense sinusoidal rotation stimuli to produce a response, but once the threshold was reached, they showed higher gain and smaller phase lags relative to head acceleration than neurons with more regular spontaneous activity which did not respond to acceleration impulses.

The post stimulus time (PST) histogram that describes the activity of the responsive neurons was characterized by several peaks.[11] The first peak occurred at latency of 5.5 to 6.0 msec from the trigger pulse, about 3.5 msec after the start of head acceleration. This timing corresponded to that of the second wave (P2) of the far field recorded VsEPs (Fig 19–7). In general, increasing the intensity of the acceleration impulses caused a decrease in the latency of the initial peak of the PST histogram, an improvement in its definition, and an increase in the number of the peaks.

Other responsive second order vestibular neurons showed a longer latency of

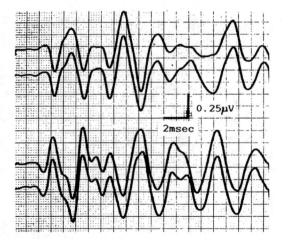

FIG 19–5.

Potentials recorded from the round window of the right ear of the cat after left labyrinthectomy and injection of 4% lidocain into the right eighth cranial nerve. These potentials are believed to represent microphonics or generator potentials. Their polarity reverses with change in direction of the rotation stimuli. *(From Elidan J, Langhofer L, Honrubia V: Recording of short-latency vestibular evoked potentials induced by acceleration impulses in experimental animals: Current status of the method and its applications.* Electroencephalogr Clin Neurophysiol *1987; 68:58–69. Used with kind permission from Elsevier Science Ireland Ltd.)*

rotational stimuli were documented as well (Fig 19–6). Most of the neurons (80%) were of type I (excitable to ipsilateral rotation). The rest (20%) were of type II (excitable to contralateral rotation).[10, 11]

Only a small fraction of the second order vestibular neurons recorded were found to respond to impulse stimuli. These neurons showed low (0 to 5 spikes/sec) and irregular spontaneous discharge (coefficient of variation greater than 0.3) (see Fig 19–6). These neurons also re-

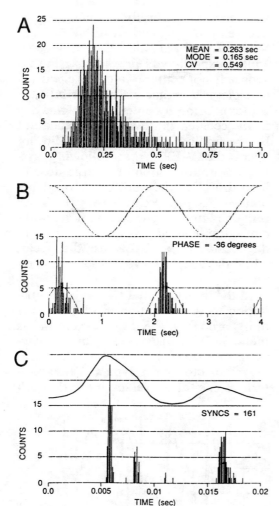

FIG 19–6.
Firing pattern of a kinetic type I second-order vestibular neuron in the cat. **A,** interspike time interval histogram. **B,** neural response to sinusoidal stimuli of 0.5 Hz. **C,** post-stimulus time histogram of the neural response to the acceleration impulses. *(From Elidan J, Langhofer L, Honrubia V: The firing properties of second order vestibular neurons in correlation with the far-field recorded vestibular evoked responses. Laryngoscope 1989; 99:92–99. Used by permission.)*

The phase lag of the neurons, which did not respond to acceleration impulses, was greater than 90°.[11]

The Effect of Various Drugs on the Vestibular Evoked Potentials

Using this method of induction and recording of VsEPs in experimental animals allows, for the first time, the direct assessment of vestibular function in a noninvasive way, with separate representation of the vestibular nerve and nucleus. We have used this method to evaluate the effect of loop diuretics and of aminoglycosides on the vestibular sys-

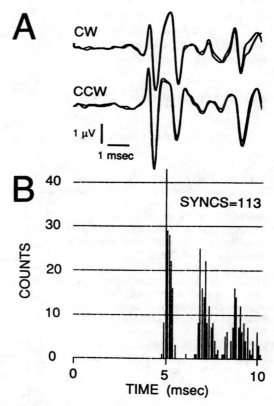

FIG 19–7.
Vestibular evoked potentials **(A)** and post-stimulus time (PST) histogram of a second order kinetic vestibular neuron **(B)** to the same acceleration impulses in the cat. Note the correspondence in timing of the second wave of the VsEPs and the first peak of the PST histogram. *(From Elidan J, Langhofer L, Honrubia V: The firing properties of second order vestibular neurons in correlation with the far-field vestibular evoked responses. Laryngoscope 1989; 99:92–99. Used by permission.)*

the first peak of the PST histogram. The range of the latency of the first peak was 3.0 to 10.0 msec with respect to the start of head acceleration. A significant positive correlation ($r = 0.699$; $P > .001$) was found between the latency of the first peak of the PST histogram and the phase lag in response to sinusoidal rotations (ranged between $-35°$ and $-80°$).

tem. Ethacrynic acid and furosemide injected intravenously into cats caused a complete disappearance of the auditory evoked response, whereas the VsEPs were not affected.[13] Following systemic administration of gentamicin, the VsEPs were altered and later disappeared, whereas the ABR remained unchanged. Histopathologic examination following the gentamicin showed severe damage to the vestibular end organ, particularly on the summit of the cristae. The maculae were spared.[19]

The VsEPs disappeared after the induction of anoxia for a few minutes and recovered gradually shortly after restoration of breathing (Fig 19–8). The VsEPs were found to be more sensitive to anoxia than the auditory evoked potentials.[9, 19]

Summary of Animal Studies

Induction and recording of VsEPs has been demonstrated to be an effective tool for experimentally assessing vestibular end organ and vestibular nerve function in animals. Carefully controlled experiments proved that the response is not contaminated by electrical or biological artifacts. The possibility of contamination by potentials originating in the cochlear pathways was ruled out by the finding that white noise did not affect the VsEPs; that following systemic administration of a large dose of loop diuretics the auditory evoked potentials disappeared, whereas the VsEP remained unchanged; and that gentamicin administered systemically for 14 days caused the VsEPs to disappear, while the auditory evoked potentials remained.

In the intact animal the major contribution to the initiation of the VsEPs is most probably the SCCs, each in its plane of responsiveness. This is suggested by the fact that after unilateral labyrinthectomy the typical VsEPs pattern of excitation versus inhibition fol-

FIG 19–8.
Effect of anoxia on the VsEPs of the cat. The potentials disappeared after 3 minutes, 45 seconds and recovered gradually shortly after restoration of respiration. However, even after 8 minutes, the latency of the response was still longer than before the anoxia. *(From Elidan J, Langhofer L, Honrubia V: Recording of short-latency vestibular evoked potentials induced by acceleration impulses in experimental animals: Current status of the method and its applications. Electroencephalogr Clin. Neurophysiol 1987; 68:58–69. Used with kind permission from Elsevier Science Ireland Ltd., Bay 15K, Shannon Industrial Estate, Co. Clare, Ireland)*

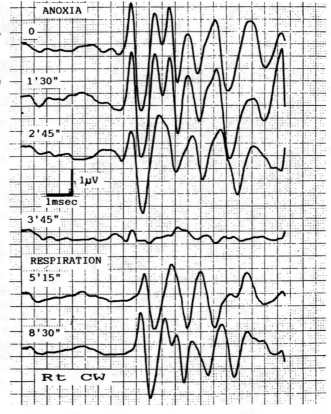

lows Ewald's laws of SCC physiology.[9, 19]

Moreover, the VsEPs disappeared following systemic administration of gentamicin, and this was associated with an affect on type I hair cells on the summit of the cristae. This suggests that these cells are responsible for the initiation of the VsEPs. They are innervated by caliceal endings corresponding to large neurons that have irregular spontaneous discharge, high-frequency phase leads, and rapid conduction time.[21, 44] These fibers probably influence the responses of the kinetic second order afferents,[22] which were shown in our studies to respond to the acceleration impulses with short latencies.[10, 11] Therefore, it is possible that loss of type I hair cells results in a disappearance of the VsEPs, whereas other vestibular functions, less dependent on these hair cells, may persist.

In the intact animal the VsEPs are the result of synchronous electrical events in both labyrinths and vestibular pathways. Each SCC relates synergistically to a canal on the contralateral side as a "push-pull" system. Thus, in the intact animal the VsEPs do not change significantly whether CW or CCW rotational stimuli are used or whether the recording electrode is on the right or left ear. In the unilateral labyrinthectomized animal, on the other hand, because the response of the remaining ear is not opposed by the synergistic contralateral one, changes in the direction of rotation or position of the head cause a large change in the VsEPs. Still, after unilateral labyrinthectomy, the VsEPs in response to inhibitory stimuli of the remaining ear are characterized by the absence of P1 and P2 waves, and by the presence of longer latency smaller waves. The source of these waves is still unknown. One possibility is that after synchronous inhibition of the firing of many nerve fibers, these neurons start firing again synchronously, which produces the delayed potentials. Another explanation is that inhibition of the nor-

mal side causes activation of the vestibular nuclei on the side in which labyrinthectomy was performed, and that this initiates the late response (Chapter 5, in reference 43). Further experiments are needed to clarify this point.

The main contributors to the longer latency waves of the VsEPs are in more rostral parts of the brain stem, most probably in the third, fourth, and sixth cranial nerve nuclei, which have close connections with the vestibular nuclei. The generator potentials (similar to cochlear microphonic potentials),[9, 42, 40] which may represent the vibration of the cupula and the hairs in response to intense acceleration impulses, became obvious after the elimination of the neurogenic potentials, which were much larger.

It was shown in our experiments that the main contributions to the first and second waves of the VsEPs are the vestibular nerve and nuclei, respectively. However, both of these generators are the source of additional smaller potentials that are embedded in the final configuration of the VsEPs. These smaller potentials are generated presumably by repeated firing of neurons in these generators in response to the intense stimuli. These repeated firings have been demonstrated in our recordings from second order vestibular neurons. Thus, the situation is much more complex than a simple correlation between a certain peak of the VsEPs and a particular site in the brain. Most probably, evoked potentials from different sources have similar latencies and are overlapping in the VsEPs.

The responses of several components of the vestibular pathways to angular acceleration impulses have been shown to be very rapid. Both the generator potentials in the peripheral terminals of the primary afferents[40] and the discharge rate of the second order neurons[37, 38] increased rapidly to a peak and then declined exponentially. However, since the authors of these studies did not provide the exact specification of their impulse stimuli, it is impossible to compare them with the stimuli used in our studies for the VsEPs. The ultrashort rise time of our impulse stimuli and their very high intensity produce a high degree of synchronization in the firing of the vestibular nerve fibers and then in the second order vestibular neurons, which makes possible the recording of gross potentials with surface electrodes.

Although the gain of the vestibular neurons to stimuli of high frequency should be extremely low (according to the torsion pendulum model), some studies[20, 41] have shown that the gain of neurons with irregular spontaneous activities increase with frequencies between 1 and 8 Hz. Yet, the highest frequency used in these studies was less than 10 Hz, which is far lower than the frequency equivalent to that of the stimuli used for the VsEPs (about 150 Hz).

Studies of Other Groups

Bohmer et al.[4] induced and recorded middle latency potentials in awake Rhesus monkeys. They used the primate rotating chair to produce angular acceleration stimuli of 2,000°/sec². The recording electrodes were implanted deeply over the bone of the mastoid and the occiput. The evoked potential consisted of a mastoid positive potential at latency of 44 msec after the start of the trace. The real latency with regard to the head acceleration could not be determined, as there was no sharp onset of acceleration. This wave was absent in two monkeys with nonfunctioning horizontal SCCs. The second wave at latency of 84 msec was present also in animals with no vestibular response.

Dechesne and Sans[7] showed that brief pressure pulses (1 msec duration) to a cannulated lateral SCC of a cat evoked potentials in both the eighth cranial nerve and the lateral vestibular nucleus. Later, Dechesne et al.[6] used the same method to demonstrate the pharmacologic effect of various drugs and neurotransmitters on vestibular function.

Latkowski and Puzio,[29] working on guinea pigs, constructed a special device and a head holder to induce short acceleration impulses. The waveform of their stimuli is lacking in their article, but the maximal acceleration of the mechanical device is mentioned to be 255°/sec² (which is not necessarily identical with the acceleration of the animal's head, which was not determined). The response to 256 stimuli was recorded between two mastoid electrodes, with another gluteal electrode serving as ground. The response was composed of several potentials, with the latency of the first being 5.8 to 6.2 msec from the beginning of the trace (the latency with respect to head acceleration is not given). No control experiments were included in this study to confirm the vestibular origin of these potentials.

Coale et al.[5] produced vestibular evoked potentials in cats by direct mechanical stimulation of the cannulated horizontal semicircular canal. The stimuli were fluid pressure pulses in a closed hydraulic system that was coupled to the lateral semicircular canal near the ampulla. Field potentials were recorded differentially by subdermal mastoid and nasal electrodes. The evoked potential produced was a high-fidelity copy of the pressure stimulus waveform, and reflected, probably, depolarization and hyperpolarization of the hair cells.

Hoffman et al.[25] recorded short latency VsEPs by means of chronically implanted electrodes into the fallopian canal of the chinchilla. The stimuli were linear acceleration impulses with maximum intensity of 8 g, with rise time of 1 msec. The response consisted of a negative going wave (N1) followed by an additional series of waves. The response disappeared after introduction of potassium chloride into the perilymph. Acoustic masking caused the abolishment of all the waves except the N1 wave, which is believed to be generated by the vestibular nerve fibers. The mean amplitude and latency of N1 in response to 8 g stimuli were 46.1 µV and 1.26 msec, respectively, and its threshold 0.125 g.

VESTIBULAR EVOKED POTENTIALS IN HUMANS

Long Latency Potentials—Review of the Literature

Molinari and Mingrino[32] have tried to develop a method to evoke vestibular potentials in humans in response to galvanic stimulation. The exciting electrode was placed near the external auditory canal and produced pulses of 1 to 6 mA and 10 msec duration. The response from the scalp was made up of a series of positive-negative waves beginning at 60 to 80 msec and continuing for 400 to 500 msec. The response was absent in patients with bilateral absence of vestibular function. It was still preserved in patients with isolated lesions of the cochlea and after curarization.

For several decades, several groups have tried to induce and record evoked potentials of the vestibular system in humans by using various types of rotational stimuli, which had relatively long rise time and duration, and low intensity. Greiner et al.[23] used rotational stimuli of a few seconds with maximal acceleration of 400°/sec². The response, which was recorded by temporal and occipital electrodes, was inconsistent, and composed of two broad negative-positive potentials at latencies of 3.8 and 7.3 sec with respect to the start of the rotational stimuli (in sitting position), and a maximal amplitude of 30 µV.

Spiegel et al.[39] used acceleration stimuli of about 120°/sec² for about 1 second generated by sudden cessation of the rotating chair. From both cats and humans, they recorded long latency potentials, 300 to 600 msec from the cessation of rotation, but as they pointed out, the exact latency was not clear since the timing of the triggering of the averager was not determined. In the cat, the disappearance of this evoked potential was induced by thiopentone sodium (Pentothal) anesthesia or bilateral labyrinthectomy, but paralysis of the animal or sectioning of the spinal cord above the upper cervical segments did not affect the potentials.

Bodo et al.[2, 3] developed a system for producing acceleration stimuli by sudden stop and reversal of the direction of a rotating chair. The stimuli were 20 to 50°/sec² and 300 to 600 msec in duration. Twenty stimuli in both directions were used to elicit the evoked potentials which consisted of several waves. The first wave (N1) had a latency of 60 msec (with respect to the reversal of the rotating chair) when recorded from the vertex. Decreasing the stimulus intensity caused a prolongation of the latency of the response. This response, however, was not specific to vestibular stimuli and a similar one could be evoked with even shorter latency by visual and acoustic stimuli.

Salamy et al.[35] recorded, in 20 human subjects, long latency responses to angular acceleration stimuli (maximum 50°/sec²) produced by a torsion swing chair. The evoked potentials occurred during the first 400 msec, at which time the chair rotation was 4°. The most prominent potential was a negative-positive complex with peaks at about 193 and 345 msec, respectively, and several microvolts in amplitude. On the basis of these latencies, it was argued that the potentials were of vestibular rather than somatosensory origin.

Hofferberth and Rothenberger[24] used angular acceleration stimuli caused by sudden stop of a revolving chair. A late response evoked by 64 stimuli was recorded in 30 normal adults (with a mean latency of 219.4 msec), while no response was present in two labyrinthectomized patients. In children with minimal brain damage, a higher range of response variability and longer latency compared to normal children was found.

Hood[26] used angular velocity stimuli of a rotating chair, with a peak angular velocity of 120°/sec and 2 seconds duration. The subjects were asked to fixate on a small light target to minimize the possibility of corneoretinal potential contamination. The response recorded by vertex and mastoid electrodes from 10 normal subjects consisted of an initial negative deflection at a latency of 150 msec, followed by a larger positive wave whose peak coincided with the time of maximal acceleration. The response could not be recorded in patients with bilateral vestibular damage. However, a response with similar latencies and waveform could be evoked by optokinetic stimuli alone, thus it was not a specific response to vestibular stimulation.

In a more recent study by the same group,[27] the stimuli were sinusoidal rotations with a peak of 1,000 °/sec^2 and 2 seconds duration. The evoked potential to 15 to 20 stimuli was recorded by means of vertex versus nasal electrodes and consisted of several slow negative-positive waves, starting at latencies of 250 msec. The response was absent in patients with complete bilateral vestibular loss.

Pirodda et al.[33] used whole body rotational stimuli of 90° clockwise or counterclockwise, with a peak acceleration of 800 to 3,400°/sec^2 (rise time of about 150 msec). The response (which was recorded by vertex and earlobe electrodes) to a series of 10 stimuli consisted of several (2 to 6) potentials starting at a latency of about 200 msec with respect to the start of the acceleration, and with amplitude of about 20 μV. The duration of each wave was about 150 to 200 msec. The potentials were absent in patients suffering from a complete loss of bilateral vestibular function, and markedly reduced in amplitude in patients with unilateral vestibular loss.

Kast and Lankford[28] described evoked potentials to head-drop stimuli, which they suggested originate in the otolithic organs. The acceleration stimuli lasted for 200 msec with peak deceleration of 1.1 g (the waveform of the stimuli as not provided). Twenty such

drops were used for each test, and the response was recorded by vertex and mastoid electrodes. The response consisted of several potentials: the first negative wave (N1) at a latency of 67 to 97 msec (changing with age) and amplitude of about −16 to −28 μV, followed by a positive wave at a latency of about 156 to 190 msec and amplitude of about 9 to 21 μV. Later appearing potentials were irregular and inconsistent.

Durrant and Furman[8] used acceleration-deceleration stimuli of 200 to 400°/sec^2, ranging in duration from 50 to 900 msec, produced by abrupt reversal in direction of a rotating chair. The recording electrodes were vertex referred to mastoid. Potentials evoked by acceleration and deceleration were averaged together. The response to 16 repetitive stimuli consisted of a positive-going wave followed by a negative deflection at latencies of about 100 and 200 msec, respectively, and amplitude of some 25 μV. However, the responses from subjects with vestibular loss did not differ markedly from those of the normal subjects. The authors therefore concluded that the long latency rotational evoked potential is not of vestibular origin.

In conclusion of this section, it is obvious from the survey of the literature that there is much confusion with regard to the methods and a considerable discrepancy between the results of the different investigators that claim to have evoked long latency vestibular potentials. This discrepancy can be attributed to the difference in acceleration stimuli (which in most of the articles were not defined accurately, nor were acceleration waveforms provided) and to triggering problems. As the stimuli were relatively long, there were difficulties in the synchronization of the averager sweep with a particular phase of the stimulus. In any case, the evoked potentials were in the middle and long latency range. Different recording sites were used, and in most of the investigations, contamination by somatosensory, auditory, and ocular potentials were not excluded. In two investigations[8, 26] it was even demonstrated that long latency potentials were not specific to vestibular stimulation.

Short and Middle Latency Potentials

On a theoretical basis, it is clear that the success of a technique of induction of reliable short latency vestibular evoked potentials is dependent on the following conditions: (1) the acceleration stimuli used to evoke the response should be of short rise time with respect to the latency, after which the response is expected; and (2) the stimuli should be intense enough to excite synchronously a sufficient number of vestibular nerve fibers, which would facilitate the recording of compound action potentials by scalp electrodes.

In view of the disappointing results in the literature, it was obvious that the most promising way would be to apply to humans the same acceleration stimuli which we used to evoke short latency VsEPs in experimental animals.

The application of this method to humans was associated with many technological obstacles.[12, 15, 30] In experimental animals, the efficient transfer of the mechanical stimulus to the anesthetized animal's head was achieved by tight clamping of the head with a special holder. This, of course, is not applicable to humans, and another method had to be developed. In addition, special procedures had to be taken to eliminate various electrical artifacts that are more easily induced in humans than in experimental animals (due to the larger and stronger motor, larger size of the head, wire displacement, and other factors).

Stimulus System[12, 15, 30]

The transfer of the stimulus from the motor to the human head is achieved by a drum (patent pending) which was spe-

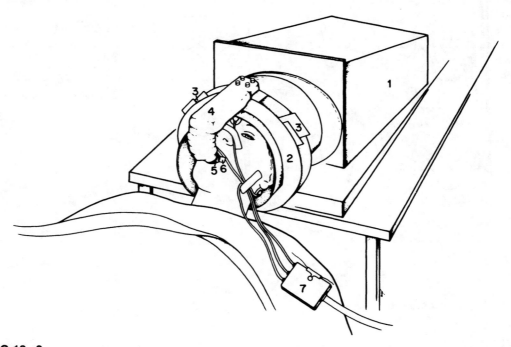

FIG 19–9.
The mechanical stimulation system: *1*, the motor (shielded); *2*, metallic drum; *3*, holders for acrylic pads; *4*, acrylic rod; *5*, acrylic dental plate; *6*, accelerometer; *7*, pre-amplifier. *(From Elidan J, Sela M, Leibner E, et al: Short latency vestibular evoked response in animals and in humans. Otolaryngology Head Neck Surg 1991; 105:353–359. Used by permission.)*

cially designed and constructed. The head is inserted into the drum and secured by two acrylic pads in the front of the drum, in an angle for maximal stimulation of the lateral SCCs. The drum is connected to the shaft of a powerful motor capable of producing intense and short acceleration stimuli. A strong acrylic rod is attached to the rim of the drum and is connected to an acrylic dental plate that is constructed individually to fit the teeth of the upper jaw of each subject (Fig 19–9).

Thus, the acceleration impulses (either CW or CCW) are effectively transmitted to the skull of the subject. The acceleration impulse starts about 1.5 msec after the trigger pulse, and reaches a maximum of some 12,000°/sec^2 with a rise time of 1.5 to 2 msec. Each step of the drum (1.8°) is followed by a much slower return step, after which the head comes to a complete stop before the

next stimulus. Usually the stimulus is repeated twice per second. The acceleration is measured by a small linear accelerometer attached to the acrylic rod close to the dental plate. The drum is equipped with special brakes which prevent rotation beyond several degrees in each direction.

The recording of the evoked potentials are done differentially by electrodes on the mastoid and the forehead, with the other ear serving as ground. Disposable pediatric electrocardiographic electrodes are used. They were found to provide a larger contact area with the skin, reduced slippage and movement artifacts, and lower impedance (1-3 kΩ) and DC contact potentials (about 10 mV).

The recorded VsEPs are analyzed in two separate post-stimulus windows: short latency (12.7 msec), and middle latency (63 msec). The analysis is done by

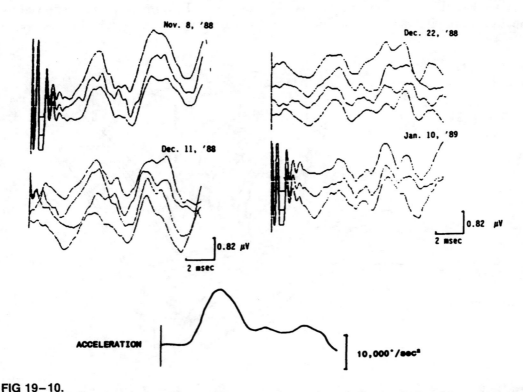

FIG 19–10.
Short latency VsEPs in two normal subjects. Note the good response replicability and the similarity of the waves in the two subjects. *Lower trace* is the acceleration waveform. *(From Elidan J, Sela M, Leibner E, et al: Short latency vestibular evoked response in animals and in humans.* Otolaryngology Head Neck Surg *1991; 105:353–359. Used by permission.)*

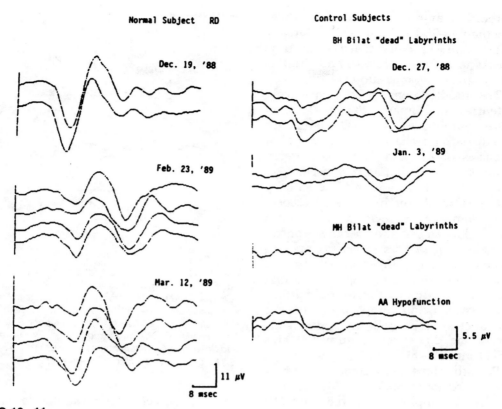

Normal Subject   RD

Dec. 19, '88

Feb. 23, '89

Mar. 12, '89

11 μV

8 msec

Control Subjects

BH Bilat "dead" Labyrinths

Dec. 27, '88

Jan. 3, '89

MH Bilat "dead" Labyrinths

AA Hypofunction

5.5 μV

8 msec

FIG 19–11.
Left: Middle latency VsEPs recorded repeatedly in three different sessions. *Right,* recordings from three control subjects. Note the absence of clear potentials. *(From Elidan J, Sela M, Leibner E, et al: Short latency vestibular evoked response in animals and in humans.* Otolaryngology Head Neck Surg *1991; 105:353–359. Used by permission.)*

Micro-Shev 2000 evoked response system with digital filtering. For the short latency VsEPs the bandpass is 200 to 2,000 Hz, and 500 to 2,000 impulses are needed to obtain a response with good signal-to-noise ratio. For the middle latency VsEPs, the bandpass is 30 to 300 Hz, and usually 64 to 128 stimuli are sufficient for a good response. Forehead positivity is displayed upward.

Permission to conduct these experiments was obtained from the Committee for Human Experimentation of our Medical Center, and informed consent was obtained from each subject. The stimulus is well tolerated by the subjects, with some even falling asleep. There is no evidence of immediate or late side effects or complications caused by the intense acceleration impulses. Thus far, 30 normal subjects have been tested, most of them several times, on different dates. As a control, we selected three students from the local School for the Deaf in whom the bithermal caloric test showed either bilateral absence of response (two students) or severe bilateral hypofunction (one student). The age range of all subjects was 16 to 28 years. Each of the subjects had to be free of dental or cervical spine problems.

The short latency VsEPs in humans were composed of several waves during the first 10 msec.[12, 15, 30] The first upward wave (P1, forehead positive) had a latency of about 3.0 msec with respect to the onset of head acceleration (Fig 19–10). The second upward wave (P2) was seen about 1.5 msec later, and a prominent negative deflection, at a latency of about 6 msec with respect to the onset of head acceleration, followed. The amplitude of the waves was less than 1 μV. The human short latency VsEPs showed consistency over time (weeks to months interval) and similarity between different subjects.

The middle latency vestibular evoked potentials in humans (Fig 19–11) had larger amplitudes (10 to 20 μV) with two upward (forehead positive) waves at latencies of 8.8 and 26.8 msec and a downward deflection at 18.8 msec.

Both the short and middle latency VsEPs were absent in repeated recordings from the subjects with bilateral "dead" labyrinths and in other control recordings (cadavers, inert conducting masses, and so forth). Thus, the grand average for the recordings of normal subjects accentuated the normal pattern of the response in comparison with the lack of clear response in the grand average of the three control subjects (Figs 19–12 and 19–13).

Both the short and the middle latency VsEP were not affected by white noise of 70 dB HL applied near the subject's ears.

Figure 19–14 demonstrates the intensity function of the human VsEPs which shows that lowering the stimulus intensity caused a decrease in the amplitude and increase of the latencies of P1 and other waves. The threshold of the response was determined to be around 2,000°/sec².

Similar to what was shown in the cat, we believe that the short latency VsEPs represent the neurogenic activity of the vestibular nerve (P1), the vestibular nucleus (P2), and higher centers in the vestibular pathways.

The sources of the human middle latency VsEPs are still not clear. It is obvious that they are originated in the vestibular pathways, since they were absent in the control experiments and they were not influenced by white noise. We assumed that these potentials are of myogenic origin following vestibular stimulation, but we failed to demonstrate electromyographic activity in any of the cervical muscles which could

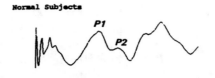

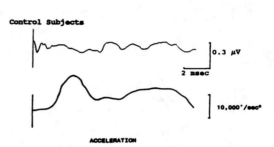

FIG 19–12.
Grand average of the short latency VsEPs. *Upper trace* is from 32 recordings obtained in eight normal subjects. *Middle trace* is from nine recordings in three control subjects. *Lower trace* shows the acceleration waveform. *(From Elidan J, Sela M, Leibner E, et al: Short latency vestibular evoked response in animals and in humans. Otolaryngology Head Neck Surg 1991; 105:353–359. Used by permission.)*

be the source of the middle latency VsEPs. Similarly, synchronous recordings of VsEPs and electronystagmography showed that corneoretinal potentials do not contribute significantly to the generation of the middle latency VsEPs.

PLANS AND PROSPECTS FOR THE FUTURE

The objectives of this project in the near future are to improve and simplify our ability to induce and record VsEPs in humans and to develop a better understanding of the physiologic basis of the VsEPs and the pathophysiology of deviations from the normal patterns in humans.

The mechanical stimulation system is being improved and refined from both the mechanical and electronic aspects. Until now, the head holder could stimulate the lateral SCCs only, and a special dental plate had to be produced for each subject specifically. Recently, our team

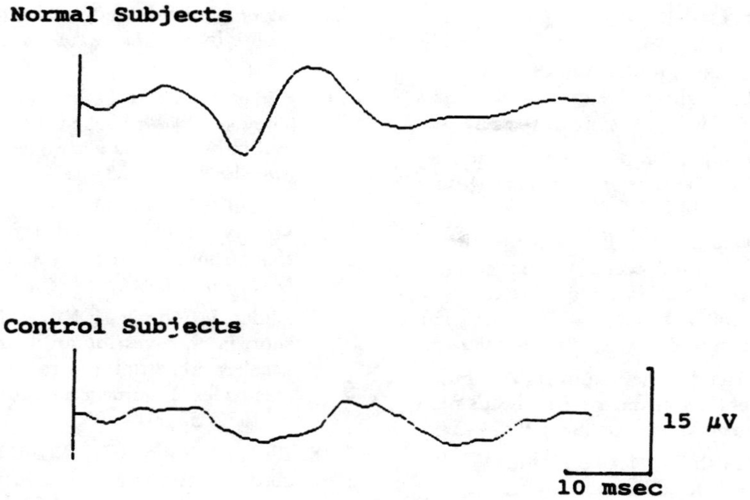

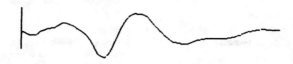

Normal Subjects

Control Subjects

15 μV

10 msec

FIG 19–13.
Grand average of the middle latency VsEPs. *Upper trace* is from 51 recordings in nine normal subjects. *Lower trace* is from 11 recordings in three control subjects. *(From Elidan J, Sela M, Leibner E, et al: Short latency vestibular evoked response in animals and in humans.* Otolaryngology Head Neck Surg *1991; 105:353–359. Used by permission.)*

has designed a new head holder that can transmit the acceleration impulses produced by the motor to the subject's head at an angle appropriate for stimulation of the vertical SCCs also. Moreover, it is

ACCELERATION
X100
deg/sec²

124

112

83

69

48

0.31 μV

1.27 msec

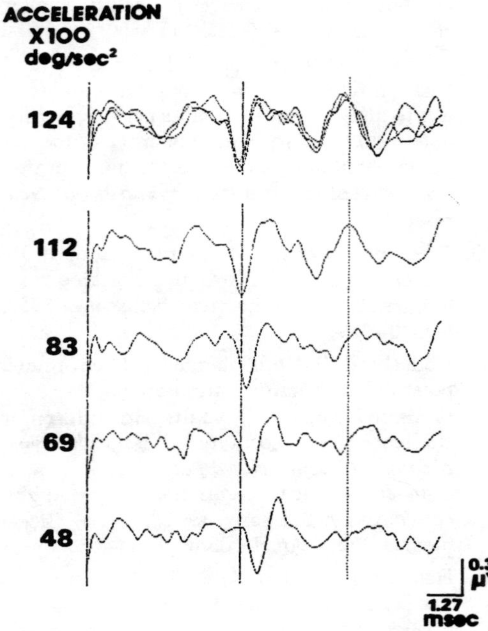

FIG 19–14.
Intensity function of the short latency VsEPs in a normal subject. On the *left* are the intensities of the acceleration impulses (in degrees/sec²).

likely that a personal dental plate will not be required, so that the preparations for the test would be much simpler. This would be a passage from the stage of experimentation with the prototype to an advanced system that would be appropriate for clinical use.

We plan to test subjects with known lesions in various locations in the vestibular pathways in order to try to correlate the clinical diagnosis (as determined by imaging and clinical tests) to the deviations from the normal pattern of the VsEPs.

Should such a correlation be established, the recording of VsEPs will improve our ability to determine the site of lesion in the vestibular pathways of vertigenous patients, which is usually impossible today with the conventional vestibular tests.

Acknowledgments

The authors thank Dr. M. Nitzan, Dr. S. Freeman, Dr. V. Honrubia, L. Langhofer, and E. Leibner for their important contribution to the success of this project. The human data are part of a doctoral thesis of E. Leibner.

REFERENCES

1. Blanks RHI, Curthoys IS, Markham, CH: Plannar relationships of semicircular canals in the cat. *J Physiol* 1972; 223:55–62.

2. Bodo G: Examination of the vestibular system by short-time acceleration. *Laryngoscope* 1976; 86:874–878.

3. Bodo G, Rozsa L, Antal P: Scalp electrical response evoked by acceleration in young healthy men, in Surjan L (ed): *Proceedings of the 12th ORL World Congress*. Budapest, Hungary, Akademiai Nyomda, 1981, pp 389–392.

4. Bohmer A, Henn V, Lehmann D: Vestibular evoked potentials in the awake Rhesus monkey. *Adv Otorhinolaryngol* 1983; 30:54–57.

5. Coale FS, Walsh EJ, McGee J, et al: Vestibular evoked potentials in response to direct unilateral mechanical stimulation. *Otolaryngol Head Neck Surg* 1989; 100:177–186.

6. Dechesne C, Reymond J, Sans A: Action of glutamate in the cat labyrinth. *Ann Otol Rhinol Laryngol* 1984; 93:163–165.

7. Dechesne C, Sans A: A new stimulation technique of the crista ampullaris of the lateral canal in the adult cat: Study of action potential of the vestibular nerve. *Experientia* 1978; 36:846–847.

8. Durrant JD, Furman JMR: Long-latency rotational evoked potentials in subjects with and without bilateral vestibular loss. *Electroencephalogr Clin Neurophysiol* 1988; 71:251–256.

9. Elidan J, Langhofer L, Honrubia V: Recording of short-latency vestibular evoked potentials induced by acceleration impulses in experimental animals: Current status of the method and its applications. *Electroencephalogr Clin Neurophysiol* 1987; 68:58–69.

10. Elidan J, Langhofer L, Honrubia V: The neural generators of the vestibular evoked response. *Brain Res* 1987; 423:385–390.

11. Elidan J, Langhofer L, Honrubia V: The firing properties of second order vestibular neurons in correlation with the far-field recorded vestibular evoked responses. *Laryngoscope* 1989; 99:92–99.

12. Elidan J, Leibner E, Freeman S, et al: Short and middle latency vestibular evoked responses to acceleration in man. *Electroencephalogr Clin Neurophysiol* 1991; 80:140–145.

13. Elidan J, Lin J, Honrubia V: The effect of loop diuretics on the vestibular system. Assessment by recording the vestibular evoked response. *Arch Otolaryngol Head Neck Surg* 1986; 112:836–839.

14. Elidan J, Lin J, Honrubia V: Vestibular ototoxicity of gentamicin assessed by the recording of a short-latency vestibular-evoked response in cats. *Laryngoscope* 1987; 97:865–870.

15. Elidan J, Sela M, Leibner E, et al: Short latency vestibular evoked response in animals and in humans. *Otolaryngology Head Neck Surg* 1991; 105:353–359.

16. Elidan J, Sohmer H, Lev S, et al: Short latency vestibular evoked response to acceleration stimuli recorded by skin electrodes. *Ann Otol Rhinol Laryngol* 1984; 93:257–261.

17. Elidan J, Sohmer H, Nitzan M: Recording of short latency vestibular evoked potentials to acceleration stimuli in rats by means of skin electrodes. *Electroencephalogr Clin Neurophysiol* 1982; 53:501–505.

18. Elidan J, Sohmer H, Nitzan M: A surface recorded vestibular evoked response to acceleration in cats. *J Laryngol Otol* 1984; (Suppl 9):111–119.

19. Elidan J, Sohmer H, Nitzan M, et al: Vestibular evoked potentials, in Cracco J (ed): *Evoked Potentials* (Frontiers in Clinical Neuroscience). New York, Allan R. Liss, 1986, pp 165–173.

20. Fernandez C, Goldberg JM: Physiology of peripheral neurons innervating semicircular canals of the squirrel monkey. II: Response to sinusoidal stimulation and dynamics of peripheral vestibular system. *J Neurophysiol* 1971; 34:661–675.

21. Goldberg JM, Fernandez C: Conduction times and background discharge of vestibular afferents. *Brain Res* 1977; 122:545–550.

22. Goldberg JM, Fernandez C, Highstein SM: Differential projections of regularly and irregularly discharging vestibular nerve afferents onto individual secondary neurons of the superior vestibular nucleus in the barbiturate-anesthetized squirrel monkey. *Abstr Soc Neurosci* 1981; 7:39.

23. Greiner GF, Collard M, Conreaux C, et al: Recherche de potentiels evoques d'origine vestibulaire chez l'homme. *Acta Otolaryngol* 1967; 63:320–329.

24. Hofferberth B, Rothenberger A: Event-related potentials to rotatory stimulation—preliminary results in adults and children, in Rothenberger A (ed): *Proceedings of the Symposium on Event Related Potentials in Children—Basic Concepts and Clinical Application*. Essen Germany, 1982, Elseviez Biomedical Press, Amsterdam, p 463–470.

25. Hoffman L, Bohmer A, Beykirch K, et al: Far-field potentials evoked by pulsed linear accelerations in the chinchilla. Abstracts of the Association for Research in Otolaryology Midwinter Meeting, St Petersburg, Fla., 1991.

26. Hood JD: Vestibular and optokinetic evoked potentials. *Acta Otolaryngol* 1983; 95:589–593.

27. Hood JD, Kayan A: Observations upon the evoked responses to natural vestibular stimulation. *Electroencephalogr Clin Neurophysiol* 1985; 62:266–276.

28. Kast R, Lankford JE: Otolithic evoked potentials: A new technique for vestibular studies. *Acta Otolaryngol* 1986; 102:175–178.

29. Latkowski B, Puzio J: Recording of electrical-evoked response from a remote field in the vestibular part of the eighth nerve. *Audiology* 1989; 28:111–116.

30. Leibner E, Elidan J, Freeman S, et al: Vestibular evoked potentials with short and middle latencies recorded in humans. *Electroencephalog Clin Neurophysiol*, suppl 41, 1990, pp 119–123.

31. Louie AW, Kimm J: The response of 8th nerve fibers to horizontal sinusoidal oscillation in the alert monkey. *Exp Brain Res* 1976; 24:447–457.

32. Molinari GA, Mingrino SM: Cortical evoked responses to vestibular stimulation in man. *J Laryngol Otol* 1974; 88:515–521.

33. Pirodda E, Ghedini S, Zemeti MA: Investigations into vestibular evoked responses. *Acta Otolaryngol* 1987; 104:77–84.

34. Precht W, Shimazu H: Functional connections of tonic and kinetic vestibular neurons with primary vestibular afferents. *J Neurophysiol* 1965; 28:1014–1028.

35. Salamy J, Potvin A, Jones K, et al: Cortical evoked responses to labyrinthine stimulation in man. *Psychophysiology* 1975; 12:55–61.

36. Schmidt CL: Electrically evoked computer-averaged vestibular brainstem potentials in the cat. *Arch Otolaryngol* 1979; 222:199–204.

37. Shimazu H, Precht W: Tonic and kinetic responses of cat's vestibular neurons to horizontal angular acceleration. *J Neurophysiol* 1965; 28:991–1013.

38. Shinoda Y, Yoshida K: Dynamic characteristics of responses to horizontal head angular acceleration in vestibulo-ocular pathway in the cat. *J Neurophysiol* 1974; 37:653–673.

39. Spiegel EH, Szekely EG, Moffet R: Cortical responses to rotation. *Acta Otolaryngol* 1968; 66:181–185.

40. Taglietti V, Rossi ML, Casella C: Adaptive distortions in the generator potential of semicircular canal sensory afferents. *Brain Res* 1977; 123:41–57.

41. Tomko DL, Peterka RJ, Schor RH, et al: Response dynamics of horizontal canal afferents in barbiturate-anesthetized cats. *J Neurophysiol* 1981; 45:376–396.

42. Valli P, Zucca G: The origin of the slow potentials in semicircular canals of the frog. *Acta Otolaryngol* 1976; 81:395–405.

43. Wilson VJ, Melvill Jones G: *Mammalian Vestibular Physiology*. New York, Plenum Press, 1979.

44. Yagi T, Simpson NE, Markham CH: The relationship of conduction velocity to other physiological properties of the cat's horizontal canal neurons. *Exp Brain Res* 1977; 30:587–600.

Index